Encyclopaedia of Antibiotics

Second Edition

Encyclopaedia of Antibiotics

Second Edition

JOHN S. GLASBY
ICI (Organics) Limited,
Hexagon House, Blackley,
Manchester

A Wiley-Interscience Publication

JOHN WILEY & SONS Chichester • New York • Brisbane • Toronto

Copyright © 1979, by John Wiley & Sons Ltd.

All rights reserved.

No part of this book may be reproduced by any means, nor transmitted, nor translated into a machine language without the written permission of the publisher.

Library of Congress Cataloging in Publication Data:

Glasby, John Stephen.
   Encyclopaedia of antibiotics.
   'A Wiley–Interscience publication.'
   1. Antibiotics—Dictionaries. I. Title.
RS161.G56 1979   615'.329   78-13356
ISBN 0 471 99722 6

Printed and bound at
William Clowes & Sons Limited
Beccles and London

Preface

Since the first edition of this encyclopaedia two years ago a large number of new antibiotics have been described in the scientific and patent literature and these have been included in the present volume. In addition the structures of several of the antibiotics previously described have been elucidated and others have been revised in the light of further examination.

    The author also wishes to thank those research chemists and medical consultants who have provided him with additional data on the antibiotic activity of several important members of this class of compounds, particularly on their present use in human medicine.

Woodhouses, Manchester,
May, 1978
                                    J. S. GLASBY

AABOMYCIN
$C_{39-40}H_{65-68}O_{11}N$
M.p. 144–145°C

This antibiotic is elaborated by *Streptomyces hygroscopicus* var. *aabomyceticus* when cultivated on a medium consisting of glucose, dried beer yeast, defatted soybean flour, meat extract and sodium chloride at 26–27°C and pH 7·0 for 4 days. The compound is isolated by extraction of the culture filtrate with AcOEt and purified by chromatography on an alumina column. Aabomycin forms colourless needles when crystallized from a variety of solvent systems including $EtOH-H_2O$, $(CH_3)_2CO-H_2O$, $CHCl_3-C_6H_6$ and $C_6H_6-AcOEt$. It is dextrorotatory with a specific rotation of $[\alpha]_D^{26}$ + 93·5° (c 1·0, $CHCl_3$) and gives an ultraviolet spectrum in EtOH consisting of a single absorption maximum at 280 nm. The antibiotic is weakly acidic and soluble in EtOH but insoluble in H_2O. It is not active against bacteria but is effective against *Piricularia oryzae* and *Trichophyton rubrum*. Mice tolerate a dose of 100 mg/kg when administered intravenously.

Aizawa *et al., J. Antibiotics* (Japan), **22**, 457 (1969)
Yamaguchi *et al., ibid.*, **22**, 463 (1969)
Misato *et al., Japanese Patent*, 7,121,794 (1971)

ABIKOVIROMYCIN *(Latumcidin)*
$C_{10}H_{11}ON$

Both *Streptomyces abikoensis* and *S. rubescens* produce this antibiotic possessing antiviral properties. The compound is isolated from the broth culture by chromatography on an alumina column. So far, it has not been obtained in the pure state since it is highly unstable and, even at temperatures as low as −50°C, it rapidly polymerizes. Some difficulty is experienced when freeze-drying the antibiotic since it sublimes readily even under these extreme conditions. Dilute solutions are, however, reasonably stable and the substance may be conveniently handled in this form. The ultraviolet spectrum in 0·1 N-KOH or EtOH exhibits two absorption maxima at 218 and 244 nm and a pronounced shoulder at 289 nm, while that in 0·1 N-HCl has absorption maxima at 236 and 341 nm. The sulphate is stable but decomposes at 140–141°C. This salt is dextrorotatory with a specific rotation of $[\alpha]_D$ + 24° (c 1·0, H_2O). The picrate is also stable and crystalline, decomposing at 137–140°C. Reduction of the antibiotic with $LiAlH_4$ or $NaBH_4$ furnishes the dihydro derivative, m.p. 60–61°C.

Abikoviromycin has been shown to be active against both Eastern and Western equine encephalomyelitis viruses when dilutions of 1:8,000,000 are mixed with the virus suspensions and administered intracerebrally into mice. It is not, however, effective against the Venezuelan type virus. The antibiotic has only a slight activity against bacteria or fungi. The LD_{50} is 1·0 mg (subcutaneous) and 0·1 mg (intravenous) per 12 g mouse. It has a limited use in medicine as an antimicrobial.

Umezawa *et al., Japan. Med. J.*, **4**, 331 (1951)
Umezawa *et al., Japanese Patent*, 6200 (1952)
Identity with latumcidin
Sakagami *et al., J. Antibiotics* (Japan), **11A**, 231 (1958)
See also
Gurevitch *et al., Dokl. Akad. Nauk SSSR*, **182**, 828 (1968)

ABKHAZOMYCIN
Russian workers have described this antibiotic which has been obtained from cultures of *Streptomyces badiocolor* var. *abkhasus*. The antibiotic has been isolated by extraction of the mycelium followed by column chromatography. Abkhazomycin has only weak activity against bacteria and yeasts but is effective against a number of fungi.

Barashkova *et al., Antibiotiki*, **20**, 195 (1975)

ABLASTMYCIN
$C_{18}H_{33}O_{10}N_2$
M.p. Indefinite

When *Streptomyces aburaviensis* var. *ablastmyceticus* is freshly isolated from soil and cultivated in a common nutrient medium at 28°C for 3 days, this antibiotic may be obtained by extraction of the culture filtrate with an organic solvent and purified by treatment with an ion exchange resin. Ablastmycin is a basic compound, soluble in H_2O but virtually insoluble in most organic solvents. It gives a negative ninhydrin reaction and has no activity against bacteria but is highly active against both *Piricularia oryzae* and *Helminthosporium oryzae* in the presence of rice juice. It has found some use in the treatment of rice blast.

Umezawa *et al.*, *Japanese Patent*, 7,207,059 (1972)

ABURAMYCIN A
See Chromomycin A_2

ABURAMYCIN B
See Chromomycin A_3

ABURAMYCIN C
$C_{57}H_{84}O_{25}$
M.p. Indefinite

One of the large number of antibiotics elaborated by *Streptomyces* species, this compound is an amorphous powder, yellowish in colour, with no definite melting point. It has a specific rotation of $[\alpha]_D - 17°$ (c 1·0, EtOH) and gives a complex ultraviolet spectrum having absorption maxima at 228, 282, 318, 351 and 415 nm. When treated with Ac_2O it gives a peracetate, m.p. 219–221°C and $[\alpha]_D - 18°$ ($CHCl_3$). Aburamycin C has shown some promise as a cancerostatic agent.

Berlin *et al.*, *Nature*, **218**, 193 (1968)

ABURAMYCIN D
See Chromomycin A_4

ACETOMYCIN
$C_{10}H_{14}O_5$
M.p. 115°C

A simple antibiotic produced by *Streptomyces ramulosus*, this substance forms colourless rods and sublimes at 70°C. It is laevorotatory with a specific rotation of $[\alpha]_D - 167°$ (c 1·0, EtOH). Acetomycin is active against gram-positive bacteria.

Ettlinger *et al.*, *Helv. Chim. Acta*, **41**, 216 (1958)

2-ACETYL-2-DECARBOXAMIDO-OXYTETRACYCLINE
(*Terramycin X*)
$C_{23}H_{25}O_9N$

A tetracycline antibiotic, this compound is produced by *Streptomyces rimosus*. It is usually obtained as the crystalline hydrochloride which forms yellow crystals and has m.p. 201–203°C and $[\alpha]_D^{25} - 46·6°$ (c 0·9, 0·1 N-HCl). It is a broad spectrum antibiotic, active against both gram-positive and gram-negative bacteria.

Hochstein *et al.*, *J. Amer. Chem. Soc.*, **82**, 5934 (1960)
Frolova, Rozenfel'd, Listvinova, *Antibiotiki*, **16**, 687 (1971)

β-N-ACETYLRACEMOMYCIN
$C_{21}H_{36}O_9N_8$

An acetyl derivative of racemomycin (q.v.), this antibiotic substance has been prepared by Japanese workers by a series of selective chemical reactions. The minimum inhibitory concentration of the antibiotic for *Staphylococcus aureus* is given as 400 µg/ml compared with only 10 µg/ml for the parent antibiotic. From this observation it has been concluded that the β-amino group of the β-lysine side chain in racemomycin is of significant importance as a site for antimicrobial activity.

Sawada, Taniyama, *Yakugaku Zasshi*, **94**, 264 (1974)

ACIDOPHILIN

This antibiotic substance has been obtained from *Lactobacillus acidophilus* by fermentation in a medium containing sterilized skim milk. The antibiotic is isolated by extraction of the culture filtrate with EtOH, evaporation under reduced pressure, extraction of the residue with $(CH_3)_2CO$, evaporation and chromatography. It is normally employed as an aqueous suspension and is active against gram-positive bacteria.

Shahani, Vakil, Chandan, *U.S. Patent*, 3,689,640 (1972)

ACHROMYCIN

See Puromycin

ACLACINOMYCIN A

$C_{42}H_{53}NO_{15}$

One of two structurally similar glycosidic antibiotics isolated from an unclassified microorganism, this substance has been separated from the accompanying aclacinomycin B by chromatographic methods. It is a broad spectrum antibiotic possessing bacteriostatic, fungistatic, antiviral and antileukemic properties. The structure has been elucidated from chemical and spectroscopic examination.

Oki et al., *J. Antibiotics*, (Japan), **28**, 830 (1975)

ACLACINOMYCIN B

$C_{42}H_{51}NO_{15}$

A second antibiotic isolated by Oki and his colleagues from an unclassified microorganism, this compound possesses similar properties to the preceding antibiotic. It has been assigned the structure shown above on the basis of chemical degradations, hydrolysis experiments and a study of the infrared, NMR and mass spectra.

Oki et al., *J. Antibiotics*, (Japan), **28**, 830 (1975)

ACRYLAMIDINE

An unstable antibiotic, acrylamidine is produced by a species of *Streptomyces* allied to *S. eurythermus*. It has a maximum stability in neutral solution and is normally isolated as the hydrochloride which forms colourless crystals from H_2O. Acrylamidine has no activity against bacteria but is weakly active against species of *Candida*.

Yagishita et al., *J. Antibiotics* (Japan), **21**, 444 (1968)

ACTIDIONE *(Cycloheximide, Naramycin A)*
$C_{15}H_{23}O_4N$
M.p. 115–116·5°C (119·5–121°C)

Streptomycin-producing strains of *Streptomyces griseus* have been found to yield a second antibiotic which, although not active against bacteria, is highly effective against several yeasts. Crude actidione is purified by countercurrent distribution between C_6H_6 and H_2O and, when recrystallized from amyl acetate, gives colourless plates, m.p. 115–116·5°C. When crystallized from H_2O containing a little CH_3OH it has the higher melting point given above. The substance is laevorotatory having the following specific rotations: $[\alpha]_D^{25} - 2·8°$ (c 9·6, CH_3OH) and $[\alpha]_D^{29} - 3·38°$ (c 9·47, EtOH). The antibiotic forms a number of crystalline derivatives including the biologically inactive acetate, m.p. 150–152°C; $[\alpha]_D^{25} + 24·6°$ (c 3·7, CH_3OH); the semicarbazone monohydrate, m.p. 187–188°C (*dry*) and the *p*-nitrobenzoyl derivative, m.p. 215–220°C (*dec.*). Catalytic reduction with PtO_2 in AcOH furnishes dihydroactidione, m.p. 137–139°C, the latter characterized as the diacetate, m.p. 72–5°C and the N-methyl derivative, m.p. 129–132°C. Oxidation of the antibiotic with CrO_3 in glacial AcOH yields dihydroactidione as colourless crystals, m.p. 177–180°C. Determination of the absolute configuration of actidione has shown that it possesses the (R)(−) configuration.

When tested against a number of representative bacteria it fails to inhibit even at concentrations up to 1 mg/ml but even in concentrations as low as 0·002 mg/ml it inhibits *Cryptococcus neoformans*, a pathogenic fungus which is the cause of cryptococcosis, a rare but normally fatal disease. This high activity suggests its usefulness in the treatment of this disease. Actidione has a toxicity, given intravenously in mice, of LD_{50} of approximately 150 mg/kg.

Whiffen, Bohonos, Emerson, *J. Bact.*, **52**, 610 (1946)
Leach, Ford, Whiffen, *J. Amer. Chem. Soc.*, **69**, 474 (1947)
Ford, Leach, *ibid.*, **70**, 1223 (1948)
Kornfield, Jones, *Science*, **108**, 437 (1948)
Kornfield, Jones, Parks, *J. Amer. Chem. Soc.*, **71**, 150 (1949)
Okuda, *Chem. Pharm. Bull.*, **7**, 659 (1959)
Hawkins, Hainton, *Exp. Cell. Res.*, **65**, 258 (1971)
Evans, Smith, *J. Biol. Chem.*, **246**, 6144 (1971)

Cho, *Han'guk Saenghwahakhoe Chi*, **5**, 1 (1972)
Oddoux, Porte, Shaw, *Bull. Trav. Soc. Pharm. Lyon*, **16**, 153 (1972)
Muromtsev, Davydova, Klyagina, *Soviet Patent*, 378,409 (1973)
Verbin, Diluios, Farber, *Cancer Res.*, **33**, 2086 (1973)
Szabo et al., *Hung. Teljes*, 7931 (1974)
Absolute configuration
Sharkovsky, Johnson, *Tetrahedron Lett.*, 919 (1964)
Total synthesis
Johnson et al., *J. Amer. Chem. Soc.*, **86**, 118 (1964)

ACTILIN
See Neomycin B

ACTINOBOLIN
$C_{13}H_{20}O_6N_2$
M.p. Indefinite

This antibiotic has been isolated from *Streptomyces griseoviridus* var. *atrofaciens* and forms a fluffy amorphous powder with no definite melting point. It is hygroscopic and very soluble in H_2O in which it is amphoteric with a weakly acidic pK_a of 8·8 and a basic function pK_a of 7·5. In a phosphate buffer of pH 7·0 it gives an ultraviolet spectrum with a single absorption maximum of 263 nm.

Acid hydrolysis furnishes actinobolamine whereas hydrolysis with alkalies yields L-alanine, 1-(2:5-dihydroxyphenyl)propan-2-ol, ammonia and carbon dioxide. The sulphate forms colourless crystals from aqueous EtOH with $[\alpha]_D^{22} + 54·5°$ (c 1·0, H_2O), the ultraviolet spectrum at pH 7·0 having an absorption peak at 264 nm. The acetate furnishes colourless needles from EtOH, partially melting at 130°C followed by resolidification and decomposition at 263–266°C. This salt is also dextrorotatory with $[\alpha]_D^{26} + 58°$ (c 1·0, H_2O) and its ultraviolet spectrum is virtually identical with that of the sulphate. It is readily soluble in warm CH_3OH, EtOH and $(CH_3)_2CO$ but only sparingly soluble in AcOEt. The N-acetyl derivative, formed as white needles from EtOH, has m.p. 254–255°C (*dec.*) and $[\alpha]_D^{26} + 30°$ (c 3·8, H_2O). The ultraviolet spectra of the antibiotic have been extensively studied. In H_2O there is a single absorption maximum at 261 nm; in 0·1 N-NaOH this is shifted to 288 nm, while in 0·1 N-HCl it is at 262 nm.

The antibiotic has found some use in medicine, principally as a broad spectrum antimicrobial.

Haskell, Bartz, *Antibiotics Annual*, 505 (1958–1959)
Haskell et al., *U.S. Patent*, 3,043,830 (1962)
Struck et al., *Tetrahedron Lett.*, 1589 (1967)
Monk et al., *J. Amer. Chem. Soc.*, **90**, 1087 (1968)

ACTINOCARCIN
A complex antibiotic, actinocarcin is produced by *Streptomyces cinnamomeus* when grown on a common nutrient medium. Acid hydrolysis with N HCl for 20 hours at 110°C furnishes arginine, aspartic acid, histidine, isoleucine, leucine, lysine, phenylalanine, serine, threonine and tyrosine. Actinocarcin is inactive against bacteria, fungi and yeasts but injections with a dose of 1 mg/kg/day for six days it prolonged the survival period of mice inoculated with cells of Ehrlich sarcoma. The LD_{50} for mice was approximately 40–50 mg/kg given for six days.

Kihora et al., *J. Antibiotics* (Japan), **27**, 994 (1974)

ACTINOFLAVIN
See Actinomycin J_1

ACTINOMYCELIN
This antibiotic is produced by a culture which is related to *Streptomyces antibioticus*. It forms yellowish-green crystals which are soluble in H_2O and EtOH with an intense green fluorescence, somewhat less soluble in $CHCl_3$ and $(CH_3)_2CO$. The antibiotic is most stable at neutral reaction, less so under acid or alkaline conditions. It has been shown to be active against gram-positive bacteria but not against mycobacteria or fungi. The toxicity in rats is LD_{50} of 25 mg/kg when administered subcutaneously.

Cercos, *Publ. Tech. Fitotecnia* (Buenos Aires), **16**, 147 (1948)

ACTINOMYCES LYSOZYME
This substance has been described by Kriss who obtained it from *Streptomyces violaceus* and classified it as a lysozyme.

Kriss, *Mikrobiologiya* (USSR), **9**, 32 (1940)

ACTINOMYCETIN

Produced by *Streptomyces albus* cultures in beef-bouillon, this lytic substance is stated to be protein-like in nature. The structure is not yet known although it is said to consist of an enzyme, actinozyme, and a lipoid antibacterial fatty acid fraction. The compound is soluble in H_2O from which it is precipitated by various protein precipitants such as $(CH_3)_2CO$, EtOH and ammonium sulphate. Strong acid destroys the substance and it is also rapidly deactivated by heating to 60–70°C. It is appreciably more stable at pH 10·0 than at pH 4·0. Ultraviolet light below 300 nm destroys the antibiotic. Electromicrographs show it to be composed of particles with a diameter of about 4 millimicrons.

In its action, actinomycetin dissolves such organisms as *Staphylococcus aureus* in aqueous suspension and also dead gram-negative organisms. Dissolution of dead gram-positive organisms takes place too, but with more difficulty. No data on its toxicity has been reported.

Gratia, Alexander, *Compt. Rend. Soc. Biol.*, **91**, 1442 (1924)
Gratia, *Bull. Mem. Acad. Chir.*, **56**, 344 (1930)
Welsch, *J. Bact.*, **42**, 801 (1941)
Ghuysen, *Belgian Patents*, 517,191 and 521,114 (1953)
See also
Hoogerheide, Welsch, *Botan. Rev.*, **10**, 599 (1944)
Hoogerheide, Welsch, *J. Bact.*, **53**, 101 (1947)

ACTINOMYCIN A (*Actinomycin B, Actinomycin X*)

This antibiotic has been obtained and described under various synonyms—Actinomycin A (Waksman and Woodruff), Actinomycin B (Lehr and Berger) and Actinomycin X (Linge). Since the last worker has demonstrated that the substance can be fractionated into at least two closely related compounds, Actinomycins X_1 and X_2, these are described below in more detail. See Actinomycins X_1 and X_2.

ACTINOMYCIN A_{II}
See Actinomycin F_8

ACTINOMYCIN A_{III}
See Actinomycin F_9

ACTINOMYCIN A_V
See Actinomycin X_2

ACTINOMYCIN B
See Actinomycin A

ACTINOMYCIN B_V
See Actinomycin X_2

ACTINOMYCIN C_1
See Actinomycin D

ACTINOMYCIN C_2 (*Actinomycin I_2, VI*)

$C_{63}H_{88}O_{16}N_{12}$
M.p. 237–239°C

This antibiotic from *Streptomyces antibioticus* and *S. chrysomallus* is separated from the accompanying components by countercurrent distribution methods, having a higher R_f value than actinomycin D (q.v.). When purified by recrystallization from C_6H_6 or EtOH, the antibiotic forms red needles or bipyramids. It is laevorotatory with a specific rotation of $[\alpha]_D -325° \pm 10°$ (CH_3OH). The structure is similar to that of actinomycin D, which may be regarded as the basic structure of the actinomycins, but with D-valine in the β-peptide chain replaced by D-*allo*-isoleucine. It is therefore usually referred to as an anisoactinomycin since the pentapeptide residues are different. This antibiotic has been synthesized, but in order to obtain it free of the isomeric actinomycin C_{2a} (q.v.), separation of the intermediate actinomycinic acid monolactones must be carried out prior to the final cyclization of the second peptide ring.

The biological activity and toxicity of actinomycin C_2 are virtually identical to those given for actinomycin D (q.v.). The concentration required to inhibit the growth of *Bacillus subtilis* has been given as 0·25 μg/ml by Reich and his colleagues. The activity against *B. subtilis* diminishes with any change in the chromophore, e.g. 7-hydroxyactinomycin C_2 has only about 0·2 per cent of the activity of actinomycin C_3 (taken as the standard), 7-aminoactinomycin C_2 has <1·0 per cent and 7-nitroactinomycin C_2 has 40 per cent relative activity.

Brockmann, Pfennig, *Naturwiss.*, **39**, 429 (1952)
Brockmann, Grone, *Chem. Ber.*, **87**, 1036 (1954)
Brockmann, *Angew. Chem.*, **72**, 944 (1960)
Brockmann, Boldt, Petras, *Naturwiss.*, **47**, 62 (1960)
Brockmann, Petras, *ibid*, **48**, 218 (1961)
Brockmann, Boldt, *ibid*, **50**, 19 (1963)
Structure
Brockmann, Petras, *Naturwiss.*, **48**, 218 (1961)
Brockmann *et al.*, *Chem. Ber.*, **99**, 3672 (1966)
Synthesis
Brockmann, Lackner, *Tetrahedron Lett.*, 3517 (1964)
Biological activity
Brockmann, Muller, Peterssen-Borstel, *Tetrahedron Lett.*, 3531 (1966)

ACTINOMYCIN C_{2a} (*Actinomycin i-C_2*)

$C_{63}H_{88}O_{16}N_{12}$
M.p. 233–235°C

When separated chromatographically from the actinomycin C mixture isolated from *Streptomyces chrysomallus*, this component has an R_f value intermediate between actinomycins C_2 and C_3. The antibiotic forms red crystals from EtOH and is laevorotatory having a specific rotation of $[\alpha]_D^{18} - 297°$ (c 0·267, CH_3OH). It is an anisoactinomycin, isomeric with actinomycin C_2, the structure being the same but with the D-*allo*-isoleucine and D-valine aminoacids being transposed. In the first attempts to synthesize actinomycin C_2, this isomer was present in the final product and the two compounds cannot be separated. A pure product can only be obtained by separating the intermediate monolactones prior to the final cyclization. This antibiotic has not been studied in as much detail as either actinomycin C_3 or D but the toxicity and biological activity appear to be similar to those of these two compounds.

Brockmann, Frank, *Naturwiss.*, **47**, 15 (1960)
Synthesis
Brockmann, Lackner, *Tetrahedron Lett.*, 3517 (1964)

ACTINOMYCIN i-C_2
See Actinomycin C_{2a}

ACTINOMYCIN C_3 (*Actinomycin VII*)

$C_{64}H_{90}O_{16}N_{12}$
M.p. 234°C

This component of the actinomycin C mixture obtained from *Streptomyces chrysomallus* and *S. antibioticus* forms reddish crystals from C_6H_6. It is, however, more readily obtained in the crystalline form from AcOEt on addition of CS_2. The antibiotic is laevorotatory with $[\alpha]_D^{20} - 357°$ (C_6H_6). Structurally, actinomycin C_3 is an isoactinomycin, both the α- and β-peptide chains consisting of the aminoacids L-threonine, D-*allo*-isoleucine, L-proline, sarcosine and L-N-methylvaline. The first synthesis of an actinomycin was based upon the observation by Sunderkotter that actinomycin C_3 is hydrolytically cleaved between sarcosine and L-N-methylvaline to yield bis-(seco-actinomycin C_3), the latter being synthesized through oxidative coupling which brings about dimerization. The bis-(seco-actinomycin C_3) readily reforms the natural antibiotic.

X-ray studies have shown that actinomycin C_3 may have a pseudo-two-fold axis of symmetry in the plane of the phenoxazine ring. Solutions in organic solvents contain only monomers, but in aqueous solution molecular weight determinations found by sedimentation equilibrium show that dimers predominate between concentrations of 10^{-5} and 10^{-3} molar. At higher concentrations oligomers are formed. It is now generally accepted that the presence of the nonpolar aminoacids in the molecule produces a hydrophobic effect which explains the stability of the dimers in water.

Actinomycin C_3 is active against gram-positive bacteria and inhibits the growth of *Bacillus subtilis* at a concentration of 0·25 µg/ml. It is also, like actinomycin D, highly effective against rhabdonyosarcoma, Wilm's tumour and trophoblastic tumours. Clinical use, however, is limited by its high toxicity; 50 mg/kg being lethal to mice when given orally. Investigation has shown that the antibiotic complexes with DNA and inhibits the synthesis of RNA although it does not complex with the latter. Several complexes of actinomycin C_3 with various purine bases have been investigated and compared with that formed with DNA. The entropy change for the former is not favourable for interaction and these complexes are about 1000 times weaker than that with DNA where the entropy change is both large and positive. There is now little doubt that this antibiotic acts in the same manner as actinomycin D (q.v.) and recently a small angle X-ray scattering study on the interaction between actinomycin C_3 and calf thymus DNA has been reported by Zipper and his co-workers.

    Brockmann et al., *Naturwiss.*, **47**, 230 (1960)
    Brockmann, Lackner, *ibid.*, **48**, 555 (1961)
    Brockmann, Boldt., *ibid.*, **50**, 19 (1963)
Synthesis
    Brockmann, Sunderkotter, *Naturwiss.*, **47**, 229 (1960)
  X-ray studies
    Perutz, *Nature*, **201**, 814 (1964)
    Marsh Jnr, Goodman, *Can. J. Chem.*, **44**, 799 (1966)
  Solution studies
    Berg, *J. Electroanal. Chem.*, **10**, 371 (1965)
    Muller, Ennie, *Z. Naturforsch.*, **20B**, 835 (1965)
    Gellert et al., *J. Mol. Biol.*, **11**, 445 (1965)
    Crothers et al., *Biochemistry*, **7**, 1817 (1968)
Complexes with nucleic acids
    Muller, Spatz, *Z. Naturforsch.*, **20B**, 842 (1965)
    Crothers, Ratner, *Biochemistry*, **7**, 1823 (1968)
    Schara, Muller, *Eur. J. Biochem.*, **29**, 210 (1972)
Complex with calf thymus DNA
    Zipper et al., *Fed. Eur. Biochem. Soc. Lett.*, **25**, 123 (1972)

ACTINOMYCIN D (*Actinomycin C_1, D_{IV}, I, IV, X, Dactinomycin*)
$C_{62}H_{86}O_{16}N_{12}$
M.p. 235·5–236·5°C (*dec.*)

Extraction of the dry mycelium of various species of *Streptomyces*, particularly *S. antibioticus* and *S. chrysomallus*, with C_6H_6 yields an antibiotic substance, actinomycin C, which has been shown by countercurrent distribution and chromatography to consist of a number of components. These have been designated actinomycins C_1 (actinomycin D), C_2, C_{2a} and C_3 where the subscript refers to an increasing R_f value. Actinomycin D forms red crystals which are freely soluble in C_6H_6, $(CH_3)_2CO$ and $CHCl_3$, less so in EtOH and only slightly soluble in H_2O. The antibiotic is laevorotatory with $[\alpha]_D^{23} - 262°$ (c 0·25, 95 per cent EtOH) and gives an ultraviolet spectrum with an absorption maximum at 242 nm and negative Cotton effects centered at 269 and 213 nm. The visible spectrum in H_2O exhibits an absorption at 441 nm, while in less polar solvents such as C_6H_6, CH_3OH and AcOEt, there are two absorptions at 425 and 445 nm. X-ray studies do not completely differentiate between a decapeptide dilactone and a bis-pentapeptide lactone structure, but Brockmann has proved the latter structure both by degradation and synthesis.

Like the accompanying components, actinomycin D is active against gram-positive bacteria but has only a limited activity against gram-negative organisms. The minimum inhibitory concentration against *Bacillus subtilis* of pure actinomycin D has been given by Formica and his colleagues as 0·02 µg/ml. Like all of the actinomycins, this antibiotic is highly toxic. When given at a dosage of 5 mg/kg intraperitoneally, or 50 mg/kg orally, mice die within 24 hours. Nevertheless it possesses a marked antineoplastic effect in non-toxic doses and, like actinomycin C_3 (q.v.), is highly effective as a chemotherapeutic in the treatment of carcinoma, particularly of the lymphatic system. It therefore has a use in treating Hodgkin's disease, rhabdomyosarcoma, trophoblastic tumours and Wilm's tumour.

Actinomycin D is one of the most effective antitumour agents known at the present time, but owing to its high toxicity it finds only limited clinical use. The cytostatic properties of the antibiotic are due to its complexing with DNA and the consequential inhibition of RNA synthesis. Actinomycin D also interferes with those reactions in which DNA is modified, e.g. by methylation. Four molecular models for the actinomycin D-DNA complex have been put forward, two in which the chromophore of the antibiotic is intercalated between two successive base pairs and two in which the antibiotic is bound to the outside of the double-stranded DNA helix.

Support for all four models comes from a wide variety of physical and spectroscopic measurements, but the model described by Sobell and Jain explains most of the data pertaining to the binding of the antibiotic with DNA and is most widely accepted at the present time. This model combines the specificity of the guanine 2-amino group of the two 'outside-bound' models with the intercalative feature of the 'inner-bound' models.

Although numerous synthetic actinomycins have been prepared in the hope of improving the chemotherapeutic index and increasing the biological activity, it is now apparent that the efficiency of actinomycin D requires a precise and unique fit between the antibiotic and DNA. Even a small change in the actinomycin D molecule interferes with the structural geometry of the complex and renders the system less active. Most experimental work is now directed towards improving the chemotherapeutic index which is related to the difference in permeability in the cell wall of the normal and malignant cell.

Waksman, Woodruff, *Proc. Soc. Exp. Biol. Med.*, **45**, 609 (1940)
Waksman, Tishler, *J. Biol. Chem.*, **142**, 519 (1942)
Vining, Waksman, *Science*, **120**, 389 (1954)
Johnson, *Chem. Soc. Spec. Publ.*, No. 5, 82 (1956)
Roussos, Vining, *J. Chem. Soc.*, 2469 (1956)
Bullock, Johnson, *ibid.*, 3280 (1957)
Brockmann, Boldt, Petras, *Naturwiss.*, **47**, 62 (1960)
Biosynthesis
Katz, Weissbach, *J. Biol. Chem.*, **237**, 882 (1962)
Weissbach et al., *ibid.*, **240**, 4377 (1965)
Weissbach et al., *Biochem. Biophys. Res. Commun.*, **19**, 524 (1965)
Katz, Weissbach, *Develop. Ind. Microbiol.*, **8**, 67 (1967)
Katz, *Antibiotics II, Biosynthesis*, Ed. Gottlieb, Shaw, p. 276, Springer-Verlag, New York (1967)
Katz, *Actinomycin*, Ed. Waksman, Chap. 4, Wiley, New York (1968)
Synthesis
Brockmann, Petras, *Naturwiss*, **48**, 218 (1961)
Woodward, Olofson, Mayer, *J. Amer. Chem. Soc.*, **83**, 1010 (1961)
Staab, *Angew. Chem.*, **74**, 407 (1962)
Brockmann, Mangegold, *Naturwiss.*, **51**, 382 (1964)
Brockmann, Lackner, *ibid.*, **51**, 384, 407 (1964)
Brockmann et al., *Chem. Ber.*, **99**, 3672 (1966)
Brockmann, Lackner, *ibid.*, **101**, 1312 (1968)
Meienhofer, *Experientia*, **24**, 776 (1968)
Meienhofer, *J. Amer. Chem. Soc.*, **92**, 3771 (1970)

CR/ORD Studies
  Courtois, Guschibauer, Fromageot, *Eur. J. Biochem.*, **6**, 106 (1968)
  Crothers et al., *Biochemistry*, **7**, 1817 (1968)
  Ascoli et al., *Nature*, **227**, 1237 (1970)
  Ascoli et al., *Biopolymers*, **11**, 1173 (1972)
X-ray Studies
  Palmer, Palmer, Dickerson, *Nature*, **202**, 1052 (1964)
  Marsh Jnr, Goodman, *Can. J. Chem.*, **44**, 799 (1966)
  Ponnuswamy, McGuire, Scheraga, *Int. J. Peptide Protein Res.*, **5**, 73 (1973)
NMR Studies
  Victor et al., *Tetrahedron Lett.*, 4721 (1969)
  Victor et al., *Nature*, **223**, 302 (1969)
  Lackner, *Tetrahedron Lett.*, 2807 (1970)
  Danyluk, Victor, *Jerusalem Symp. Quant. Chem. Biochem.*, **2**, 394 (1970)
  Arison, Hoogsteen, *Biochemistry*, **9**, 3976 (1970)
  Conti, de Santis, *Nature*, **227**, 1239 (1970)
  Lackner, *Tetrahedron Lett.*, 2221 (1971)
  Lackner, *Proc. of 3rd Amer. Peptide Symp.*, p. 147, Ann Arbor, Mich. (1972)
Conformation
  De Santis, *Jerusalem Symp. Quant. Chem. Biochem.*, **5**, 493 (1973)
Biological Activity
  Meienhofer, *Experientia*, **24**, 776 (1968)
  Meienhofer, *J. Amer. Chem. Soc.*, **92**, 3771 (1970)
  Sobell, *Proc. Nucl. Acid Res. Mol. Biol.*, **13**, 153 (1973)
  Cancer Chemother. Rep., Part I, **58**, 1 (1974)
Complex with DNA
  Goldberg, Rabinowitz, Reich, *Proc. Nat. Acad. Sci. U.S.*, **48**, 2094 (1962)
  Reich, Goldberg, *Proc. Nucl. Acid. Res.*, **3**, 183 (1964)
  Reich, *Symp. Soc. Study Develop. Growth*, **23**, 73 (1964)
  Cerami et al., *Proc. Nat. Acad. Sci. U.S.*, **57**, 1030 (1967)
  Hartman et al., *Angew. Chem. Int. Ed. Eng.*, **7**, 693 (1968)
  Wells, Larson, *J. Mol. Biol.*, **49**, 319 (1970)
  Hyman, Davidson, *ibid.*, **50**, 421 (1970)
  Goldberg, Friedman, *Ann. Rev. Biochem.*, **40**, 772 (1971)
  Goldberg, Friedman, *Pure. Appl. Chem.*, **28**, 499 (1971)
  Gale et al., *The Molecular Basis of Antibiotic Action*, p. 220, Wiley, New York (1972)
  Sobell, *Prog. Nucl. Acid Res. Mol. Biol.*, **13**, 153 (1973)
Models of Actinomycin D-DNA Complex
  Hamilton, Fuller, Reich, *Nature*, **198**, 538 (1963)
  Muller, Crothers, *J. Mol. Biol.*, **35**, 251 (1968)
  Gurskii, *Mol. Biol.*, **3**, 749 (1969)
  Gurskii, *Mol. Biol. (USSR)*, **3**, 292 (1970)
  Sobell, Jain, *J. Mol. Biol.*, **68**, 21 (1972)
  Sobell, *Prog. Nucl. Acid Res. Mol. Biol.*, **13**, 153 (1973)
Stereochemistry with DNA
  Sobell, *Jerusalem Symp. Quant. Chem. Biochem.*, **4**, 149 (1972)
Biological activity
  French, Casida, *J. Anim. Sci.*, **37**, 1218 (1973)
  Henry, *U.S. Nat. Tech. Inform. Serv.*, PB Rep., No. 225594/1GA (1973)
  Valeriote, Vietti, Tolen, *Cancer Res.*, **33**, 2658 (1973)
  Bouloy, Hannoun, *Ann. Microbiol.* (Paris), **124B**, 547 (1973)
  Dolzhanskii, *Probl. Tuberk*, **68**, (1974)
  Modest, Sengupta, *Cancer Chemother. Rep.*, Part I, **58**, 35 (1974)
  Goldin, Johnson, *ibid.*, **58**, 63 (1974)
  Kwon, *Kalullik Taehak Uihakpu Nonmunjip*, **27**, 187 (1974)
  Stephan-Dubois, Biver, *C.R. Seances Soc. Biol. Ses Fil.*, **168**, 1068 (1974)
  De Azevedo e Silva et al., *Mem. Inst. Biocienc., Univ. Fed. Pernambuco*, **1**, 37 (1974)
  Bader et al., *Acta Biol. Med. Ger.*, **32**, 91 (1974)
  Finn, Downie, *J. Endocrinol.*, **65**, 259 (1975)
  Henry, Roesler, DiDomenico, *Cancer Chemother. Rep.*, Part I, **59**, 447 (1975)
  Tattersall et al., *Clin. Pharmacol. Ther.*, **17**, 701 (1975)
See also
  Hollstein, *Chem. Rev.*, **74** (6), 625 (1974)

ACTINOMYCIN D_0

This new actinomycin has recently been described by Russian workers. It differs from the previously known actinomycins in that one of the sarcosine units is replaced by glycine.

Devan, Orlova, Silaev, *Antibiotiki*, **19**, 107 (1974)

ACTINOMYCIN D_{IV}
  See Actinomycin D

ACTINOMYCIN E₁
$C_{64}H_{96}O_{16}N_{12}$

```
         CH(CH₃)₂      CH(CH₃)C₂H₅
OC────────CH      HC────────CO
          |           |
          NCH₃        NCH₃
          |           |
       Sarcosine   Sarcosine
          |           |
       L-Proline   L-Proline
          |           |
   D-allo-Isoleucine  D-allo-Isoleucine
          |           |
          CO          CO
          |           |
CH₃HC─────CH      HC────────CHCH₃
          |           |
          NH          NH
          |           |
          CO          CO
           \         /
            phenoxazinone
            (—NH₂, =O, CH₃, CH₃)
```

One method of predetermining the structure of an antibiotic is controlled biosynthesis. Here, specific chemical precursors are fed to the particular microorganism in the culture medium and these compete with the endogenously synthesized aminoacid and are incorporated into the peptide chain. When DL-*iso*leucine is included in the medium in which *Streptomyces antibioticus* is grown, two new actinomycins are formed designated E₁ and E₂. This particular antibiotic has the same structure as actinomycin C₃ but with one of the L-N-methylvaline groups replaced by L-methyl-*allo*-isoleucine.

Gunther, Schmidt-Kastner, *Naturwiss.*, **43**, 131 (1956)
Brockmann, *Angew. Chem.*, **72**, 945 (1960)

ACTINOMYCIN E₂
$C_{65}H_{98}O_{16}N_{12}$

Also isolated in small amounts from cultures of *Streptomyces antibioticus* and *S. chrysomallus* when DL-*iso*leucine is added to the culture medium, this antibiotic belongs to the isoactinomycin class, both the α- and β-chain consisting of the aminoacids L-threonine, D-*allo*-isoleucine, L-proline and L-methyl-*allo*-isoleucine. It forms reddish crystals when crystallized from C_6H_6.

Gunther, Schmidt-Kastner, *Naturwiss.*, **43**, 131 (1956)
Brockmann, *Angew. Chem.*, **72**, 945 (1960)

ACTINOMYCIN F₁ (*Actinomycin KS4:KS4*)
$C_{58}H_{88}O_{16}N_{12}$

```
         CH(CH₃)₂      CH(CH₃)₂
OC────────CH      HC────────CO
          |           |
          NCH₃        NCH₃
          |           |
       Sarcosine   Sarcosine
          |           |
       Sarcosine   Sarcosine
          |           |
       D-Valine    D-allo-Isoleucine
          |           |
          CO          CO
          |           |
CH₃HC─────CH      HC────────CHCH₃
          |           |
          NH          NH
          |           |
          CO          CO
           \         /
            phenoxazinone
            (—NH₂, =O, CH₃, CH₃)
```

Actinomycin F$_2$

This antibiotic is obtained from *Streptomyces chrysomallus* and from other actinomycin C-elaborating strains such as *Streptomyces* BOP 476 (NRRL 2580). Actinomycin F$_1$ is an anisoactinomycin with one peptide chain containing L-threonine, D-valine, two moles of sarcosine and one of L-N-methylvaline, the other being similar but with D-valine replaced by D-*allo*-isoleucine.

Gunther, Schmidt-Kastner, *Naturwiss.*, **43**, 131 (1956)
Brockmann, *Angew. Chem.*, **72**, 939 (1960)

ACTINOMYCIN F$_2$
$C_{60}H_{90}O_{16}N_{12}$

Also isolated from *Streptomyces chrysomallus* and *Streptomyces* BOP 476, this anisoactinomycin has one peptide chain consisting of L-threonine, D-valine, L-proline, sarcosine and L-methyl-*allo*-isoleucine and the other containing L-threonine, D-*allo*-isoleucine, sarcosine, sarcosine and L-N-methylvaline.

Gunther, Schmidt-Kastner, *Naturwiss.*, **43**, 131 (1956)
Brockmann, *Angew. Chem.*, **72**, 939 (1960)

ACTINOMYCIN F$_3$
$C_{59}H_{90}O_{16}N_{12}$

An isoactinomycin isolated from *Streptomyces chrysomallus* and *Streptomyces* BOP 476, the peptide chains in this compound consist of L-threonine, D-*allo*-isoleucine, sarcosine, sarcosine and L-N-methylvaline.

Gunther, Schmidt-Kastner, *Naturwiss.*, **43**, 131 (1956)
Brockmann, *Angew. Chem.*, **72**, 939 (1960)

ACTINOMYCIN F$_4$
$C_{61}H_{92}O_{16}N_{12}$

A fourth component of the antibiotic mixture obtained from *Streptomyces chrysomallus* and *Streptomyces* BOP 476, the structure of this compound is identical with that of actinomycin E$_2$ but with one of the sarcosine groups replaced by L-proline.

Gunther, Schmidt-Kastner, *Naturwiss.*, **43**, 131 (1956)
Brockmann, *Angew. Chem.*, **72**, 939 (1960)

ACTINOMYCIN F$_8$ (*Actinomycin II, A$_{II}$*)

C$_{57}$H$_{86}$O$_{16}$N$_{12}$
M.p. 215–218°C

ACTINOMYCIN F$_9$ (*Actinomycin III, A$_{III}$*)

C$_{60}$H$_{84}$O$_{16}$N$_{12}$
M.p. 237–238°C

An antibiotic produced by *Streptomyces antibioticus*, this substance forms red plates when crystallized from $(CH_3)_2CO$—CS_2. It is laevorotatory having a specific rotation of $[\alpha]_D^{17} - 157°$ (c 0·24, CHCl$_3$). The antibiotic is an isoactinomycin, each peptide chain consisting of L-threonine, D-valine, sarcosine, sarcosine and L-N-methylvaline.

Johnson, Mauger, *Biochem. J.*, **73**, 535 (1959)
Brockmann, *Angew. Chem.*, **72**, 939 (1960)
Goss, Katz., *Antibiotics & Chemotherapy*, **10**, 221 (1960)

Also formed by *Streptomyces antibioticus*, this antibiotic crystallizes from $(CH_3)_2CO$ as red prisms. It has a specific rotation of $[\alpha]_D^{19} - 205°$ (c 0·22, CHCl$_3$). The minimal inhibitory concentration against *Bacillus subtilis* is given by Brockmann and Manegold as 0·7 times that of actinomycin C$_3$, the latter being taken as the standard. It has also been shown that this antibiotic is identical with actinomycin X$_{0\gamma}$.

Johnson, Mauger, *Biochem. J.*, **73**, 535 (1959)
Brockmann, *Angew. Chem.*, **72**, 939 (1960)
Brockmann, Manegold, *Chem. Ber.*, **95**, 1081 (1962)

ACTINOMYCIN KS4 = KS$_4$
See Actinomycin F$_1$

ACTINOMYCIN J$_1$ (*Actinoflavin*)
This antibiotic has been isolated from *Streptomyces flavus* and is closely related to actinomycin C$_1$ if not actually identical with it. It forms red crystals from (CH$_3$)$_2$CO or Et$_2$O and has the same biological activity as actinomycin C$_1$. The toxicity is very high and so far it has found no use in medicine.

Umezawa *et al.*, *J. Antibiotics* (Japan), **1**, 129 (1947)
Hirata, Nakaniski, *ibid.*, **2**, 181 (1948)
Hirata, Nakaniski, *Bull. Soc. Chem. Japan*, **22**, 121 (1949)

ACTINOMYCIN J$_2$
The preparation described as actinomycin J$_2$ has been shown to be a mixture of actinomycin J$_1$ with duodecyl 5-ketostearate, the latter compound having no antibiotic activity whatsoever.

Hirata, Nakaniski, *Bull. Soc. Chem. Japan*, **22**, 121 (1949)

ACTINOMYCIN Pip 1α

When grown in the presence of pipecolic acid, *Streptomyces antibioticus* yields three 'new' actinomycins, designated actinomycin Pip 1α, Pip 1β and Pip 2, in which L-proline is progressively replaced by pipecolic acid. This particular antibiotic contains 4-oxopipecolic acid in addition to pipecolic acid in the peptide chains. The minimal inhibitory concentration against *Bacillus subtilis* is given as 0·25 µg/ml.

Formica, *Diss. Abstr.*, **28B** (8), 3398 (1967)
Formica, Shatkin, Katz, *J. Bact.*, **95**, 2139 (1968)
Formica, Katz, *J. Biol. Chem.*, **248**, 2066 (1973)

ACTINOMYCIN Pip 1β

This antibiotic is also produced when *Streptomyces antibioticus* is grown in the presence of pipecolic acid. In this substance only one L-proline group is replaced by pipecolic acid. The minimal inhibitory concentration against *Bacillus subtilis* is 0·02 µg/ml.

Formica, *Diss. Abstr.*, **28B** (8), 3398 (1967)
Formica, Shatkin, Katz, *J. Bact.*, **95**, 2139 (1968)
Formica, Katz, *J. Biol. Chem.*, **248**, 2066 (1973)

ACTINOMYCIN Pip 2

The third antibiotic formed when *Streptomyces antibioticus* is grown in a culture medium containing pipecolic acid has both of the L-proline groups replaced by pipecolic acid. The minimal inhibitory concentration against *Bacillus subtilis* is 0·1 μg/ml.

Formica, *Diss. Abstr.*, **28B** (8), 3398 (1967)
Formica, Shatkin, Katz, *J. Bact.*, **95**, 2139 (1968)
Formica, Katz., *J. Biol. Chem.*, **248**, 2066 (1973)

ACTINOMYCIN $X_{0\alpha}$
$C_{60}H_{84}O_{17}N_{12}$

From the culture medium and mycelium of *Streptomyces antibioticus*, a fraction designated actinomycin X_0 has been obtained which, on further separation, yields various components with increasing R_f values. Since other fractions, actinomycins X_1 and X_2 had already been identified, these components have a further greek subscript to differentiate them. Actinomycin $X_{0\alpha}$ forms reddish crystals from C_6H_6. One of the peptide chains consists of L-threonine, D-valine, sarcosine, sarcosine and L-N-methylvaline and the other, L-threonine, D-valine, L-hydroxyproline, sarcosine and L-N-methylvaline. It has not yet been fully established in which chain the L-hydroxyproline moiety is located. The antibiotic inhibits *Bacillus subtilis* at a concentration of only 0·15 that of actinomycin C_3 taking the latter as the standard.

Brockmann, Linge, Grone, *Naturwiss*, **40**, 224 (1953)
Brockmann, Manegold, *Chem. Ber.*, **95**, 1081 (1962)

ACTINOMYCIN X
See Actinomycin A

ACTINOMYCIN $X_{0\beta}$ (*Actinomycin I*)
$C_{62}H_{86}O_{17}N_{12}$
M.p. 244–245°C

A number of *Streptomyces* species elaborate this antibiotic which forms reddish crystals from $CHCl_3$—light petroleum. It has specific rotations of $[\alpha]_D^{22} - 265°$ (c 0·2, $(CH_3)_2CO$) and $[\alpha]_D^{22} - 308°$ (c 0·2, CH_3OH). It forms crystalline derivatives, e.g. the monoacetate, m.p. 242–243°C; $[\alpha]_D^{21} - 283°$ (c 0·2, CH_3OH) and $[\alpha]_D^{21} - 260°$ (c 0·2, $(CH_3)_2CO$) and the monopalmitate, m.p. 200–201°C; $[\alpha]_D^{22} - 238° \pm 5°$ (c 0·2, CH_3OH) and $[\alpha]_D^{22} - 221° \pm 5°$ (c 0·2, $(CH_3)_2CO$). It contains the same chromophore as the other actinomycins, one peptide chain consisting of L-threonine, D-valine, L-proline, sarcosine and L-N-methylvaline and the other of L-threonine, D-valine, L-hydroxyproline, sarcosine and L-N-methylvaline.

Actinomycin $X_{0\gamma}$

The minimal inhibitory concentration against *Bacillus subtilis* is 0·25 times that of actinomycin C_3.

Brockmann, Linge, Grone, *Naturwiss.*, **40**, 224 (1953)
Brockmann, Grone, *Chem. Ber.*, **87**, 1036 (1954)
Brockmann, Pampus, *Angew. Chem.*, **67**, 419 (1955)
Brockmann, Pampus, Manegold, *Chem. Ber.*, **92**, 1249 (1959)
Brockmann, Manegold, *ibid.*, **93**, 2971 (1960)
Brockmann, Boldt, Petras, *Naturwiss.*, **47**, 62 (1960)
Brockmann, Manegold, *Chem. Ber.*, **95**, 1081 (1962)

ACTINOMYCIN $X_{0\gamma}$
See Actinomycin F_9.

ACTINOMYCIN $X_{0\delta}$
$C_{62}H_{86}O_{17}N_{12}$
M.p. 245–246°C

A synthetic antibiotic produced by reduction of actinomycin X_1 with aluminium isopropoxide, the compound crystallizes from $CHCl_3$-light petroleum as red prisms. It is laevorotatory having a specific rotation of $[\alpha]_D^{20} - 297°$ (c 0·2, CH_3OH) or $- 241°$ (c 0·2, $(CH_3)_2CO$). It may be characterized as the monoacetate, m.p. 249–250°C with $[\alpha]_D^{18} - 310°$ (c 0·2, CH_3OH) and $-279°$ (c 0·2, $(CH_3)_2CO$) and the monopalmitate with m.p. 200–201°C and specific rotations of $[\alpha]_D^{21} - 256°$ (c 0·2, CH_3OH) and $[\alpha]_D^{21} - 224°$ (c 0·2, $(CH_3)_2CO$). Like all of the actinomycins, the antibiotic has a high toxicity. The minimal inhibitory concentration against *Bacillus subtilis* is 0·4 times that of actinomycin C_3.

Brockmann, Manegold, *Chem. Ber.*, **93**, 2971 (1960)
Brockmann, Manegold, *ibid.*, **95**, 1081 (1962)

ACTINOMYCIN X_{1a}
$C_{60}H_{82}O_{17}N_{12}$

A minor antibiotic obtained from *Streptomyces* species, this substance forms red crystals from a mixture of $CHCl_3$ and light petroleum. The structure is similar to that of actinomycin D (q.v.) but with the two proline groups replaced by sarcosine and L-γ-oxoproline. The minimal inhibitory concentration against *Bacillus subtilis* is 0·7 times that of actinomycin C_3.

Brockmann, Grone, *Chem. Ber.*, **87**, 1036 (1954)
Brockmann, Manegold., *ibid.*, **93**, 2971 (1960)
Brockmann, Manegold, *ibid.*, **95**, 1081 (1962)

Actinomycin X₂

ACTINOMYCIN X₂ (*Actinomycin V, A$_V$, B$_V$*)

$C_{62}H_{84}O_{17}N_{12}$

M.p. 249·5–250·5°C

Structure (upper): two peptide chains attached to the phenoxazinone chromophore:
- Chain 1: D-Valine – Sarcosine – Sarcosine – L-threo-(CH(CH₃)₂)... with CH₃HC–CH terminus
- Chain 2: D-Valine – L-Oxoproline – Sarcosine – ... with CHCH₃ terminus

Structure (lower, labelled ACTINOMYCIN X₂):
- Chain 1: D-Valine – L-Proline – Sarcosine
- Chain 2: D-Valine – L-Oxoproline – Sarcosine

Actinomycin Z₅

The original actinomycin X obtained from various *Streptomyces* species, has now been separated into at least two components. This particular antibiotic crystallizes as red needles from light petroleum. It has specific rotations of $[\alpha]_D^{24} - 359°$ (c 0·2, CH_3OH) and $[\alpha]_D^{24} - 288°$ (c 0·2, $(CH_3)_2CO$). Reduction with aluminium isopropoxide furnishes actinomycin D and actinomycin $X_{0\delta}$. The structure is the same as that of actinomycin D with one of the L-proline groups oxidized to L-γ-oxoproline. The minimal inhibitory concentration against *Bacillus subtilis* is 1·5 times that of actinomycin C_3.

Brockmann, Linge, Grone, *Naturwiss.*, **40**, 224 (1953)
Brockmann, Grone, *Chem. Ber.*, **87**, 1036 (1954)
Brockmann, Manegold, *ibid.*, **93**, 2971 (1960)
Brockmann, Boldt, Petras, *Naturwiss.*, **47**, 62 (1960)
Brockmann, Manegold, *Chem. Ber.*, **95**, 1081 (1962)

ACTINOMYCIN Z

A recently discovered member of the actinomycin group of antibiotics, this substance has been shown to contain 3-hydroxy-4-oxo-5-methylproline in the molecule.

Brockmann, Staehler, *Tetrahedron Lett.*, 3685 (1973)

ACTINOMYCIN Z₁

The structure of this anisoactinomycin is not yet known with certainty. It has been found to contain L-threonine, sarcosine, D-valine, L-N-methylalanine, L-N-methylvaline, 5-methyl(?)4-L-γ-oxoproline and a hydroxyaminoacid which has not yet been identified. The order in which these aminoacids are present in the peptide chains has still to be established. The minimal inhibitory concentration against *Bacillus subtilis* is 50 times that of actinomycin C_3.

Brockmann, Staehler, *Naturwiss.*, **52**, 391 (1965)
Brockmann, Manegold, *Hoppe-Seyler's Z. Phys. Chem.*, **343**, 86 (1966)

ACTINOMYCIN Z₅

A further newly discovered actinomycin, this substance contains L-N-methylproline, L-4-oxo-5-methylproline and L-N-methylalanine in the peptide chains. The L-N-methylproline in this compound has been shown to have the cis-configuration.

Brockmann, Staehler, *Tetrahedron Lett.*, 2567 (1973)
Katz, Mason, Mauger, *Biochem. Biophys. Res. Commun.*, **52**, 819 (1973)

ACTINOMYCIN I
See Actinomycin $X_{0\beta}$

ACTINOMYCIN I_2
See Actinomycin C_2

ACTINOMYCIN II
See Actinomycin F_8

ACTINOMYCIN III
See Actinomycin F_9

ACTINOMYCIN IV
See Actinomycin D

ACTINOMYCIN V
See Actinomycin X_2

ACTINOMYCIN VI
See Actinomycin C_2

ACTINOMYCIN VII
See Actinomycin C_3

ACTINOMYCIN (Ser-Val-Pro-Sar-MeVal)
$C_{60}H_{82}O_{16}N_{12}$
M.p. 269–273°C (dec.)
A synthetic actinomycin, this antibiotic is obtained as deep red crystals from AcOEt-hexane. It is laevorotatory having $[\alpha]_D^{21} - 435°$ (c 0·25, CH_3OH) and gives an ultraviolet spectrum with a single absorption maximum at 450 nm. It has a minimal inhibitory concentration against *Bacillus subtilis* eight times that of actinomycin C_3.

Brockmann, Lackner, *Tetrahedron Lett.*, 3523 (1964)

ACTINONE A
This antibiotic is the Et_2O-soluble component of actinone, isolated from a species of *Streptomyces* closely related to *S. antibioticus*. It is soluble in $CHCl_3$ and is active against *Trichophyton* and *Saccharomyces* species but has no activity against other fungi or bacteria. The LD_0 in mice when administered intravenously is 1000 mg/kg.

Ikeda, Hirai, Nishimaki, *J. Antibiotics* (Japan), **3**, 724 (1950)

ACTINONE B
Also obtained from a *Streptomyces* species allied to *S. antibioticus*, this antibiotic is insoluble in both Et_2O and $CHCl_3$. Its biological activity and toxicity are similar to those of the preceding compound.

Ikeda, Hirai, Nishimaki, *J. Antibiotics* (Japan), **3**, 724 (1950)

ACTINONIN
$C_{19}H_{35}O_5N_3$
M.p. 148–149°C
Actinonin is isolated from the culture filtrate of a strain of *Streptomyces*, Cutter C/2 (NCIB 8845), by extraction into BuOH from which, after

concentration *in vacuo*, it is purified further by a series of partitions between H$_2$O and CHCl$_3$ at different pH values to give the final CHCl$_3$ concentrate. From this, the antibiotic is precipitated by the addition of Et$_2$O at 0°C. Treatment in hot EtOH with activated carbon and recrystallization from EtOH—Et$_2$O gives fine white needles or colourless rods. The antibiotic is stable in cold alkalies and not readily affected by cold dilute acids. It is soluble in H$_2$O, the lower alcohols and pyridine and active against both gram-positive and gram-negative bacteria including *Bacillus anthracis*, *Klebsiella pneumoniae*, *Mycobacterium phlei*, *M. smegmatis*, *Salmonella enteritidis*, *S. typhosa*, *Staphylococcys aureus* and *Streptococcus pyogenes*. It has also been shown to inhibit the phages of a number of strains of *Staphylococcus aureus* at concentrations down to 0·25 μg/ml. It shows no apparent toxicity in mice at doses up to 400 mg/kg. Activity *in vivo* is comparatively low, possibly due to cleavage of the antibiotic into inactive products.

Gordon, Kelly, Miller, *Nature*, **195**, 701 (1962)
Broughton *et al.*, *J. Chem. Soc.*, *Perkin I*, 857 (1975)
Synthesis
Anderson *et al.*, *Chem. Commun.*, 420 (1974)
Devlin *et al.*, *ibid.*, 421 (1974)

ACTINORHODINE
C$_{32}$H$_{36}$O$_{14}$
Decomp. 270°C

An antibiotic pigment, this substance has been isolated from *Streptomyces coelicolor* discovered in the woods near Gottingen in Germany. The organism is grown on a culture medium at pH 7·0 containing corn extract, glycerol or sucrose, glycine and potassium nitrate and the antibiotic obtained from the mycelium. Actinorhodine crystallizes from dioxan as bright red needles which decompose without melting. It is freely soluble in EtOH, AcOH and (CH$_3$)$_2$CO. In aqueous acids, the antibiotic is virtually insoluble but it dissolves in aqueous alkalies with a bright blue colour. Similar coloured solutions are obtained in (CH$_3$)$_2$CO in which it forms a red solution and in pyridine when it gives a blue colouration. The solution in (CH$_3$)$_2$CO changes to a violet-blue with a red fluorescence when heated with boric-acetic anhydride. In dioxan, the antibiotic gives a visible spectrum consisting of two absorption peaks at 523 and 560 nm. The tentative structure given above, which is based upon chemical and spectroscopic evidence, shows it to be a dimeric quinone. Actinorhodine inhibits *Staphylococcus aureus* at a concentration of 1:100,000.

Plotho, Brockmann, Pini, *Naturwiss.*, **34**, 190 (1947)
Brockmann *et al.*, *Ber.*, **83**, 161 (1950)
Structure
Brockmann, Hieronymus, *Ber.*, **88**, 1379 (1955)
Brockmann *et al.*, *Naturwiss.*, **49**, 131 (1962)
Brockmann, *Angew. Chem.*, **76**, 863 (1964)
Brockmann *et al.*, *Annalen*, **698**, 209 (1966)

ACTINORUBIN
C$_6$H$_{14}$O$_3$N$_2$ (C$_9$H$_{22}$O$_4$N$_5$)
M.p. Indefinite

Produced by a species of *Actinomyces*, this antibiotic is closely related to streptothricin (q.v.). It is a basic polypeptide which is stable to heat and dialyzes through cellophane. Crude actinorubin, when dried *in vacuo*, forms a brownish hygroscopic powder with no definite melting point. It is soluble in H$_2$O and CH$_3$OH but insoluble in Et$_2$O. Actinorubin reduces both KMnO$_4$ and Fehling's solution and gives a positive biuret reaction but negative Molisch and Sakaguchi reactions. It may be characterized as the helianthate which forms clusters of small reddish-orange needles with m.p. 206–214°C (*dec.*).

The antibiotic is active against gram-positive, gram-negative and acid-fast bacteria and also shows some activity against certain fungi. It has, however, only a limited activity against streptococci and *Bacillus cereusmycoides*. Using a serial dilution assay by streak test with *Escherichia coli* as the test organism, crude actinorubin has 0·5–0·6 γ/unit and the helianthate 0·5 γ/unit. Typical inhibition concentrations (units/ml) *in vitro* are:

Escherichia coli (1·05); *Aerobacter aerogenes* (0·25); *Bacillus anthracis* (2·0–4·0); *B. cereus* (32); *Brucella abortus* (4·0); *B. suis* (16); *Diplococcus pneumoniae* (>132); *Gaffkya tetragena* (0·03); *Klebsiella pneumoniae* (0·125); *Micrococcus auranticus* (0·007); *Mycobacterium tuberculosis bovis* (8·0); *Proteus vulgaris* (1·0); *Staphylococcus aureus* (0·06); *Streptococcus pyogenes* (128) and *Vibrio comma* (0·6). When given to mice intraperitoneally, 0·2 per *E. coli* unit gives complete protection against experimental infection with *Klebsiella pneumoniae*. The toxicity in mice has been given as LD_{50} 0·68 mg/kg when administered intraperitoneally. Following such administration, the antibiotic has been detected in the blood whereas it is not so detected following oral administration.

Kelner *et al.*, *J. Bact.*, **51**, 591 (1946)
Kelner, Morton, *ibid.*, **53**, 695 (1947)
Morton, *Proc. Soc. Exptl. Biol. Med.*, **64**, 327 (1947)
Junowicz-Kocholaty, Kocholaty, *J. Biol. Chem.*, **168**, 757 (1947)

ACTINOSPECTACIN (*Spectinomycin*)
$C_{14}H_{24}O_7N_2$
M.p. 65–72°C

Actinospectacin was first isolated from cultures of *Streptomyces spectabilis* and subsequently from *S. flavopersicus* and *S. hygroscopicus* var. *sagamiensis* ATCC 21,703. The anhydrous antibiotic is an amorphous powder but, when crystallized from $(CH_3)_2CO$—H_2O, it forms colourless crystals of the hexahydrate having the melting point given above. This form is dextrorotatory with a specific rotation of $[\alpha]_D^{25}$ + 7·6° (c 1·0, H_2O) and reverts to the amorphous powder on drying. The sulphate crystallizes from $(CH_3)_2CO$—H_2O with m.p. 185°C (*dec. dry*), having $[\alpha]_D^{25}$ + 17° (c 1·0, H_2O). Acid hydrolysis furnishes actinamine, $C_8H_{18}O_4N_2$.

Actinospectacin is active against both gram-positive and gram-negative bacteria, being inhibitory against most strains of *Enterobacter*, *Escherichia coli*, *Klebsiella* and *Staphylococcus epidermidis*. The minimum inhibition concentration against *Klebsiella pneumoniae* is 2·6 μg/ml. When administered to healthy human volunteers at a dose of 0·5–8·0 g intravenously per day for 5 days, no indications of hepatotoxicity, nephrotoxicity, ototoxicity or local intolerance were observed. In veterinary medicine it has found some use in the treatment of bacterial enteritis and coccidiosis of dogs.

Mason, Dietz, Smith, *Antibiotics & Chemotherapy*, **11**, 118 (1961)
Bergy, Eble, Hess, *ibid.*, **11**, 661 (1961)
Chapman *et al.*, *Proc. Nat. Acad. Sci. U.S.*, **48**, 1108, 1693 (1962)
Washington, Yu, *Antimicrobial Agents & Chemotherapy*, **2**, 427 (1972)
Nara *et al.*, *German Patent*, 2,233,555 (1973)
Novak *et al.*, *J. Clin. Pharmacol.*, **14**, 442 (1974)
Nara *et al.*, *U.S. Patent*, 3,819,485 (1974)
Novak, Gray, Pfeifer, *J. Inf. Diseases*, **130**, 50 (1974)
Structure
Hoeksema, Argoudelis, Wiley, *J. Amer. Chem. Soc.*, **84**, 3212 (1962)
Hoeksema, Argoudelis, Wiley, *ibid.*, **85**, 2652 (1963)
Biosynthesis
Mitscher *et al.*, *J. Chem. Soc.*, D, 1541 (1971)

ACTINOTIOCIN
M.p. 247–249°C

This antibiotic has recently been described by Japanese workers. It is obtained from *Actinomadura pusilla* by cultivation on a medium containing maltose, soybean flour, soybean oil, neat extract and inorganic salts at 30°C for 7 days. The compound is isolated by extraction of the culture broth and mycelium with AcOEt and purified by chromatography on silica gel. Actinotiocin forms colourless columnar crystals and is dextrorotatory with a specific rotation of $[\alpha]_D^{20}$ + 164° (c 0·77, dioxan). It is soluble in CH_3OH—$CHCl_3$, $EtOH$—$CHCl_3$, dioxan and $(CH_3)_2SO$, slightly soluble in CH_3OH, $EtOH$, $(CH_3)_2CO$, $AcOEt$ and $CHCl_3$, insoluble in C_6H_6, H_2O and hexane. The antibiotic is stable in neutral and alkaline solutions but unstable in acids. It is active against gram-positive bacteria, mycobacteria and mycoplasma, but not against gram-negative bacteria, *Candida*, *Trichophyton* or *Trichomonas*. It is also active *in vivo* affording 70 per cent and 100 per cent protection to mice infected with *Staphylococcus aureus* and *Diplococcus pneumoniae* respectively when given at 100 mg/kg intraperitoneally. A dose of 1 g/kg given either orally or intraperitoneally to mice produced no adverse effects.

Tamura *et al.*, *J. Antibiotics* (Japan), **26**, 343 (1973)
Tamura *et al.*, *Japanese Patent*, 7,328,692 (1973)

ACTITHIAZIC ACID (*Mycobacidin*)
$C_9H_{15}O_3NS$
M.p. 139–140°C

An antibiotic elaborated by *Streptomyces lavendulae* and *S. virginiae*, this substance forms colourless crystals from BuOH. It is laevorotatory with $[\alpha]_D^{25} - 60.5°$ (EtOH). The antibiotic is soluble in alkaline solutions and in the lower alcohols but insoluble in H_2O, C_6H_6, and $CHCl_3$. It shows no typical absorptions in the ultraviolet spectrum and the structure has been determined as 4-thiazolidone-2-caproic acid.

Actithiazic acid is largely active against mycobacteria at a level of 0·02–0·5 μg/ml, having only a limited activity against other bacteria. The development of resistance is slow, while the toxicity in mice, both intravenous and subcutaneous, is 1·5 gm/kg. Being inactive *in vivo*, with no chemotherapeutic effect in experimental tuberculosis in mice, it has found no application in medicine.

Grundy et al., *Antibiotics & Chemotherapy*, **2**, 399 (1952)
Schenck, DeRose, *Arch. Biochem. Biophys.*, **40**, 263 (1952)
Clark, Schenck, *ibid.*, **40**, 270 (1952)
Hwang, *Antibiotics & Chemotherapy*, **2**, 453 (1952)
Sobin, *J. Amer. Chem. Soc.*, **74**, 2247 (1952)
McLamore et al., *ibid.*, **74**, 2246 (1952)
Tejera et al., *Antibiotics & Chemotherapy*, **2**, 233 (1952)

ACULEACINS
Aspergillus aculeatus M 4217 (FERM-P 2324) yields an antibiotic complex when cultured aerobically at 26°C and pH 6·5 for 96 hours on a medium containing peptone, sucrose, dextrin, KH_2PO_4, $MgSO_4$ and $FeSO_4 \cdot 7H_2O$. The cells are extracted with MeOH by stirring for 20 hours and the extract concentrated *in vacuo* and then extracted with BuOH. The extract is decolourized with activated carbon, concentrated, and the concentrate treated with hexane forming a precipitate which, after further washing with hexane and drying, yields a dark brown powder. This crude preparation is washed with AcOEt, dissolved in MeOH and reprecipitated with AcOEt, giving a pale brown powder. Fractionation by silica gel chromatography yields aculeacins B, C, D, E, F and G. Molecular weight determinations of these peptide-like substances give values of 1145–1300. The antibiotics are soluble in the lower alcohols and insoluble in Me_2CO, AcOEt, hexane, $CHCl_3$, petroleum ether and HO. They are effective against fungi and yeasts but show very little activity towards bacteria.

Mizuno et al., *Japanese Patent*, 76 98,387 (1976)

ACUMYCIN
$C_{38}H_{61}O_{12}N$
M.p. 233–237°C (*dec.*)

One of several antibiotics obtained from *Streptomyces griseoflavus*, this compound forms colourless crystals from $CHCl_3$. It is laevorotatory having $[\alpha]_D^{25} - 92°$ (c 1·0, $CHCl_3$) and gives an ultraviolet spectrum consisting of a single absorption maximum at 241 nm. Hydrolysis yields mycaminose.

Bicket et al., *Helv. Chim. Acta*, **45**, 1396 (1962)

ADICILLIN
See Penicillin N

ADRIAMYCIN (*Doxorubicin, 14-Hydroxydaunomycin*)
$C_{27}H_{29}O_{11}N$

A semi-synthetic antibiotic, adriamycin possesses marked antitumour and antileukemic properties and is similar in this respect to daunomycin (q.v.). When hydrolysed with dilute acids it yields daunosamine and adriamycinone, the latter having an anthraquinone structure, m.p. 223–224°C; $[\alpha]_D^{23} + 188°$ (c 1·0, dioxan) and giving a crystalline pentaacetate, m.p. 166°C; $[\alpha]_D^{23} - 94°$ (c 1·0, $CHCl_3$).

Adriamycin is not a potent antimicrobial agent although one strain of *Streptococcus fecalis* 6-MP/R, resistant to 6-mercaptopurine, is inhibited by the antibiotic. Adriamycin markedly decreases the mitotic index in a culture of HeLa cells containing hydroxyurea at 0·1 and 0·5 µg/ml. It also inhibits RNA synthesis but exerts no effect upon protein synthesis. Massimo *et al.* have demonstrated that 0·05–5·0 µg/ml inhibits blastogenesis when added to human lymphocytes *in vitro* in the presence of phytohemaglutinin. Several alterations to the chromosomes in the lymphocytes were also found including fragmentations, rearrangements, polyradial figures, rupture of centromeres and chromatid exchanges. The antibiotic appears to exert a mutagenic effect.

A number of 14-O-acyl derivatives of adriamycin have been prepared by the reaction of 14-bromodaunorubicin hydrochlotide with the appropriate sodium or potassium salt in $(CH_3)_2CO$ and examined for their biological activity. All have been found to possess antiviral, cytotoxic and antitumour activity, the most active antitumour compound being adriamycin 14-octanoate hydrochloride when tested in mice. All of these acyl derivatives have activities equal to or greater than that of adriamycin. However, Price and his coworkers have also shown that when given at a non-toxic dose, the antibiotic not only failed to protect rat embryo cells *in vitro* from transformation by 3-methylcholanthrene but also acted on its own as a transforming agent.

Arcamone *et al.*, *Tetrahedron Lett.*, 1007 (1969)
Pittillo, Woolley, *Cancer Chemother. Rep., Part I*, **55**, 221 (1971)
Vig, *Cancer Res.*, **31**, 32 (1971)
Arena *et al.*, *Arzneim.-Forsch.*, **21**, 1258 (1971)
Lambertenghi-Deliliers, *Int. Symp. Adriamycin*, 26 (1971)
Boll, *ibid.*, 23 (1971)
Di Marco, *ibid.*, 53 (1971)
Massimo *et al.*, *ibid.*, 35 (1971)
Goldin, *ibid.*, 64 (1971)
Isetta, Intini, Soldati, *Experientia*, **27**, 202 (1971)
Negishi, Takahiri, *Yakugaku Zasshi*, **93**, 1498 (1973)
Liss, Ifrim, *Proc. Electron Microsc. Soc. Amer.*, **31**, 542 (1973)
Arcamone *et al.*, *J. Med. Chem.*, **17**, 335 (1974)
Blum, Carter, *Ann. Intern. Med.*, **80**, 249 (1974)
Barranco, Novak, *Cancer Res.*, **34**, 1616 (1974)
Iwamoto *et al.*, *Biochem. Biophys. Res. Commun.*, **58**, 633 (1974)
Arcamone *et al.*, *J. Med. Chem.*, **17**, 335 (1974)
Biondo *et al.*, *IRCS Med. Sci., Libr. Compend.*, **3**, 155 (1975)
Price *et al.*, *Science*, **187**, 1200 (1975)
See also
Skovsgaard, Nissen, *Dan. Med. Bull.*, **22**, 62 (1975)

AEROSPORIN
See Polymyxin A

AERUGINOIC ACID
$C_{10}H_7O_3NS$

When cultivated in an aqueous medium containing kerosine, peptone, Tween-20 and inorganic salts, *Pseudomonas aeruginosa* elaborates this antibiotic substance which is active against gram-positive bacteria and also has antiinflammatory and hypotensive properties. The structure has been determined by chemical and spectroscopic methods.

Imai *et al.*, *German Patent*, 2,045,819 (1971)

AFSILLIN
See Procaine Penicillin G

AGROCYBIN
$C_8H_5O_2N$
M.p. 140°C (*dec.*)

$HOCH_2-C{\equiv}C-C{\equiv}C-C{\equiv}C-CONH_2$

This antibiotic is elaborated by the basidiomycete *Agrocybe dura*. It forms colourless crystals from 20 per cent aqueous EtOH or from Et_2O and deflagrates at the melting point. It is relatively unstable, turning black and becoming insoluble in Et_2O on standing for 1 day in air. Agrocybin is soluble in EtOH, Et_2O, $(CH_3)_2CO$, $CHCl_3$ and methyl *iso*butyl ketone, slightly soluble in H_2O and insoluble in hexane. It is active against gram-positive bacteria, particularly *Escherichia coli* and *Staphylococcus aureus* and also against a number of pathogenic fungi. Care must be taken in handling this substance since it causes dermatitis. It is highly toxic and inactivated by blood and for this reason no *in vivo* tests have been carried out.

Kavanagh *et al.*, *Proc. Nat. Acad. Sci., U.S.*, **36**, 102 (1950)
Structure and synthesis
Bu'Lock *et al.*, *Chem. & Ind.*, 990 (1954)
Ashworth *et al.*, *J. Chem. Soc.*, 950 (1958)

AKLAVINE
$C_{30}H_{37}O_{11}N$
M.p. Indefinite

Streptomyces galilaeus produces three antibiotics when grown on a common nutrient medium at 28–30°C and pH 7·0. This compound forms a reddish powder and on hydrolysis furnishes aklavinone I (q.v.). Aklavine forms a number of crystalline salts, e.g. the hydrochloride as orange crystals with m.p. 197°C, giving an ultraviolet spectrum in EtOH with absorption maxima at 228, 258 and 288 nm, the helianthate, m.p. 197°C and the picrate, m.p. 168°C. It is active against a number of gram-positive bacteria.

Strelitz *et al.*, *J. Bact.*, **72**, 90 (1956)
Gordon *et al.*, *Tetrahedron Lett.*, 28 (1960)

AKLAVINONE I
$C_{22}H_{20}O_8$
M.p. 169–170°C

A further antibiotic isolated from cultures of *Streptomyces galilaeus*, this substance crystallizes from EtOH in the form of bright red needles. It is also produced by the acid hydrolysis of aklavine. It has a similar antibiotic spectrum to that of aklavine.

Eckardt, Tresselt, *Z. Chem.*, **14**, 57 (1974)

AKLAVINONE II
$C_{22}H_{20}O_8$
M.p. 186–188°C

A further pigment antibiotic isolated from the culture filtrate of *Streptomyces galilaeus*, aklavinone II is a stereoisomer of the preceding antibiotic. It also forms bright red needles when crystallized from EtOH and is active against a number of gram-positive bacteria.

Eckardt, Tresselt, *Z. Chem.*, **14**, 57 (1974)

ALAMETHICIN

A broad-spectrum antibiotic, alamethicin is elaborated by *Trichoderma viride* grown on a nutrient medium containing molasses, dextrin, cottonseed meal and fish meal at 25°C for 5 days with shaking. The antibiotic is isolated by adding diatomaceous earth to the culture broth, filtering, extracting the residue with $(CH_3)_2CO$, evaporating the solvent and lyophilizing the residual aqueous fraction. Further purification is carried out by transforming the dry powder into the H_2O-soluble sodium salt. Alamethicin is active against gram-positive bacteria, fungi, protozoa and KB cells in tissue culture.

Coats, Meyer, Reusser, *French Patent*, 1,511,185 (1968)

ALANOSINE
$C_3H_7O_4N_3$
Dec. 190°C

A simple propionic acid derivative, this antibiotic from *Streptomyces alanosinicus* forms a microcrystalline powder from dilute HCl. It is laevorotatory with a specific rotation of $[\alpha]_D^{25} - 37·8°$ (c 0·5, H_2O) or $[\alpha]_D - 46°$ (c 1·0, 0·1 *N*-NaOH). The ultraviolet spectrum in 0·1 *N*-HCl has an absorption maximum at 228 nm, shifted to 250 nm in 0·1 *N*-NaOH. It is slightly soluble in H_2O and insoluble in common organic solvents. The ($\pm$)-form has been prepared as colourless crystals from H_2O with m.p. 185°C (*dec.*). The structure of the natural compound has been established as L-2-amino-3-(N-hydroxy-N-nitrosoamino)-propionic acid. Alanosine is active against gram-positive bacteria and is reported to also have antiviral and antineoplastic activity.

Coronelli *et al.*, *Il Farmaco Ed. Sci.*, **21**, 269 (1966)
Murthy *et al.*, *Nature*, **211**, 1198 (1966)
Synthesis
Lancini, Diena, Lazzari, *Tetrahedron Lett.*, 1769 (1966)

ALAZOPEPTIN
$C_{15}H_{21}O_6N_7$?
M.p. Indefinite

Streptomyces griseoplanus produces this antitumour antibiotic which has the probable structure of L-allyl-(6-diazo-5-oxo)-L-norleucyl-(6-diazo-5-oxo)-L-norleucine. When purified by crystallization from aqueous $(CH_3)_2CO$ it forms colourless crystals of the monohydrate which is relatively unstable and has no definite melting point. Alazopeptin is dextrorotatory with a specific rotation of $[\alpha]_D^{25} + 9.5°$ (c 4.7, H_2O) and gives an ultraviolet spectrum in neutral phosphate buffer with absorption maxima at 242 and 274 nm. It is readily soluble in H_2O, moderately so in AcOH, $(CH_3)_2SO$, formamide and aqueous alcohols, insoluble in anhydrous $(CH_3)_2CO$, alcohols, Et_2O and AcOEt. It inhibits experimental tumours and is comparatively toxic with LD_{50} in mice of 150 mg/kg given intravenously.

De Voe *et al.*, *Antibiotics Annual*, 730 (1956–1957)

ALBIMYCIN
See Hondamycin

ALBOCYCLINE
$C_{18}H_{28}O_4$
M.p. Indefinite

A macrocyclic antibiotic isolated from cultures of a number of *Streptomyces* species, this compound crystallizes from EtOH as colourless plates with no definite melting point. It has been characterized as the acetate, m.p. 84°C. The structure has been determined by chemical and spectroscopic methods. Albocycline is active against gram-positive and some gram-negative bacteria.

Nagahama *et al.*, *Chem. Pharm. Bull.*, **19**, 649 (1971)
Nagahama, Takamori, Suzuki, *ibid.*, **19**, 655, 660 (1971)

ALBOMYCIN A_1
M.p. Indefinite

Actinomyces subtropicus elaborates an iron-containing antibiotic complex consisting of at least six components of which this is the active constituent, the others apparently being degradation products of this particular antibiotic. Albomycin A_1 is employed in the form of the sulphate which is an amorphous red powder having no definite melting point. It gives an ultraviolet spectrum consisting of a single absorption maximum at 283 nm. The salt is freely soluble in H_2O, slightly soluble in CH_3OH and insoluble in all other organic solvents. It has a pronounced activity against penicillin-resistant pneumococci and staphylococci and has a low toxicity comparable to that of penicilllin.

Gause, Braznikova, *Novosti Med.*, **23**, 3 (1951)
Braznikova *et al.*, *Biokhimiya*, **22**, 111 (1959)
Turkova *et al.*, *Antibiotiki*, **7**, 878 (1962)
Structure
Turkova *et al.*, *Collect. Czech. Chem. Commun.*, **27**, 591 (1962)
Mikes *et al.*, *ibid.*, **28**, 1747 (1963)
Mikes *et al.*, *Experientia*, **19**, 633 (1963)
Turkova *et al.*, *Collect. Czech. Chem. Commun.*, **30**, 118 (1965)
Elnaggar, Poddubnaya, *Zhur. Obshch. Khim.*, **36**, 1604 (1966)

ALBONOURSIN
$C_{15}H_{16}O_2N_2$
M.p. 275–276°C

Isolated from cultures of *Streptomyces noursei* and *S. albus* var. *fungatus*, this antibiotic has been shown to be identical with Component 2 obtained by Brown and Kelley and also with Compound B-73 isolated by Rao and Cullen. When crystallized from AcOEt it forms colourless plates. The ultraviolet spectrum consists of two absorption maxima at 234 and 318 nm. Chemical and spectroscopic investigations have shown the structure to be 3-benzylidene-6-*iso*butylidene-piperazine-2:5-dione. It is active against gram-positive and some gram-negative bacteria.

Brown, Kelley, *Ann. Rep. New York State Dept. Health Albany*, 10 (1957); 47 (1958); 52 (1959); 50 (1960); 40 (1961)
Rao, Cullen, *J. Amer. Chem. Soc.*, **82**, 1127 (1960)

Vondrack, Vanek, *Chem. Ind.* (London), 1686 (1964)
Khokhlov, Lokshin, *Tetrahedron Lett.*, 1881 (1963)
Brown, Kelley, Wiberley, *J. Org. Chem.*, **30**, 277 (1965)

ALBORIXIN
$C_{48}H_{84}O_{12}$
M.p. 100–115°C

A polyether antibiotic, alborixin has been isolated from cultures of *Streptomyces albus*. It forms an amorphous white powder and has an optical rotation of $[\alpha]_{578}^{20} - 7.0°$ (c 4·0, Me_2CO). It has been characterized as the methyl ester, m.p. 67–68°C; the potassium salt with m.p. 209–210°C and the triacetate, m.p. 70–75°C. The structure has been established by an X-ray crystallographic study.

Alleaume *et al.*, *Chem. Commun.*, 411 (1975)

ALDGAMYCIN C
$C_{36}H_{60}O_{14}$
M.p. 150–153°C

An antibiotic elaborated by *Streptomyces lavendulae* (Lederle soil isolate AL471), the substance crystallizes from EtOH as colourless needles and is laevorotatory having $[\alpha]_D^{25} - 70°$ (c 0·67, CH_3OH). The ultraviolet spectrum shows a single absorption maximum at 217 nm.

Kunstmann, Mitscher, Bohonas, *Tetrahedron Lett.*, 839 (1966)
Ellestad *et al.*, *Tetrahedron*, **23**, 3893 (1967)

ALDGAMYCIN E
$C_{37}H_{58}O_{15}$
M.p. 158–161°C and 173–178°C

Two crystalline forms of this antibiotic from *Streptomyces lavendulae* have been obtained, as colourless needles with the lower melting point given above and as colourless plates with the higher melting point. The compound has a specific rotation of $[\alpha]_D^{25} - 56°$ (c 0·972, CH_3OH) and gives an ultraviolet spectrum having an absorption maximum at 216 nm.

Hydrolysis with barium hydroxide yields aldgamycin C (q.v.) while methanolysis furnishes methyl aldgarosides A and B and methyl mycinoside. Hydrogenation yields the dihydro derivative as colourless crystals with m.p. 118–125°C. Acetylation furnishes two diacetates, m.p. 167–171°C and 239–243°C respectively.

Kunstmann, Mitscher, Patterson, *Antimicrobial Agents & Chemotherapy*, 87 (1964)
Kunstmann, Mitscher, Bohonas, *Tetrahedron Lett.*, 839 (1966)
Ellestad *et al.*, *Tetrahedron*, **23**, 3893 (1967)

ALDGAMYCIN F
$C_{37}H_{56}O_{15}$
M.p. Indefinite

Streptomyces lavendulae elaborates this antibiotic which has been obtained as a non-crystallizable solid having no definite melting point. It is laevorotatory with a specific rotation of $[\alpha]_D^{20} - 25°$ (c 0·3, $CHCl_3$). The structure has been determined from chemical and spectroscopic evidence.

Achenbach, Karl., *Chem. Ber.*, **108**, 780 (1975)

ALLICIN
$C_6H_{10}OS_2$
B.p. Indefinite

$$C_3H_5-\overset{\overset{O}{\|}}{S}-S-C_3H_5$$

Allicin has been isolated from garlic cloves although it is not normally present in the free state in the plant. Alliin, which is the precursor, is an odourless, thermostable substance which is biologically inactive. Crushing of the cloves yields allicin, ammonia and pyruvic acid due to the action of an enzyme, alliinase. Allicin is a colourless liquid which decomposes when dry distilled. It is soluble in H_2O, EtOH, Et_2O and C_6H_6 but only slightly soluble in 'Shellysolves'. It is optically inactive, has the characteristic odour of garlic and irritates the skin. When hydrolysed it yields SO_2 and allyldisulphide indicating that it is the allyl ester of allylthiosulphinic acid. This structure has been confirmed by its synthesis from diallyl sulphide with H_2O_2 in glacial AcOH.

The antibiotic is active against both gram-positive and gram-negative bacteria. The inhibition concentration in millimoles/millimeter ($\times 10,000$) for typical organisms is: *Bacillus cereus* (0·3); *B. subtilis* (0·3–0·5); *Clostridium histolyticus* (0·6); *C. welchii* (1·0); *Diplococcus pneumoniae* (2·0); *Escherichia coli* (1·5); *Salmonella paratyphi* (1·0); *Sarcina lutea* (0·2); *Staphyloccocus albus* (1·5); *S. aureus* (0·6); *Streptococcus fecalis* (2·0); *Strep. hemolyticus* (1·0). It is also active against various fungi, e.g. *Aspergillus niger* (0·6); *Penicillium notatum* (0·9); *Microsporum audouini* (0·6) and *Trychophyton gypseum* (0·06). The LD_{50} in mice has been given as 120 mg/kg (subcutaneous) and approximately 60 mg/kg (intravenous).

Cavallito, Bailey, *J. Amer. Chem. Soc.*, **66**, 1950 (1944)
Cavallito, Bailey, Buck, *ibid.*, **67**, 1032 (1945)
Raghumandana, Srinivasa, Vankataraman, *J. Sci. Ind. Res.* (India), **1B**, 31 (1946)
Oppikofer, *Schweiz. Apoth. Ztg.*, **85**, 849 (1947)
Small, Bailey, Cavallito, *J. Amer. Chem. Soc.*, **69**, 1710 (1947)
Stoll, Seebeck, *Experimentia*, **3**, 114 (1947)
Raghunandana, Krishna, *Curr. Sci.* (India), **17**, 23 (1948)
Stoll, Seebeck, *Helv. Chim. Acta*, **31**, 189 (1948)
Stoll, Seebeck, *ibid.*, **32**, 197, 866 (1949)

ALLISTATIN
This antibiotic has been described by Indian workers. It is stated to occur with allicin (q.v.) in garlic cloves and consists of allistatins I and II with possbily a third fraction present in the mixture. From the literature it appears that this group of antibiotic substances is also formed from a precursor in the plant by the action of alliinase. The properties of these substances are said to be similar to those of allicin.

Datta, Krishnamurthi, Siddiqui, *J. Sci. Ind. Res.* (India), **7B**, No. 3, 42 (1948)

ALPHACILLIN
See Penicillin V potassium salt

ALTERNARIC ACID
M.p. 134°C

This antibiotic was first described by Brian and his colleagues in 1949 who obtained it from *Alternaria solani*. It also possibly occurs in *A. porri*. When purified by crystallization from C_6H_6 followed by several recrystallizations from EtOH or H_2O, it forms colourless crystals. It is an optically inactive, dibasic acid and is assayed by 'stunting' of the developing germ tubes in *Botrytis allii* or *Myrothecium verrucaria*. The antibiotic spectrum *in vitro* shows negligible activity against bacteria but specific antifungal activity. In concentrations of 0·1–1·0 µg/ml it inhibits the spore germination of *Absidia glauca, Myrothecium verrucaria* and *Stachybotrys atra* but shows no effect on spore germination of *Botrytis allii, Fusarium coeruleum* or *Penicillium digitatum* even at concentrations as high as 200 µg/ml. At very low concentrations of the order of 0·01 µg/ml it 'stunts' the germ tubes of *Botrytis allii*.

Brian *et al.*, *Nature*, **164**, 534 (1949)

ALTHIOMYCIN
$C_{17}H_{19}N_5O_6S_2$
M.p. 180–181·6°C (dec.)

An unidentified species of *Streptomyces* produces this antibiotic which was originally assigned the empirical formula $C_{15}H_{14}O_6N_4S_2$, later changed to that given above. The compound forms colourless crystals from EtOH or CH_2Cl_2—EtOH and has the following specific rotations: $[\alpha]_D^{20} + 20\cdot3°$ (c 1·33, methylcellosolve) and $[\alpha]_D^{25} + 37\cdot8°$ (1:1 $CHCl_3$—EtOH). When treated with Ac_2O in pyridine it yields the acetyl derivative. The antibiotic has a maximum stability in the pH range from 5·0 to 7·0.

Yamaguchi et al., *J. Antibiotics* (Japan), **10A**, 195 (1957)
Revised formula
Cram et al., *J. Amer. Chem. Soc.*, **85**, 1430 (1963)
Structure
Sakakibara et al., *J. Antibiotics* (Japan), **27**, 897 (1974)
Byercroft, Pinchin, *Chem. Commun.*, 121 (1975)
Kirst et al., *J. Antibiotics* (Japan), **28**, 286 (1976)

ALVEIN

M.p. Indefinite

This antibiotic, formed by *Bacillus alvei*, is normally produced by submerged growth in aerated bottles since surface growth is not successful unless some form of mechanical support is provided for the pellicle. The culture filtrate may be extracted with BuOH at pH 9·0 or the filtrate activity adsorbed in activated carbon at pH 7·0 and eluted with aqueous acidified BuOH, the BuOH layer separated, aqueous Et_2O added and the aqueous layer separated and neutralized. Purification is normally carried out by precipating the alvein with picric acid at 4°C, the precipitate converted into the hydrochloride after drying, precipitated from dry Et_2O and further purified by countercurrent distribution methods.

The free base is probably a polypeptide containing alanine, arginine, cystine, leucine, lysine, serine, threonine and valine. It is soluble in EtOH and BuOH, slightly so in H_2O, the solubility in the latter decreasing above pH 7·0 and on adding sodium chloride. The hydrochloride is soluble in H_2O and EtOH but insoluble in $(CH_3)_2CO$, Et_2O and $CHCl_3$. It is thermostable between pH 2·0 and 7·0 and less stable outside these limits. It is inactivated by trypsin. The assay is normally carried out in a cylinder plate with *Staphylococcus aureus*. The inhibition dilution ($\times 1000$) against typical organisms is: *Bacillus anthracis* (512); *Escherichia coli* (32); *Mycobacterium phlei* (32,000); *Myco. tuberculosis* (10–100); *Pseudomonas aeruginosa* (16); *Staphylococcus aureus* (512) and *Streptococcus pyogenes* (128). Alvein is bactericidal to *Mycobacterium tuberculosis* and there is no increase in resistance with *Staphylococcus aureus*. The activity of the antibiotic is not affected by horse serum. Pharmacologically, alvein is hemolytic to red blood cells.

Gilliver, Holmes, Abraham, *Brit. J. Exper. Path.*, **30**, 209 (1949)

AMBRUTICIN (*Antibiotic W7783*)
$C_{28}H_{42}O_6$

Isolated from cultures of *Polyangium cellulosum fulvum*, this antibiotic is obtained from the crude AcOEt extract by column chromatography. The structure given above had been elucidated from X-ray analysis of the triformate. Ambruticin is active against both gram-positive and gram-negative bacteria and is also active *in vitro* against such pathogenic fungi as *Blastomyces dermatitidis*, *Coccidioides immitis*, *Histoplasma capsulatum* and dermatophytic filamentous fungi. The acute LD_{50} in mice for the sodium salt is 315 mg/kg when given intravenously and >100 mg/kg when administered orally.

Ringel et al., *J. Antibiotics* (Japan), **30**, 371 (1977)

AMBUTYROSINE A

Bacillus biterinus may be surface grown on agar containing glycerol-bouillon for 7 days at 37°C and then used to incubate a culture medium containing peptone, meat extract and sodium chloride at 28°C and pH 7·0 for 3 days, the seed culture then being inoculated onto a further medium consisting of glucose, meat extract, peptone and inorganic salts when two closely related antibiotics are produced, separated by column chromatography. This antibiotic is active against gram-positive bacteria.

Hasegawa et al., *Japanese Patent*, 7,362,993 (1973)

AMBUTYROSINE B

A component of the antibiotic mixture produced by cultivation of *Bacillus biterinus*, this compound is separated from the accompanying substance by chromatography on an alumina column. The structure is not yet known. Ambutyrosine B is also active against a range of gram-positive bacteria.

Hasegawa et al., *Japanese Patent*, 7,362,993 (1973)

AMEBACILIN

See Fumagillin

AMICETIN
$C_{29}H_{44}O_9N_6$
M.p. 160–165°C (243–244°C)

Amicetin is produced by several *Streptomyces* species, particularly by *S. fasciculatus*. It forms colourless crystals from H_2O, which when warmed to 50–70°C in H_2O or CH_3OH suspension, are converted into a granular form having the higher melting point given above. The specific rotation of the latter form is $[\alpha]_D^{24} + 116\cdot5°$ (c 0·5, 0·1 N-HCl). Although freely soluble in H_2O, the substance is only slightly soluble in all of the usual organic solvents. The ultraviolet spectrum in H_2O has a single absorption maximum at 305 nm, that in 0·1 N-HCl has a maximum at 316 nm and in 0·1 N-NaOH, a maximum at 322 nm.

The antibiotic is active against most gram-positive bacteria and especially against mycobacteria. When used as the citrate complex at pH 6·0 in mice, the LD_{50} is about 90 mg/kg, while the subcutaneous LD_{50} in rats is approximately 650 mg/kg. The acute intravenous LD_{50} in rats is about 200 mg/kg. Amicetin has a high toxicity towards guinea pigs being about 40 times as toxic as streptomycin when administered subcutaneously. However, it is only about 0·1 times as toxic as penicillin to the same species.

DeBoer et al., *J. Amer. Chem. Soc.*, **75**, 499 (1953)
McCormick, Hoehn, *Antibiotics & Chemotherapy*, **2**, 718 (1953)

AMICETIN B
See Plicacetin

AMICLENOMYCIN
$C_{10}H_{16}O_2N_2$
M.p. 215–216°C (*dec.*)

A comparatively simple antibiotic, amiclenomycin is elaborated by *Streptomyces lavendulae*. subsp. *amiclenomycini*. It forms a yellowish. amorphous powder and is dextrorotatory with a specific rotation of $[\alpha]_D^{25} + 10\cdot9°$ (c 0·3, H_2O). It is active against a number of gram-positive bacteria and inhibits the growth of mycobacteria, this activity being reversed by biotin and desthiobiotin.

Okami et al., *J. Antibiotics* (Japan), **27**, 656 (1974)

AMIDINOMYCIN
$C_9H_{18}N_4O$
M.p. Indefinite

In addition to producing kasugamycin (q.v.), *Streptomyces kagugaensis* also elaborates this antibiotic when fermented in a medium containing glycerol, soybean flour and inorganic salts at 27°C for 3 days. The antibiotic is isolated by adjusting the pH of the broth to 7·6, filtering, adsorbing the filtrate on an ion exchange resin, eluting with 0·5 N-HCl, concentrating the eluate and adding EtOH. The sulphate darkens at 260°C and melts at approximately 280–285°C. This salt is lævorotatory with a specific rotation of $[\alpha]_D^{25} - 2\cdot3°$.

Nakamura et al., *J. Antibiotics* (Japan), **14**, 103 (1961)
Nakamura et al., *Chem. Pharm. Bull.*, **9**, 641 (1961)
Katsube, Saito, *Japanese Patent*, 21,418 (1968)
Takesawa et al., *J. Antibiotics* (Japan), **21**, 567 (1968)

AMIDOMYCIN
$C_{40}H_{58}O_{12}N_4$
M.p. 192°C

A macrocyclic peptide antibiotic elaborated by an unclassified species of *Streptomyces*, amidomycin forms colourless crystals from petroleum ether or aqueous EtOH. It has a specific rotation of $[\alpha]_D^{26} + 19 \cdot 2°$ (c 1·0, EtOH) and can be hydrolysed to D-valine and D-2-hydroxy-3-methylbutyric acid. It is primarily active against yeasts and has only a limited activity against bacteria.

Vining, Taber, *Can. J. Chem.*, **35**, 1109 (1957)

AMIKACIN (*Antibiotic BB-K8*)
$C_{22}H_{43}O_{13}N_5$

A semi-synthetic derivative of kanamycin A, this antibiotic has a higher activity against clinical isolates of *Enterobacter* species, *Pseudomonas aeruginosa* and *Staphylococcus aureus* than gentamicin sulphate, kanamycin sulphate or tobramycin, this being associated with the fact that amikacin is a rather ineffective substrate for most of the enzymes that inactivate other aminoglycosidic antibiotics. No major toxicity has been observed with normal doses although some renal toxicity has been encountered and it is suggested that amikacin should be administered intermittently and in doses less than 50 mg in patients with extreme renal dysfunction.

Mitsuhashi *et al.*, *J. Antibiotics* (Japan), **27**, 189 (1974)
Nishimura, Takayasu, *ibid.*, **27**, 218 (1974)
Ueda *et al.*, *ibid.*, **27**, 354 (1974)
Yamasaku *et al.*, *ibid.*, **27**, 366 (1974)
Clarke *et al.*, *Clin. Pharmacol. Ther.*, **15**, 610 (1974)
Price *et al.*, *Antimicrobial Agents & Chemotherapy*, **5**, 143 (1974)
Bodey *et al.*, *ibid.*, **5**, 508 (1974)

AMIMYCIN
See Oleandomycin

L-trans-2-AMINO-4-(2-AMINOETHOXY)-3-BUTENOIC ACID
$C_6H_{12}O_3N_2$
M.p. 185–186°C

A simple antibiotic, this compound is produced by *Streptomyces* species X-11085 grown on a nutrient agar slant and then inoculated into a Trypticase soy broth medium and fermented at 27°C for 3 days. The antibiotic forms colourless crystals from EtOH and is dextrorotatory with a specific rotation of $[\alpha]_D^{25} + 85 \cdot 8°$ (c 1·0, H_2O). It is active against a number of gram-positive bacteria and also possesses anthelmintic properties.

Berger, Pruess, Scannell, *U.S. Patent*, 3,751,459 (1973)
Pruess *et al.*, *J. Antibiotics* (Japan), **27**, 229 (1974)

D-4-AMINO-4-CARBOXYBUTYL-PENICILLINIC ACID
(*Penicillin M, N, Cephalosporin N*)
$C_{14}H_{21}O_6N_3S$

A penicillin type antibiotic, this compound has been isolated from cultures of several *Cephalosporium* species. It yields a crystalline barium salt which is

7-(5-Amino-5-carboxypentamido)-3-methylthiomethyl-3-cephem-4-carboxylic acid

dextrorotatory having $[\alpha]_D^{20} + 187°$ (c 0·6, H_2O) and has pK at 2·8, 3·2 and 9·8. It is a broad spectrum antibiotic active primarily against gram-positive bacteria.

Abraham, Newton, Hale, *Biochem. J.*, **58**, 94, 103 (1954)
Olson *et al.*, *Antibiotics & Chemotherapy*, **4**, 1 (1954)
Demain, Newkirk, *Appl. Microbiol.*, **10**, 321 (1962)
Troum *et al.*, *Biochem. J.*, **84**, 157 (1962)
Cole, Batchelor, *Nature*, **198**, 383 (1963)

7-(5-AMINO-5-CARBOXYPENTAMIDO)-3-METHYLTHIOMETHYL-3-CEPHEM-4-CARBOXYLIC ACID
$C_{15}H_{21}O_6N_3S_2$

The culture broth of a mutant strain of *Cephalosporium*, No. 155, contains this cephem derivative which has been isolated as the crystalline sodium salt. It is active against a range of gram-positive bacteria and has a comparatively low toxicity. The structure has been established by comparison with the synthetic compound.

Kanzaki *et al.*, *J. Antibiotics* (Japan), **27**, 361 (1974)

7-(5-AMINO-5-CARBOXYVALERAMIDO)-3-CARBAMOYLOXYMETHYL-3-CEPHEM-4-CARBOXYLIC ACID
$C_{15}H_{20}O_8N_4S$
M.p. Indefinite

Three structurally related antibiotics have recently been isolated from a number of *Streptomyces* species. This particular substance is produced by *S. clavuligerus*. The structure has been established on the basis of chemical

7-(5-Amino-5-carboxyvaleramido)-7-methoxycephalosporanic acid

and spectroscopic investigations. It forms a crystalline sodium salt which inhibits the growth of both gram-positive and gram-negative bacteria.

Nagarajan *et al.*, *J. Amer. Chem. Soc.*, **93**, 2308 (1971)

7-(5-AMINO-5-CARBOXYVALERAMIDO)-3-CARBAMOYLOXYMETHYL-7-METHOXY-3-CEPHEM-4-CARBOXYLIC ACID
$C_{16}H_{22}O_9N_4S$

This antibiotic, which is the 7-methoxy derivative of the preceding compound, has been isolated from cultures of *Streptomyces clavuligerus* and *S. lactamdurans* MA 2908 (NRRL 3802) by addition of glycine and L-phenylalanine to the fermentation medium. The antibiotic is isolated by passing the crude broth through a cationic exchange resin, eluting with 0·5M pyridine, passing the eluate through a weakly basic exchange resin, washing with 0·5M AcOH and eluting with phosphate buffer at pH 8·0. The antibiotic and its salts are active in inhibiting the growth of both gram-positive and gram-negative organisms.

Nagarajan *et al.*, *J. Amer. Chem. Soc.*, **93**, 2308 (1971)
Inamine, Birnbaum, *German Patent*, 2,224,707 (1972)
Birnbaum, Inamine, *German Patent*, 2,224,620 (1972)
Goegelman, *U.S. Patent*, 3,709,880 (1973)

7-(5-AMINO-5-CARBOXYVALERAMIDO)-7-METHOXYCEPHALOSPORANIC ACID
$C_{17}H_{23}O_9N_3S$

Although possessing a very similar structure to the two preceding compounds, this antibiotic is elaborated by *Streptomyces lipmanii*. The structure has been elucidated from chemical and spectroscopic evidence and com-

7-(5-AMINO-5-CARBOXYVALERIMIDO)-3-(METHOXYCINNAMOYLOXYMETHYL)-7-METHOXY-3-CEPHEM-4-CARBOXYLIC ACID
$C_{25}H_{29}O_{10}N_3S$

This antibiotic is produced by culturing Actinomycete NRRL 3851 in a nutrient medium at pH 7·0 and 20–37°C for 3 days. It is isolated from the culture broth by adsorption on activated carbon, eluting with EtOH followed by chromatography on an alumina column. It is active against a range of gram-positive and gram-negative organisms.

Stapley, Mata, *German Patent*, 2,166,462 (1974)

L-(αS, 5S)-α-AMINO-3-CHLORO-4:5-DIHYDRO-5-ISOXAZOLEACETIC ACID
$C_5H_7O_3N_2Cl$

A synthetic antibiotic substance, this compound has been shown to be a powerful inhibitor of many bacterial reactions involving the transfer of nitrogen from the α-carboxamide of L-glutamine. Treatment of L1210 cells growing in a low L-glutamine medium with the substance produced an arrest in the G_1 or early S phase. Only L-glutamine, of all the aminoacids tested antagonized such inhibition of bacterial growth.

Jarayam et al., *Cancer Chemother. Rep. Part 1*, **59**, 481 (1975)

AMINOCHLORTHENOXYCYCLINE
$C_{32}H_{34}O_{10}N_4Cl.2H_2SO_4$

A semi-synthetic antibiotic having both antimicrobial and antiinflammatory properties, this compound is useful in the treatment of burns of the respiratory tract caused by the inhalation of toxic vapours, the antibiotic attaining much higher concentrations in this region than in normal tissues.

Rognoni, Ariano, Lucca, *Arch. Sci. Med.*, **130**, 148, 151 (1973)

5″-AMINO-5″-DEOXYBUTIROSIN
$C_{21}H_{42}O_{11}N_6$

This semi-synthetic antibiotic has been prepared from butirosin (q.v.). It has a greater bactericidal activity than the parent butirosins and a somewhat lower toxicity.

Culbertson, Watson, Haskell, *J. Antibiotics* (Japan), **26**, 790 (1973)

5″-AMINO-4′:5″-DIDEOXYAMBUTYROSIN A
$C_{21}H_{42}O_{10}N_6$

A further semi-synthetic antibiotic, this substance is prepared from 4′-deoxyambutyrosin A and has a marked activity against gram-positive and gram-negative bacteria.

Naito et al., *Japanese Patent*, 7,535, 132 (1975)

1-N-(S-4-AMINO-2-HYDROXYBUTYRYL) 3':4'-DIDEOXYKANAMYCIN B
$C_{22}H_{44}O_{10}N_6$

One of a number of kanamycin derivatives synthesized and examined for their antibiotic properties. This compound is highly active against kanamycin-resistant bacteria which produce kanamycin-phosphotransferases I and II and kanamycin-nucleotidyl-transferase.

Kondo et al., J. Antibiotics (Japan), **26**, 412 (1973)
Kondo et al., ibid., **26**, 705 (1973)

1-N-(S-AMINO-2-HYDROXYBUTYRYL)-KANAMYCIN B
$C_{22}H_{44}O_{12}N_6$

A further kanamycin derivative prepared from the parent antibiotic, this substance has an activity against kanamycin-resistant bacteria similar to that of the preceding compound.

Kondo et al., J. Antibiotics (Japan), **26**, 412 (1973)
Kondo et al., ibid., **26**, 705 (1973)

1-N-(S-4-AMINO-2-HYDROXYBUTYRYL)-LIVIDOMYCIN A
$C_{33}H_{62}O_{19}N_6$

A semi-synthetic antibiotic, this substance has a broader antibiotic spectrum than lividomycin A (q.v.) and is also effective against a number of bacteria which are resistant to the parent compound, e.g. *Escherichia coli* strains K-12 ML1629, K-12 ML1630 and J-5 R 11-2.

Watanabe et al., J. Antibiotics (Japan), **26**, 310 (1973)

N¹-(L-γ-AMINO-α-HYDROXYBUTYRYL)-PAROMOMYCIN

$C_{27}H_{52}O_{16}N_6$

An antibiotic prepared by a series of selective chemical reactions from carboxybenylparomomycin, this compound has been shown to possess a higher antimicrobial activity than the parent antibiotic. The toxicity is similar to that of paromomycin.

Naito, Nakagawa, Toda, *German Patent*, 2,322,576 (1973)

6-D-(−)-α-AMINO-(p-HYDROXYPHENYL)ACETAMIDO PENICILLANIC ACID

$C_{16}H_{19}O_5N_3S$

A new semi-synthetic antibiotic, the structure of this compound is similar to that of ampicillin (q.v.). Given orally to healthy subjects, it is well absorbed and produces significantly higher concentrations in serum than ampicillin accompanied by a greater degree of urinary excretion.

Neu, Winshell, *Antimicrobial Agents & Chemotherapy*, 423 (1970)

L-2-AMINO-4-METHOXY-*trans*-3-BUTENOIC ACID

$C_5H_9O_3N$
M.p. 240–245°C

When cultured under submerged aerobic conditions in a common nutrient medium, *Pseudomonas aeruginosa* ATCC 7700 elaborates this simple antibiotic substance. Both it and its metal salts are bactericidal against a number of gram-positive and gram-negative bacteria.

Demny, Scannell, *U.S. Patent*, 3,739,022 (1973)

2-AMINO-4-METHYL-5-HEXENOIC ACID

$C_7H_{15}O_2N$
M.p. 260°C (*dec.*)

A simple aminoacid, this antibiotic is produced by cultivating *Streptomyces* species UC-5159 in a medium containing phytone, starch, mannitol and inorganic salts at 32°C for 4–5 days. The activity of the culture filtrate is adsorbed on activated carbon, eluted with 5 per cent aqueous $(CH_3)_2CO$, the solvent evaporated and the residue dissolved in H_2O and chromatographed on an ion exchange resin. It is finally purified by crystallizing from 95 per cent EtOH when it forms colourless crystals. The antibiotic gives a violet colour with ninhydrin and is assayed by serial dilution with *Escherichia coli*, grown in a synthetic medium, as the test organism. It is active against gram-positive bacteria, particularly *Bacillus subtilis*, *Sarcina lutea* and *Staphylococcus aureus*. The activity is lost in the presence of leucine.

Kelly, Martin, Hanka, *Can. J. Chem.*, **47**, 2504 (1969)

6-DL-2-AMINO-2-(2-METHYL-4-THIAZOLYL)ACETAMIDO PENICILLANIC ACID

$C_{14}H_{18}O_4N_4S_2$

A large number of heterocyclic analogues of ampicillin have been synthesized and, of those derived from 4-thiazolylglycines, this has proved to be the most potent. Minimum inhibitory concentrations which have been determined *in vitro* are 0·037 µg/ml against *Bacillus subtilis* and *Staphylococcus aureus* and 0·62 µg/ml against *Shigella dysenteriae*. The compound has a toxicity comparable with ampicillin (q.v.).

Hatanaka, Ishimaru, *J. Med. Chem.*, **16**, 978 (1973)

5″-AMINO-3′,4′,5″-TRIDEOXYBUTIROSIN A
$C_{21}H_{42}N_6O_9$

A semi-synthetic antibiotic, this substance exhibits an enhanced antibiotic activity compared with other butirosin antibiotics. It is particularly active against strains of *Pseudomonas aeruginosa* and *Escherichia coli* which are highly resistant to gentamicin, butirosin and 5″-amino-5″-deoxybutirosin.

Woo, *J. Antibiotics* (Japan), **28**, 522 (1975)
Saoki *et al.*, **28**, 530 (1975)

AMINOMYCIN
See Perimycin A

AMIPURIMYCIN
$C_{20}H_{29}N_7O_8$

A recently discovered antibiotic, amipurimycin has been isolated from cultures of *Streptomyces novoguineensis* nov. sp. It has been purified by a combination of ion-exchange and adsorption chromatography based upon its amphoteric water-soluble characteristics. A study of the ultraviolet and NMR spectra indicates that amipurimycin is structurally similar to 2-aminopurine-9-β-D-riboside.

Harada, Kishi, *J. Antibiotics* (Japan), **30**, 11 (1977)

AMOXYCILLIN
$C_{16}H_{19}O_5N_3S$

A semi-synthetic penicillin antibiotic, this compound has been extensively examined by numerous workers. Normally employed as the crystalline sodium salt, it is highly effective *in vitro* and *in vivo* against a wide range of gram-positive and gram-negative bacteria including *Citrobacter*, *Diplococci*, *Enterobacter*, *Escherichia coli*, *Neisseria gonorrhoeae*, *Klebsiella*, *Pneumococci*, *Proteus vulgaris*, *Ps. maltophila*, *Salmonella*, *Shigella* and *Bacteroides fragilis* is, however, insensitive to the antibiotic.

Amoxycillin may be assayed by the cup method using *Bacillus subtilis* or *Sarcina lutea* as the test organism or by the superposition assay method with *Streptococcus hemolyticus* S-8 or *Bacillus subtilis*. Following oral administration of the trihydrate to rats, the blood and skin levels of amoxycillin are higher than with ampicillin. The maximum serum concentration is normally reached 2 hours after oral administration.

Mitsuhashi, Odakura, Yaginuma, *Chemotherapy* (Tokyo), **21**, 1355 (1973)
Kozakai, Oguri, *ibid.*, **21**, 1359 (1973)
Watanabe *et al.*, *ibid.*, **21**, 1369 (1973)
Nakazawa *et al.*, *ibid.*, **21**, 1375 (1973)
Mine *et al.*, *ibid.*, **21**, 1409 (1973)
Kato *et al.*, *ibid.*, **21**, 1415 (1973)
Matsumoto *et al.*, *ibid.*, **21**, 1427 (1973)
Shimizu, Kunii, *ibid.*, **21**, 1436 (1973)
Mashimo *et al.*, *ibid.*, **21**, 1441 (1973)
Ueda *et al.*, *ibid.*, **21**, 1446 (1973)
Nakagawa *et al.*, *ibid.*, **21**, 1455 (1973)
Kishikawa *et al.*, *ibid.*, **21**, 1487 (1973)
Morita, Usami, *ibid.*, **21**, 1493 (1973)
Okubo *et al.*, *ibid.*, **21**, 1497 (1973)
Miki *et al.*, *ibid.*, **21**, 1504 (1973)
Hara *et al.*, *ibid.*, **21**, 1522 (1973)
Shibata *et al.*, *ibid.*, **21**, 1611 (1973)
Ishii *et al.*, *ibid.*, **21**, 1619 (1973)
Kondo, *ibid.*, **21**, 1638 (1973)
Ishibashi *et al.*, *ibid.*, **21**, 1649 (1973)

Sasaki et al., *ibid.*, **21**, 1655 (1973)
Ishigami et al., *ibid.*, **21**, 1687 (1973)
Kondo et al., *ibid.*, **21**, 1697 (1973)
Ohi et al., *ibid.*, **21**, 1723 (1973)
Cho et al., *ibid.*, **21**, 1759 (1973)
Harima, Tanaka, Yameda, *ibid.*, **21**, 1777 (1973)
Seiga et al., *ibid.*, **21**, 1780 (1973)
Yakushiji, Takahashi, *ibid.*, **21**, 1787 (1973)
Arata, Tanioku, *ibid.*, **21**, 1808 (1973)
Mishima et al., *ibid.*, **21**, 1825 (1973)
Iwasawa, *ibid.*, **21**, 1830 (1973)
Tan, Bannister, Phair, *J. Inf. Diseases*, **129**, Suppl., S144 (1974)
Vitti, Gurwith, Ronald, *ibid.*, **129**, Suppl., S147 (1974)
Lode et al., *ibid.*, **129**, Suppl., S154 (1974)
Motta, Malberti, *Farmaco, Ed. Prat.*, **30**, 357 (1975)

AMPHOMYCIN

An acidic, surface-active antibiotic, this substance has been isolated from *Streptomyces canus* obtained from soil found near Syracuse in the United States. It belongs to the polypeptide class of antibiotics and is slightly dextrorotatory at pH 6·0 with $[\alpha]_D^{25} + 7·5°$. It is readily soluble in H_2O, CH_3OH, EtOH, PrOH, iso-PrOH and BuOH, but virtually insoluble in nonpolar solvents. Being acidic, it forms stable calcium and sodium salts, the LD_{50} for the calcium salt being 120·2 mg/kg on intravenous injection. When given intravenously it induces hemolysis but, as an active agent against gram-positive bacteria it is sometimes employed for certain skin infections. Its use has been suggested as a topical agent for plant and animal infections.

Heinemann et al., *Antibiotics & Chemotherapy*, **3**, 1239 (1953)
Heinemann et al., *U.S. Patent*, 3,126,317 (1964)

AMPHOTERICIN A

One of the two complex antibiotics produced by *Streptomyces nodosus*, this substance is dextrorotatory having the following specific rotations: $[\alpha]_D^{24} + 36°$ (dimethylformamide), $+93°$ (AcOH) and $+163°$ (pyridine). It gives a comparatively complex ultraviolet spectrum in CH_3OH with absorption maxima at 228, 291, 304 and 318 nm. It has only weak antibacterial activity but is active against a number of pathogenic fungi.

Gold et al., *Antibiotics Annual*, 579 (1955–1956)
Vandeputte, Wachtel, Stiller, *ibid.*, 587 (1955–1956)

Dutcher et al., *ibid.*, 866 (1956–1957)
Olin Mathieson Chem. Corp., *British Patent*, 795,482 (1959)
Dutcher et al., *U.S. Patent*, 2,908,612 (1959)

AMPHOTERICIN B (*Fungizone*)

$C_{47}H_{73}O_{17}N$
Dec. 170°C

A second antibiotic of the polyene group produced by *Streptomyces nodosus*, this compound forms deep yellow needles or prisms when crystallized from dimethylformamide which gradually decompose when heated above 170°C. It has specific rotations of $[\alpha]_D^{24} + 333°$ (acidic dimethylformamide) and $[\alpha]_D^{24} - 33·6°$ (0·1 N-CH_3OH—HCl). When stored at low temperatures out of contact with air or light, the solutions are stable for long periods between pH 4·0 and 10. When given within 5 days postinoculation, experimental exogenous endophthalmitis induced by *Candida albicans* is reversed by a single intravitreal dose of 5 mg of the antibiotic. When injected intravitreally into normal rabbits, a dose of 5·0–10·0 µg caused no toxic changes in the eye although doses of 25 µg and higher brought about retinal necrosis and detachment. Yaremenko and his colleagues have shown that when given intravenously to rats beginning 24 hours after a transplantation of a metastasizing Pliss lymphosarcoma, the antibiotic inhibited tumour development, this effect being significantly increased in combination with 5-fluorouracil. Amphotericin B binds to a great extent to organ homogenates from tumour-bearing rats than to those obtained from control animals. In addition, the levels of the antibiotic are higher in tumour metastases than in the primary tumour.

Amphotericin B is relatively non-toxic, the LD_{50} in mice being 280 mg/kg. It has found some use in medicine as an antifungal agent both for topical and intravenous administration although it is toxic when given intravenously. In veterinary work it has been used in cases of coccidiomycosis, histoplasmosis and nocardioses.

Gold et al., Antibiotics Annual, 579 (1955–1956)
Vandeputte et al., ibid., 587 (1955–1956)
Dutcher et al., ibid., 866 (1956–1957)
Walters et al., J. Amer. Chem. Soc., **79**, 5076 (1957)
Dutcher et al., U.S. Patent, 2,908,611 (1959)
Axelrod et al., Amer. J. Ophthalmol., **76**, 578, 584 (1973)
Kasumov, Liberman, Etingov, Biofizika, **18**, 1020 (1973)
Keim et al., Science, **179**, 584 (1973)
Yaremenko, Kharitonenko, Golubeva, Antibiotiki, **20**, 433 (1975)
Structure
Borowski et al., Tetrahedron Lett., 473 (1965)
Cope et al., J. Amer. Chem. Soc., **88**, 4228 (1966)

AMPICILLIN
$C_{16}H_{19}O_4N_3S$
M.p. 202°C (dec.)

This semi-synthetic antibiotic is normally prepared from penicillanic acid and (+)-2-aminophenylacetic acid and occurs in various hydrated forms, e.g. the monohydrate as colourless crystals from H_2O, decomposing at 202°C, having $[\alpha]_D^{21} + 281°$ (c 1·0, H_2O); the sesquihydrate, decomposing at 199–202°C; $[\alpha]_D^{20} + 283·1°$ (c 1·0, H_2O) and the trihydrate, colourless crystals, m.p. 200–202°C. The anhydrous form (ampicillin B, Omnipen) has a specific rotation of $[\alpha]_D^{23} + 287·9°$ (c 1·0, H_2O) and is more stable on storage, less soluble in H_2O and $(CH_3)_2SO$, and has a different crystal structure to those of the hydrated forms. Hydration converts it to the monohydrate. Ampicillin is known under a variety of pseudonyms and Trade names including Amblosin, Ampicin, Amplital, Austnapen, Binotal, Britacil, Doktacillin, Penbristol, Penbritin, Penbrock, Penicline, Pentrex, Pentrexyl, Polycillin and Totapen. The preparation of the antibiotic is covered by numerous patents.

Ampicillin is acid stable and finds use in medicine as an antimicrobial being active against a wide range of gram-positive and gram-negative bacteria and mycobacteria although it is not used in human medicine against mycobacteria. The normal dose is 250–500 mg given orally, the sodium salt being used for injections. Side effects include diarrhoea, nausea, vomiting and skin rashes. In veterinary medicine it has been used against staphylococci, streptococci, Escherichia coli and various other pathogens.

Doyle et al., Nature, **191**, 1091 (1961)
Doyle et al., J. Chem. Soc., 440 (1962)
Dane, Dockner, Chem. Ber., 789 (1965)
Greenwood, O'Grady, J. Med. Microbiol., **2**, 435 (1969)
Lochovsky et al., Advan. Antimicrob. Antineoplast. Chemother., Proc. Int. Conf. Chemother., 7th, 1413 (1971)
Smith, Bremner, Datta, Antimicrobial Agents & Chemotherapy, **6**, 418 (1974)
Vietor et al., Z. Kinderheilkd., **117**, 175 (1974)
Scheer, Foerster, Hoffmann, Berl. Muench. Tieraeztl. Wochenschr., **88**, 141 (1975)
Zaremba et al., Med. Wter., **31**, 141 (1975)
Patents
Doyle et al U.S. Patent, 2,985,648 (1961)
Doyle et al., British Patent, 902,703 (1962)
Kaufmann, Bauer, U.S. Patent, 3,079,307 (1963)
Johnson, Wolfe, Johnson, U.S. Patents, 3,140,282 and 3,157,640 (1964)
Grant, Alburn, U.S. Patent, 3,144,445 (1964)
Fujii et al., Japanese Patent, 7,412,098 (1974)

AMUDOL
$C_7H_7O_3Cl$
M.p. 146–147°C

A simple antibiotic, amudol is produced by the cultivation of Penicillium martensii on a semi-synthetic medium containing corn starch, glucose, lactose, carrot extract and inorganic salts. The antibiotic is isolated from the dried mycelium and separated from the accompanying amudane, m.p. 219–220°C, amudene, m.p. 270–272°C, mannitol and ergosterol. The structure has been shown from chemical and spectroscopic evidence to be 2:5-dihydroxy-4-chlorobenzyl alcohol. Amudol is active against Bacillus anthracis, B. subtilis, Escherichia coli, Salmonella paratyphi A and B, S. typhosa, Sarcina lutea and Staphylococcus aureus.

Kamal et al., Pak. J. Sci. Ind. Res., **13**, 236 (1970)

ANEMONIN
$C_{10}H_8O_4$
M.p. 158°C

Isolated from plants of the Ranunculaceae, including *Anemone pratensis, A. pulsatilla, Ranunculus acer, R. alpester, R. arvensis, R. bulbosus, R. japonicum, R. montanus* and *R. sceleratus*, this antibiotic substance is obtained by steam distilling the macerated plant material, saturating with sodium chloride and extracting with $CHCl_3$, C_6H_6 or Et_2O when protoanemonin is obtained on evaporation *in vacuo* as a pale yellow, irritating oil. This polymerizes within a few hours on standing at room temperature to form anemonin as colourless crystals. Anemonin forms odourless, tasteless prisms, plates, needles or rhomboids when recrystallized from EtOH. It is more soluble in hot H_2O than in cold, moderately soluble in EtOH and freely so in $CHCl_3$, aqueous alkalies and aliphatic fatty oils. On exposure to air it polymerizes, while heating partially depolymerizes it to form protoanemonin. With aqueous alkalies it gives a deep yellow colour. The unsaturated nature of the molecule is shown by its reduction of Fehling's solution, silver nitrate solution, gold and platinum chlorides.

Anemonin is not active against bacteria, e.g. *Escherichia coli, Staphylococcus aureus* nor against *Candida albicans*. It is, however, active against various fungi and yeasts having the following inhibition dilutions: *Aspergillus niger* (25,000–50,000); *Mycoderma* (30,000); *Oidium lactis* (30,000) and *Saccharomyces cerevisiae* (50,000–10,000). A 2 mg/ml solution in H_2O at pH 3·5–4·0 produces an irritation of the throat.

Bekurts, *Arch. Pharm.*, **230**, 182 (1892)
Asahina, Fujita, *Acta phytochim.* (Japan), **1**, 1 (1922)
Muskat, Becker, Loewenstein, *J. Amer. Chem. Soc.*, **52**, 326 (1930)
Boas, *Ber. deut. bot. Ges.*, **52**, 126 (1934)
Boas, Steude, *Biochem. Ztschr.*, **279**, 417 (1935)
Kipping, *J. Chem. Soc.*, **1**, 145 (1935)
Baehr, Holden, Seegal, *J. Biol. Chem.*, **162**, 65 (1946)
Brodersen, Kjaer, *Acta Pharmacol. Toxicol.*, **2**, 109 (1946)

ANGUSTMYCIN A (*Decoyinine*)
$C_{11}H_{13}O_4N_5$
M.p. 130–133°C (*dec.* 156–159°C)

Isolated from *Streptomyces hygroscopicus*, this antibiotic forms colourless needles of the monohydrate which soften at 125°C, melt at 130–133°C and then resolidify before decomposing at 156–159°C. Angustmycin A has a specific rotation of $[\alpha]_D^{26} + 43·8°$ (c 1·0, H_2O). The ultraviolet spectrum in H_2O has an absorption maximum at 259 nm which is shifted to 261 nm at pH 11·0. Treatment of the antibiotic with Ac_2O yields the triacetate, m.p. 188–189°C, the tetraacetate, m.p. 63–67°C and the pentaacetate, m.p. 152–153°C. The structure has recently been revised and confirmed by synthesis.

Yüntsen *et al.*, *J. Antibiotics* (Japan, **9A**, 195 (1956)
Yüntsen, Yonehara, *Bull. Agr. Chem. Soc.* (Japan, **21**, 261 (1957)
Yüntsen, *J. Antibiotics* (Japan), **11A**, 79 (1958)
Hoeksema, Slomp, van Tamelen, *Tetrahedron Lett.*, 1787 (1964)
Synthesis
McCarthy *et al.*, *J. Amer. Chem. Soc.*, **90**, 4993 (1968)

ANGUSTMYCIN C
See Psicofuranine

ANTHELMYCIN
$C_{25}H_{44}O_{16}N_5$
Dec. ca. 200°C

This antibiotic possessing anthelmintic activity has been isolated from a strain of *Streptomyces longissimus* (ATCC-14562). It crystallizes as white needles which decompose over a fairly wide range of temperature. It is dextrorotatory with $[\alpha]_D + 17·5°$ (c 1·58, H_2O). In aqueous solution it has pK_a 3·3, 6·8 and 7·9 while in a 66 per cent solution of dimethylformamide it has pK_a 3·3, 6·8 and 8·2. The ultraviolet spectrum in alkali has two absorption maxima at 234 and 267 nm, while that in dilute acid has only a single absorption maximum at 274 nm. The antibiotic may be characterized as the crystalline hydrochloride which decomposes at about 205°C and the *p*-(*p'*-hydroxyphenylazo)-benzenesulphonyl derivative which forms colourless crystals from H_2O with m.p. 218°C (*dec.*).

Hamill, Hoehn, *J. Antibiotics* (Japan), **17A**, 100 (1964)

ANTHRAMYCIN
$C_{16}H_{17}O_4N_3$
M.p. 188–194°C

An antibiotic isolated from cultures of *Streptomyces refuineus* var. *thermotolerans* (NRRL-3143), this substance has marked antitumour activity. It forms small yellow crystals from aqueous $(CH_3)_2CO$ and is strongly dextrorotatory having $[\alpha]_D^{25} + 930°$ (c 1·0, dimethylformamide). The ultraviolet spectrum in CH_3CN consists of two absorption maxima at 235 and 333 nm. The methyl ether is formed as light yellow needles of the monohydrate, decomposing above 120°C, when the antibiotic is crystallized from hot aqueous CH_3OH. This derivative is also strongly dextrorotatory in dimethylformamide with $[\alpha]_D^{25} + 1002°$. When crystallized from hot $(CH_3)_2CO$, anthramycin forms yellow plates of the anhydro derivative which may be CH_3CN as yellow needles, m.p. 205–206°C; $[\alpha]_D^{25} +$ 1796° (c 1·0, dimethylformamide). This derivative also yields the methyl ether when crystallized from hot aqueous CH_3OH.

Leimgruber *et al.*, *J. Amer. Chem. Soc.*, **87**, 5791 (1965)
Leimgruber, Batcho, Schenker, *ibid.*, **87**, 5793 (1965)

Synthesis
Leimgruber, Batcho, Czajowski, *J. Amer. Chem. Soc.*, **90**, 5641 (1968)

ANTIAMOEBIN
M.p. 192–195°C

A neutral polypeptide antibiotic, antiamoebin is produced by aerobic submerged culture of *Cephalosporium pimprina* ATCC 16,541, *Emericellopsis poonensis* ATCC 16,411 or *Emer. synnematicola* ATCC 16,540 in a common nutrient broth at 28°C for 3–5 days. Antiamoebin forms colourless crystals from $CH_3OH—(CH_3)_2CO$ and is slightly dextrorotatory with a specific rotation of $[\alpha]_D^{25} + 10°$ (c 1·02, CH_3OH). It possesses antiprotozoal and anthelmintic properties. It inhibits *Paramecium* species at a concentration of 60 µg/ml and *Tetrahymena* species at 40 µg/ml in H_2O. Cyclops are completely destroyed by an aqueous solution containing only 20 µg/ml of the antibiotic.

Thirumalachar, *U.S. Patent*, 3,657,419 (1972)

ANTIAMOEBIN I
$C_{82}H_{127}N_{17}O_{20} \cdot 2H_2O$
M.p. 194–196°C

The antibiotic antiamoebin isolated from *Cephalosporium pimprina* Thirum, *Emericellopsis poonensis* Thirum and *Emer. synnematicola* Mathur and Thirum has been shown to consist of two components, antiamoebins I and II. This substance is the major component and forms colourless crystals of the dihydrate. It is dextrorotatory with a specific rotation of $[\alpha]_D^{25} + 17\cdot8°$ (c 2·1, MeOH). The structure given above has been determined by chemical and spectroscopic techniques. Antiamoebin I is active against protozoa and helminths.

Thirumalachar, *Hindustan Antibiotics Bull.*, **10**, 287 (1968)
Deshmukh, *ibid*, **10**, 299 (1968)
Vaidya, Deshmukh, *ibid.*, **11**, 81 (1968)
Revised structure
Pandey *et al.*, *J. Amer. Chem. Soc.*, **99**, 5203 (1977)

ANTIAMOEBIN II

A minor component of the antibiotic antiamoebin, this substance has not been fully investigated and the structure has not yet been elucidated.

Thirumalachar, *Hindustan Antibiotics Bull.*, **10**, 287 (1968)
Deshmukh, *ibid.*, **10**, 299 (1968)
Vaidya, Deshmukh, *ibid.*, **11**, 81 (1968)

ANTIBIOTIC 5

Japanese workers have recently obtained this antibiotic by aerobic fermentation of *Streptomyces* species No. 5 on a medium containing starch, meat extract, and inorganic salts incubated at 30°C for 2 days. The active material is extracted from the cells with $(CH_3)_2CO$ or from the culture filtrate with Et_2O. Antibiotic 5 is stated to be active against rice blast disease. The structure is not yet known.

Takeda *et al.*, *Japanese Patent*, 7,330,397 (1973)

ANTIBIOTIC 6-MFA

M.p. Indefinite

A thermolabile, high molecular weight, non-dialysable antibiotic, this compound is elaborated by *Aspergillus flavus* strain 6-MFA by cultivation in a common nutrient medium at 28°C and pH 6·8 for 3 days. It forms a white amorphous powder with no definite melting point and is stable to freeze-drying. It is also stable *in vitro* between pH 6·0 and 7·0. The antibiotic is primarily an antiviral agent and gives a significant protection to mice against Semliki Forest virus. It is relatively non-toxic, the maximum tolerated dose in mice being about 300 mg/kg. A large increase in the antiviral activity is produced when used in conjunction with actidione (q.v.).

Maheshwari, Gupta, *J. Antibiotics* (Japan), **26**, 320, 328, 335 (1973)

ANTIBIOTIC 13 (*Gliotoxin?*)

This antibiotic is produced by *Aspergillus fumigatus* grown in Cottinger medium containing 5 per cent lactose at 37°C for 2 days. The physical and chemical characteristics, together with its chromatographic behaviour in a number of solvent systems indicate that it is almost certainly identical with gliotoxin (q.v.). It possesses antibacterial and antiviral activity against a number of bacteria and viruses and also exerts antitumour activity against Ehrlich adenocarcinoma in mice.

Plotnikov *et al.*, *Antibiotiki*, **13**, 316 (1968)

ANTIBIOTIC 18-45

One of a number of weakly acidic antibiotics elaborated by *Streptomyces* species, this tetraene compound is separated from the accompanying substances by paper chromatography. It has no effect against yeasts but inhibits the growth of *Candida albicans* and *Verticillium dahliae*.

Tokhtamuratov, Silaev, *Antibiotiki*, **12**, 887 (1967)

ANTIBIOTIC 18-80

This tetraene antibiotic accompanies the preceding compound and is separated from it by paper chromatography. It has a similar biological activity and is also a weak acid. The structure is not known with certainty.

Tokhmuratov, Silaev, *Antibiotiki*, **12**, 887 (1967)

ANTIBIOTIC 30 504 RP

Streptomyces gullinarius NRRL 5785 yields this antibiotic when cultured at 27°C and pH 6·4 for 116 hours on a medium consisting of sucrose, distillers solubles and inorganic salts with aeration and agitation. The culture is filtered, washed with H_2O and MeOH and the filtrate extracted with CH_2Cl_2, from which the crude product is crystallized and finally purified by recrystallization from C_6H_6. The antibiotic is effective against coccidia.

Florent, Lunel, Mancy, *German Patent*, 2,508,914 (1975)

ANTIBIOTIC 34

An antibiotic substance isolated from cultures of *Penicillium crustosum*, this complex compound is isolated by extraction of the mycelium with $(CH_3)_2CO$, evaporation of the solvent, dissolving the residue in AcOEt and purified by chromatographing on an alumina column. Hydrolysis experiments shown that it contains octadecadienoic and octadecenoic acids together with a number of other fatty acids. When administered intravenously to mice it is active against Ehrlich ascites sarcoma.

Tamura et al., *Japanese Patent*, 7,119,590 (1971)

ANTIBIOTIC 35-NT
Streptomyces strain 35-NT produces this antibiotic which is primarily active against gram-positive bacteria, particularly resistant strains of *Staphylococcus aureus*. The inhibition concentration *in vitro* has been given as 0·25–0·5 µg/ml and the activity is not affected by the presence of human serum. When tested *in vivo* it is effective against *Staphylococcus* infections in mice at 10 mg/kg given intraperitoneally, but ineffective when administered orally. The LD_{50} in mice, both intravenously and intraperitoneally is 540 mg/kg.

Tanaka, *Hakko Kogaku Zasshi*, **44**, 784 (1966)

ANTIBIOTIC 54
An antibiotic pigment, this compound occurs in cultures of *Streptomyces nitrosporeus* No. 54. It is a weakly basic, orange-red crystalline material which is freely soluble in $CHCl_3$ and C_6H_6 but insoluble in H_2O and the lower alcohols. Antibiotic 54 is active against *Mycoplasma hominis*, *Staphylococcus aureus* and inhibits the growth of sarcoma 180 in mice. It is comparatively toxic with LD_{50} in mice of 170 mg/kg.

Kikuchi, Yamamoto, Tanaka, *Japanese Patent*, 7,310,293 (1973)

ANTIBIOTIC 60-6
Bacillus cereus strain 60-6 elaborates this antibiotic when cultured aerobically at 28°C and pH 7·0 for 44 hours in a medium consisting of glucose, glycerol, meat extract, peptone and NaCl. Antibiotic 60–6 has been shown to be active against gram-positive bacteria. It is relatively non-toxic with LD_{50} in mice of 500 mg/kg when given subcutaneously.

Shoji et al., *German Patent*, 2,420,103 (1974)

ANTIBIOTIC 61-26
$C_{50}H_{93}N_{11}O_{17}$
M.p. 170–180°C (*dec.*) and 193–200°C (*dec.*)
An amorphous white powder, antibiotic 61-26 has been obtained from cultures of an unclassified *Bacillus* species. It has been characterized as the hydrochloride which has the higher of the two melting points given above and is dextrorotatory with a specific rotation of $[\alpha]_D^{24} + 51°$ (c 0·494, Me_2SO). This substance possesses an intensely bitter taste and is active against gram-positive bacteria.

Shoji et al., *J. Antibiotics* (Japan), **28**, 129 (1975)

ANTIBIOTIC 66-40B
$C_{18}H_{35}N_5O_7$
M.p. 91–102°C

Micromonospora inyoensis yields this aminoglycosidic antibiotic which forms an amorphous powder. It is strongly dextrorotatory with a specific rotation of $[\alpha]_D + 152·8°$ (c 0·3, H_2O). Antibiotic 66-40B is a broad spectrum antibiotic and has been characterized as the dihydro derivative which is also an amorphous powder with m.p. 135–145°C. The structure has been established from chemical and spectroscopic data.

Davis et al., *J. Chem. Soc., Perkin I*, 814 (1975)

ANTIBIOTIC 66-40D
$C_{18}H_{35}N_5O_7$
M.p. 92–103°C

An isomer of antibiotic 66-40B, this compound is a minor constituent of the extract from the culture broth of *Micromonospora inyoensis*. It is an amorphous powder and has a specific rotation of $[\alpha]_D + 47·3°$ (c 0·3, H_2O). The dihydro derivative forms a gum which softens at about 100°C and decomposes above 180°C. Like antibiotic 66-40B, this compound is a broad spectrum antibiotic.

Davis et al., *J. Chem. Soc., Perkin I,* 814 (1975)

ANTIBIOTIC 67-121

An antibiotic complex produced from *Actinoplanes caerulans* when cultured at 28°C for 3 to 4 days with stirring on a medium consisting of dextrose, soybean meal and $CaCO_3$. Extraction of the broth extract with saturated aqueous BuOH followed by column and thin layer chromatography separates the complex into four components, antibiotics 67-121A, B, C and D.

Weinstein et al., *U.S. Patent* 4,027,015 (1977)

ANTIBIOTIC 67-694

$C_{31}H_{51}O_9N$
M.p. 110–114°C

An antibiotic derived from *Micromonospora rosaria* NRRL 3718, this compound is produced by aerobic fermentation of the organism in a medium containing yeast extract, beef extract, tryptose, potato starch, dextrose and calcium carbonate at pH 6·0–8·5 and 27–37°C for 2–7 days. The antibiotic is isolated by adjusting the pH to 9·5 and extracting with AcOEt, the extract being concentrated *in vacuo*, and then re-extracted with 0·1 N-H_2SO_4. The acid extract is then adjusted to pH 9·5, re-extracted with AcOEt, concentrated *in vacuo*, and added to a mixture of Et_2O and hexane when a precipitate forms which is discarded. The filtrate is then evaporated *in vacuo*, the residue dissolved in EtO, filtered, and added to petroleum ether. The precipitate which forms is filtered, washed with petroleum ether, dried *in vacuo* at 40°C and purified by chromatography on a silica gel column. Antibiotic 67-694 forms colourless crystals and is laevorotatory with a specific rotation of $[\alpha]_D^{25} - 33·4°$ (c 3·0, EtOH). It is active against a range of gram-positive bacteria and has LD_{50} in mice of 155 mg/kg (intravenous), 350 mg/kg (intraperitoneal) and 625 mg/kg (subcutaneous).

Weinstein, Wagman, Marquez, *S. African Patent,* 7,100,402 (1971)
Weinstein, Wagman, Marquez, *German Patent,* 2,102,718 (1971)
Weinstein, *French Patent,* 2,081,448 (1972)

ANTIBIOTIC 84-B-3

M.p. Indefinite

Streptomyces species ATCC 21,273 yields this antibiotic substance when grown in a medium containing peptone, starch, meat extract, soybean oil and inorganic salts at 26°C for 2–3 days. The activity of the culture filtrate is adsorbed on activated carbon, eluted with NH_4OH—CH_3OH and purified by chromatography on alumina and silica gel columns. The antibiotic is soluble in H_2O and has a specific rotation of $[\alpha]_D^{25} + 60°$. It is unstable under acid conditions. Antibiotic 84-B-3 has no activity against bacteria but is effective against plant viruses, particularly tobacco mosaic virus which is almost completely eliminated at a concentration of 0·1 mg/ml.

Harada et al., *Japanese Patent,* 7,119,593 (1971)

ANTIBIOTIC 99

An acidic antibiotic, this compound is produced by *Penicillium tardum* grown in a common nutrient medium at 27°C for 3 days. Structurally, it closely resembles antibiotic 34 (q.v.) containing octadecadienoic and octadecenoic acids and other fatty acids. It is extracted from the mycelium with $(CH_3)_2CO$, the solvent evaporated, the residue dissolved in hexane at pH 3·0 and purification carried out by chromatography. Antibiotic 99 is an oily substance with no definite boiling point. It has no activity against bacteria but is effective against Ehrlich ascites sarcoma.

Tamura et al., *Japanese Patent,* 7,119,591 (1971)

ANTIBIOTIC 136

Streptomyces lavendulae produces this antibiotic which is very similar to streptothricin (q.v.). It is a basic substance precipitated from solution in CH_3OH with $(CH_3)_2CO$. Soluble in CH_3OH and H_2O, it is insoluble in $(CH_3)_2CO$ and is most stable in acid solution. It is not inactivated by cysteine.

Biologically, antibiotic 136 is active against gram-positive and gram-negative bacteria, mycobacteria and fungi and is most active in alkaline solution. The presence of glucose decreases the activity. It is highly toxic with LD_{50} in mice, both intravenous and subcutaneous, of 10 mg/kg.

Bohonos et al., *Arch. Biochem.,* **15**, 215 (1947)

ANTIBIOTIC 156

An antibiotic isolated from *Streptomyces* strain 156, this compound has been obtained by growing the organism on a medium containing starch as the carbon source and soybean flour as the nitrogen source. The medium is incubated at pH 5·0–8·0 for 3 days at 30°C. Antibiotic 156 is isolated from the culture filtrate by extraction with BuOH or from the cells with $(CH_3)_2CO$. It has been shown to be effective against *Piricularia oryzae*.

Takeda *et al.*, *Japanese Patent*, 7,329,159 (1973)

ANTIBIOTIC 175

This weakly acidic antibiotic is elaborated by *Pseudomonas fluorescens* strain 175 grown under aerobic conditions in a medium containing glucose, corn steep liquor and inorganic salts at 28°C and pH 7·0. The antibiotic is isolated by successive extraction of the culture filtrate with Et_2O at pH 4·5 and H_2O at pH 8·5, followed by removal of Et_2O from the aqueous fraction and freeze-drying. The antibiotic is assayed against *Staphylococcus aureus* and is active against a number of gram-positive and gram-negative bacteria although certain resistant strains of *Escherichia coli* have been encountered. It is stable over a wide range of pH and is comparatively non-toxic but inactivated by serum and haemolytic at high concentrations. Its use has been proposed in agricultural applications.

Woolford, *J. Appl. Bacteriol.*, **35**, 221 (1972)

ANTIBIOTIC 185
See Neomycin B

ANTIBIOTIC 243
Russian workers have isolated this aromatic heptane antibiotic, similar in structure to levorin (q.v.) from cultures of *Actinomyces levoris*. Although inactive against bacteria, it inhibits the growth of a number of yeasts.

Peikrishvili *et al.*, *Antibiotiki*, **17**, 15 (1972)

ANTIBIOTIC 255H
M.p. Indefinite
Streptomyces hygroscopicus B-255 produces an antibiotic complex when grown in a medium containing glucose, corn extract and ammonium nitrate at 28°C for 3 days. The complex is extracted from the culture filtrate with organic solvents and has chemical and biological properties very similar to those of hydromycins A and B (q.v.). It is active against gram-positive bacteria and also has anthelmintic activity.

Georgieva-Borisova *et al.*, *Kongr. Mikrobiol., Mater. Kongr. Mikrobiol. Bulg.*, *2nd*, **4**, 125 (1969)

ANTIBIOTIC 289-E
Streptomyces phaeoverticillatus var. *takatsukiensis* yields this antitumour antibiotic when grown on a medium containing anthraquinone sulphonic acid or its salts. The antibiotic is highly toxic although the toxicity may be reduced by acetylation without significant loss of the antitumour activity.

Kanda *et al.*, *Japanese Patent*, 7,328,079 (1973)

ANTIBIOTIC 289-F
M.p. 211·4–213°C
This antibiotic has recently been isolated from a culture of *Streptomyces phaeoverticillatus* var. *takatsukiensis*. The structure has not yet been elucidated.

Kanda *et al.*, *Japanese Patent*, 7,328,079 (1973)

ANTIBIOTIC 289-FO
M.p. 183–194°C (*dec.*)
Also obtained from cultures of *Streptomyces phaeoverticillatus* var. *takatsukiensis*, this antibiotic forms colourless crystals from CH_3OH. Its structure has not yet been determined.

Asano, Furukawa, Kando, *German Patent*, 1,939,045 (1970)

ANTIBIOTIC 339-29
A basic peptide antibiotic, this substance has been isolated from cultures of *Bacillus pumilus*. It has been obtained as the hydrochloride which is soluble in H_2O and aqueous alcohols. The antibiotic has been shown to contain a fatty acid in the molecule together with isoleucine, leucine, lysine, tyrosine and valine in molar proportions of 1:2:3:1:3. Antibiotic 339-29 is active against a range of gram-positive bacteria.

Shoji *et al.*, *J. Antibiotics* (Japan), **29**, 809 (1976)

ANTIBIOTIC 340-19-II
Bacillus lacterosporus No. 340–19 (FERM-P 2361) yields this antibiotic when cultured aerobically at 28°C for 41 hours at pH 7·0 on a medium consisting of glucose, glycerol, peptone, soybean powder and NaCl. The active compound is adsorbed on activated carbon, extracted with Me_2CO at pH 2·0, concentrated, and the impurities removed by extraction with BuOH. The antibiotic is finally purified by paper chromatography. It forms a colourless hygroscopic powder which is soluble in H_2O and the lower alcohols but insoluble in Me_2CO, $CHCl_3$, AcOEt and Et_2O. It is effective

against *Klebsiella pneumoniae* and *Staphylococcus aureus* in vivo and has LD_{50} in mice of 50 mg/kg when given intraperitoneally.

Shoji *et al.*, *Japanese Patent*, 76 35,492 (1976)

ANTIBIOTIC 417A
$C_7H_8O_3$
M.p. Indefinite
A *Penicillium* antibiotic, this compound is produced by culturing *P. claviforme*, freshly obtained from soil, in a medium consisting of glucose and corn steep liquor at 24°C for 5 days. The antibiotic is isolated by treating the culture filtrate with activated carbon, extracting the cake with CH_3OH and chromatographing the extract. The antibiotic forms colourless crystals, soluble in H_2O, and is dextrorotatory with a specific rotation of $[\alpha]_D^{22}$ + 114·3° (EtOH). It gives an ultraviolet spectrum in EtOH or AcOEt with a single absorption maximum at 280 nm. The minimum inhibition concentration against *Pseudomonas aeruginosa* and *Trichophyton asteroides* (*Trich. mentagrophytes*) is 100 µg/ml.

Yamamoto *et al.*, *Japanese Patent*, 7,228,191 (1972)

ANTIBIOTIC 534
This antibiotic substance is formed when *Cephalosporium diospyri* is grown in a common nutrient medium at 27°C for 3 days. Extraction of the mycelium with $(CH_3)_2CO$ followed by $CHCl_3$ yields the compound which gives a mixture of unsaturated fatty acids on hydrolysis. The mixture is active against Ehrlich ascites sarcoma.

Tamura *et al.*, *Japanese Patent*, 7,119,596 (1971)

ANTIBIOTIC 583
$C_{19}H_{27}O_3N_9$
M.p. Indefinite
Streptomyces orientalis elaborates this antibiotic when grown in a common nutrient medium. It has been characterized as the crystalline hydrochloride with m.p. 177–181°C. It is active against a number of gram-positive bacteria.

Mochizuki *et al.*, *Japanese Patent*, 7,017,596 (1970)

ANTIBIOTIC 593A
$C_7H_{11}ON_2Cl$
M.p. Indefinite
An antibacterial and antitumour antibiotic, this substance is produced by *Streptomyces griseoluteus* grown upon a dextrose medium. The antibiotic is basic in character, soluble in H_2O, the lower alcohols and $CHCl_3$ and yields a crystalline acetate, m.p. 228–229°C. It is active in inhibiting the growth of a number of bacteria including *Brucella bronchisepta*, *Proteus vulgaris*, *Pseudomonas stutzeri* and *Vibrio percolans*. It also possesses antitumour properties, inhibiting 60 per cent of the growth of human adenocarcinomas implanted in the chorioallantois of eggs with 9-day embryos.

Gitterman *et al.*, *German Patent*, 2,029, 768 (1971)

ANTIBIOTIC 695
This antibiotic substance has been investigated by Russian and Bulgarian workers. It is elaborated by *Actinomyces* species 695 grown upon a nutrient medium at 28°C for 7 days. Few details concerning its biological activity have been reported.

Kominkov *et al.*, *Kongr. Mikrobiol., Mater. Kongr. Mikrobiol. Bulg.*, 2nd, **4**, 121 (1969)

ANTIBIOTIC 737
An antibiotic substance, this compound appears to be a mixture of the α-monoglycerides of octadecadienoic and octanoic acids. It is produced by fermenting a *Cercospora* species in a common nutrient medium at 26·5°C for 4 days. The compound shows activity in inhibiting the growth of Ehrlich ascites sarcoma in mice.

Tara *et al.*, *Japanese Patent*, 7,119,597 (1971)

ANTIBIOTIC 768
$C_{18}H_{22}O_6N_5$?
M.p. 276–278°C
A recently discovered antibiotic, this substance is produced by *Streptomyces davawensis* (FERM-P 1402). It is isolated from the culture filtrate by extraction with pyridine, adsorption on activated carbon and purified by countercurrent distribution. It forms deep red needles and is soluble in H_2O, CH_3OH, EtOH, pyridine, $(CH_3)_2SO$, BuOH, $(CH_3)_2CO$ and dimethylformamide but insoluble in C_6H_6, AcOEt, Et_2O, $CHCl_3$, hexane and petroleum ether. It is sensitive to light, air and acids. The antibiotic inhibits the growth of a number of bacteria including *Bacillus*, *Sarcina* and *Staphylococcus* species. It is relatively non-toxic, mice tolerating 300 mg/kg of the crude material.

Otani *et al.*, *Japanese Patent*, 7,396,793 (1973)

ANTIBIOTIC 810 A$_1$
$C_{25}H_{29}O_{14}N_3S_2$

Streptomyces griseus MA-2837 and *S. lactamdurans* MA-2908 both yield a number of antibiotics when grown in an aqueous nutrient medium containing sucrose, glycerol and mono-sodium glutamate together with inorganic salts at 27°C and pH 5·5–8·0 for 3 days. This particular compound is a component of antibiotic 810 A complex and has the structure given above which is based upon chemical and spectroscopic data. It is active against a number of gram-positive and gram-negative bacteria.

Stapley, Martinez Mata, *German Patent*, 2,109,854 (1971)

ANTIBIOTIC 810 A$_2$
$C_{25}H_{29}O_{11}N_3S$

A component of the antibiotic 810 A complex elaborated by *Streptomyces griseus* MA-2837 and *S. lactamdurans* MA-2908, this compound has a similar antibiotic spectrum to the preceding antibiotic.

Stapley, Martinez Mata, *German Patent*, 2,109,854 (1971)

ANTIBIOTIC 842 A
$C_{16}H_{22}O_9N_4S$

In addition to the above complex, *Streptomyces griseus* MA-2837 and *S. lactamdurans* MA-2908 also yield this antibiotic which has a similar structure to the two preceding antibiotics. It is active against a range of gram-positive and gram-negative bacteria both *in vitro* and *in vivo* in mice.

Stapley, Martinez Mata, *German Patent*, 2,109,854 (1971)

ANTIBIOTIC 890A$_1$
$C_{13}H_{18}N_2O_5S$

Both *Streptomyces flavogriseus* ATCC 8139 and ATCC 8140 elaborate this antibiotic, the structure of which has been determined from chemical and spectroscopic examination. It has been shown to be active against both gram-positive and gram-negative bacteria.

Cassidy, Goegelman, *German Patent*, 2,652,677 (1976)

ANTIBIOTIC 890A$_3$
$C_{13}H_{18}N_2O_5S$

A stereoisomer of antibiotic 890A$_1$, this antibiotic has been isolated only from cultures of *Streptomyces flavogriseus* strain ATCC 8140. It has a similar antibiotic spectrum as the preceding substance against gram-positive and gram-negative bacteria.

Cassidy, Goegelman, *German Patent*, 2,652,677 (1976)

ANTIBOTIC 924A1
$C_{13}H_{18}O_5N_2S$

This antibiotic which has been obtained from cultures of *Streptomyces cattleya* NRRL 8057 has been shown to be N-acetylthienamycin and may also be conveniently prepared by acetylation of thienamycin. It is active *in vitro* and *in vivo* against both gram-positive and gram-negative organisms in mice.

Sawyer Kahan *et al.*, *German Patent*, 2,652,681 (1976)

ANTIBIOTICS 1004
$C_{24}H_{31}NO_{12}$
Decomp. > 245°C

Streoptomyces tanashiensis var. 1004 (FERM-P 1804) yields this antibiotic when cultured at 30°C for 45 hours at pH 10·0 on a starch, glucose, dried yeast, gluten meal medium. The culture filtrate is extracted with AcOEt at pH 8·2–8·4 and the antibiotic purified by chromatographic methods to give yellow crystals that decompose without melting.

Arima *et al.*, *Japanese Patent*, 74 102,893 (1974)

ANTIBIOTIC 1037
$C_{105}H_{217}N_{23}O_{53}$
M.p. 260–262°C

A highly complex antibiotic, this compound has recently been isolated from cultures of *Trichoderma viride* 1037 (FERM-P 3333). It forms colourless crystals and is laevorotatory having a specific rotation of $[\alpha]_D - 8.0°$. The antibiotic is soluble in the lower alcohols and hot $CHCl_3$ and pyridine but insoluble in hexane, CS_2, CCl_4, dioxan, Me_2CO, AcOEt, petroleum and H_2O. Hydrolysis furnishes L-alanine, L-proline, L-leucine, L-valine, glycine, L-glutamic acid, L-phenylalaninol and α-aminobutyric acid. The antibiotic is effective against gram-positive bacteria and in controlling coccidiosis.

Ooka, *Japanese Patent*, 77 72,891 (1977)

ANTIBIOTIC 1085 I
Japanese workers have isolated two antitumour antibiotic substances from *Sepedonium ampullosporum* grown in a normal medium at 26·5°C for 4 days. The mycelium is extracted and the extract chromatographed on an alumina column. This compound is an oil which contains octadecadienoic and octadecenoic acids together with a number of other unsaturated fatty acids. It is effective in inhibiting Ehrlich ascites sarcoma.

Tamura *et al.*, *Japanese Patent*, 7,119,595 (1971)

ANTIBIOTIC 1085 II
Sepedonium ampullosporum also elaborates this antibiotic compound which is separated from the preceding substance by chromatography. It forms a white waxy solid and has been shown to contain monoglycerides of a number of unsaturated fatty acids. It also possesses inhibitory activity against Ehrlich ascites sarcoma.

Tamura *et al.*, *Japanese Patent*, 7,119,595 (1971)

ANTIBIOTIC 1233 A
$C_{18}H_{28}O_5$
M.p. 76–77°C

One of two structurally similar antibiotics isolated from various species of *Cephalosporium*, this compound forms colourless prisms when crystallized from Et_2O-light petroleum. The structure has been shown to be 12-hydroxy-13-hydroxymethyl-3:5:7-trimethyltetradeca-2:4-diene-1:14-dioic acid (12 → 14) lactone.

Aldridge, Giles, Turner, *J. Chem. Soc.*, C, 3888 (1971)

ANTIBIOTIC 1233 B
$C_{18}H_{30}O_6$
M.p. 88–94°C

Also derived from *Cephalosporium* species, this antibiotic crystallizes from Et_2O. The structure is 12-hydroxy-13-hydroxymethyl-3:5:7-trimethyltetradeca-2:4-diene-1:14-dioic acid.

Aldridge, Giles, Turner, *J. Chem. Soc.*, C, 3888 (1971)

ANTIBIOTIC 1294B-Z
An antibacterial antibiotic, this substance has been obtained from *Nocardia formica* var. *Kurihasiensis* by culturing the organism at 30°C and pH 6·5 for

4 days aerobically on a medium consisting of glycerol, glucose, gluten meal, peptone and NaCl. The antibiotic is separated and purified chromatographically.

Arima *et al.*, *Japanese Patent*, 74 32,229 (1974)

ANTIBIOTIC 1308
M.p. 128–132°C
This antibiotic has been isolated from both the mycelium and culture filtrate of *Streptomyces* 1308 (NRRL 5318) and is purified by chromatography on activated carbon and silica gel. It is laevorotatory with a specific rotation of $[\alpha]_D^{18} - 50.5°$ (c 2·0, $CHCl_3$). Antibiotic 1308 has proved useful as a fungicide, particularly against rice blast disease.

Takeda *et al.*, *U.S. Patent*, 3,780,172 (1973)

ANTIBIOTIC 1719
See Azotomycin

ANTIBIOTIC 1754-Z3
Streptomyces komoroensis elaborates an antibiotic complex when grown on a common nutrient medium. The complex has been separated into three compartments, antibiotics 1754-Z3 A, 1754-Z3 B and 1754-Z3 Bw by silica gel chromatography. Physical and antibiotic characteristics indicate that component 1754-Z3 B is identical with staphylomycin S. All three constituents are broad spectrum antibiotics against gram-positive bacteria and components A and B exhibit a synergistic effect.

Oka *et al.*, *Yamanouchi Seiyaku Kenkyu Hokoku*, **2**, 173 (1974)

ANTIBIOTIC 1998
Bacillus brevis strain AS 1998 (NRRL B-8029) yields this antibiotic when cultured on a variety of nutrient media at pH 5·0–8·0 and between 27°C and 40°C for 12–72 hours. It has been isolated as the hydrochloride, $C_{23}H_{34}N_3O_8Cl_2$ having a melting point of 142–145°C. This salt is freely soluble in the lower alcohols, Me_2CO and H_2O, moderately soluble in AcOEt and $CHCl_3$ and insoluble in C_6H_6, hexane and petroleum ether. It is active against gram-positive bacteria, particularly *Escherichia coli*, *Staphylococcus aureus* and *Vibrio metschnikovii*.

Shimojima *et al.*, *German Patent*, 2,424,707 (1975)

ANTIBIOTIC 2305
$C_{10}H_{10}N_4O_6$
M.p. 248°C
A comparatively simple antibiotic elaborates by *Streptomyces murinus* strain 2305 (FERM-P 1807), this substance has been prepared by cultivating the organism at 30°C for 45 hours in a medium of glucose, dried yeast, gluten meal and inorganic salts. The antibiotic has been isolated by extraction of the culture filtrate with BuOH and purified by silica gel chromatography. It is active against a range of gram-positive bacteria.

Arima *et al.*, *Japanese Patent*, 74 102,894 (1974)

ANTIBIOTIC 2315
Actinoplanes philippinensis NRLL 5462 elaborates this antibiotic complex which has been separated into three components, antibiotics 2315 A, 2315 B and 2315 C by silica gel chromatography. The complex is active against cariogenic bacteria and is also effective as a growth promoter in chickens.

Hamill, Stark, *U.S. Patent*, 3,923,980 (1975)

ANTIBIOTIC 2368
A heptaenic antibiotic, this compound is produced by an unclassified *Streptomyces* species, together with antibiotics 18-45 and 18-80 (q.v.). The maximum concentration of this antibiotic is elaborated under conditions of decreased aeration. Antibiotic 2368 is inhibitive towards mycelial fungi including *Candida albicans* and *Verticillium dahliae*.

Tokhtamuratov, Silaev, *Antibiotiki*, **12**, 887 (1967)

ANTIBIOTIC 2725
M.p. Indefinite
A polypeptide antibiotic, this compound accompanies bacitracin and licheniformin in cultures of *Bacillus licheniformis* strain 2725 when grown in a medium containing glycerol, soybean flour, fish meal and inorganic salts at 28°C and pH 7·0. The antibiotic is isolated by adsorption on activated carbon and eluted with acidified C_6H_6-industrial methylated spirits. It is purified by precipitation from solution with picric acid, conversion into the hydrochloride and freeze-drying. Hydrolysis furnishes alanine, aspartic acid, arginine, glutamic acid, glycine, histidine, isoleucine, lysine, leucine, phenylalanine, serine, threonine and valine. The antibiotic is active against

a range of gram-positive and gram-negative bacteria. It is almost certainly a mixture of more than one biologically-active material.

Woolford, *J. Appl. Microbiol.*, **35**, 227 (1972)

ANTIBIOTIC 3002
Two very similar antitumour antibiotics are elaborated by *Streptomyces luridus* and *S. primycini*. The structure of this compound is not yet known. It inhibits the ascites tumour forms Ehrlich ascites tumour, NK/LY lymphodenoma and S-37 sarcoma in mice but exerts no action against the corresponding solid forms.

Rossolimo *et al.*, *Antibiotiki*, **16**, 320 (1971)

ANTIBIOTIC 3008B
$C_9H_{11}NO_5$

An antibiotic isolated from *Streptomyces jumonjiensis* No. 3008, this compound has been obtained by the aerobic culture of the organism on a medium of glycerol, starch, fish meal and $CaCO_3$ at 28°C for about 90 hours. The antibiotic is adsorbed on activated carbon and eluted at pH 4·0 with H_2O. It is soluble in dioxan, tetrahydrofuran and H_2O, insoluble in $CHCl_3$, AcOEt, CCl_4, C_6H_6, Et_2O and hexane. Antibiotic 3008B is optically active with specific rotation of $[\alpha]_D + 49\cdot4°$ ($CHCl_3$). It is effective against both gram-positive and gram-negative bacteria and against bacteria resistant to most other antibiotics. It is relatively non-toxic, mice injected with 200–400 mg/kg intravenously showing no abnormal symptoms.

Arai, Terehara, Haneishi, *Japanese Patent*, 76 118,890 (1976)

ANTIBIOTIC 3853
This antibiotic accompanies the preceding compound, being isolated from cultures of *Streptomyces luridus* and *S. primycini*. It has a similar inhibitory effect against ascites tumour forms.

Rossolimo *et al.*, *Antibiotiki*, **16**, 320 (1971)

ANTIBIOTIC 4418
An antibiotic belonging to the iomycin-pluramycin class, this compound occurs in the culture filtrate of *Streptomyces griseorubiginosus* var. *spiralis*. The antibiotic consist of a number of components and is active against Ehrlich ascites sarcoma.

Kudinova *et al.*, *Antibiotiki*, **13**, 201 (1968)

ANTIBIOTIC 5879 (*Aizumycin*)
A new antibiotic, aizumycin is elaborated by *Streptomyces aizunensis*, this compound has biological and physicochemical characteristics which are identical with those of bicyclomycin (q.v.) and it appears that the two compounds are identical.

Miyamura *et al.*, *J. Antibiotics* (Japan), **26**, 479 (1973)

ANTIBIOTIC 6640
See Sisomycin

ANTIBIOTIC 8327B
Cultures of a new strain of *Actinoplanes teichomyceticus*, ATCC 31,121, yield, besides the teichmycins (q.v.), two minor antibiotics, 8327B and 8327C. The components have been separated and purified by extraction of the filtered complex with BuOH followed by paper and thin layer chromatography. Antibiotic 8327B is principally active against gram-positive bacteria.

Coronelli *et al.*, *German Patent*, 2,608,216 (1976)

ANTIBIOTIC 8327C
A second antibiotic isolated from cultures of *Actinoplanes teichomyceticus* ATCC 31,121, this substance has a similar antibiotic activity against gram-positive bacteria as the preceding compound.

Coronelli *et al.*, *German Patent*, 2,608,216 (1976)

ANTIBIOTIC 9488
Sporocytophaga cauliformis type II NCIB 9488 produces this antibiotic when grown on a peptone-agar culture at 22°C for 3 days at pH 7·0. The compound is isolated by extraction of the culture with $(CH_3)_2CO$ followed by precipitation of the proteinous matter, drying of the supernatant liquor and purification by chromatography of the residue on alumina. It is active against both gram-positive and gram-negative bacteria.

Graef, Sukatsch, *German Patent*, 1,467,923 (1972)

ANTIBIOTIC 18887 R.P.
M.p. 215°C

Isolated from *Streptomyces caelicus*, this antibiotic is obtained in the form of a white, amorphous powder. It is laevorotatory having a specific rotation of $[\alpha]_D^{20} - 21°$ (c 1·0, H_2O). The antibiotic is active against a number of gram-positive bacteria.

Mancy, Ninet, Preud'homme, *German Patent*, 1,942,832 (1970)

ANTIBIOTIC 19402 R.P.
M.p. Indefinite

A complex antibiotic, this compound is produced by growing *Streptomyces peruviensis* aerobically in a nutrient medium at 30°C and pH 6·0–7·5 for 5 days. The pH of the broth is adjusted to 4·0–5·0 and filtered, the antibiotic remaining in the filter cake from which it is removed by washing with 70 per cent aqueous CH_3OH at pH 3·0–7·0 and chromatographed on silica gel, eluting with NH_4OH—PrOH. It is purified through the sodium salt which forms a white, amorphous powder, soluble in H_2O, CH_3OH, EtOH, PrOH, iso-PrOH, insoluble in C_6H_6, Et_2O, $CHCl_3$, $(CH_3)_2CO$, hexane and AcOEt. It is active against gram-positive bacteria, particularly *Streptococcus hemolyticus*, shows some activity against *Brucella abortus bovis* and *Neisseria gonorrhoeae* but little against other gram-negative bacteria. When administered intravenously or subcutaneously to mice infected with staphylococcus or streptococcus infections it exhibits some preventative activity. It is relatively non-toxic, the LD_{50} in mice being given as 600 mg/kg when administered intraperitoneally.

Mancy, Ninet, Preud'homme, *South African Patent*, 6,801,120 (1968)

ANTIBIOTIC 20798 R.P. (*Daunorubicinol*)

This antitumour antibiotic is obtained by microbial reduction of daunorubicin with cultures of *Bacterium cyclooxydans*, *Corynebacterium simplex*, *Streptomyces lavendulae* or *S. roseochromogenes*. It exhibits some activity against experimental tumours.

Florent, Lunel, Renaut, *German Patent*, 2,456,139 (1975)

ANTIBIOTIC 21544

Streptomyces kitakiensis ATCC 21413 produces this antibiotic when shake cultured in a common nutrient medium at 27°C and pH 7·0 for 5 days. The compound is isolated from the culture filtrate by adsorption on an ion exchange resin and purified by formation of the crystalline picrate. It inhibits a number of gram-positive bacteria.

Ishida, Kikuchi, Tanimoto, *Japanese Patent*, 7,215,751 (1972)

ANTIBIOTIC 23671 R.P.

Two closely related antibiotics are elaborated by *Streptomyces chryseus* DS 12370 (NRRL 3892) or one of its mutants when the organism is cultured in a common medium under aerobic conditions. Separation is carried out by chromatography on an alumina column. The antibiotic is active against gram-positive bacteria.

Mancy, Florent, Lunel, *German Patent*, 2,209,067 (1972)

ANTIBIOTIC 23672 R.P.

This antibiotic is produced, together with the preceding substance by *Streptomyces chryseus* DS 12370 (NRRL 3892) and is separated from it chromatographically. It is also active against a number of gram-positive bacteria.

Mancy, Florent, Lunel, *German Patent*, 2,209,067 (1972)

ANTIBIOTIC 24010
Dec. 210°C

A strain of *Streptomyces*, designated 24010, elaborates this antibiotic which decomposes, without melting, above 210°C. It has a specific rotation of $[\alpha]_D^{20} + 4\cdot3°$ (c 0·2, aqueous BuOH). In many respects, antibiotic 24010 is similar to tunicamycin (q.v.). It depresses germination and mycelial growth of *Piricularia oryzae* and in concentrations of less than 1 ppm causes morphological changes in the mycelia of *Alternaria kikuchiana*, *Glomerella lagenarium*, *Pelliculiriasa sasakii* and *Piricularia oryzae*.

Mizuno et al., *J. Antibiotics* (Japan), **24**, 896 (1971)

ANTIBIOTIC 26771B

Pencicillium turbatum yields this antibiotic which has been isolated by extraction of the mycelium with AcOEt followed by crystallization and purification by thin layer chromatography. The antibiotic exhibits a moderate activity against gram-positive bacteria, mycoplasmas and a number of fungi. It also inhibits K-dependent ATPase in rat liver mitochondria. It is moderately toxic with LD_{50} in mice of 62 mg/kg when administered intraperitoneally.

Michel, Demarco, Nagarajan, *J. Antibiotics* (Japan), **30**, 571 (1977)

ANTIBIOTIC 32999 R.P.
$C_{26}H_{29}NO_{10}$

An antitumour antibiotic, this substance is produced by the reduction of carminomycin (q.v.) by *Corynebacterium simplex* ATCC 6946. The organism is cultured in a medium consisting of brewers yeast autolyzate, glucose and potassium phosphates at pH 6·9 and fermented with agitation at 30°C for

Antibiotic 35763

2 days. The carminomycin is then added and the culture fermented for a further 48 hours at 26°C. The pH is then adjusted to 9·0 with borate buffer, the culture filtrate extracted with CH_2Cl_2-BuOH and the organic phase dried with anhydrous sodium sulphate. The antibiotic is separated and purified by thin layer chromatography.

Florent, Lunel, Renaut, *German Patent*, 2,610,557 (1977)

ANTIBIOTIC 35763

An antibiotic produced by aerobic submerged culture of *Actinoplanes auranticolor*, this substance is formed together with antibiotics 37277 and 37932 (q.v.). It has been obtained by extraction of the broth extract with isobutylketone, defatting of the extract with petroleum ether, drying *in vacuo* and separation by counter-current distribution techniques. The antibiotic is active against gram-positive bacteria and has found some use in the control of swine dysentery and as a growth stimulent in swine and chicks.

Celmer *et al.*, *U.S. Patent*, 4,038,383 (1977)

ANTIBIOTIC 37277

A constituent of the antibiotic complex produced by the aerobic submerged fermentation of *Actinoplanes auranticolor* in a medium of glucose, yeast extract, corn steep liquor and the enzymatic digest of casein for 20–30 hours at 28–36°C. It has been separated from the accompanying antibiotics by counter-current distribution methods. It is effective against gram-positive bacteria and also active in controlling swine dysentery and a growth stimulant.

Celmer *et al.*, *U.S. Patent*, 4,038,383 (1977)

ANTIBIOTIC 37932

A third component of the mixture of antibiotics elaborated by *Actinoplanes auranticolor* grown in submerged culture under aerobic condition, this antibiotic is also active against gram-positive bacteria and effective in controlling swine dysentery and as a growth stimulent.

Celmer *et al.*, *U.S. Patent*, 4,038,383 (1977)

ANTIBIOTIC 41012

A polypeptide antibiotic, this compound has been obtained by culturing *Actinoplanes nipponensis* ATCC 31,145 on a medium containing common nutrients at 24–36°C for 30–66 hours after pre-culturing on a sterile medium at 28°C for 3–4 days. It is purified chromatographically. The antibiotic is active primarily against gram-positive bacteria.

Celmer *et al.*, *U.S. Patent*, 4,001,397 (1977)

ANTIBIOTIC 41043

This antibiotic has been prepared by the submerged aerobic fermentation of *Pseudonocardia fastidiosa* in a medium of glucose, starch, enzymatic digest of casein, $CaCO_3$ and $CoCl_2$ at 28–36°C and pH 7·1 for 40–60 hours with with aeration and stirring. The antibiotic is precipitated with heptane and separated from the accompanying antibiotics by chromatography on silica gel. It is active against both gram-positive and gram-negative bacteria.

Celmer *et al.*, *U.S. Patent*, 4,031,206 (1977)

ANTIBIOTIC 41494

A second component of the antibiotic mixture isolated from submerged cultures of *Pseudonocardia fastidiosa*, this antibiotic is prepared in the same manner as the preceding compound and separated from it by silica gel chromatography. It is also effective against gram-positive and gram-negative bacteria.

Celmer *et al.*, *U.S. Patent*, 4,031,206 (1977)

ANTIBIOTIC 42752

Micromonospora saitamica yields a mixture of at least three antibiotics when cultured under submerged aerobic conditions in a medium consisting of casein, glucose, starch, yeast extract, $CaCO_3$ and $CoCl_2$ at 30°C and pH 7·2–7·3 for 48–72 hours. Extraction of the culture broth with methylisobutyl-ketone, re-extraction with $CHCl_3$, concentration to precipitate the antibiotic mixture followed by silica gel chromatography yields the pure antibiotics. This antibiotic is active against gram-positive bacteria.

Celmer et al., U.S. Patent, 4,032,631 (1977)

ANTIBIOTIC 43038
A component of the antibiotic complex produced by *Micromonospora saitamica*, this antibiotic has been separated from the accompanying substances by silica gel chromatography. It possesses a similar antibiotic spectrum to antibiotic 42752.

Celmer et al., U.S. Patent, 4,032,631 (1977)

ANTIBIOTIC 43139
This antibiotic is also produced, together with the two preceding substances, by the aerobic submerged culture of *Micromonospora saitamica* in a medium comprising casein, glucose, starch, yeast extract, $CaCO_3$ and $CoCl_2$. It is active against a range of gram-positive bacteria.

Celmer et al., U.S. Patent, 4,032,631 (1977)

ANTIBIOTIC 43334
Isolated from cultures of *Streptosporangium koreanum* and *S. cinnabarinum*, this antibiotic has been obtained by culturing the organism on a medium consisting of glucose, starch, yeast extract, enzymatic digest of casein, $CaCO_3$ and $CoCl_2$ at 30°C for 2–33 days with aeration and stirring. It has been purified by chromatography and inhibits both gram-positive and gram-negative bacteria.

Celmer et al., U.S. Patent, 4,032,632 (1977)

ANTIBIOTIC 43596
This antibiotic accompanies the preceding compound in cultures of *Streptosporangium koreanum* and *S. cinnabarinum*. It has been separated and purified by column chromatography. It is also active in inhibiting gram-positive and gram-negative bacteria.

Celmer et al., U.S. Patent, 4,032,632 (1977)

ANTIBIOTIC A-2 (*4:15-Diacetylverrucarol*)
$C_{19}H_{26}O_6$
M.p. 147–178°C
Antibiotic A-2 has been isolated from the fermentation broth of a strain of *Myrothecium verrucaria*. When purified by crystallization from EtOH it forms colourless prisms and has the sesquiterpene structure given above which is based upon chemical and spectroscopic evidence. The antibiotic is highly active against *Trichophyton rubrum*.

Okuchi et al., J. Antibiotics (Japan), **26**, 562 (1973)

ANTIBIOTIC A-60
Streptomyces strain A-60 yields this antibiotic when grown on a culture medium rich in $MgSO_4$. When purified chromatographically it forms brown-orange crystals. Antibiotic A-60 has a pronounced activity against gram-positive organisms but is only weakly active against gram-negative bacteria.

Ogata, Osawa, Yoshiki, J. Ferment. Technol., **55**, 285 (1977)

ANTIBIOTIC A-128-OP
M.p. Indefinite
A polypeptide antibiotic, this substance forms one component of the cyclopeptide lactone antibiotic A-128. It is soluble in H_2O and forms a white amorphous powder with no definite melting point. It is not readily separated from the accompanying antibiotic A-128-P (q.v.) since both have very similar chromatographic and electrophoretic behaviours and almost the same solubilities in various solvents. Five hydroxyl groups, one amino group and one carboxylic acid group are present in the molecule which contains eleven aminoacids. Three of these acids have the D-configuration, namely D-aspartic acid, D-serine and D-*allo*-threonine.

Trifonova et al., Khim. Prir. Soedin., **7**. 815 (1971)

ANTIBIOTIC A-128-P
M.p. Indefinite
The second component of the antibiotic mixture A-128, this compound has a structure similar to that of the preceding antibiotic, containing eleven aminoacids but only four hydroxyl groups in the molecule.

Trifonova et al., Khim. Prir. Soedin., **7**, 815 (1971)

ANTIBIOTIC A-130
$C_{47}H_{78}O_{13}$

An antibiotic of the nigericin group, antibiotic A-130 has been isolated from cultures of *Streptomyces hygroscopicus* strain A-130. It has been shown to be active against gram-positive organisms.

Kubota *et al.*, *J. Antibiotics* (Japan), **28**, 931 (1975)

ANTIBIOTIC A-130-A
M.p. Indefinite

A polycyclic polyester antibiotic, this compound is obtained by the cultivation of several strains of *Streptomyces*, in particular *S. hygroscopicus* strain A-130, ATCC 21840, on a nutrient medium incubated at 29°C for 65 hours with aeration of 15 litres/minute. It is normally obtained in the form of the sodium salt. Antibiotic A-130-A inhibits the growth of gram-positive bacteria, acid-fast bacteria and protozoa. It is particularly useful as a feed additive for the inhibition of *Eimeria tenella* infestation of chickens.

Kubota, Kawamura, *Japanese Patent*, 7,304,558 (1973)
Oikawa *et al.*, *British Patent*, 1,356,080 (1974)
Oikawa, Kawaguchi, Kawamura, *German Patent*, 2,261,570 (1974)

ANTIBIOTIC A-150-A
$C_{40}H_{65}O_{11}N$
M.p. Indefinite

A crystalline antibiotic, this compound is produced by *Streptomyces hygroscopicus* NRRL 3444 when cultivated under submerged aerobic conditions. It is isolated by filtration of the culture broth and extracted from both the filtrate and the mycelium. Evaporation of the organic extracts gives a crude, oily material and this is purified by chromatography over silica gel followed by crystallization from Et_2O or C_6H_6. It is a broad spectrum antibiotic, active against gram-positive and gram-negative bacteria, fungi and protozoa.

Hamill, Haney, Hoehn, *U.S. Patent*, 3,711,605 (1973)

ANTIBIOTIC A-201A
M.p. Indefinite

Streptomyces capreolus NRRL 3817 yields two antibiotics when cultured by submerged aerobic techniques in a medium containing dextrose, Blackstrap molasses, soybean flour and a defoaming agent at 30°C for 2 days. The culture filtrate is adjusted to pH 8·5 and extracted with $CHCl_3$, the residue being dissolved in CH_3OH, concentrated, redissolved in $CHCl_3$ and finally precipitated with petroleum ether. This particular component forms whitish crystals and is active against a range of bacteria, particularly *Diplococcus pneumoniae*, *Staphylococcus aureus* and *Streptococcus pyogenes*. The LD_{50} in mice is 400 mg/kg given intraperitoneally.

Hamill, Hoehn, *German Patent*, 2,164, 564 (1972)

ANTIBIOTIC A-201B

This component of the antibiotic mixture produced by cultivating *Streptomyces capreolus* under submerged aerobic conditions is an oily liquid, light brown in colour, which decomposes on heating. It has a similar antibiotic spectrum to that of the preceding antibiotic.

Hamill, Hoehn, *German Patent*, 2,164,565 (1972

ANTIBIOTIC A-204-A
$C_{49}H_{84}O_{17}$
M.p. 96–98°C

This complex antibiotic has been isolated from cultures of *Streptomyces albus*. It forms colourless cyrstals when crystallized from CH_3OH and has a specific rotation of $[\alpha]_D^{25} + 68\cdot1°$ (c 2·0, CH_3OH). The structure has been established from chemical and spectroscopic data.

Jones *et al.*, *J. Amer. Chem. Soc.*, **95**, 3399 (1973)

ANTIBIOTIC A-218
$C_{46}H_{80}O_{15}$
M.p. Indefinite

A complex antibiotic derived from *Streptomyces hygroscopicus* A-218 (FERM-P924), this substance is produced by fermentation in a medium containing soybean powder, potato starch, glycerol, corn steep liquor, glucose, sodium chloride and calcium carbonate at 27°C for 90 hours. It may be extracted from both the filtrate and cells with AcOEt and is purified by chromatography of the concentrated extract over silica gel, eluting with $CHCl_3$ containing 2 per cent of CH_3OH and recrystallizing from petroleum ether. The sodium salt forms colourless prisms, m.p. 186–187°C and has an acid reaction. It is soluble in CH_3OH, EtOH, Et_2O, AcOEt, $CHCl_3$ and $(CH_3)_2CO$, insoluble in H_2O and petroleum ether. With Dragendorff reagent it gives a pronounced orange colour.

Antibiotic A-218 is active against gram-positive bacteria and is comparatively toxic with an LD_{50} in mice of 10–20 mg/kg when given intravenously.

Tsuji *et al.*, *Japanese Patent*, 7,380,793 (1973)

ANTIBIOTIC A-246
See Lagosin

ANTIBIOTIC A-300-I
$C_{17}H_{22}O_3N_2$

Streptomyces hygroscopicus A-300 yields two closely related antibiotics. The mixture is obtained by fermentation in a medium containing soybean powder, potato starch, glycerol, corn steep liquor, calcium carbonate and sodium chloride at pH 7·0 for 88 hours at 28°C. The culture filtrate is extracted with AcOEt, washed with petroleum ether, extracted with $CHCl_3$, dissolved in AcOEt and then adsorbed on a polyamide column. Elution with AcOEt gives this antibiotic which is purified by thin layer chromatography with silica gel. The antibiotic is effective primarily against dermatophytes.

Tsuji *et al.*, *Japanese Patent*, 7,414,691 (1974)

ANTIBIOTIC A-300-II
$C_{51}H_{63}O_9N_6Fe$

Also derived from *Streptomyces hygroscopicus* A-300, this iron-containing antibiotic is obtained together with the preceding substance and is isolated by eluting the material adsorbed on the polyamide column with $CHCl_3$ followed by crystallization from CH_3OH. It is normally obtained in this manner as the crystalline trihydrate. Like the preceding antibiotic it is active against dermatophytes.

Tsuji *et al.*, *Japanese Patent*, 7,414,691 (1974)

ANTIBIOTIC A-396-I
M.p. 185–195°C (*dec.*).

An antibiotic produced by *Streptoverticillium eurocidicus* A-396 (FERM-P501). The precultured organisms are grown on a medium containing soybean powder, starch, corn steep liquor, glycerol, potassium dihydrogen and potassium hydrogen phosphates and sodium chloride. When purified by preparative thin layer chromatography, lyophilization and crystallization via the Reinecke salt, the pure antibiotic is obtained as colourless crystals. Antibiotic A-396-I is active against gram-positive bacteria and is comparatively toxic, the LD_{50} in mice being 12·5 mg/kg when administered intravenously. This antibiotic is believed to be identical to Antibiotic ss-56D (q.v.).

Sayama, Shoji, *Japanese Patent*, 7,139,073 (1971)

ANTIBIOTIC A-477
An antibiotic produced by preculturing *Actinoplanes* species NRRL 3884 on a common nutrient medium followed by aerobic cultivation in a medium consisting of starch, dextrose, mannitol, soybean flour, autolysed yeast and inorganic salts at 30°C and pH 7·3–7·4 for 5 days. The antibiotic has basic properties and has been characterized as the crystalline hydrochloride, sulphate, methyl orange salt and picrate. The compound is useful as a feed additive, disinfectant and in dentifrices. The hydrochloride has LD_{50} in mice of 350 mg/kg when administered intraperitoneally.

Hamill, Haney, Stark, *German Patent*, 2,252,937 (1973)

ANTIBIOTIC A-661-I
$C_{47}H_{79}NO_{16}$

Streptomyces diastatochromogenes strain A-661 elaborates this complex antibiotic when cultured for 2 days in a medium consisting of glycerol, starch, corn steep liquor, soybean powder, $CaCO_3$ and NaCl at 28°C and pH 7·0. It is purified by silica gel chromatography. The antibiotic is effective against fungi.

Shoji *et al.*, *Japanese Patent*, 74 126,896 (1974)

ANTIBIOTIC A-2315
$C_{26}H_{39}O_7N_3$

A macrocyclic antibiotic, this substance is obtained by the aerobic fermentation of *Actinoplanes philippinensis* NRRL 5462 of a range of common nutrient media. The probable structure is that given above which is based upon chemical and spectroscopic examination. Antibiotic A-2315 is active against a range of bacteria, particularly gram-positive organisms.

Hamill, Stark, *German Patent*, 2,336,811 (1974)
Chamberlain, Chen, *J. Antibiotics* (Japan), **30**, 197 (1977)

ANTIBIOTIC A-4696
Produced by *Actinoplanes* species ATCC 23,342, this antibiotic has been used by itself, or in the form of its various salts, as an animal growth promoting substance and as an ingredient in dentrifices for its anticarious activity.

Hamill, Stark, DeLong, *German Patent*, 2,209,018 (1972)

ANTIBIOTIC A-4993A
One of two closely related nitrogenous antibiotics obtained from *Streptomyces kentuckensis* NRRL 3552 grown on an aqueous nutrient medium. The activity of the culture filtrate is adsorbed on a cationic exchange resin and eluted with $0.1\ N\text{-}H_2SO_4$. Separation of the two components of the mixture thus obtained is carried out by chromatography on an alumina column followed by crystallization from various solvents. This antibiotic is normally characterized as the crystalline sulphate. Antibiotic A-4993A is active, either alone or in admixture with the following compound, against a large number of bacteria, fungi and trypanosoma. It is particularly useful as an anthelmintic and in the treatment of trypanosomiasis in mammals and it also has a high activity against pleuropneumonia-like organisms.

Hamill, Hoehn, *U.S. Patent*, 3,629,405 (1971)

ANTIBIOTIC A-4993B
This component from the mixture obtained from the culture filtrate of *Streptomyces kentuckensis* NRRL 3552 has a biological spectrum almost identical with that given for the preceding antibiotic.

Hamill, Hoehn, *U.S. Patent*, 3,629,405 (1971)

ANTIBIOTIC A-9145
M.p. Indefinite

Streptomyces griseolus NRRL 3739 produces this antibiotic which is obtained in the form of the crystalline hydrochloride, colourless crystals with m.p. 195–197°C. The antibiotic is soluble in H_2O and possesses basic properties. It contains adenine and possibly a sugar moiety. It is active against pathogen plant fungi, *Candida* species, *Saccharomyces pastorianus* and *Trypanosoma* species. Although the activity *in vitro* against *Candida albicans* is not pronounced in Sabouraud's medium, it is very high in chemically-defined media and it is also active against the same species *in vivo*, there also being an additive effect against *C. albicans in vivo* when used with amphotericin B (q.v.).

Hamill, Hoehn, *J. Antibiotics* (Japan), **26**, 463 (1973)
Gordee, Butler, *ibid.*, **26**, 466 (1973)
Boeck *et al.*, *Antimicrobial Agents & Chemotherapy*, **3**, 49 (1973)
Hamill, Hoehn, *U.S. Patent*, 3,758,681 (1973)

ANTIBIOTIC A-16316-C
$C_{21}H_{39}O_{13}N_3 \cdot 0.5\ H_2O$
M.p. 175–185°C (*dec.*)

A basic white powder, this antibiotic has been obtained by culturing *Streptoverticillium eurodicus* on a medium containing starch, glucose, peptone, meat extract, soybean powder, soybean oil and inorganic salts at 30°C for 94 hours. The antibiotic is isolated from the supernatant liquor by ion-exchange chromatography followed by thin layer chromatography. It is dextrorotatory with a specific rotation of $[\alpha]_D + 7.5°$ (c $1.0\ H_2O$) and on acid hydrolysis it yields destomic acid, N,N'-dimethyl-2-deoxy-streptamine and D-mannose. It is soluble in H_2O and MeOH but insoluble in the higher alcohols, $CHCl_3$, Me_2CO, AcOEt, Et_2O, C_6H_6 and hexane. The antibiotic action of this substance is similar to that of destomycin B, being effective against *Staphylococcus aureus*, *Escherichia coli* K-12 and *Mycobacteria smegmatus* 607.

Tamura, Furuta, Kotani, *J. Antibiotics* (Japan), **28**, 260 (1975)
Tamura, Furuta, Kotani, *Japanese Patent*, 76 82,793 (1976)

ANTIBIOTIC A 16884
$C_{16}H_{21}O_8N_3S$
M.p. Indefinite

A broad spectrum antibiotic, this compound is produced by the aerobic cultivation under submerged conditions of *Streptomyces lipmanii* NRRL 3584 incubated at 30°C for 3 days. The antibiotic is active against a range of gram-positive and gram-negative bacteria and also possesses anthelmintic activity.

Hamill, Hoehn, Higgens, *German Patent*, 2,039,184 (1971)
Hamill, Higgens, Hoehm, *U.S. Patent*, 3,973,015 (1976)

ANTIBIOTIC A 16886A
See Antibiotic A 16886 I

ANTIBIOTIC A 16886B
See Antibiotic A 16886 II

ANTIBIOTIC A 16886 I (*Antibiotic A 16886A*)
$C_{16}H_{23}O_7N_3S$

A β-lactam antibiotic produced by *Streptomyces clavuligerus*, this compound has the structure given above. It is formed by cultivation of the organism on a nutrient medium containing carbohydrates, a source of nitrogen and inorganic salts at 25–27°C for 1–3 days under submerged aerobic conditions. It is active against gram-positive and gram-negative bacteria and also has anthelmintic properties.

Gorman *et al.*, *German Patent*, 2,040,141 (1971)
Brannon *et al.*, *Antimicrobial Agents & Chemotherapy*, **1**, 242 (1972)
Whitney *et al.*, *ibid.*, **1**, 247 (1972)

ANTIBIOTIC A 16886 II (*Antibiotic A 16886B*)
$C_{15}H_{22}O_7N_4S$

This second β-lactam antibiotic produced by *Streptomyces clavuligerus* NRRL 3585 has a structure very similar to that of the preceding compound, from which it is separated by chromatography on an alumina column. It is active against gram-positive and gram-negative bacteria and also has marked anthelmintic properties.

Gorman, Higgens, Nagarajan, *German Patent*, 2,040,141 (1971)
Brannon *et al.*, *Antimicrobial Agents & Chemotherapy*, **1**, 242 (1972)
Whitney *et al.*, *ibid.*, **1**, 247 (1972)

ANTIBIOTIC A 21101 I
$C_{24}H_{28}H_2O_7S_2$

Arachniotus aureus NRRL 3205 yields an antibiotic complex when incubated in a medium consisting of corn steep liquor, molasses, sucrose, malt extract, peptone and K_2HPO_4 and cultured for about 120 hours at 25°C. The culture filtrate is extracted with AcOEt to yield the crude material which has been separated into antibiotics A 21101, I, II, III and IV by silica gel chromatography. This substance has been shown to possess the structure given above from chemical and spectroscopic evidence.

Delong, Lively, Neuss, *U.S. Patent*, 3,907,988 (1975)

ANTIBIOTIC A 21101 II
$C_{21}H_{22}N_2O_7S_2$
A second component of the antibiotic A 21101 complex isolated from cul-

Antibiotic A 21101 III

tures of *Arachniotus aureus* NRRL 3205, this substance has the above structure determined from chemical analysis and a study of the infrared, NMR and mass spectra.

Delong, Lively, Neuss, *U.S. Patent*, 3,907,988 (1975)

ANTIBIOTIC A 21101 III
$C_{20}H_{20}N_2O_6S_2$

A further antibiotic obtained by silica gel chromatography of the A 21101 complex produced by *Arachniotus aureus* NRRL 3205, the structure of this compound has been established from chemical and spectroscopic data.

Delong, Lively, Neuss, *U.S. Patent*, 3,907,988 (1975)

ANTIBIOTIC A 21101 IV
$C_{20}H_{16}N_2O_6S_2$

A fourth constituent of the antibiotic A 21101 complex obtained from cultures of *Arachniotus aureus*, this compound has been assigned the above structure on the basis of chemical and spectroscopic examination.

Delong, Lively, Neuss, *U.S. Patent*, 3,907,988 (1975)

ANTIBIOTIC A-22082
$C_{52}H_{81}N_7O_{18}.H_2O$

An antifungal peptide antibiotic, this compound occurs in cultures of *Aspergillus nidulans* NRRL 8112 and has been isolated from the culture medium by extraction with polar organic solvents followed by column chromatography. Hydrolysis yields hydroxyproline, threonine and three unidentified aminoacids.

Higgens, Michel, *German Patent*, 2,643,487 (1976)
Higgens, Michel, *U.S. Patent*, 4,024,246 (1977)

ANTIBIOTIC A-23187
$C_{29}H_{37}O_6N_3$
M.p. 181–182°C

A novel antibiotic isolated from cultures of *Streptomyces chartreusensis*, antibiotic A-23187 forms colourless crystals and is dextrorotatory with a specific rotation of $[\alpha]_D^{25} + 362°$ (c 1·0, $CHCl_3$). The above structure has been established from chemical and spectroscopic data.

Chaney et al., *J. Amer. Chem. Soc.*, **96**, 1932 (1974)
Gale, Higgens, Hoehn, *U.S. Patent*, 3,923,823 (1975)

ANTIBIOTIC A-23812
See Pyrazomycin

ANTIBIOTIC A25822A
$C_{30}H_{49}NO$
M.p. 147°C

Geotrichum flavo-brienneum yields a number of azasteroid antibiotics having similar structures which have been isolated from the culture medium and purified by column and thin layer chromatography. This component forms white crystals, is laevorotatory with a specific rotation of $[\alpha]_D^{25} - 72°$ (c 1·15, MeOH), and gives an ultraviolet spectrum consisting of a single absorption maximum at 239 nm. The structure has been elucidated from chemical and spectroscopic data. This range of antibiotics is highly active against fungi but only marginally active against bacteria.

Chamberlain et al., *J. Antibiotics* (Japan), **27**, 992 (1974)
Boeck et al., *ibid.*, **28**, 95 (1975)
Michel et al., *ibid.*, **28**, 102 (1975)

ANTIBIOTIC A25822B
$C_{28}H_{45}NO$
M.p. 115–118°C

The major component of the antibiotic complex isolated from cultures of *Geotrichum flavo-brienneum*, this substance has been obtained as white crystals having a specific rotation of $[\alpha]_D^{25} - 20°$ (c 0·775, MeOH). The ultraviolet spectrum has a single absorption maximum at 238 nm. The structure has been established from chemical evidence and a study of the infrared, NMR and mass spectra.

Chamberlain et al., *J. Antibiotics* (Japan), **27**, 992 (1974)
Boeck et al., *ibid.*, **28**, 95 (1975)
Michel et al., *ibid.*, **28**, 102 (1975)

ANTIBIOTIC A25822D
$C_{28}H_{45}NO_2$
M.p. Indefinite

Isolated from cultures of *Geotrichum flavo-brienneum* under submerged aerobic conditions, this constituent of the antibiotic complex is an amorphous powder which has no definite melting point. It is dextrorotatory with a specific rotation of $[\alpha]_D^{55} + 39°$ (c 0·722, MeOH).

Boeck et al., *J. Antibiotics* (Japan), **28**, 95 (1975)
Michel et al., *ibid.*, **28**, 102 (1975)

ANTIBIOTIC A25822H
M.p. Indefinite
A minor constituent of the group of antibiotics obtained by the submerged

aerobic fermentation of *Geotrichum flavo-brienneum*, this antibiotic forms an amorphous white powder having no definite melting point and a specific rotation of $[\alpha]_D^{25} + 15°$ (c 0·147, MeOH).

Boeck et al., *J. Antibiotics* (Japan), **28**, 95 (1975)
Michel et al., *ibid.*, **28**, 102 (1975)

ANTIBIOTIC A25822L
$C_{28}H_{43}NO_2$
M.p. Indefinite

An amorphous white powder, this antibiotic has also been isolated from submerged aerobic cultures of *Geotrichum flavo-brienneum*. It is dextrorotatory with specific rotation of $[\alpha]_D^{25} + 75°$ (c 0·072, MeOH) and has the probable structure given above based upon chemical and spectroscopic evidence.

Boeck et al., *J. Antibiotics* (Japan), **28**, 95 (1975)
Michel et al., *ibid.*, **28**, 102 (1975)

ANTIBIOTIC A25822M
$C_{30}H_{47}NO_2$
M.p. Indefinite

Submerged aerobic cultures of *Geotrichum flavo-brienneum* also contain this azasteroid antibiotic which has been shown to be an acetyl derivative of antibiotic A25822B. It is laevorotatory having a specific rotation of $[\alpha]_D^{25} - 15°$ (c 0·021, MeOH). It is active against fungi but almost inactive against bacteria.

Chamberlain et al., *J. Antibiotics* (Japan), **27**, 992 (1974)
Boeck et al., *ibid.*, **28**, 95 (1975)
Michel et al., *ibid.*, **28**, 102 (1975)

ANTIBIOTIC A25822N
$C_{28}H_{43}NO$
M.p. 165°C

A crystalline antibiotic isolated from the culture medium of *Geotrichum flavo-brienneum*, this compound has a specific rotation of $[\alpha]_D^{25} - 14°$ (c. 0.05, MeOH). The ketonic structure given above has been established from chemical and spectroscopic data.

Boeck et al., *J. Antibiotics* (Japan), **28**, 95 (1975)
Michel et al., *ibid.*, **28**, 102 (1975)

ANTIBIOTIC A-26771-A
$C_{14}H_{16}O_3N_2S_2$
M.p. 105°C

Penicillium turbatum yields a number of structurally related antibiotics, most containing sulphur. This compound crystallizes well from Et_2O and is laevorotatory with a specific rotation of $[\alpha]_D^{27} - 88°$ (c 0·15, CH_3OH). The structure is 3-benzyl-6-(hydroxymethyl)-1:4-dimethyl-3:6-epidithio-2:5-piperazinedione. It is active in inhibiting the growth of a number of gram-positive bacteria and also certain viruses.

Michel et al., *J. Antibiotics* (Japan), **27**, 57 (1974)
Michel, Hoehn, *U.S. Patent*, 3,883,561 (1975)

ANTIBIOTIC A-26771-B
$C_{20}H_{30}O_6$

A further component of the antibiotic A-26771 complex produced by *Penicillium turbatum*, this compound differs in structure from the two accompanying compounds. It is active against a number of gram-positive bacteria but has no antiviral activity.

Michel et al., *J. Antibiotics* (Japan), **27**, 57 (1974)
Michel, Hoehn, *U.S. Patent*, 3,883,561 (1975)
Michel, De Marcs, Nagarajan, *J. Antibiotics* (Japan), **30**, 571 (1977)

ANTIBIOTIC A-26771-C
$C_{14}H_{16}O_3N_2S_4$
M.p. 130°C

Also elaborated by *Penicillium turbatum* NRRL 5630, this antibiotic is the tetrasulphide corresponding to antibiotic A-26771-A. It crystallizes from a mixture of Et_2O, $(CH_3)_2CO$ and pentane and is also laevorotatory with a specific rotation of $[\alpha]_D^{27} - 187°$ (c 0·04, CH_3OH). It possesses both antibacterial and antiviral activity.

Michel et al., *J. Antibiotics* (Japan), **27**, 57 (1974)
Michel, Hoehn, *U.S. Patent*, 3,883,561 (1975)

ANTIBIOTIC A-26771-E
$C_{16}H_{22}O_3N_2S_2$
M.p. 135°C

Cultures of *Penicillium turbatum* also yield this sulphur-containing antibiotic which crystallizes from $(CH_3)_2CO$ and has a specific rotation of $[\alpha]_D^{27} - 47°$ (c 0·13, CH_3OH). Unlike antibiotics A-26771-A and A-26771-C it does not possess a bridge-structure. It is active against a range of gram-positive bacteria.

Michel et al., *J. Antibiotics* (Japan), **27**, 57 (1974)

ANTIBIOTIC A-28695-A
This antibiotic is produced by cultivation of *Streptomyces albus* NRRL 3883 on a common nutrient medium at 30°C for 5 days. Extraction of the culture filtrate with AcOEt followed by chromatography on an alumina column yields two antibiotics A-28695-A and B. These are separated as their sodium salts and converted into the free acids by hydrolysis with dilute HCl. This antibiotic is active against a number of gram-positive and gram-negative bacteria, viruses, fungi and insects. It has shown promise in the treatment of coccidiosis of chickens. The LD_{50} in mice is 41·1 mg/kg when given orally.

Hamill, Hoehn, *German Patent*, 2,262,501 (1973)

ANTIBIOTIC A-28695-B

A component of the antibiotic mixture elaborated by *Streptomyces albus* NRRL 3883, this compound is obtained by chromatography of the mixed sodium salts of the two components. It has bactericidal, fungicidal, insecticidal and virucidal properties similar to those of the preceding antibiotic. The LD_{50} in mice when administered orally is 43·5 mg/kg.

Hamill, Hoehn, *German Patent*, 2,262,501 (1973)

ANTIBIOTIC A-30641
$C_{12}H_9N_2O_5S_2Cl$

An antibiotic isolated from submerged cultures of *Aspergillus tamarii* NRRL 8101, this substance has been obtained by chromatography, eluting with MeOH, concentrating the eluate to an oil, precipitating with hexane and drying. It has been shown to contain an epidithioketopiperazine moiety and is active against gram-positive bacteria and fungi *in vitro*. It also possesses some antiviral activity.

Berg et al., *J. Antibiotics* (Japan), **29**, 394 (1976)
Berg, Hamill, Hoehn, *U.S. Patent*, 3,991,052 (1977)

ANTIBIOTIC A-30912

This peptide antibiotic has been obtained from cultures of *Aspergillus rugulosus* NRRL 8113. It is isolated from the culture broth by extraction with polar organic solvents and separated into seven components antibiotics A-30912 A–G by chromatography. This series of antibiotics is active principally against fungi, possessing little activity against bacteria.

Hoehn, Michel, *German Patent*, 2,643,485 (1976)

ANTIBIOTIC A 32204

An antifungal antibiotic isolated from cultures of *Aspergillus echinulatus* strain A 32,204, this substance is produced by fermenting the organism on a medium of glucose, soybean meal and NaCl with shaking and aeration at 29°C for approximately 60 hours. It is particularly effective against *Candida albicans*.

Neusch et al., *Swiss Patent*, 568,386 (1975)

ANTIBIOTIC A-32390A
$C_{13}H_{19}NO_8$

Culture of a Pyrenochaete NRRL 5786 on a medium comprising glucose, sucrose, cottonseed flour and inorganic salts for 4 days at 25°C with aeration and agitation yields this antibiotic together with three additional factors which have not been investigated further. This antibiotic has been isolated by extraction of the filtered broth with AcOEt which yields the crude antibiotic on concentration and cooling. Purification has been carried out by slurrying in C_6H_6, adsorption on a silica gel column, elution with AcOEt and crystallization from Me_2CO. The antibiotic possesses antifungal, antibacterial and hypotensive activity.

Marconi, Hoehn, *U.S. Patent*, 3,986,928 (1977)

ANTIBIOTIC AB-22
M.p. Indefinite

A glucosidic polypeptide antibiotic, this substance has been obtained from *Pichia polymorpha*, the organism being used when freshly isolated from soil. It is shake-cultured in a glucose-polypeptone medium for 4 days at 28°C and the antibiotic isolated from the culture filtrate by adsorption on an ion exchange resin. It is laevorotatory with a specific rotation of $[\alpha]_D^{20} - 204°$ and has an estimated molecular weight of approximately 10,000. It is active against *Piricularia oryzae* and *Trichophyton rubrum*.

Hironaka et al., *Japanese Patent*, 7,140,194 (1971)

ANTIBIOTIC AB-64
$C_{26}H_{21}O_9N$
M.p. 275–277°C (dec.)

This antibiotic has been obtained from *Actinomadura roseoviolacea* var. *rubescens* and *A. roseoviolacea* var. *hikamiensis*. The latter organism is grown on a medium of soybean powder, starch, glucose, yeast extract, meat extract and inorganic salts at pH 8·0 for 10 days at 30°C. The antibiotic is isolated by extraction of the broth precipitate, formed by adjusting to pH 4·0 and centrifuging, with 80 per cent $(CH_3)_2CO$, the extract then being re-extracted with BuOH at pH 6·0 and the solvent evaporated. Purification was carried out by dissolving the crude material in $0·01N$ ammonium hydroxide and gel filtering with Sephadex G-25. The pure material is a red, amorphous powder which is active against gram-positive bacteria.

Tamura et al., *J. Antibiotics* (Japan), **26**, 492 (1973)
Tamura et al., *Japanese Patent*, 7,419,090 (1974)

ANTIBIOTIC AB-65
$C_{61}H_{91}N_3O_{23}Cl_2$
M.p. 262–263°C (*dec.*)
Saccharomonospora viride yields this antibiotic which has been obtained as an amorphous white powder which decomposes at the melting point. It is laevorotatory having a specific rotation of $[\alpha]_D^{20} - 65.3°$ (c 1.0, Me_2SO). The structure has not yet been fully established.

Tamura, Takeda, *J. Antibiotics* (Japan), **28**, 395 (1975)

ANTIBIOTIC AB-74
$C_{21}H_{39}N_3O_{13}$
An antibiotic isolated from cultures of *Streptomyces aquacanus* A-14317, this substance has been shown to be related to destomycin C. It is active against gram-positive bacteria.

Tamura, Furuta, Naruto, *J. Antibiotics* (Japan), **29**, 590 (1976)

ANTIBIOTIC AB-161-2
M.p. 170°C (**dec.**)
A number of unclassified *Streptomyces* species yield this antibiotic which is crystallized from EtOH. It is dextrorotatory with a specific rotation of $[\alpha]_D^{30} + 31°$. The structure is not yet known.

Tanaka et al., *Japanese Patent*, 7,387,088 (1973)

ANTIBIOTIC AH272α_2
Streptomyces platensis produces two closely related antibiotics when cultivated in a medium consisting of molasses, corn starch, soybean flour and calcium carbonate at pH 6·9 and 28°C for 114 hours. The mixture of antibiotics is isolated by extraction of the culture medium with $CHCl_3$ followed by separation and purification on a silica gel column. This antibiotic is active *in vitro* against a number of *Staphylococcus* and *Streptococcus* strains and *in vivo* against two human pathogenic strains in mice.

Evans, Thomas, *U.S. Patent*, 3,592,925 (1971)

ANTIBIOTIC AH272β_2
Also elaborated by *Streptomyces platensis*, this antibiotic inhibits both pathogenic and laboratory strains of *Staphylococcus* and *Streptococcus* *in vitro* and certain strains *in vivo* in mice.

Evans, Thomas, *U.S. Patent*, 3,592,925 (1971)

ANTIBIOTIC AM-684
M.p. 172–174·5°C
One of a number of antibiotics produced by *Streptomyces hygroscopicus*, this compound is obtained by fermenting the organism aerobically in a medium consisting of lactose, Proflo and inorganic salts at 28°C for 150 hours. After adjusting the pH of the culture broth to 7·0 it is filtered, the filtrate extracted with $CHCl_3$, the extract concentrated *in vacuo*, petroleum ether added, the mixture centrifuged, decanted and the residue dissolved in $CHCl_3$ and chromatographed on silica gel using $CHCl_3$—CH_3OH as the developer. Antibiotic Am-684 forms colourless crystals and is laevorotatory with a specific rotation of $[\alpha]_D^{25} - 48.7°$ (c 0·906, CH_3OH). It is characterized as the hydrochloride, m.p. 139·5–142°C and $[\alpha]_D^{25} - 39.6°$ (c 1·14, CH_3OH). The antibiotic inhibits the growth of gram-positive bacteria.

Whaley et al., *U.S. Patent*, 3,344,024 (1967)

ANTIBIOTIC AO-341
M.p. 225–230°C
Submerged, aerobic cultivation of *Streptomyces candidus* NRRL 3147 in a medium containing glucose, molasses and bacto-peptone at 20–35°C for 1–10 days, yields this antibiotic which is isolated by separating the solids in the culture with diatomaceous earth and eluting with aqueous $(CH_3)_2CO$. The eluate is concentrated *in vacuo*, BuOH added, the butanol fraction is washed with dilute sodium hydroxide, then with H_2O and concentrated under reduced pressure to yield the crude crystals. These are then purified by recrystallization from $(CH_3)_2CO$—CH_3OH. Antibiotic AO-341 forms colourless crystals and is laevorotatory with a specific rotation of $[\alpha]_D^{25} - 104°$ (c 1·1, aqueous CH_3OH). The ultraviolet spectrum has absorption maxima at 222, 275 and 338 nm with a shoulder at 289 nm. The crystalline hydrochloride decomposes at 238–241°C and the N-subcinyl derivative has m.p. 230–235°C (*dec.*). The antibiotic is active *in vivo* in mice infected with *Diplococcus pneumoniae*, *Staphylococcus aureus* Smith and *Streptococcus pyogenes* C-203.

Whaley et al., *U.S. Patent*, 3,377,244 (1968)

ANTIBIOTIC AP-191-γ
M.p. Indefinite

A strain of *Streptomyces candidus*, NRRL 3110 elaborates this antibiotic when grown by submerged aerobic fermentation. It is isolated from the culture filtrate by extraction with AcOEt and adsorbed at pH 9·0 on diatomaceous earth followed by elution with aqueous $(CH_3)CO$ and extraction of the organic fraction with HCl at pH 4·0. This antibiotic forms a yellow powder and is laevorotatory with $[\alpha]_D^{25} - 116°$ (c 0·516, $CHCl_3$). The ultraviolet spectrum has an absorption maximum at 271 nm and a shoulder at 289 nm. It is unstable in alkalies but stable under acid conditions. The powder is soluble in $CHCl_3$, moderately so in AcOEt, EtOH, $(CH_3)_2CO$ and H_2O and insoluble in hydrocarbons. The antibiotic is active against gram-positive and gram-negative bacteria *in vitro* and *in vivo*. It gives complete protection to mice experimentally infected with a lethal dose of *Streptococcus pyogenes* C-203 at a dose of 1·25 mg/kg given subcutaneously.

Whaley, Patterson, Thomas, *U.S. Patent*, 3,344,025 (1967)

ANTIBIOTIC AR-110
Decomp. 192–197°C

This antibiotic has been produced by culturing *Bacillus polymyxa* strain AR-110 (FERM-P 3000) at 27°C for 3 days at pH 7·0 with agitation in a medium consisting of glucose, glycerol, starch, meat extract, soybean powder and inorganic salts. The culture filtrate is adjusted to pH 2·5, filtered at 70°C and the filtrate extracted with BuOH, the extract washed with dilute alkali, acid and H_2O, concentrated to a syrup and mixed with Me_2CO to yield a powder which is purified by silica gel chromatography and isolated as the hydrochloride. The antibiotic is soluble in H_2O, dilute acids and alkalis and aqueous MeOH, insoluble in alcohols, CHCl, BuOH and Me_2CO. It forms an amphoteric white powder which yields glycine, glutamic acid, alanine, alloisoleucine, valine, phenylalanine, trytophan, 2,4-diaminobutyric acid, ammonia and an unidentified fatty acid on hydrolysis. It is effective against gram-positive bacteria but relatively toxic with LD_{50} of 12·5–25 mg/kg when administered intraperitoneally to mice.

Shoji *et al.*, *Japanese Patent*, 76 114,796 (1976)

ANTIBIOTIC ASK-753
M.p. 120°C (*dec.*)

A comples polypeptide antibiotic produced by *Streptomyces* strain AS-K-753, this compound forms buff-coloured plates from EtOH. Hydrolysis with dilute acids furnishes citric, fumaric, gluconic and α-ketoglutaric acids together with at least eight aminoacids of which alanine, aspartic acid, glutamic acid, glycine, leucine and lysine have been identified. It possesses a high degree of inhibitory activity against gram-positive bacteria and cocci, e.g. *Corynebacterium hoffmanii* and *Pseudomonas aeruginosa*, *Saccharomyces cerevisiae*, *Staphylococcus aureus* resistant to most other antibiotics and a limited activity against gram-negative organisms. The activity is not antagonized by ferrioxamine B. The LD_{50} in Swiss mice is 58 mg/kg given intraperitoneally.

Shimi *et al.*, *J. Antibiotics* (Japan), **22**, 106 (1969)

ANTIBIOTIC AT-125
$C_5H_7O_3N_2Cl$

Aerobic cultivation of *Streptomyces sviceus* NRRL 5439 in common media yields this simple antibiotic which is isolated by filtering the broth, adsorbing on an ion exchange resin, eluting with CH_3OH, followed by recrystallization from CH_3OH. Antibiotic AT-125 has proved useful as a bactericide and fungicide.

Hanks, Martin, *German Patent*, 2,311,655 (1973)

ANTIBIOTIC AV-290
Streptomyces candidus elaborates this antibiotic which is recovered from the fermentation broth by the addition of syntan, a synthetic tanning agent which forms a complex with the antibiotic. The precipitated complex is dissolved in H_2O at pH 6·0–9·0, adsorbed on CM-Sephadex, eluted with aqueous H_2SO_4 at pH 1·4–2·5, the eluate neutralized with barium hydroxide and the eluate then freeze-dried.

Shu, Dann, *U.S. Patent*, 3,819,836 (1974)

ANTIBIOTIC B-41
When *Streptomyces* strain B-41-146 is cultivated on a common medium at 28° for 6 days it yields an antibiotic mixture designated antibiotic B-41. This material has been shown to possess acaricidal and insecticidal activity against a number of plant pests. Both column and paper chromatography have now shown that B-41 may be separated into a number of individual

ANTIBIOTIC B-41-A$_1$
C$_{32}$H$_{46}$O$_7$

This macrocyclic antibiotic has been isolated from the mixture produced by *Streptomyces* strain B-41-146 and separated from the accompanying constituents by chromatography. The structure has been deduced from chemical and spectroscopic data.

Aoki *et al.*, *German Patent*, 2,329,486 (1973)

ANTIBIOTIC B-41-A$_2$
A minor constituent of the antibiotic mixture B-41, the structure of this component has not yet been elucidated.

Aoki *et al.*, *German Patent*, 2,329,486 (1973)

ANTIBIOTIC B-41-A$_3$
C$_{31}$H$_{46}$O$_7$

The structure of this macrocyclic antibiotic produced by *Streptomyces* strain B-41-146 is very similar to that of antibiotic B-41-A$_1$ (q.v.), differing only in having a secondary hydroxyl group in place of the methoxyl group and one of the double bonds fully hydrogenated.

Aoki *et al.*, *German Patent*, 2,329,486 (1973)

ANTIBIOTIC B-41-A$_4$
C$_{32}$H$_{48}$O$_7$

This antibiotic has been shown to be a higher homologue of the preceding compound. It is separated from the associated antibiotics by chromatographic techniques.

Aoki *et al.*, *German Patent*, 2,329,486 (1973)

ANTIBIOTIC B-41-B$_1$
A further component of the antibiotic mixture B-41- elaborated by *Streptomyces* strain B-41-146, the structure of this compound is not yet known.

Aoki *et al.*, *German Patent*, 2,329,486 (1973)

ANTIBIOTIC B-41-B$_2$
C$_{32}$H$_{48}$O$_7$

The structure of this antibiotic from B-41- has been shown to be a dihydro derivative of antibiotic B-41-A$_1$.

Aoik et al., German Patent, 2,329,486 (1973)

ANTIBIOTIC B-41-B$_3$
C$_{33}$H$_{50}$O$_7$

Also separated from the original antibiotic mixture from *Streptomyces* strain B-41-146, this component has the structure given above which is based upon chemical and spectroscopic evidence.

Aoki et al., German Patent, 2,329,486 (1973)

ANTIBIOTIC B-41-C$_1$
C$_{36}$H$_{47}$O$_9$N

This antibiotic and the following compound, isolated from B-41, have structures similar to those of the preceding antibiotics but contain nitrogen in the form of a 2-pyrrolylcarbonyloxymethyl group.

Aoki et al., German Patent, 2,329,486 (1973)

ANTIBIOTIC B-41-C$_2$
C$_{37}$H$_{49}$O$_9$N

The structure of this antibiotic is identical with that of the preceding compound but with an ethyl group in place of one of the methyl substituents.

Aoki et al., German Patent, 2,329,486 (1973)

ANTIBIOTIC B-43

This substance is a peptide antibiotic complex which had been obtained from cultures of *Bacillus circulans*. It has been shown to contain aspartic acid, isoleucine, leucine, phenylalanine, valine and 2,4-diaminobutyric acid. The available evidence indicates that it is related to the antibiotic complex 4205 polypetin but differs from these in the presence of aspartic acid in the molecule. It is effective against both gram-positive and gram-negative bacteria.

Shoji et al., *J. Antibiotics* (Japan), **29**, 813 (1976)

ANTIBIOTIC B-2847-αH
M.p. Indefinite
One of a number of antibiotics isolated from cultures of *Streptomyces tolypophorus* (IFO 13146). The antibiotic is isolated by adsorption on a weak acidic cation exchange resin when it forms an orange amorphous powder. The compound is effective against *Staphylococcus albus*, *Staph. aureus* and acid-fast bacteria.

Hasegawa et al., *Japanese Patent*, 7,329,154 (1973)

ANTIBIOTIC B-2847-αL
A further antibiotic isolated from a culture of *Streptomyces tolypophorus* (IFO 13146). The compound is produced by incubation at 28°C for 3 days at pH 7·0 and extracted from the filtrate with a number of organic solvents including BuOH, CHCl$_3$, AcOEt and (CH$_3$)$_2$CO. So far, the antibiotic has been obtained as a raw powder which is active against gram-positive bacteria and acid-fast organisms.

Hasegawa, Iwasaki, Shibata, *Japanese Patent*, 7,329,153 (1973)

ANTIBIOTIC B-2847-R
C$_{43}$H$_{56}$O$_{14}$N$_2$
M.p. >300°C (*dec.*)
Isolated from *Streptomyces tolypophorus*, this antibiotic crystallizes from C$_6$H$_6$ as orange–red crystals which begin to decompose when heated above 300°C. It has the following specific rotations: $[\alpha]_D^{22}$ + 345° (CHCl$_3$) and $[\alpha]_D^{20}$ + 242° (EtOH). It has been found to be active against gram-positive and acid-fast bacteria.

Shibata et al., *Japanese Patent*, 7,025,275 (1970)

ANTIBIOTIC B-2847y
C$_{43}$H$_{54}$O$_{14}$N$_2$
M.p. 120–5°C (*dec.*)
An antibiotic isolated from cultures of *Streptomyces tolypophorus*, this substance crystallizes as yellow needles from EtOH. It is dextrorotatory with a specific rotation of $[\alpha]_D^{22}$ + 325° (c 1·0, EtOH). The ultraviolet spectrum in EtOH exhibits absorption maxima at 232, 290 and 337 nm. The antibiotic is active against a number of gram-positive bacteria.

Shibata et al., *Japanese Patent*, 7,014,877 (1970)

ANTIBIOTIC B-5050-A
C$_{42}$H$_{67}$O$_{15}$N

Certain strains of *Streptomyces hygroscopicus*, e.g. *S. hygroscopicus* ATCC 21,582, B-5050-RV-124 and B-5050-RL-318 produce an antibiotic complex consisting of at least six components when cultured on a medium containing glucose, corn steep liquor, meat extract and inorganic salts at 28°C for 2 days. The antibiotics are isolated by extraction of the culture filtrate with organic solvents and separated by chromatographic techniques. All are macrocyclic compounds having very similar structures and are active against gram-positive and gram-negative bacteria, particularly *Bacillus cereus*, *B. subtilis* and *Staphylococcus aureus*. This compound, and the following antibiotics, have so far been isolated in states of reasonably purity.

Higashide et al., *German Patent*, 2,039,990 (1971)
Kishi et al., *German Patent*, 2,132, 445 (1972)
Kishi et al., *Japanese Patent*, 7,349,990 (1973)
Suzuki, Miyakawa, Uchida, *Japanese Patent*, 7,564,495 (1975)

ANTIBIOTIC B-5050-B
C$_{41}$H$_{65}$O$_{15}$N
M.p. Indefinite

This component of the antibiotic B-5050 complex produced by certain strains of *Streptomyces hygroscopicus* has the structure given above. It has been obtained as a white amorphous powder with no definite melting point. Its antibiotic activity is similar to that of the preceding compound.

Higashide *et al.*, *German Patent*, 2,039,990 (1971)
Kishi *et al.*, *German Patent*, 2,132,445 (1972)
Kishi *et al.*, *Japanese Patent*, 7,349,990 (1973)
Suzuki *et al.*, *Japanese Patent*, 7,535,391 (1975)

ANTIBIOTIC B-5050-C
$C_{40}H_{63}O_{15}N$
M.p. Indefinite

A further antibiotic isolated from the complex B-5050 elaborated by a number of *Streptocymes hygroscopicus* strains, this antibiotic is also active against gram-positive and some gram-negative bacteria.

Higashide *et al.*, *German Patent*, 2,039,990 (1971)
Kishi *et al.*, *German Patent*, 2,132,445 (1972)
Kishi *et al.*, *Japanese Patent*, 7,349,990 (1973)
Suzuki, Miyakawa, Uchida, *Japanese Patent*, 7,564,496 (1975)

ANTIBIOTIC B-5050-D
$C_{39}H_{61}O_{15}N$

This antibiotic component of the mixture B-5050 has the structure given above. The biological activity is similar to that of the accompanying antibiotics.

Higashide *et al.*, *German Patent*, 2,039,990 (1971)
Kishi *et al.*, *German Patent*, 2,132,445 (1972)
Kishi *et al.*, *Japanese Patent*, 7,349,990 (1973)

ANTIBIOTIC B-5050-E
$C_{39}H_{61}O_{15}N$
M.p. Indefinite

Another macrocyclic antibiotic isolated from the culture filtrate of species of *Streptocymes hygroscopius*, this compound is a positional isomer of the preceding substance. The structure has been determined by chemical and spectroscopic data.

Higashide *et al.*, *German Patent*, 2,039,990 (1971)
Kishi *et al.*, *German Patent*, 2,132,445 (1972)
Kishi *et al.*, *Japanese Patent*, 7,349,990 (1973)

ANTIBIOTIC B-5050-F
$C_{38}H_{59}O_{15}N$
M.p. Indefinite

Also present in the antibiotic complex B-5050 elaborated by *Streptomyces hygroscopius* strains, this macrolide substance forms a white amorphus powder and is active in inhibiting the growth of gram-positive and gram-negative bacteria.

Higashide *et al.*, *German Patent*, 2,039,990 (1971)
Kishi *et al.*, *German Patent*, 2,132,445 (1972)
Kishi *et al.*, *Japanese Patent*, 7,349,990 (1973)

ANTIBIOTIC B-14437
$C_{12}H_{15}O_5N_5$
M.p. 248–250°C

From cultures of *Streptomyces purpureofuscus*, Japanese workers have isolated this antibiotic which forms colourless crystals of the monohydrate when crystallized from aqueous $(CH_3)_2CO$. It is laevorotatory with a specific rotation of $[\alpha]_D^{26} - 53°$ (dimethylformamide). It is active against a range of gram-positive bacteria.

Shibata *et al.*, *Japanese Patent*, 7,019,638 (1970)

ANTIBIOTIC B-15565-A
M.p. 110–120°C

Streptomyces species B-15565, found in soil from Nepal, elaborates two antibiotics which have a non-polyene structure similar to endomycin (q.v.). This compound forms colourless crystals and is dextrorotatory with a specific rotation of $[\alpha]_D^{23} + 21·0°$ (c 1·0, CH_3OH). It is a broad spectrum antibiotic active against a range of gram-positive bacteria, yeasts and both saprophytic and phytopathogenic fungi.

Iwasa *et al.*, *Ann. Rep. Takeda Res. Lab.*, **27**, 74 (1968)

ANTIBIOTIC B-15565-B
M.p. 130–140° C

A further crystalline antibiotic of the non-polyene class isolated from cultures of *Streptocymes* strain B-15565, this compound is also dextrorotatory with $[\alpha]_D^{23} + 30·0°$ (c 1·0, CH_3OH). It has a similar antibiotic spectrum to that of the preceding compound.

Iwasa *et al.*, *Ann. Rep. Takeda Res. Lab.*, **27**, 74 (1968)
Iwasa *et al.*, *Japanese Patent*, 7,031,358 (1970)

ANTIBIOTIC B-15645
$C_{11}H_{13}O_5N_3$
M.p. 175–180° C

This antibiotic is produced by *Streptomyces griseolus*. It forms colourless needles when crystallized from EtOH and has a specific rotation of $[\alpha]_D^{21} - 47°$. It inhibits the growth of gram-positive bacteria.

Yamamoto *et al.*, *Japanese Patent*, 7,020,559 (1970)

ANTIBIOTIC B-21085
M.p. 255–260°C

Streptomyces collinus var. *albescens* produces this antibiotic which forms yellow crystals when purified by recrystallization from EtOH. It is laevorotatory having a specific rotation of $[\alpha]_D^{23} - 217°$ (c 0·5, $(CH_3)_2SO$).

Higashide *et al.*, *Japanese Patent*, 7,100,271 (1971)

ANTIBIOTIC B-28963
Decomp. 250–255°C

A white amorphous powder, this antibiotic has been obtained from cultures of *Streptomyces* species FERM-P 1714. It is soluble in H_2O and insoluble in organic solvents, gives positive ninhydrin and Grieg–Leabach reactions but a negative Sakaguchi test. It is effective against antibiotic-resistant *Micrococcus* species and has a low toxicity with LD_{50} of >400 mg/kg in mice when administered intravenously.

Higashide *et al.*, *Japanese Patent*, 74 80,294 (1974)

ANTIBIOTIC B-58941
$C_{37}H_{59}O_{12}N$
M.p. 229°C

A100

A macrocyclic antibiotic elaborated by a strain of *Streptomyces fradiae*, this compound forms colourless crystals from EtOH and is laevorotatory with a specific rotation of $[\alpha]_D^{22} - 88 \cdot 4°$ (c 1·0, $CHCl_3$). The ultraviolet spectrum in EtOH consists of a single absorption maximum at 240 nm.

Suzuki, *Bull. Chem. Soc., Japan*, **43**, 292 (1970)

ANTIBIOTIC BA-180265-A
See Kanchanomycin

ANTIBIOTIC BB-K8
See Amikacin

ANTIBIOTIC BD-12
$C_{19}H_{35}O_{12}N_7$

An antibiotic isolated from various species of *Streptomyces*, this compound is produced mainly by *S. luteocolor*. It is characterized as the crystalline dihydrochloride with m.p. 200·5–201·5°C; $[\alpha]_D^{25} - 75°$ (c 1·0, H_2O) and the picrate, pale yellow needles, m.p. 160–165·5°C (*dec.*).

Ito *et al.*, *Japanese Patent*, 7,009,837 (1970)

ANTIBIOTIC BH-890α
Streptomyces misionensis yields a mixture of two closely related antibiotics when grown aerobically on a medium containing starch, corn steep liquor, corn flour, casein, cottonseed flour and inorganic salts, incubated at 28°C for 3 days. This particular component is obtained by dissolving the crude mixture in dimethylformamide, precipitating with AcOEt and recrystallizing from AcOEt. Antibiotic BH-890 is an effective antifungal agent, active against *Candida albicans*, *Cryptococcus neoformans* and *Microsporum audouini*.

Martin, *German Patent*, 2,021,436 (1971)

ANTIBIOTIC BH-890β
This component of the antibiotic mixture isolated from cultures of *Streptomyces misionensis* is separated from the preceding antibiotic and purified by countercurrent distribution. It is active against *Candida albicans*, *Cryptococcus neoformans* and *Microsporum audouini*. The minimum inhibition concentration against *C. neoformans* E 138 is given as 2 µg/ml.

Martin, *German Patent*, 2,021,436 (1971)

ANTIBIOTIC BK-217α
This antibiotic is one of three produced by culturing *Streptoverticillium cinnamoneus* strain NRRI 3594 aerobically on a nutrient medium at 28°C for 3 days. The compound is isolated by washing the mycelium with $CHCl_3$, extracting with CH_3OH, centrifuging and suspending the material in $(CH_3)_2CO$. The antibiotic is purified by extracting with *iso*PrOH, evaporating the solvent *in vacuo*, dissolving the residue in EtOH, chromatographing on an alumina column and eluting with EtOH. Antibiotic BK-217α is active against *Cryptococcus neoformans* and *Trichophyton tonsurans*.

Shu, Barbatschi, *German Patent*, 2,021,434 (1971)

ANTIBIOTIC BK-217β
This antibiotic is produced by *Streptoverticillium cinnamoneus* strain NRRL 3594 by the same method as described for the preceding compound. It is isolated by extraction of the crude suspension in $(CH_3)_2CO$ with CH_3OH and precipitation with Et_2O. The crude antibiotic thus obtained is purified in the same manner as antibiotic BK-217α. This compound is highly active against fungi, particularly *Cryptococcus neoformans* and *Trichophyton tonsurans*. The minimum inhibition concentration against the

former organism is 0·5 µg/ml. The LD_{50} in mice is approximately 100 mg/kg when administered subcutaneously.

Shu, Barbatschi, *German Patent*, 2,021,434 (1971)
Shu, Barbatschi, *S. African Patent*, 7,002,463 (1971)

ANTIBIOTIC BK-217γ

A third antifungal antibiotic isolated from cultures of *Streptoverticillium cinnamoneus* strain NRRL 3594. The crude antibiotic is isolated from the $(CH_3)_2CO$ suspension by drying the residue. It is purified by extraction with *iso*PrOH, evaporation of the solvent *in vacuo*, dissolving in EtOH, passing through an alumina column and elution with EtOH. It is also highly active against *Cryptococcus neoformans* and *Trichophyton tonsurans*, the minimum inhibition concentration against *C. neoformans* being 0·5 µg/ml.

Shu, Barbatschi, *German Patent*, 2,021,434 (1971)
Shu, Barbatschi, *S. African Patent*, 7,002,463 (1971)

ANTIBIOTIC BL-S217
$C_{18}H_{20}O_6N_3S_2$

A semi-synthetic antibiotic of the cephalosporin class, this compound has the structure given above. It possesses a high *in vitro* activity against gram-negative bacteria and gram-positive cocci, including strains of *Staphylococcus aureus* which are resistant to penicillin G. The antibiotic inhibits 77 per cent of *Escherichia coli* isolates, 83 per cent of *Klebsiella* isolates and 67 per cent of *Proteus mirabilis* at a concentration of 12·5 µg/ml.

Casey, Bodey, *J. Antibiotics* (Japan), **27**, 520 (1974)

ANTIBIOTIC BL-580α

One of two closely related antibiotics obtained from the culture broth of *Streptomyces hygroscopicus*. The filtered broth is extracted with AcOEt and evaporated to give an oily residue which is then passed through a silica gel column in CH_2Cl_2 and eluted with a mixture of CH_2Cl_2 and AcOEt and then chromatogrammed on a diatomaceous earth partition column using a mixture of AcOEt, CH_3OH, hexane and H_2O. This particular compound is the first to elute and is purified by countercurrent distribution. It forms an amorphous powder which is dextrorotatory with a specific rotation of $[\alpha]_D^{25} + 15\cdot6°$ (c 1·08, CH_3OH). The antibiotic is active against gram-positive bacteria.

Martin, Kantor, *U.S. Patent*, 3,812,249 (1974)

ANTIBIOTIC BL-580β

This antibiotic accompanies the preceding substance in the culture broth of *Streptomyces hygroscopicus*. It is obtained in a similar manner but has a higher R_f value and is also purified by countercurrent distribution. Like the related antibiotic, it forms an amorphous powder with no definite melting point.

Martin, Kantor, *U.S. Patent*, 3,812,249 (1974)

ANTIBIOTIC BL-617

M.p. Indefinite

When cultivated under submerged aerobic conditions in a medium containing common carbon and nitrogen sources and inorganic salts at 25–9°C for 40–96 hours, *Streptomyces luteoverticillatus* IFO 3840 yields this antibiotic which is isolated by extraction of the filtrate with an organic solvent followed by countercurrent distribution. It is dextrorotatory with $[\alpha]_D^{25} + 169°$ (c 0·2, dimethylformamide). The antibiotic is active against a number of gram-positive bacteria and also inhibits the growth of a range of pathogenic fungi.

Kunstmann, Williamson, Porter, *U.S. Patent*, 3,728,488 (1973)

ANTIBIOTIC BLP-1654
$C_{18}H_{22}O_5N_6S$

A synthetic antibiotic, this substance is active against gram-positive bacteria and particularly against *Pseudomonas* species. Tube dilution studies show large discrepancies between the inhibitory and bactericidal concentrations of this antibiotic against various species of *Pseudomonas*, and it has been shown that these are due to the presence of small numbers of resistant cells covering a wide range of concentrations. Such resistant cells can only be detected by susceptible subculturing methods. The kinetics of the bactericidal effect are characteristic of the penicillins with killing of the bacteria initiating simultaneously with growth.

Sanders, Sanders, *Antimicrobial Agents & Chemotherapy*, **7**, 435 (1975)

ANTIBIOTIC BL-S786
$C_{21}H_{22}N_6O_6S_2$

A semi-synthetic cephalosporin, this antibiotic has the structure shown above. It possesses a broader antibiotic spectrum than cephalothin and has significantly lower inhibition concentrations against members of the Enterobacteriaceae.

Jones *et al.*, *J. Antibiotics* (Japan), **30**, 576 (1977)

ANTIBIOTIC BM-123
Nocardia species NRRL 5646 yields a complex of antibiotics from which antibiotics BM 123α, BM 123β and BM 123γ have been isolated. The proportions of these components produced is dependent upon the particular culture medium used. All three compounds, and the mixture, are active against a range of gram-positive and gram-negative bacteria.

Martin, Tresner, Porter, *German Patent*, 2,351,344 (1974)

ANTIBIOTIC BN-7
Dec. 237–240°C
A polypeptide antibiotic produced by *Bacillus circulans* BN-7 (FERM-P 1154), this compound is isolated as the sulphate which, when purified by gel filtration with Sephadex LH-20, forms colourless needles. The antibiotic is soluble in CH_3OH and AcOH, slightly soluble in $(CH_3)_2CO$ and C_6H_6 and insoluble in AcOEt, Et_2O and $CHCl_3$. It gives positive ninhydrin and biuret reactions and negative Benedict and $FeCl_3$ reactions. Hydrolysis shows that it contains the aminoacids α,γ-diaminobutyric acid, isoleucine leucine, phenylalanine, threonine and valine together with an unidentified organic acid. It is active against gram-positive and gram-negative bacteria and fungi. The LD_{50} for mice is approximately 10 mg/kg when given intraperitoneally.

Ezaki *et al.*, *Japanese Patent*, 7,356,895 (1973)

ANTIBIOTIC BN-103
Isolated from cultures of *Bacillus pumilis* BN-103, this antibiotic is obtained from the culture filtrate by extraction with AcOEt. It is active against gram-positive bacteria.

Miyado *et al.*, *Japanese Patents*, 7,569,295–6 (1975)

ANTIBIOTIC BN-130
Pseudomonas stutzeri strain BN-130 yields this antibiotic which is a colourless oil having a specific rotation of $[\alpha]_D^{25} - 19 \cdot 2°$ and giving an ultraviolet spectrum in ethanolic solution having two absorption maxima at 227 and 233 nm. It has been characterized as the methyl ester which forms colourless crystals with m.p. 86°C. The antibiotic is active against a wide range of gram-positive and gram-negative bacteria.

Ezaki *et al.*, *German Patent*, 2,516,615 (1975)

ANTIBIOTIC BN-175
A species of *Bacillus*, BN-175 (FERM-P 3145) elaborates this antibiotic when cultured with agitation at 28°C for 20 days on a medium containing glucose, peptone, soybean flour and NaCl. The crude material has been purified by column chromatography. The antibiotic is a basic colourless powder which is soluble in H_2O but insoluble in $CHCl_3$, Me_2CO and AcOEt. Acid hydrolysis furnishes glycine and two unidentified aminoacids. The antibiotic is effective against gram-positive bacteria and *Candida*. The LD_{50} in mice has been reported as greater than 30 mg/kg when administered intravenously.

Ezaki *et al.*, *Japanese Patent*, 77, 18,894 (1977)

ANTIBIOTIC BN-183
Decomp. 213°C
A white basic powder, this antibiotic is produced by *Pseudomonas* strain

BN-183 (FERM-P 3332). It is laevorotatory having a specific rotation of $[\alpha]_D - 35 \cdot 8°$. The organism is cultured with agitation on a medium of glucose and powdered bouillon at 28°C for 3 days and the antibiotic adsorbed from the culture filtrate onto activated carbon, eluted with 70 per cent Me_2CO at pH 2·0, the eluated concentrated *in vacuo* and the product column chromatographed. Antibiotic BN-183 is soluble in H_2O and MeOH but insoluble in AcOEt, $CHCl_3$ and Me_2CO. It is active against gram-positive and gram-negative bacteria.

Ito *et al.*, *Japanese Patent*, 77,105,292 (1977)

ANTIBIOTIC BT-3-3
See Thermorubin A

ANTIBIOTIC BU-1709-E$_1$
$C_{21}H_{40}O_{13}N_4$
M.p. Indefinite

One of a number of antibiotic that have been isolated from cultures of *Bacillus circulans*, this compound is similar to the butirosins (q.v.). It forms an amorphous powder with no definite melting point and is dextrorotatory with $[\alpha]_D + 28°$ (c 1·47, H_2O). It has a similar activity against gram-positive bacteria as the butirosins, but not as pronounced.

Tsukiura *et al.*, *J. Antibiotics* (Japan), **26**, 386 (1973)

ANTIBIOTIC BU-1709-E$_2$
$C_{21}H_{40}O_{13}N_4$
M.p. Indefinite

This antibiotic is a stereoisomer of the preceding compound and has also been isolated from cultures of *Bacillus circulans*. It, too, forms an amorphous white powder and has a specific rotation of $[\alpha]_D + 33°$ (c 1·3, H_2O). Its antibacterial activity is very like that of antibiotic BU-1709-E$_1$.

Tsukiura *et al.*, *J. Antibiotics* (Japan), **26**, 386 (1973)

ANTIBIOTIC BU-1880
M.p. 239–242°C

One of a number of antibiotics produced by *Bacillus circulans*, this compound is produced by *B. circulans* strain BU-1880 (ATCC 21,828). It has been obtained by culturing the organism aerobically at 28°C and pH 8·0–8·5 for 2–3 days on a common nutrient medium and extracting the medium with BuOH followed by chromatography. Antibiotic BU-1880 is a basic peptide containing phenylalanine, leucine, α,γ-diaminobutyric acid and 8-methyldecanoic acid in molar ratios of 1:2:5:1. It is soluble in dilute mineral acids, H_2O, the lower alcohols and dioxan but insoluble in AcOEt and Me_2CO. Tests have shown it to be more effective than colistin against gram-positive bacteria but less so against gram-negative organisms. The LD_{50} in mice are 37 mg/kg when given intravenously and 300 mg/kg when administered intramuscularly.

Kawaguchi *et al.*, *Japanese Patent*, 74 85,295 (1974)

ANTIBIOTIC BU-1975-A$_1$
This antibiotic, isolated from cultures of *Bacillus circulans croceus*, *B. biotinicus* and *B. proteophilus* is identical with ambutyrosin A.

Hiroshi *et al.*, *Japanese Patent*, 74 66,981 (1974)

ANTIBIOTIC BU-1975-A$_2$

This antibiotic, isolated with the preceding compound is identical with ambutyrosin B.

Hiroshi *et al.*, *Japanese Patent*, 74 66,981 (1974)

ANTIBIOTIC BU-1975-C$_1$
$C_{21}H_{41}O_{11}N_5$

The antibiotic complex BU-1975 is produced by various strains of *Bacillus circulans*, e.g. *B. circulans* var. *biotinicus*, *B. circulans* var. *croceus* and *B. circulans proteophilus* when grown aerobically on nutrient media. The culture filtrate is then passed through an alumina column when the two components of the mixture can be separated. The antibiotic inhibits the growth of both *Escherichia coli* and *Klebsiella pneumoniae*. It has found some use clinically for preoperative sterilization of the intestines.

Kawaguchi *et al.*, *German Patent*, 2,346,243 (1974)

ANTIBIOTIC BU-1975-C$_2$
$C_{21}H_{41}O_{11}N_5$

This component of the antibiotic complex BU-1975 is a stereoisomer of the preceding compound. It also inhibits *Escherichia coli* and *Klebsiella pneumoniae*.

Kawaguchi *et al.*, *German Patent*, 2,346,243 (1974)

ANTIBIOTIC C20-12
$C_{47}H_{82}O_{15}$

Produced by *Streptomyces* species C20-12 (FERM-P 2736), this antibiotic is formed when the organism is cultured aerobically at 30°C for 90 hours on a medium consisting of glycerol, sucrose, soybean powder, yeast and $CaCO_3$. It has been isolated in the pure state as the sodium salt which forms colourless needles when crystallized from H_2O, decomposing at 184–189°C and having a specific rotation of $[\alpha]_D$ + 22·6°. Both the antibiotic and the sodium salt are effective against gram-positive bacteria.

Seino *et al.*, *Japanese Patent*, 76 91,396 (1976)

ANTIBIOTIC C-43-219
$C_{19}H_{28}N_4O_8S_2$
Decomp. 155–165°C

Cephalosporium acremonium strain C-43-219 (FERM-P 2826) elaborates this antibiotic when cultured at 24°C for 190 hours in a sucrose-corn steep liquor medium, containing cottonseed oil, soybean powder, DL-methionine and $CaCO_3$. It has been separated and purified by chromatography on ion-exchange resin columns. Antibiotic C-43-129 forms an amorphous white powder and is active against gram-positive organisms.

Kanzaki *et al.*, *Japanese Patent*, 76 76,488 (1976)

ANTIBIOTIC C-1051
$C_8H_{19}O_5N_3 \cdot 2HCl$
M.p. Indefinite

Streptomyces akayamaensis Furukawa produces this antibiotic which is obtained from the culture filtrate by adsorbing the activity on a strong acid cation exchange resin and eluting with strong acids, e.g. $2N$-HCl or HNO_3. The eluate is concentrated *in vacuo*, CH_3OH added and the solution filtered, followed by precipitation with $(CH_3)_2CO$. Purification is carried out by chromatography followed by crystallization from CH_3OH. Antibiotic C-1051 forms a colourless, amorphous powder which is basic in nature. It is freely soluble in H_2O and CH_3OH, moderately so in EtOH, slightly soluble in $(CH_3)_2CO$ and insoluble in Et_2O, C_6O_6, $CHCl_3$, AcOEt and hexane. The substance is stable in neutral or acid solutions, but unstable under alkaline conditions. It is thermostable, being unchanged by heating at 100°C for 10 minutes. Antibiotic C-1051 is active against parasitic ticks and plant diseases caused by *Botrytis*, *Sclerotina* and plant viruses.

Sasaki *et al.*, *Japanese Patent*, 7,373,395 (1973)

ANTIBIOTIC C-2801X
$C_{24}H_{27}N_3O_{11}$

Cultures of *Streptomyces heteromorphus* and *S. panayensis* yield this antibiotic in addition to cephamycins A and B. It has been separated from the latter by column chromatography on Amberlite XAD-2 and obtained in the pure form as the monosodium salt. It is active against gram-positive and gram-negative bacteria including those insensitive to cephamycins A and B.

Fukase *et al.*, *J. Antibiotics* (Japan), **29**, 113 (1976)

ANTIBIOTIC C-2554 A-I
$C_8H_{10}O_5$

A component of the antibiotic C-2554 complex produced by culturing *Streptomyces lavenduligriseus* strain C-2554 on a common nutrient medium, this substance has the structure given above which has been elucidated from chemical and spectroscopic evidence. It is active against *Klebsiella pneumoniae*, *Proteus vulgaris* and *Staphylococcus aureus*. A dose of 200 mg/kg given intraperitoneally or intravenously to mice did not prove lethal.

Hatano *et al.*, *Japanese Patent*, 75 70,597 (1975)

ANTIBIOTIC C-2554 A-II
$C_8H_{10}O_5$

A positional isomer of the preceding antibiotic, this constituent of the C-2554 complex has the structure given above which has been established from chemical and spectroscopic data. The antibiotic spectrum and toxicity is virtually identical to that for antibiotic C-2554 A-I.

Hatano *et al.*, *Japanese Patent*, 75 70,597 (1975)

ANTIBIOTIC C-2554 B
$C_6H_8O_4$

The simplest of the three antibiotics isolated by silica gel chromatography of the C-2554 complex, this compound has been assigned the structure given on the basis of chemical analysis and a study of the infrared, NMR and mass spectra.

Hatano *et al.*, *Japanese Patent*, 75 70,597 (1975)

ANTIBIOTIC C-7819B

Streptomyces parvullus C-7819 yields this antibiotic when cultured aerobically in a medium containing glucose, peptone and soybean flour at 28°C for 140 hours. It is particularly effective in controlling *Eimeria tenella*.

Imada *et al.*, *Japanese Patent*, **77** 83,801 (1977)

ANTIBIOTIC C-9154
$C_{12}H_{12}N_2O_3$

This antibiotic has been described by Japanese workers and has the structure shown above. It possesses both antibacterial and antifungal activity. The structure has been elucidated from chemical and spectroscopic evidence.

Hasegawa *et al.*, *J. Antibiotics* (Japan), **28**, 713 (1975)

ANTIBIOTIC CGP 9000
$C_{16}H_{19}O_5N_3S$

A semi-synthetic antibiotic, this substance possesses an antibacterial action *in vitro* similar to that of cephalexin (q.v.) but it has a superior bacterial efficacy. When administered orally to mice infected with a range of bacteria it has been shown to be between two and seven times more effective than either cephalexin or cephadrine. As an orally active broad-spectrum cephalosporin antibiotic CGP 9000 exhibits a number of advantages over these two antibiotics.

Zak *et al.*, *J. Antibiotics* (Japan), **29**, 653 (1976)

ANTIBIOTIC CP-21,635
$C_{36}H_{45}O_9N_9S$
M.p. Indefinite

A complex antibiotic derived from *Streptomyces olivaceus*, this substance is prepared by aerobic fermentation of the organism in a medium containing corn starch, soybean flour, cerelose, distillers solubles, sodium chloride and calcium carbonate at 28°C for 3 days. The antibiotic is purified by gel filtration followed by chromatography on a Sephadex LH-20 column, elution with CH_3OH, further chromatography on alumina and a final elution with AcOEt. Antibiotic CP-21,635 has a minimum inhibition concentration against *Staphylococcus aureus* of 12·5 μg/ml.

Sciavalino *et al.*, *German Patent*, 2,138,588 (1972)

ANTIBIOTIC CP 35587
$C_{15}H_{18}N_6O_3S$

A semi-synthetic antibiotic, this substance has the above structure and is a broad spectrum antibiotic active against a wide range of gram-positive cocci except penicillin G-resistant *Staphylococcus aureus*. It also inhibits a number of gram-negative bacteria. Tests have shown that it is more active against *Klebsiella* than the other penicillins examined.

Bodley, Weaver, Pan., *J. Antibiotics* (Japan), **30**, 724 (1977)

ANTIBIOTIC CS-1170
$C_{15}H_{19}N_7O_5S_3$

A semi-synthetic antibiotic, this substance has the structure of 7α-methoxy-cephalosporin. It has been shown to possess enhanced activity against gram-positive and gram-negative bacteria compared with cefoxitin and cephalothrin.

Nakao et al., *J. Antibiotics* (Japan), **29**, 554 (1976)

ANTIBIOTIC CYL-2
$C_{32}H_{46}O_7N_4$

A unique cyclotetrapeptide antibiotic, this substance has been obtained from cultures of *Cylindrocladium scoparium*. The structure given above has been determined by mass spectrometry. It is active against a range of bacteria.

Hirota et al., *Agr. Biol. Chem.*, **37**, 955 (1973)

ANTIBIOTIC DB-2073
$C_{15}H_{24}O_2$
M.p. 86–88°C

An organism freshly obtained from soil, *Pseudomonas* strain B-9004, gives this antibiotic when cultivated in a common medium at 30°C for 90 hours. The substance is isolated by extracting the cells with CH_3OH at pH 2·0, re-extracting with $CHCl_3$ and chromatographing on an alumina column. Antibiotic DB-2073 forms colourless crystals. It is active against *Diplococcus pneumoniae* and *Trichophyton gypseum* and is comparatively non-toxic, mice tolerating an intraperitoneal dose up to 800 mg/kg.

Kanda, Ishizaki, Inoue, *Japanese Patent*, 7,305,995 (1973)

Kanda et al., *J. Antibiotics* (Japan), **28**, 935 (1975)
Kitahara, Kanda, *ibid.*, **28**, 943 (1975)

ANTIBIOTIC DE-3936
$C_{44}H_{76}O_{14}$
M.p. (sodium salt) 173–176°C

Cultures of Streptomyces hygroscopicus 9375-1 (FERM-P 3159) yield this polyether antibiotic which has been obtained by extraction of the wet cells with MeOH, concentrating the extract, and re-extracting with C_6H_6, concentrating the C_6H_6 extract to give an oil. Purification has been carried out by alumina, Sephadex LH-20 and silica gel chromatography and crystallization from C_6H_6-petroleum ether. The antibiotic is soluble in the lower alcohols, esters, $CHCl_3$, CCl_4, C_6H_6, Et_2O, hexane, cyclohexane and petroleum ether and insoluble in H_2O. It is effective against gram-positive bacteria, *Erwinia carotovora*, plasmodia and pathogenic protozoa such as *Eimeria* and *Toxoplasma*. The LD_{50} in mice is 13·0 mg/kg given intraperitoneally.

Ooshima et al., *Japanese Patent*, 77 12,990 (1977)
Ooshima et al., *ibid.*, 77 12,915 (1977)

ANTIBIOTIC E-212
See Toyocamycin

ANTIBIOTIC E-749-C
See Antibiotic LL-AC541

ANTIBIOTIC EM-2
$C_{91}H_{146}O_{26}N_{18}$
M.p. 261–264°C

A polypeptide antibiotic, this complex substance is obtained from cultures of *Emericelliopsis microspora* 333 NRRL 5648 grown in the presence of

4(R)-propyl-L-proline, the latter being added to the culture liquor 24 hours after the fermentation process begins. The culture is incubated at 28°C and pH 7·2 for 6 days. After filtration, the culture liquor is chromatographed on silica gel which affords separation of the three individual components of the initial mixture.

Argoudelis, Johnson, *German Patent*, 2,352,693 (1974)

ANTIBIOTIC EM-3
$C_{68}H_{109}O_{19}N_{13}$
M.p. 256–259°C
A second complex polypeptide antibiotic isolated from cultures of *Emericelliopsis microspora* 333 NRRL 5648 to which 4(R)-propyl-L-proline has been added. The antibiotic is separated from the accompanying components by chromatography on a silica gel column.

Argoudelis, Johnson, *German Patent*, 2,352,693 (1974)

ANTIBIOTIC EM-4
$C_{81}H_{127}O_{22}N_{17}$
M.p. 239·8°C
This crystalline polypeptide antibiotic is a third component of the mixture isolated from the culture filtrate of *Emericelliopsis microspora* 333 NRRL 5648. Like the two preceding antibiotics, this substance has bactericidal and protozoacidal activity.

Argoudelis, Johnson, *German Patent*, 2,352,693 (1974)

ANTIBIOTIC EM-49
M.p. 263–5°C
This complex polypeptide antibiotic obtained from *Bacillus circulans* ATCC 21,656 has been shown to consist of three structurally related components which differ only in the nature of the amido side chain. The complex is prepared by the aerobic fermentation of a nutrient medium at 37°C and is separated and purified by countercurrent distribution. The structure has been determined by Edman degradation studies and deacylation. It is a very hygroscopic material and forms a crystalline hydrochloride, m.p. 180–207°C (*dec*.) and a tetraamidino derivative which, like the parent antibiotic, is active against a number of bacteria, fungi and protozoa.

Meyers *et al.*, *J. Antibiotics* (Japan), **26**, 444 (1973)
Parker, Rathnum, *ibid.*, **26**, 449 (1973)
Parker, Meyers, *German Patent*, 2,357,858 (1974

Structure
Parker, Rathnum, *J. Antibiotics* (Japan), **28**, 379 (1975)

ANTIBIOTIC EM-98
An antibiotic derived from *Streptomyces venezuelae*, this compound is obtained by fermentation on a common medium and has been characterized as the crystalline hydrochloride and picrate. Antibiotic EM-98 has bactericidal activity and has been examined *in vivo*, giving complete protection to mice against *Escherichia coli* infections when a dose of 250 mg/kg is administered subcutaneously 1 hour after intraperitoneal infection with 500 LD_{50} doses of *Escherichia coli*.

Meyers, Slusarchyk, Liu, *German Patent*, 2,316,893 (1973)

ANTIBIOTIC F-1028
$C_8H_{17}O_4N_3$
M.p. Indefinite

Streptomyces kagawaensis, freshly isolated from soil, elaborates this cyclic antibiotic when cultivated aerobically on a medium containing glucose, peptone, yeast extract, meat extract and inorganic salts at 27°C for 2 days. The culture filtrate is treated with Amberlite IRC-50 and eluted with dilute HCl, the eluate evaporated, treated with $(CH_3)_2CO$ and the residue chromatographed on activated carbon to yield colourless crystals of the hydrochloride. The antibiotic and its hydrochloride are active against *Botrytis cinerea* and *Sclerotinia sclerotiorum*. The LD_{50} in mice is 160 mg/kg given intravenously and 750 mg/kg when administered orally.

Hata *et al.*, *Japanese Patent*, 7,310,292 (1973)
Hata *et al.*, *German Patent*, 2,231,979 (1973)

ANTIBIOTIC FA-252-C
M.p. 159–161°C
Streptomyces acropoliensis strain FA-252 (FERM-P 2675) elaborates this antibiotic when cultured at 28°C and pH 7·0 for 72 hours on a culture medium of starch, soybean powder, corn steep liquor and inorganic salts.

The antibiotic is adsorbed from the culture filtrate on ion-exchange resins and purified chromatographically. It forms a white amorphous powder and is effective against gram-positive and gram-negative bacteria and also acidophilic bacteria. It is non-toxic, the LD_{50} in mice being 500–1000 mg/kg when given intraperitoneally.

Ichihashi *et al.*, *Japanese Patent*, 76 35,496 (1976)

ANTIBIOTIC FA-313
M.p. 172–175°C

Isolated from aerobically fermented cultures of *Streptomyces chromovarius* FA-313, this antibiotic forms a weakly basic red powder. It is dextrorotatory with a specific rotation of $[\alpha]_D^{25} + 20°$. The antibiotic has been obtained from both the supernatant liquor and the cells. It is soluble in the lower alcohols, AcOEt, $CHCl_3$, C_6H_6 and Et_2O, insoluble in hexane, petroleum ether and H_2O. Antibiotic FA-313 is active against gram-positive and gram-negative bacteria, acidophilic bacteria, and also has antitumour activity. The LD_{50} in mice is about 1 mg/kg administered intraperitoneally.

Ichihashi *et al.*, *Japanese Patent*, 77,12,992 (1977)

ANTIBIOTIC FL-1060
$C_{15}H_{23}O_3N_3S$

A new β-lactam antibiotic derived from penicillanic acid, this compound has the structure 6β-(hexahydro-1*H*-azepin-1-methyleneamino) penicillanic acid. The antibiotic shows a high activity against ampicillin-sensitive strains of *Escherichia coli*. At low osmolality it is more active than ampicillin against sensitive strains of *E. coli* under conditions which simulate bacterial growth in the urinary bladder. At high osmolality, the two antibiotics have similar activities.

Greenwood *et al.*, *J. Clin. Pathol.*, **27**, 192 (1974)

ANTIBIOTIC FR-O2A
This antibiotic is found in the cells of *Streptomyces lactamdurans* and also extracted from the fermentation liquor by $CHCl_3$ after adjusting the pH to 5·0. The extract is evaporated to dryness, redissolved in petroleum ether and air-dried. The structure is unknown but the compound has a molecular weight of approximately 1000. It shows inhibitory activity against both gram-positive and gram-negative bacteria and is of particular value in the treatment of mycoplasma (PPLO) in cattle, chickens and pigs.

Wax, Maiese, *German Patent*, 2,450,813 (1975)

ANTIBIOTIC Fr-1923
M.p. Indefinite

Nocardia uniformis ATCC 21,806 elaborates this antibiotic substance which is obtained by cultivation in an aqueous medium containing cottonseed flour, glycerol, yeast and inorganic salts at 30°C for 3 days. The culture filtrate is extracted with $CHCl_3$ and chromatographed to yield the crystalline sodium salt. Antibiotic Fr-1923 is amphoteric and freely soluble in alkaline solutions. It is highly active against gram-negative bacteria, the minimum inhibition concentration against *Corynebacterium* diphtheriae PW-8 being 12·5 µg/ml. The LD_{50} in rats is 5100 mg/kg when given subcutaneously.

Aoki *et al.*, *German Patent*, 2,242,699 (1973)

ANTIBIOTIC FR-3383
An antibiotic produced by the aerobic culture of *Streptomyces odainensis* 1271 at 30°C for 72 hours in a medium containing gluten meal, glucose, cottonseed meal and $CaCO_3$. The broth yields the antibiotic on filtration followed by column and thin layer chromatography.

Okuhara., *Japanese Patent*, 77 93,701 (1977)

ANTIBIOTIC FR-29038
$C_{23}H_{28}N_4O_7$

One of a number of structurally similar antibiotics isolated from cultures of *Nocardia uniformis* subsp. *tsuyamanensis* when fermented aerobically at 30°C for 96 hours, this substance has been purified by chromatographic methods. It has been found to be effective against *Bacillus*, *Escherichia*, *Klebsiella*, *Pseudomonas*, *Salmonella* and *Shigella* species.

Hosoda, Aoki, Imanaka, *Japanese Patent*, 77 44,291 (1977)

ANTIBIOTIC FR-29055
$C_{23}H_{25}N_3O_8$

A colourless, crystalline antibiotic isolated, together with the preceding substance from aerobically cultured *Nocardia uniformis* subsp. *tsuyamanensis*, this antibiotic has a similar spectrum of activity to antibiotic FR-29038. Doses of 500 mg/kg show no abnormal symptoms in mice when administered intravenously.

Hosoda, Aoki, Imanaka, *Japanese Patent*, 77 44,292 (1977)

ANTIBIOTIC FR-29644
Nocardia uniformis subsp. *tsuyamensis* (FERM-P 971) yields this crystalline antibiotic when cultured aerobically at 30°C for 96 hours at pH 6·0 on a medium of dried yeast, cottonseed cake, starch, glycine, L-tyrosine and mineral salts. It has been isolated from the culture filtrate by selective extraction and purified by column chromatography on Diaion HP-20, activated carbon and cellulose. The antibiotic is soluble in H_2O and dimethylsulphoxide but insoluble in alcohols, hexane, Et_2O and Me_2CO.

Hosoda, Aoki, Imanaka, *Japanese Patent*, 77 94,496 (1977)

ANTIBIOTIC FR-900012
This antibiotic has been isolated from cultures of *Streptomyces carnoses* 1668. Antibiotic FR-900012 is active against *Bacillus subtilis, Escherichia coli, Proteus vulgaris, Pseudomonas aeruginosa* and *Staphylococcus aureus*. It is relatively non-toxic having an LD_{50} in mice of greater than 500 mg/kg when administered intravenously.

Kuroda *et al.*, *Japanese Patent*, 77 118,402 (1977)

ANTIBIOTIC FS-351A
M.p. Indefinite
When *Streptomyces platensis* (FERM-P 1361 is cultivated on a medium containing glucose, starch, dried yeast, ammonium sulphate and other inorganic salts at 27°C for 4 days, a mixture of two antibiotics is obtained. The activity of the filtrate is adsorbed on active carbon, eluted, concentrated *in vacuo*, re-adsorbed on active carbon, chromatographed on cellulose and separated with Biogel P-6. A dose of 0·25 mg of the antibiotic given subcutaneously to mice infected with *Staphylococcus aureus* gave a complete cure. The LD_{50} in mice is 200 mg/kg when administered intraperitoneally.

Hayashi, Okazaki, Harada, *Japanese Patent*, 7,407,495 (1974)

ANTIBIOTIC FS-351B
M.p. Indefinite
This antibiotic is also obtained from cultures of *Streptomyces platensis* (FERM-P 1361) and is separated from the foregoing compound with Biogel P-6. It gives a similar protection to mice against *Staphylococcus aureus* and has LD_{50} of 100 mg/kg when given intraperitoneally.

Hayashi, Okazaki, Harada, *Japanese Patent*, 7,407,495 (1974)

ANTIBIOTIC G-15-I
M.p. Indefinite
Bacillus cereus G-15 (FERM-P 2488) yields two similar antibiotics when cultured aerobically at 28°C for 3 days at pH 7·0 on a medium containing glycerol, glucose, soybean powder, peptone and NaCl. The antibiotics have been obtained by extraction of the cells with 70 per cent Me_2CO, concentration of the extract under vacuum at pH 7·0, extraction with BuOH, concentration, washing with dilute hydrochloric acid, H_2O, dilute sodium bicarbonate solution, H_2O and concentration to a syrup. Extraction with $CHCl_3$-MeOH, followed by a further concentration to a syrup and precipitation with Et_2O yields the crude preparation which has been purified by silica gel chromatography and thin layer chromatography. Antibiotic G-15-I is a colourless neutral powder, soluble in Me_2SO, tetrahydrofuran and a mixture of $CHCl_3$ and MeOH, but insoluble in alcohols, Me_2CO, $CHCl_3$, C_6H_6, Et_2O and H_2O. It gives positive Dragendorff and potassium permanganate reactions. It is similar in physical properties to micrococcin P but may be distinguished from this antibiotic by the thin layer chromatographic characteristics. Antibiotic G-15-I is effective against gram-positive bacteria and is comparatively non-toxic having LD_{50} in mice greater than 500 mg/kg when given intraperitoneally.

Shoji *et al.*, *Japanese Patent*, 76 79,789 (1976)

ANTIBIOTIC G-15-II
M.p. Indefinite.
An antibiotic isolated together with the preceding substance from cultures of *Bacillus cereus* G-15 (FERM-P 2488) and separated from it by silica gel

and thin layer chromatography. It forms a neutral, colourless powder having no definite melting point and has similar physical and antibiotic properties to antibiotic G-15-I.

Shoji et al., *Japanese Patent*, 76 79,789 (1976)

ANTIBIOTIC G 41

Aspergillus strain G-41, grown on a medium prepared from wheat bread at 20–26°C and pH 3·5 for 8–12 days, yields this non-toxic antibiotic which is stated to be active against bacteria causing tuberculosis of the kidneys and lungs when given orally. The structure of the compound is still unknown.

Grigorescu et al., *German Patent*, 2,205,096 (1973)

ANTIBIOTIC G-52
$C_{20}H_{39}O_7N_5$
M.p. Indefinite

This antibiotic is produced, with sisomycin (q.v.), by submerged aerobic culture of the second *Micromonospora zionensis* inoculate in an aqueous nutrient medium incubated at 35°C and pH 7·2 for 2–4 days. It is isolated by adjusting the culture filtrate to pH 2·0 with $6N$-H_2SO_4 and oxalic acid, treating with Amberlite IRC-50 and $2N$ ammonium hydroxide and freeze-drying the extract. Antibiotic G-52 is separated from the accompanying sisomycin by chromatography on silica gel, the lower phase of a 2:1:1 (by volume) mixture of $CHCl_3$, isoPrOH and concentrated ammonium hydroxide. The antibiotic is active *in vivo*, in mice, against *Escherichia*, *Pseudomonas* and *Staphylococcus* infections.

Weinstein, Wagman, Marquez, *German Patent*, 2,334,923 (1974)

ANTIBIOTIC G-418
$C_{20}H_{40}O_{10}N_4$

An antibacterial and protozoacidal antibiotic, this compound is produced by fermentation of *Micromonospora rhodorangea*. It is also obtained from *M. grisea* cultures together with sisomycin and gentamycin A. The antibiotic is characterized as the sulphate which has a minimum inhibitory concentration against *Staphylococcus aureus* 209P of 0·8 µg/ml and LD_{50} in mice of 140 mg/kg when given intravenously.

Weinstein et al., *German Patent*, 2,239,964 (1973)

ANTIBIOTIC G2201-C
$C_6H_6O_4$

A simple antibiotic, this substance has been isolated from the culture broth of *Streptomyces cattleya*. The structure has been determined from chemical and spectroscopic examination. It is active against gram-positive bacteria, only weakly active against gram-negative bacteria and inactive against fungi. It is toxic to mice.

Noble, Noble, Fletton, *J. Antibiotics* (Japan), **31**, 15 (1978)

ANTIBIOTIC G7063-2
$C_7H_6O_4N_2$

A simple epoxy derivative, this antibiotic occurs in the culture broth of a *Streptomyces* species isolated from soil. It has been purified by chromatography on Sephadex LH20 and forms yellow crystals. Moderately soluble in organic solvents it is readily soluble in mineral acids. Antibiotic G7063-2 has a moderate degree of activity against gram-positive and gram-negative bacteria, particularly *Escherichia coli* and *Staphylococcus aureus*. It is, however, only marginally active against fungi. It is quite toxic to mice having an $LD_{50} \sim 17$ mg/kg when administered intraperitoneally.

Noble, Noble, Sykes, *J. Antibiotics* (Japan), **30**, 455 (1977)

ANTIBIOTIC Gp-3

This antibiotic is elaborated by *Bacillus cereus* strain Gp-3 (ATCC 21,928) when grown on a neutral medium consisting of glucose, glycerol, meat extract, peptone and NaCl for 24 hours at 28°C. It has been shown to be effective against gram-positive bacteria and has LD_{50} in mice of 100 mg/kg when administered intraperitoneally.

Shoji et al., *German Patent*, 2,420,104 (1974)

ANTIBIOTIC H 537 SY2
$C_{19}H_{33}N_5O_{11}$

This antibiotic from an unclassified *Streptomyces* species has been described by Japanese workers. It is only weakly active against bacteria but effective against many yeasts.

Kondo et al., *J. Antibiotics* (Japan), **29**, 847 (1976)

ANTIBIOTIC H-2609
$C_{34}H_{76}O_{45}$

A complex antibiotic, this compound has been obtained by culturing *Streptomyces hachijoensis* strain H-2609 aerobically at 27–30°C for 4–5 days on a medium comprising glucose, starch, peptone, meat extract, protease peptone and NaCl. The culture broth is centrifuged and the supernatant liquor treated with chilled MeOH to precipitate the active principle. The precipitate is dissolved in dilute potassium phosphate solution at pH 7·0–9·0, the extract filtered and freeze-dried. The antibiotic shows little activity against bacteria but has anticarcinoma properties.

Soeda, *German Patent*, 2,615,099 (1976)

ANTIBIOTIC H-3787
Decomp. 285–9°C

A strain of *Streptomyces* H-3787 (FERM-P 1400) yields this antibiotic when cultured at 27°C for 66 hours on a medium consisting of glucose, glycerol, soybean powder, yeast extract and inorganic salts. It is soluble in dilute mineral acids and alkalis, insoluble in alcohols, AcOEt, C_6H_6 and Me_2CO. At a concentration of 125 ppm it inhibited the growth of *Staphylococcus aureus* strain FDA-209P but in laboratory tests with mice an injection of 1 g/kg resulted in death after 7 days.

Seino et al., *Japanese Patent*, 76 76,493 (1976)

ANTIBIOTIC HA-9
$C_7H_6O_2N_2S_2$
M.p. 178–180°C

A *Streptomyces* species related to *S. lipmanii* furnishes this antibiotic which has properties very like those of tioaurin (q.v.). It forms yellow needles when crystallized from AcOEt and is neutral in reaction. In glacial AcOH the substance in optically inactive and the ultraviolet spectrum in MeOH has a single absorption maximum at 370 nm. It is soluble in CH_3OH, slightly soluble in AcOEt and virtually insoluble in $CHCl_3$ and H_2O. Biologically it is active against both gram-positive and gram-negative bacteria and shows a slight activity against fungi. It is not deactivated by serum. So far, it has shown little promise in medicine due to its relatively high toxicity with LD_{50} in mice of 15 mg/kg on intravenous injection and 20 mg/kg when administered subcutaneously.

Eiserman et al., *Antibiotics & Chemotherapy*, **3**, 385 (1953)

ANTIBIOTIC I-337A
M.p. 148–149°C

One of three antibiotics elaborated by *Kitasatoa kauaiensis*, this compound has been shown to be identical with chloramphenicol (q.v.).

Abe, Hata, *J. Antibiotics* (Japan), **21**, 545 (1968)

ANTIBIOTIC I-337B
M.p. Indefinite

A second antibiotic isolated from cultures of *Kitasatoa kauaiensis*, the physicochemical and biological properties of this substance indicate that it is bottromycin (q.v.).

Abe, Hata, *J. Antibiotics* (Japan), **21**, 545 (1968)

ANTIBIOTIC I-337C

This compound obtained from *Kitasatoa kauaiensis* has been shown to be identical with fradicin (q.v.).

Abe, Hata, *J. Antibiotics* (Japan), **21**, 545 (1968)

ANTIBIOTIC IN-183-T
$C_{15}H_{33}O_9N_6$

Isolated from cultures of *Streptomyces lavendulae* strain IN-183-T, this antibiotic is obtained as the sulphate which is soluble in H_2O and active against *Xanthomonas oryzae*. It is relatively non-toxic, mice tolerating a dose of 200 mg/kg given intravenously.

Kado et al., *Japanese Patent*, 7,123,040 (1971)

ANTIBIOTIC JI-20A
$C_{19}H_{39}O_9N_5$

The structure of this glycosidic antibiotic is very similar to that of antibiotic G-52 (q.v.). It has been obtained by culturing mutant strains of *Micromonospora purpurea* on a medium consisting of dextrin, cerulose, soybean flour, calcium carbonate and conalt chloride at 34°C with stirring. The antibiotic is isolated as the complex with oxalic acid, purified by adsorption on an ion exchange resin and resolved by chromatography on silica gel to give two components, this antibiotic and the methyl derivative described below.

Ilavsky, Bayan, Charney, *German Patent*, 2,329,012 (1973)

ANTIBIOTIC JI-20B
$C_{20}H_{41}O_9N_5$

An aminoglycosidic antibiotic, this substance accompanies the preceding compound in the antibiotic mixture isolated from cultures of a nutant strain of *Micromonospora purpurea*. It is separated from the accompanying component by chromatography on silica gel.

Ilavsky, Bayan, Charney, *German Patent*, 2,329,012 (1973)

ANTIBIOTIC K-6-6-A

A colourless oily substance, this antibiotic is produced by culturing *Streptomyces shimizuensis* var. *isomyceticus* aerobically at 30°C for 30 hours in a medium comprising starch, soybean powder, dried yeast and inorganic salts. It has been purified by chromatography of the culture filtrate on ion exchange and silical gel columns.

Koyama et al., *Japanese Patent*, 74 34,840 (1974)

ANTIBIOTIC K-13-1A

This antibiotic is obtained from *Streptomyces bikiniensis* var. *medermyceticus* cultured on a medium containing meat extract, starch, peptone, sodium chloride and calcium carbonate at 30°C and pH 7·0 for 2 days. The broth is acidified to pH 2·0, filtered and then extracted with C_6H_6, $CHCl_3$, AcOEt or BuOH, followed by evaporation of the solvent *in vacuo*. The antibiotic is active mainly against gram-positive bacteria.

Koyama et al., *Japanese Patent*, 7,330,394 (1973)
Koyama et al., *British Patent*, 1,402,392 (1975)

ANTIBIOTIC K-16
$C_{13}H_{18}O_9N_4$
M.p. Indefinite

Streptomyces rimosus yields this antibiotic which forms a white microcrystalline powder with no definite melting point, It is laevorotatory with a specific rotation of $[\alpha]_{577}^{20} - 64°$ (c 1·0, H_2O). It is active against gram-positive organisms.

Batelaan et al., *Tetrahedron Lett.*, 3103, 3107 (1972)

ANTIBIOTIC K-41
$C_{48}H_{82}O_{19}$
M.p. 196–198°C

A crystalline antibiotic, this compound has been obtained by culturing *Streptomyces* species K-41 on a nutrient medium at 27°C and pH 7·0 for 4 days. The antibiotic is extracted from the filtrate and the mycelium with

AcOEt, concentrated *in vacuo*, dissolved in $CHCl_3$, adsorbed on silica gel and eluted with $CHCl_3$ containing 2 per cent CH_3OH. The antibiotic forms colourless crystals when crystallized from $CHCl_3$ and is slightly dextrorotatory with a specific rotation of $[\alpha]_D^{23} + 1.9° \pm 0.4°$. It is active against gram-positive bacteria and is moderately toxic with LD_{50} in mice of 53 mg/kg when given intraperitoneally.

Tsuji *et al.*, *Japanese Patent*, 7,414,692 (1974)
Tsuji *et al.*, *J. Antibiotics* (Japan), **29**, 10 (1976)

ANTIBIOTIC K-73A
$C_{24}H_{29}NO_8 \cdot HCl$
Decomp. 180°C
Streptomyces strain KW-75 elaborates this crystalline antibiotic which is dextrorotatory having a specific rotation of $[\alpha]_D^{25} + 177°$. It is soluble in H_2O, MeOH, EtOH, AcOEt, Me_2CO and C_6H_6 but insoluble in hexane and petroleum ether. Antibiotic K-73A is active against *Bacillus*, *Sarcina*, *Shigella*, *Staphylococcus* and *Xanthomonas*. It has LD_{50} in mice of 8.8 mg/kg when administered intravenously.

Koyama *et al.*, *Japanese Patent*, 77 15,895 (1977)

ANTIBIOTIC K-231
M.p. Indefinite
Streptomyces albus var. *coleimyceticus* elaborates this antibiotic when cultivated on a medium containing glucose, peptone, meat extract, dry yeast and inorganic salts at 28°C for 24 hours followed by fermentation in fresh medium for 2 days. After extraction, the crude material is purified by dissolving in CH_3OH, adsorbing on activated carbon, eluting with CH_3OH and chromatographing on alumina in $CHCl_3$. It is active against gram-positive bacteria.

Inoue *et al.*, *Japanese Patent*, 7,227,046 (1972)

ANTIBIOTIC K-231F-1
M.p. Indefinite
This antibiotic derived from *Streptomyces albus* var. *coleimyceticus* has also been described by Japanese workers. It is obtained by cultivating the organism on a medium consisting of starch, soybean flour and sodium chloride at 30°C for 45 hours. The compound is active against *Sarcina lutea* and *Staphylococcus aureus*, particularly against those strains which are resistant to erythromycin and oleandomycin. It is comparatively non-toxic with LD_{50} in mice of 925 mg/kg when given intraperitoneally.

Kanda, Abe, *Japanese Patent*, 7,225,391 (1972)

ANTIBIOTIC K-5610
$C_{33}H_{59}O_{10}Na$
M.p. 158–160°C
Antibiotic K-5610 is produced by a mutant strain of *Streptomyces cacaoi* var. *asoensis*. The culture filtrate is acidified to pH 2.0 with HCl and the precipitate thus formed is suspended in $(CH_3)_2CO$ and extracted with BuOH, $(CH_3)_2CO$ and CH_3OH in succession. The substance forms colourless needles from CH_3OH and is dextrorotatory with a specific rotation of $[\alpha]_D^{25} + 11.5°$. It is soluble in CH_3OH, EtOH, BuOH, $(CH_3)_2CO$, C_6H_6, $CHCl_3$ and pyridine but insoluble in H_2O. The antibiotic is active against gram-positive bacteria and is comparatively toxic with LD_{50} in mice of 70 mg/kg administered intraperitoneally.

Kasahara *et al.*, *Japanese Patent*, 7,310,797 (1973)

ANTIBIOTIC KM-214
$C_{35}H_{54}O_9$
M.p. 139–140°C
This antibiotic has been obtained by culturing *Bacillus aurantinus* aerobically at 27°C for 60 hours on a medium comprising glucose, yeast extract and mineral salts. It has been purified by centrifuging the supernatant liquor, extracting with BuOH at pH 2–3, evaporating to dryness and column chromatographing. Antibiotic KM-214 is active against both bacteria and fungi.

Omura *et al.*, *J. Antibiotics* (Japan), **29**, 477 (1976)
Omura *et al.*, *Japanese Patent*, 77 100,401 (1977)

ANTIBIOTIC LA-7017
See Aureolic acid

ANTIBIOTIC LL-AB664
$C_{18}H_{30}O_8N_8$
M.p. Indefinite
Isolated from a variant strain of *Streptomyces candidus*, the structure of this antibiotic is still somewhat uncertain regarding the location of the amide group in the molecule. It belongs to the streptothricin group of compounds and is relatively stable in acid and neutral solutions but degraded by alkalies.

The compound has a specific rotation of $[\alpha]_D^{25} - 59°$ (c 1·004, H_2O). It is active *in vivo*, protecting mice against experimental infections due to *Escherichia coli*, *Klebsiella pneumoniae*, *Salmonella typhosa* and *Staphylococcus aureus* when given subcutaneously.

Sax *et al.*, *Antimicrobial Agents & Chemotherapy*, 442 (1967)
Structure
Borders *et al.*, *Tetrahedron*, **26**, 3123 (1970)

ANTIBIOTIC LL-AC541 (*Antibiotic E-749-C*)
$C_{17}H_{28}O_8N_8$
M.p. 210–240°C (*dec.*)

This antibiotic is elaborated by a strain of *Streptomyces hygroscopicus* and has also been shown to be identical with antibiotic E-749-C produced by the same organism. Dilute acids hydrolyse it to a number of compounds, e.g. streptolidine, formic acid, N-methyl-2-amino-deoxygulose, N-methyl-N-*guan*-streptolidylgulosaminide, ammonia and carbon dioxide. Structurally it is the N-demethyl analogue of the preceding antibiotic and, again, the exact location of the amide group is still uncertain. It is active against both gram-positive and gram-negative bacteria.

Borders *et al.*, *Tetrahedron Lett.*, 4187 (1967)
Shoji *et al.*, *J. Antibiotics* (Japan), **21**, 509 (1968)
Structure
Borders *et al.*, *Tetrahedron*, **26**, 3123 (1970)

ANTIBIOTIC LL-AF283
The antibiotic substance isolated from cultures of a strain of *Streptomyces filipinensis* consists of two components, LL-AF283α and LL-AF283β. So far, they have been found to be active only against *Corynebacterium xerosis*.

Martin *et al.*, *Antimicrobial Agents & Chemotherapy*, 422 (1967)

ANTIBIOTIC LL-AM31α
$C_{12}H_{27}N_3O_8$

Three homologous antibiotics have been isolated from cultures of a *Streptoverticillium* species and separated and purified by ion-exchange chromatography. This component has been shown to possess the structure given above based on chemical and spectroscopic evidence.

Kirby *et al.*, *J. Antibiotics* (Japan), **30**, 344 (1977)

ANTIBIOTIC LL-AM31β
$C_{15}H_{31}H_3O_9$
A further antibiotic obtained from cultures of an unclassified *Streptoverticillium* species, this component has the above structure.

Kirby *et al.*, *J. Antibiotics* (Japan), **30**, 344 (1977)

ANTIBIOTIC LL-AM31γ
$C_{14}H_{29}N_3O_9$

Also produced by an unclassified *Streptoverticillium* species, this antibiotic is the N-acetyl derivative of antibiotic LL-AM31α. The structure has been established from chemical correlations and spectroscopic data.

Kirby *et al.*, *J. Antibiotics* (Japan), **30**, 344 (1977)

ANTIBIOTIC LL-AV290
See Avoparicin

ANTIBIOTIC LL-BM123α
$C_{30}H_{54}N_9O_{17}$

A water-soluble, basic antibiotic isolated from a culture of an unidentified species of *Nocardia*, antibiotic LL-BM123 is moderately active against gram-negative bacteria but has the advantage of being very non-toxic. The structure has been elucidated from chemical and spectroscopic evidence.

Ellestad *et al.*, *J. Antibiotics* (Japan), **30**, 678 (1977)

ANTIBIOTIC LL-BM408
$C_{17}H_{33}N_3O_{11}$

An unidentified species of *Streptomyces* yields this antibiotic which has been assigned the structure shown above based upon a study of the hydrolysis products and the NMR and mass spectra. It has been shown to be effective against bacterial infections in mice.

Kirby, Borders, Van Lear, *J. Antibiotics* (Japan), **30**, 175 (1977)

ANTIBIOTIC LL-S491α
$C_{20}H_{26}O_5$
M.p. 180–185°C

Aspergillus chevalieri elaborates two closely related antibiotics having a reduced anthracene structure. This substance forms colourless crystals and is dextrorotatory with a specific rotation of $[\alpha]_D + 112\cdot4°$ (CH_3OH).

Ellestad *et al.*, *J. Amer. Chem. Soc.*, **94**, 6206 (1972)

ANTIBIOTIC LL-S491β
$C_{20}H_{28}O_5$
M.p. 190–195°C

A second antibiotic produced by *Aspergillus chevalieri*, this compound is the secondary alcohol corresponding to antibiotic LL-S491 as the ketone. It has a specific rotation of $[\alpha]_D + 69.3°$ (CH_3OH).

Ellestad *et al.*, *J. Amer. Chem. Soc.*, **94**, 6206 (1972)

ANTIBIOTIC LL-Z1220
$C_{11}H_8O_4$
M.p. 148°C (*dec.*)

This antibiotic, produced by an unidentified fungal species, is laevorotatory with $[\alpha]_D^{25} - 123°$ (c 0.59, $CHCl_3$) and has been shown to have the structure 2-(3,4:5,6-diepoxycyclohex-1-enyl)-4*H*-pyran-4-one. It is a colourless solid and gives an ultraviolet spectrum in CH_3OH with a single absorption maximum at 269 nm.

Borders *et al.*, *Antimicrobial Agents & Chemotherapy*, 233 (1970)
Borders, Shu, Lancaster, *J. Amer. Chem. Soc.*, **94**, 2540 (1972)
Borders, Lancaster, *J. Org. Chem.*, **39**, 435 (1974)

ANTIBIOTIC M-81
Dec. 208–213°C
An antibiotic produced by *Streptomyces griseus* subsp. *psychrophilus* cultured on a common medium at 20–37°C, this substance decomposes at 208–213°C without melting. Chemical investigations show that it has a polypeptide structure. It is comparatively non-toxic with LD_{50} in mice 300 mg/kg when administered intraperitoneally.

Yoshida *et al.*, *J. Antibiotics* (Japan), **27**, 128 (1974)

ANTIBIOTIC M-4126
$C_{31}H_{24}O_{11}$
M.p. 189–191°C
A weakly acidic antibiotic, this compound has been obtained by cultivating *Chaetomium cochloides* (FERM-P1382) on a medium containing potato extract, glucose, cottonseed flour and inorganic salts and incubating at 27°C for 63 hours. The cells are extracted with $(CH_3)_2CO$, followed by back extraction with AcOEt and precipitation with petroleum ether. Antibiotic M-4126 is a yellow solid having a specific rotation of $[\alpha]_D^{23.5} + 55.3°$. It is soluble in CH_3OH, EtOH, AcOEt, $(CH_3)_2CO$, $AcOCH_3$, C_6H_6, $CHCl_3$ and pyridine, slightly soluble in hexane and insoluble in H_2O and petroleum ether. The antibiotic is unstable to light. It is active against gram-positive bacteria and has LD_{50} in mice of approximately 150 mg/kg when given intravenously.

Mizuno, Takada, Furuhashi, *Japanese Patent*, 7,401,797 (1974)

ANTIBIOTIC M-4365 A₁
$C_{31}H_{53}NO_8$

The antibiotic M-4365 complex isolated from cultures of *Micromonospora capillata* strain MCRL 0940 has been separated into six components, antibiotics M-4365 A_1, A_2, A_3, G_1, G_2, and G_3. Three of these are identical with known antibiotics (see below). This particular antibiotic has been separated from the culture filtrate by solvent extraction and purified by column chromatography. It exhibits an inhibitory action against *Klebsiella pneumoniae* and *Mycoplasma* species. Some cross-resistance with other macrocyclic antibiotics has been demonstrated.

Furumai *et al.*, *J. Antibiotics* (Japan), **30**, 443 (1977)
Structure
Kinumatsu *et al.*, *J. Antibiotics* (Japan), **30**, 450 (1977)

ANTIBIOTIC M-4365 A$_2$

This macrocyclic antibiotic isolated from cultures of *Micromonospora capillata* strain MCRL 0940 has been shown to be identical with rosamicin.

Furumai *et. al., J. Antibiotics* (Japan), **30**, 443 (1977)

ANTIBIOTIC M-4365 A$_3$

A further macrocyclic antibiotic isolated from cultures of *Micromonospora capillata* strain MCRL 0940, this substance is identical with juvenimicin A$_4$.

Furumai *et al., J. Antibiotics* (Japan), **30**, 443 (1977)

ANTIBIOTIC M-4365 G$_1$
$C_{31}H_{53}NO_7$

This component of the M-4365 antibiotic complex obtained by solvent extraction of the culture filtrate of *Micromonospora capillata* strain MCRL 0940 is a minor constituent and has the structure given above based upon hydrolysis experiments and spectroscopic data. It is active against both gram-positive and gram-negative bacteria.

Furumai *et al., J. Antibiotics* (Japan), **30**, 443 (1977)
Structure
Kinumatsu *et al., J. Antibiotics* (Japan), **30**, 450 (1977)

ANTIBIOTIC M-4365 G$_2$
$C_{31}H_{51}NO_8$

A major component of the complex of macrocyclid antibiotics isolated from cultures of *Micromonospora capillata* strain MCRL 0940, this substance has the above structure deduced from a chemical and spectroscopic examination of the hydrolysis fragments. It possesses a high activity against gram-positive and gram-negative bacteria and an inhibitory action against *Klebsiella pneumonia* and *Mycoplasma* species. Some cross-resistance with other macrocyclic antibiotics has been observed.

Furumai *et al., J. Antibiotics* (Japan), **30**, 443 (1977)
Structure
Kinumatsu *et al., J. Antibiotics* (Japan), **30**, 450 (1977)

ANTIBIOTIC M-4365 G$_3$

This component of the M-4365 complex has been shown to be identical with juvenimicin B$_1$.

Furamai *et al., J. Antibiotics* (Japan), **30**, 443 (1977)

ANTIBIOTIC MBU-18

Streptomyces species 18 produces this glucoantibiotic which is obtained from the culture filtrate by adsorption on activated carbon followed by elution with CH_3OH, chromatography on an ion exchange resin and paper chromatography. The structure has been established as 7-deoxy-L-glycero-α,β-D-glucoheptopyranose by spectroscopic examination of the substance as the crystalline acetyl derivative.

Hauser *et al., Antibiotiki*, **19**, 483 (1974)

ANTIBIOTIC MC 902-I

Aerobic culture of *Streptomyces* strain MC 902-A$_3$ produces two similar antibiotics which have been obtained by extraction of the culture filtrate with BuOH followed by purification by column chromatography and recrystallization. This antibiotic is effective against *Piricularia sasaki*, *Bacillus anthracis* and *Staphylococcus aureus*.

Umezawa *et al., Japanese Patent*, 77 102,201 (1977)

ANTIBIOTIC MC 902-I'
A second constituent of the antibiotic mixture produced by *Streptomyces* strain MC 902-A$_3$ when cultured under aerobic conditions, this substance also exhibits activity against *Bacillus anthracis*, *Piricularia sasaki* and *Staphylococcus aureus*.

Umezawa *et al.*, *Japanese Patent*, 77 102,201 (1977)

ANTIBIOTIC MD 129-C2
$C_{55-61}H_{92-99}NO_{16-20}$

A strain of *Streptomyces* FERM-P 1596 yields this complex antibiotic which has been obtained by culture of the organism at 27°C for 5 days on a medium of sucrose, soybean powder and inorganic salts, extracting the fermentation broth twice with AcOEt at pH 6·0, concentrating the combined extracts at 40°C, re-extracting with Et$_2$O and purifying the antibiotic by gel chromatography. The compound forms colourless crystals and is soluble in Me$_2$CO, Et$_2$O, AcOEt, EtOH and BuOH but insoluble in CHCl$_3$ and petroleum ether. It is very toxic with LD$_{50}$ of 1 mg/kg given intraveneously to mice.

Okami *et al.*, *Japanese Patent*, 74 85,296 (1974)

ANTIBIOTIC ML-236A
M.p. 126–132°C

A neutral white powder, this antibiotic has been isolated from the culture filtrate of *Penicillium citrinum* SANK (FERM-P 2609) by fermenting at 28°C for 96 hours with aeration. The filtrate is evaporated to dryness, extracted with AcOEt at pH 4·0 and the oily material obtained by concentration of the extract purified by chromatography. The antibiotic is soluble in AcOEt, Me$_2$CO, CHCl$_3$, alcohols and C$_6$H$_6$ but insoluble in hexane and petroleum ether. It has been shown to inhibit cholesterol biosynthesis by approximately 50 per cent at a concentration of 0·04 micrograms/millilitre. It is comparatively non-toxic with LD$_{50}$ of >400 mg/kg when administered intraperitoneally to mice.

Endo *et al.*, *Japanese Patent*, 76 136,885 (1976)

ANTIBIOTIC ML-236C
$C_{18}H_{26}O_3$
B.p. Indefinite

A colourless neutral oil, this antibiotic has been isolated from *Penicillium citrinum* SANK 18,767 by aerobic fermentation on a nutrient medium at 28°C for 96 hours. It has been obtained by concentrating the filtrate in a vacuum, extracting with AcOEt at pH 4·0, evaporating the extract to dryness giving an oil which has been purified by silica gel chromatography. Antibiotic ML-236C is soluble in the lower alcohols, Me$_2$CO, AcOEt, C$_6$H$_6$, CHCl$_3$ but insoluble in hexane and petroleum ether. It has been shown to inhibit cholesterol synthesis by approximately 50 per cent at concentrations of 0·08 micrograms/millilitre. The LD$_{50}$ in mice is greater than 400 mg/kg given intraperitoneally.

Endo *et al.*, *Japanese Patent*, 76 136,886 (1976)

ANTIBIOTIC MM-446
By cultivating *Fusarium lateritium* (ATCC 20227) aerobically in a medium containing sources of carbon and nitrogen together with inorganic salts at pH 5·0–9·0, this antibiotic is formed which has been shown to be a highly effective insecticide.

Cole, Rolinson, *U.S. Patent*, 3,793,449 (1974)

ANTIBIOTIC MM-4550
M.p. Indefinite

An antibiotic produced by *Streptomyces olivaceus* (ATCC 21379) in a medium containing glucose, soybean flour and manganous sulphate at 28°C for 2 days with aeration. The compound is isolated by adsorption on a cellulose ion exchange resin, eluted with 0·5*M*-sodium sulphate solution, the eluate concentrated *in vacuo* and purified by chromatography on an Amberlite XAD-2 column. The antibiotic is active against a number of bacteria and has a synergistic effect with cephalosporin and penicillin, inhibiting the β-lactamaze activity of bacteria.

Butterworth, Rolinson, *German Patent*, 2,146,400 (1972)

ANTIBIOTIC MM 17880
$C_{13}H_{18}O_8N_2S_2$

This antibiotic has been isolated from the glucose-soybean meal culture of *Streptomyces olivaceus* ATCC 31,126 by extraction of the filtrate with an

Antibiotic MSD 890A$_2$

organic solvent followed by gel filtration. Antibiotic MM 17880 is active against gram-positive and gram-negative bacteria and also exhibits a synergistic effect in conjunction with amoxycillin (q.v.) against *Klebsiella aerogenes* and *Staphylococcus aureus*.

Box, Hood, *German Patent*, 2,609,766 (1976)

ANTIBIOTIC MSD 890A$_2$
C$_{13}$H$_{16}$N$_2$O$_5$S

Streptomyces flavogriseus MA-4434 produces two stereoisomeric antibiotics by inoculating a medium of dextrin, tomato paste and yeast extract with a preculture of the organism and fermenting at 24°C and pH 7·3 for 101 hours with stirring. Centrifuging of the broth followed by separation of the components by chromatography of the supernatant liquor yields this and the following antibiotic. This antibiotic has a wide activity against gram-positive and gram-negative bacteria. The structure has been elucidated from chemical correlations and spectroscopic evidence.

Cassidy *et al.*, *German Patent*, 2,718,782 (1977)

ANTIBIOTIC MSD 890A$_5$
C$_{13}$H$_{16}$N$_2$O$_5$S

A stereoisomer of the preceding antibiotic, this substance is also produced by *Streptomyces flavogriseus* MA-4434. It is active against a wide range of gram-positive and gram-negative bacteria.

Cassidy *et al.*, *German Patent*, 2,718,782 (1977)

ANTIBIOTIC MT-10
C$_{19}$H$_{31}$O$_6$N$_3$
Dec. 204°C

Streptomyces indicus Chakrabarty furnishes this antibiotic which decomposes, without melting, at 204°C. In EtOH it gives an ultraviolet spectrum with two absorption maxima at 420 and 442 nm. It is laevorotatory with a specific rotation which varies from $[\alpha]_D - 205°$ to $-215°$ (c 0·25, EtOH).

Chakrabarty, Nandi, *Experientia*, **27**, 595 (1971)

ANTIBIOTIC MX-A

An antibiotic isolated from cultures of *Bacillus biterinus* Z-1159 and *B. circulans* V-7, this substance has been shown to be effective in the control of *Pseudomonas aeruginosa*.

Arai, Migami, Yamano, *Japanese Patent*, 77 83,803 (1977)

ANTIBIOTIC MYC-8003 (*Mocimycin*)
M.p. Indefinite

This antibiotic is derived from *Streptomyces ramocissimus*. When purified by chromatography on an alumina column it forms a yellow powder which is soluble in CHCl$_3$, AcOEt, CH$_3$OH, (CH$_3$)$_2$CO, butyl acetate and alkaline solutions, slightly soluble in C$_6$H$_6$ and CCl$_4$, insoluble in ligroine, Et$_2$O, H$_2$O and acid solutions. The antibiotic is laevorotatory with a specific rotation of $[\alpha]_D^{22} - 60°$ (c 1·0, CH$_3$OH). Its main use, and that of its sodium salt, is as a growth-promoting feed additive.

Vos, *German Patent*, 2,140,674 (1972)
Vos, *Netherlands Appl.*, 7,111,168 (1972)

ANTIBIOTIC N-1409

Streptomyces plumbeus yields this antibiotic as colourless crystals when cultured aerobically at 30°C for 67 hours on a medium comprising glucose and inorganic salts. The fermentation broth is filtered and the filtrate fractionated by column chromatography and the antibiotic finally purified by crystallization from EtOH. Antibiotic N-1409 is active against gram-positive bacteria.

Boku, Hirota, Sakai, *Japanese Patent*, 77 108,904 (1977)

ANTIBIOTIC NA-181
C$_{25}$H$_{43}$O$_7$N
M.p. 150–152°C

A novel antibiotic formed by aerobically cultivating *Streptomyces fungicidicus* var. *chikusanensis* with shaking in an aqueous medium containing yeast, starch, ammonium sulphate and other inorganic salts at 28°C and pH 7·4 for 2 days. The substance inhibits phytopathogenic fungi, e.g. *Helminthosporium sigmoideum* and *Piricularia oryzae*.

Akashiba, Minowa, Tsuchiyama, *Japanese Patent*, 7,200,039 (1972)

ANTIBIOTIC NA-699

This antibiotic is produced by *Streptomyces aichinensis* which is cultured aerobically in a medium containing glucose, soybean flour, starch, meat extract, peptone, sodium chloride and H_2O. The substance is isolated by extracting the culture filtrate with BuOH, the organic fraction is then extracted with dilute acid to pH 2·0, the pH adjusted to 8·0 and re-extracted with BuOH. The butanol extract is then concentrated under reduced pressure and added to CH_3OH when a precipitate of the crude antibiotic is formed. This is finally purified by chromatography on an alumina column.

Antibiotic NA-699 is highly effective in controlling a number of plant diseases due to bacteria.

Munekata, Ito, *Japanese Patent*, 7,445,599 (1974)

ANTIBIOTIC NK-1001
$C_{18}H_{35}O_{12}N_3$
M.p. 238–242°C (*dec.*)

Isolated from *Streptomyces kanamyceticus*, this antibiotic forms colourless needles when recrystallized from EtOH. It is dextrorotatory with a specific rotation of $[\alpha]_D^{21} + 132°$ (c 1·0, H_2O).

Meiji Confectionery Co. Ltd., *British Patent*, 1,181,623 (1970)

ANTIBIOTIC NK-1003
$C_{12}H_{25}O_7N_3$
M.p. 202–205°C (*dec.*)

A further antibiotic elaborated by *Streptomyces kanamyceticus*, this substance forms colourless crystals and has a specific rotation of $[\alpha]_D^{21} + 94°$ (c 1·0, H_2O).

Kawaji *et al.*, *Japanese Patent*, 7,016,792 (1970)

ANTIBIOTIC NP-023
$C_{11}H_7O_3NCl_2$
M.p. 173–175°C (*dec.*)

A chlorine-containing antibiotic, this compound is obtained by culturing *Pseudomonas pyrocianolyticus* (FERM-P2125) on a neutral medium containing n-hexadecane, inorganic salts, molasses and dead cells of *Pseudomonas aeruginosa* at 32°C for 2 days. The culture broth is extracted with $(CH_3)_2CO$, stirred and filtered, the $(CH_3)_2CO$ evaporated at 50°C and extracted with Et_2O at pH 7·0. The extract is then dried with anhydrous sodium sulphate and evaporated. The residue is then dissolved in Et_2O and chromatographed on a silica column. Antibiotic NP-023 forms yellow needles which are soluble in CH_3OH, EtOH, $(CH_3)_2CO$, AcOEt, Et_2O, $CHCl_3$ and C_6H_6 but insoluble in H_2O, petroleum ether and hexane. It is effective against gram-positive, gram-negative and acidophilic bacteria and causes lysis of the cells of *Pseudomonas aeruginosa*.

Mimura *et al.*, *Japanese Patent*, 7,525,796 (1975)

ANTIBIOTIC NRC-101
$C_{43}H_{72}O_{19}N_{20}$

A polypeptide antibiotic derived from *Streptomyces* NRC-101 isolated from Egyptian soil, this substance is a basic white, amorphous powder with no definite melting point. The ultraviolet spectrum in EtOH has a single absorption maximum at 210 nm indicative of amines while hydrolysis with dilute acids yields glycine, L-proline, L-threonine and β-alanine. The antibiotic is active against gram-positive bacteria both *in vitro* and *in vivo*, particularly against *Bacillus* and *Staphylococcus* species.

Abou-Zeid, Shehata, *Z. Allg. Mikrobiol.*, **11**, 475 (1971)

ANTIBIOTIC O-2867
$C_{14}H_{25}O_9N_3$
M.p. 161–163·5°C

An unclassified species of *Streptomyces* furnishes an antibiotic which has been shown to consist of two components. This substance is an amorphous white powder and is laevorotatory with a specific rotation of $[\alpha]_D^{24} - 43°$ (c 1·0, H_2O). It is soluble in H_2O and is amphoteric. It inhibits the growth of *Piricularia oryzae in vitro* but has no effect *in vivo* with rice infected with this pathogenic fungus.

Sato *et al.*, *J. Antibiotics* (Japan), **24**, 774 (1971)

ANTIBIOTIC O-2867
$C_{10-11}H_{17-19}O_7N_3$
M.p. 143–146°C

The second component of the antibiotic complex O-2867 forms colourless needles from H_2O. It is also laevorotatory with a specific rotation of $[\alpha]_D^{24} - 16°$ (c 0·8, H_2O). It has a similar activity against *Piricularia oryzae* as the preceding antibiotic both *in vivo* and *in vitro*.

Sato *et al.*, *J. Antibiotics* (Japan), **24**, 774 (1971)

ANTIBIOTIC OM-1
$C_{16}H_{15}O_3$
M.p. Indefinite
An antifungal antibiotic, this compound is produced by *Oudemansiella mucida* and is extracted from both the mycelium and culture filtrate by countercurrent distribution with Et_2O, $CHCl_3$, butyl acetate or $CHCl:CCl_2$. The extract is concentrated and the crude product chromatographed on alumina in petroleum ether, eluted with $CHCl_3$ and distilled or cyrstallized. Antibiotic OM-1 has no activity against bacteria but is active against a range of pathogenic fungi.

Vondracek *et al.*, *Czechoslovakian Patent*, 136,495 (1970)

ANTIBIOTIC OS-1804
$C_{18}H_{37}N_7O_2$
Isolated from the culture broth and mycelia of *Streptomyces michiganensis*, this antibiotic is active against gram-positive bacteria, some gram-negative bacteria and filamentous fungi. It is inactive against yeasts but shows some activity against such plant pathogens as *Alternaria kikuchiana*, *Piricularia oryzae* and *Sclerotinia cinerea*.

Shimada *et al.*, *J. Antibiotics* (Japan), **30**, 330 (1977)

ANTIBIOTIC OS-3256-B
M.p. Indefinite
This antitumour antibiotic has recently been described by Japanese workers. It is obtained from *Streptomyces candidus* grown aerobically on common nutrient media. It forms a white amorphous powder with no definite melting point and is active against Ehrlich ascites sarcoma.

Satoh *et al.*, *J. Antibiotics* (Japan), **27**, 620 (1974)

ANTIBIOTIC OS-3966A
$C_{16}H_{14}O_6$
M.p. 178–180°C
One of two antibiotics isolated from cultures of *Streptomyces rosanotoensis*, this compound forms colourless crystals from EtOH and is laevorotatory having a specific rotation of $[\alpha]_D^{26} - 27·5°$.

Omura *et al.*, *Japanese Patent*, 75 52,287 (1975)

ANTIBIOTIC OS-3966B
M.p. 84–86°C
A minor antibiotic isolated from *Streptomyces rosa-notoensis*, this compound is also crystalline and has a specific rotation of $[\alpha]_D^{26} - 74·5°$. The structure has not been fully elucidated.

Omura *et al.*, *Japanese Patent*, 75 52,288 (1975)

ANTIBIOTIC OS-4742
This antibiotic is produced by *Streptomyces* species OS-4742 when cultured aerobically on a medium consisting of glucose, starch, meat extract, peptone and $CaCO_3$ at 27°C for 3 days at pH 7·0. The cells are extracted with AcOEt and chromatographed on a silica gel column eluting with $CHCl_3$–MeOH. Antibiotic OS-4742 is active against gram-positive and some gram-negative bacteria. It is fairly non-toxic with LD_{50} in mice of 100–150 mg/kg given intraperitoneally.

Ohmura *et al.*, *Japanese Patent*, 77 105,101 (1977)

ANTIBIOTIC P-42-1
$C_{27}H_{24}O_9N_2$
Actinomyces tumemacerans elaborates this antitumour antibiotic which forms yellow crystals from EtOH. It has a high degree of inhibitory activity against a wide range of gram-positive bacteria and fungi but little activity against gram-negative organisms. It exhibits an inhibitory activity against Ehrlich ascites sarcoma in mice and it is cytotoxic to MeLa cells *in vitro*. Physicochemical and biological characteristics indicate that it is identical with kanchanomycin.

Fukushima *et al.*, *J. Antibiotics* (Japan), **26**, 65 (1973)

ANTIBIOTIC P-42
An antibiotic produced by cultivating *Streptomyces tumemacerans* strain P-42 in a medium containing wheat flour, this compound has been shown to possess antibacterial and cytotoxic properties. It belongs to the albofungin group of compounds.

Krasil'nikov, Skalozub, Kuimova, *Biol. Luchistykh Gribkov*, 179 (1975)

ANTIBIOTIC P-2563 I
$C_{15}H_{33}N_3O_8$

Pseudomonas fluorescens strain P-2563 elaborates an antibiotic complex from which three components have been isolated, antibiotics P-2563 I, II and III, when cultivated aerobically at 28°C and pH 6·8 for 72 hours on a medium consisting of corn steep liquor, glucose, soybean meal, cottonseed powder, yeast extract and inorganic salts. The individual antibiotics have been separated and purified by ion exchange chromatography. This compound is soluble in H_2O and insoluble in organic solvents. It is effective against gram-positive and gram-negative bacteria, especially *Pseudomonas* species. It is relatively non-toxic with LD_{50} in mice of >400 mg/kg when given intravenously. The antibiotic is optically active with a specific rotation of $[\alpha]_D$ + 60·3 to 61·3° and has the structure given above.

Nara *et al.*, *Japanese Patent*, 76 123,886 (1976)

ANTIBIOTIC P-2563 II
$C_{14}H_{29}N_3O_9$

A further component of the antibiotic complex produced by *Pseudomonas fluorescens* strain P-2563, this compound is a water-soluble powder and has a specific rotation of $[\alpha]_D$ + 76·1 to 77·1° and has the structure given above based upon chemical and spectroscopic data. It has an antibiotic spectrum similar to that of the preceding substance and has a low toxicity in mice with LD_{50} of >400 mg/kg when administered intravenously.

Nara *et al.*, *Japanese Patent*, 76 123,886 (1976)

ANTIBIOTIC P-2563 III
$C_{12}H_{27}N_3O_8$

The simplest of the three antibiotics isolated from the P-2563 complex obtained from cultures of *Pseudomonas fluorescens* strain P-2563, this substance has the structure given above. It is dextrorotatory with a specific rotation of $[\alpha]_D$ + 81·4 to 83·4° and has antibiotic and toxic properties similar to those of the two preceding antibiotics.

Nara *et al.*, *Japanese Patent*, 76 123,886 (1976)

ANTIBIOTIC P-3355
$C_7H_9NO_2$

Isolated from an unidentified organism, this antibiotic possesses both antibacterial and antifungal activity. The structure and stereochemistry have been elucidated from chemical and spectroscopic data.

Sumino *et al.*, *J. Antibiotics* (Japan), **29**, 479 (1976)

ANTIBIOTIC PA 114A
See Ostreogrycin A

ANTIBIOTIC PA-132
See Pentalenolactone

ANTIBIOTIC PBA
$C_{16}H_{17}N_3O_4$

Streptomyces spadicogriseus yields this antibiotic by fermenting an inoculum of a preculture in a medium comprising glucose, meat extract, peptone and

NaCl at pH 7·0 with agitation and aeration at 32–34°C for 2 days. The antibiotic is adsorbed from the culture filtrate onto activated carbon, eluted with Me_2CO, the eluate concentrated, taken up in BuOH, $CHCl_3$–MeOH added and finally chromatographed on silica gel. Laboratory tests showed that antibiotic PBA at 30 g/kg/day prevented the retention of ascites sarcoma 37 in mice two weeks after injection in the abdominal cavity.

Komatsu, *U.S. Patent*, 4,011,140 (1977)

ANTIBIOTIC PS46-B1

Decomp. 255–260°C

Pseudomonoas species PS46-B1 elaborates this antibiotic which is a white powder that turns brown at the temperature given above. It is soluble in H_2O but insoluble in alcohols, AcOEt, Me_2CO and $CHCl_3$. The antibiotic has an antitumour activity and is also effective against *Cochliobolus miyabeanus*. It is comparatively non-toxic with LD_{50} in mice in excess of 600 mg/kg given intraperitoneally.

Minoda, Domori, *Japanese Patent*, 76 151,395 (1976)

ANTIBIOTIC PSX-1

Penicillium stipitatum Thom. furnishes this antibiotic which has been obtained as red plates. It is dextrorotatory with a specific rotation of $[\alpha]_D^{22}$ + 182° (c 1·0, $CHCl_3$). It shows antibacterial activity.

Fuska *et al.*, *J. Antibiotics* (Japan), **27**, 123 (1974)

ANTIBIOTIC R4H

A complex antibiotic of the streptothricin type, this substance has been isolated from cultures of *Streptomyces lavendulae* strain R4 grown on a common medium and extracting the fermentation broth with AcOEt. It is active against gram-positive and gram-negative bacteria and also against mycobacteria. It exhibits no delayed toxicity *in vivo* in mice.

Sawada *et al.*, *J. Antibiotics* (Japan), **27**, 535 (1974)

ANTIBIOTIC RIT D-2214
$C_{12}H_{17}O_6N_3S_2$

A penicillin derivative, this antibiotic is obtained semi-synthetically and also from cultures of *Acremonium chrysogenum*. By the latter method it is isolated by extraction of the culture filtrate and purified by chromatography on an ion exchange resin and azeotropic distillation with *iso*PrOH. The antibiotic is active against gram-positive and gram-negative bacteria.

Troonen, Roelants, Boon, *U.S. Patent*, 3,883,511 (1975)

ANTIBIOTIC Ro 21-6150
$C_{47}H_{78}O_{13}$

A complex polyether antibiotic isolated from cultures of *Streptomyces hygroscopicus* strain X-14563, this substance is normally obtained as the crystalline sodium salt with m.p. 235°C and a specific rotation of $[\alpha]_D$ + 95° (c 1·0, $CHCl_3$). The sodium salt is active *in vitro* against a range of gram-positive bacteria.

Liu *et al.*, *J. Antibiotics* (Japan), **29**, 21 (1975)
Crystal structure
Blount *et al.*, *Chem. Commun.*, 853 (1975)

ANTIBIOTIC RP-17967

M.p. 290–300°C (*dec.*)
An antibiotic elaborated by *Streptomyces roseopullatus*, this compound has a

specific rotation of $[\alpha]_D^{20} + 103°$ (c 0·5, dimethylformamide). It is active against a range of gram-positive bacteria.

Mancy, Ninet, Preud'homme, *German Patent*, 1,924,431 (1970)

ANTIBIOTIC RP-21190
Streptomyces hygroscopicus NRRL 3576 produces this antibiotic when grown on common media. It is active against a number of gram-positive bacteria, particularly *Neisseria* species for which it has minimum inhibition concentrations of 0·6–1·26 µg/ml. It is relatively non-toxic with LD_{50} in mice of 2500 mg/kg when administered subcutaneously.

Mancy, Florent, Preud'homme, *German Patent*, 2,258,537 (1973)

ANTIBIOTIC RP-23671
When grown in common nutrient media, *Streptomyces chryseus* NRRL 3892 yields two related antibiotics which have been isolated by French workers. This compound is active against gram-positive bacteria both *in vitro* and *in vivo* and also possesses antitubercular activity.

Mancy, Florent, Lunel, *British Patent*, 1,314,657 (1973)

ANTIBIOTIC RP-23672
This antibiotic accompanies the preceding compound in the culture filtrate of *Streptomyces chryseus* NRRL 3892. It is separated from it by chromatography on an alumina column. Its antibacterial and antitubercular activity is similar to that of antibiotic RP-23671.

Mancy, Florent, Lunel, *British Patent*, 1,314,657 (1973)

ANTIBIOTIC S-4C-33
$C_{42}H_{67}O_{16}N$
M.p. 126–128°C (*dec.*)
An unclassified strain of *Streptomyces* elaborates this complex antibiotic which is laevorotatory with a specific rotation of $[\alpha]_D^{22} - 44°$ ($CHCl_3$).

Otani, Yokouchi, *Japanese Patent*, 7,000,112 (1970)

ANTIBIOTIC S 15-1
$C_{18}H_{36}O_{10}N_6$
M.p. Indefinite
Antibiotic S 15-1 has been obtained from *Streptomyces griseocarneus* S 15-1 (NRRL 5311) which is cultured in a medium at pH 7·0 containing polypeptone, starch and inorganic salts at 28°C for 50 hours. The substance is isolated by adsorbing the activity of the culture filtrate on Amberlite IRC-50, washing, eluting with dilute HCl, adjusting the pH to 7·0, concentrating the eluate and freeze-drying. The crude antibiotic thus obtained is extracted with CH_3OH and precipitated from $(CH_3)_2CO$ to give the hydrochloride. Antibiotic S 15-1 is active against gram-positive, gram-negative and acid-forming bacteria.

Arima *et al.*, *U.S. Patent*, 3,814,795 (1974)

ANTIBIOTIC S-19
Decomp. 181–182°C
Streptomyces strain S-19 (FERM-P3157) yields this antibiotic when cultured aerobically on a medium comprising glucose, starch, yeast, meat extract and soybean powder at 27°C for 72 hours. The cell extract is adsorbed on Dowex at pH 2·0, eluted with 2M-pyridine-AcOH buffer, concentrated in a vacuum and purified by column chromatography. The antibiotic forms a white, crystalline amphoteric powder having a specific rotation of $[\alpha]_D^{25} - 33·8°$ ($CHCl_3$) and contains histidine, serine and three unidentified amino-acids in the molecule. It is active against *Collectotrichum lagenarium* and *Pellicularia sasaki*. Tests with mice have shown that they survive a dose of 100 mg/kg given intraperitoneally.

Suzuki *et al.*, *Japanese Patent*, 77 12,993 (1977)

ANTIBIOTIC S-232
An antifungal antibiotic, this substance is produced by an unclassified strain of *Streptomyces*. It is stated to have a pentaene structure.

Harcsa *et al.*, *Hung. Teljes*, 6848 (1973)

ANTIBIOTIC S-491β
Aspergillus chevalieri (NRRL 5463), when cultured under carefully controlled aerobic conditions, produces two antibiotics. The mixture is isolated by extracting the fermentation mash with AcOEt, concentrating the extracts *in vacuo* and defatting by partitioning between CH_3OH and *n*-heptane. Separation and purification of the two components is carried out by chromatography and fractional crystallization. Hydrogenation of this antibiotic with sodium borohydride also yields antibiotic S-491.

The antibiotic exhibits *in vitro* activity against protozoa, particularly against *Tetrahymena pyriformis*. The acetate, diacetate, methyl ester and cyclopropyl methyl ester have been prepared and both the antibiotic and these derivatives are active against gram-positive bacteria.

Ellestad, McGahren, *U.S. Patent*, 3,775,433 (1973)

ANTIBIOTIC S-491γ

This compound is separated from the preceding antibiotic by chromatography and fractional crystallization. It also exhibits antiprotozoal activity in a broth dilution test against *Tetrahymena pyriformis* but, unlike antibiotic S-491β, it shows antiviral rather than antimicrobial activity.

Ellestad, McGahren, *U.S. Patent*, 3,775,433 (1973)

ANTIBIOTIC S-583-B

$C_{59}H_{78}O_{20}N$
M.p. Indefinite
Isolated from a culture of *Streptomyces purpurascens*, this complex antibiotic is usually obtained as the dihydrochloride which is an amorphous red powder, m.p. 184–190°C (*dec.*).

Nishimura, Otsuka, *Japanese Patent*, 7,017,600 (1970)

ANTIBIOTIC S-728

$C_{56}H_{93}O_{20}N$
M.p. Indefinite
A complex, amorphous antibiotic, this compound is produced by *Streptomyces* species S-728 (FERM-P972) which is cultured on a medium containing starch, soybean flour, corn steep liquor, glycerol, sodium chloride and calcium carbonate in a jar fermentor at 28°C for 2 days. The antibiotic is extracted from the cells with 60 per cent $(CH_3)_2CO$ and from the culture filtrate with BuOH. The former extract is concentrated under reduced pressure and extracted with BuOH, the two butanol fractions being combined and concentrated and precipitated with AcOEt. Purification is carried out by chromatography on silica gel, being eluted with a mixture of EtOH, $CHCl_3$ and H_2O. Antibiotic S-728 is a yellow powder with no definite melting point, soluble in CH_3OH, EtOH, BuOH and H_2O, insoluble in C_6H_6, AcOEt, $CHCl_3$, $(CH_3)_2CO$ and hexane. It gives a positive ninhydrin reaction and a negative $FeCl_3$ reaction. It is active *in vitro* against gram-positive bacteria and is comparatively toxic, the LD_{50} in mice being 25–50 mg/kg when given intravenously.

Shoji, Wakisaka, Mayama, *Japanese Patent*, 7,380,794 (1973)

ANTIBIOTIC S-887-B

M.p. Indefinite
An antibiotic resembling melanosporin (q.v.), this compound is produced by *Streptomyces melanosporofaciens* by culturing on a common nutrient at 27°C for 4 days. It is isolated by extraction of the culture filtrate with BuOH and the mycelium with 50 per cent aqueous $(CH_3)_2CO$ and purified by chromatography on a silica gel column and treatment with activated carbon. It is active against gram-positive bacteria and fungi and has the following minimum inhibition concentrations (μg/ml): *Candida albicans* (25); *Epidermophytum floccosum* (6·25); *Microsporum gypseum* (12·5) and *Trichophyton rubrum* (>50).

Shoji *et al.*, *Japanese Patent*, 7,322,690 (1973)

ANTIBIOTIC S-3466

This antibiotic complex, consisting of antibiotic S-3466 A, B and C is produced by cultivation of *Streptomyces aureus* ATCC 21,428 on a medium consisting of glucose, peptone, glycerol, meat extract, soybean flour, yeast and inorganic salts at 27°C for 4 days. The individual components are separated by fractionation on a silica gel column using a 2:1 mixture of $CHCl_3$—AcOEt. The complex is particularly active against mites and adult nematodes and has LD_{50} in mice of 3450 mg/kg given orally.

Ando *et al.*, *German Patent*, 2,108,739 (1971)

ANTIBIOTIC S-7481/F 1

A newly discovered antibiotic elaborated by *Cylindrocarpon lucidum* NRRL 5760, this compound as well as being active against *Aspergillus niger*, possesses valuable antiinflammatory and immunosuppressant properties which suggest its use as a treatment for rheumatic diseases and arthritis.

Härri, Ruegger, *German Patent*, 2,455,859 (1975)

ANTIBIOTIC S-7481/F 2

This antibiotic has similar properties to those of the preceding compound. It is obtained from cultures of *Trichoderma polysporum* grown in a common nutrient medium.

Härri, Ruegger, *German Patent*, 2,455,859 (1975)

ANTIBIOTIC S 9508/A-5

This antibiotic has been prepared by cultivating *Streptomyces hygroscopicus* in Pharmamedia 25 and glucose at 27°C for 2–3 days with agitation and inoculating a medium of malt extract and Pharmamedia 25 with the culture and maintaining at 27°C and pH 6·9 for 4–7 days with shaking. The antibiotic has been isolated as the sodium salt which is a white amorphous

Antibiotic SC-28762

powder soluble in organic solvents but insoluble in H_2O. It is effective against a range of gram-positive bacteria.

Keller, Juslen, King, Kis, *Swiss Patent*, 590,924 (1977)

ANTIBIOTIC SC-28762
$C_{34}H_{30}O_{14}$

A number of structurally similar antibiotics have been isolated from cultures of *Spicaria divaricata* NRRL 5771 and separated and purified by column and thin layer chromatography. This antibiotic exhibits inhibitory activity against gram-positive bacteria.

Jiu, Mizuba, *J. Antibiotics* (Japan), **27**, 760 (1974)

ANTIBIOTIC SC-28763
$C_{34}H_{30}O_{13}$

A second component of the antibiotic mixture obtained from cultures of *Spicaria divaricata* NRRL 5771, the structure of this substance is almost identical to that of the preceding antibiotic. It exhibits good antimicrobial activity against anaerobic organisms.

Jiu, Mizuba, *J. Antibiotics* (Japan), **27**, 760 (1974)

ANTIBIOTIC SC-30532
$C_{34}H_{30}O_{12}$

Spicaria divaricata NRRL 5771 also elaborates this antibiotic which has a structure very similar to those of the two preceding antibiotics. At low concentrations it inhibits *Clostridium perfringens* and *Trichomonas vaginolis*. It

possesses very little, if any, activity against aerobic or facultative anaerobic bacteria or fungi.

Mizuba *et al.*, *J. Antibiotics* (Japan), **30**, 670 (1977)

ANTIBIOTIC Sch 14342
$C_{19}H_{38}O_{10}N_4$

An aminoglycosidic antibiotic, this substance is formed as a minor component, with gentamycin (q.v.). It has the same antibacterial activity as gentamycin but is appreciably less toxic, particularly with reference to renal toxicity and ataxia potential.

Waitz *et al.*, *Antimicrobial Agents & Chemotherapy*, **2**, 464 (1972)

ANTIBIOTIC Sch 16656

Actinoplanes strain NRRL 5325 elaborates an antibiotic complex when fermented in a common nutrient medium, the complex having been obtained by extraction of the broth followed by selective precipitation. It consists of at least one major component and three minor components, the major constituent being a heptaene. This component is highly effective against *Candida albicans* and strains of *Torulopsis in vitro* and *in vivo*, being a more potent antibiotic against *C. albicans* than candicidin when taken orally.

Wagman *et al.*, *Antimicrobial Agents & Chemotherapy*, **7**, 457 (1975)

ANTIBIOTIC SE 73
$C_{73}H_{110}O_{38}$
M.p. 196–205°C

An antibiotic possessing animal growth promoting activity, this substance has been prepared by inoculating a preculture of *Actinoplanes* strain SE 73 or SE 73B into a medium consisting of glycerose, defatted soybean powder and $CaCO_3$ and fermenting with agitation at 28°C for 8 days. Extraction of the culture filtrate with Me_2CO, followed by concentration under vacuum, adjustment of the pH to 9·0, extraction with AcOEt, drying the organic phase and precipitation with cyclohexane, gave the crude antibiotic. This was purified by chromatography.

Bauer *et al.*, *German Patent*, 2,510,160 (1975)

ANTIBIOTIC SF-98
$C_{13}H_{20}O_5N_6$
M.p. Indefinite

This peptide antibiotic is derived from *Streptomyces noboritoensis* strain SF-98 which is cultivated in normal media at 27–28°C for 6 days. The activity is adsorbed on an ion exchange resin and the antibiotic isolated as the crystalline sulphate which is soluble in hot H_2O, 1·0 N-HCl and 1·0 N-NaOH, slightly soluble in cold H_2O and insoluble in organic solvents. The antibiotic gives an ultraviolet spectrum in 0·1 N-HCl with an absorption maximum at 238 nm which is shifted to 324 nm in 0·1 N-NaOH. The substance is dextrorotatory with a specific rotation of $[\alpha]_D^{20} + 25°$ (c 1.0, 1N-HCl). The sulphate is active against *Mycobacterium* 607 and *Sarcina lutea* and is comparatively non-toxic with LD_{50} in mice > 150 mg/kg when given intraperitoneally.

Shimura *et al.*, *Japanese Patent*, 7,136,197 (1971)

ANTIBIOTIC SF-666A
$C_7H_{14}O_6$
M.p. 160–170°C (*dec.*)

This antibiotic, and the following compound, have been isolated from the culture filtrate of *Streptomyces setonensis* by treating with activated carbon followed by adsorption on acid and basic ion exchange resins, extraction with CH_3OH, chromatography on a cellulose column and activated carbon, and lyophilization. The structure of this antibiotic has been shown to be that given above. It is soluble in H_2O and CH_3OH and is hygroscopic when pure, being unstable in alkaline solutions. It gives no characteristic absorption in the ultraviolet spectrum. It is dextrorotatory with a specific rotation of $[\alpha]_D^{24} + 38°$ (H_2O) and gives positive anthrone, Benedict, Barfoed and Fehling reactions, negative ninhydrin and orcinol reactions. It has been characterized as the crystalline phenylosazone, m.p. 177°C.

Ezaki *et al.*, *Meiji Seika Kenkyu Nempo*, No. 11, 15 (1970)
Ezaki *et al.*, *Japanese Patent*, 7,021,631 (1970)

ANTIBIOTIC SF-666B
$C_7H_{14}O_6$
M.p. 180–185°C (*dec.*)

$H_3C-CH-CH-CH-CH-COCH_2OH$
       $|$ $|$ $|$ $|$
       OH OH OH OH

Also produced by *Streptomyces setonensis*, this antibiotic is a white, amorphous and hygroscopic powder which is soluble in H_2O and CH_3OH and unstable in alkaline solution. The compound gives positive anthrone, Benedict, Barfoed, orcinol and Molisch reactions and a negative ninhydrin reaction. It may be obtained from the preceding antibiotic by boiling in sodium hydroxide solution at a pH > 10·0 for 20 minutes. The structure has been shown to be 1:3:4:5:6-pentahydroxyheptan-2-one. It is characterized as the phenylosazone, m.p. 175°C.

Ezaki *et al.*, *Meiji Seika Kenkyu Nempo*, No. 11, 15 (1970)

ANTIBIOTIC SF-689
$C_{60}H_{99}O_{14}N_5$
M.p. 145–150°C (*dec.*)

A highly complex antibiotic, this compound is produced by *Streptomyces platensis*, being isolated from the mycelium by extraction with CH_3OH, concentration *in vacuo*, re-extraction with BuOH and chromatography on Amberlite GC-50. The antibiotic is basic and is soluble in dilute acids and aqueous alcohols. It gives a positive $FeCl_3$ reaction and negative Benedict and ninhydrin reactions. With concentrated H_2SO_4 it gives a deep blue colour. The antibiotic is stable in neutral or alkaline solution but unstable in acids or in ultraviolet light.

Tsuruoka *et al.*, *Meiji Seika Kenkyu Nempo*, **11**, 35 (1970)

ANTIBIOTIC SF-689-B
$C_{64}H_{107}O_{15}N_5$
Dec. 142–146°C

Recently, it has been found that the antibiotic described above, when subjected to countercurrent distribution yields a second component and this may be further purified by chromatography on Sephadex G-10 eluted with aqueous BuOH. This antibiotic is weakly basic and is dextrorotatory with a specific rotation of $[\alpha]_D + 66°$ (c 1·0, CH_3OH). The ultraviolet spectrum in CH_3OH has absorption maxima at 243 and 285 nm, with a shoulder at 252–263 nm. It dissolves freely in CH_3OH, aqueous BuOH, AcOH and dilute mineral acids, is moderately soluble in EtOH and BuOH and insoluble in C_6H_6, $(CH_3)_2CO$, $CHCl_3$, AcOEt, Et_2O and H_2O. It gives a positive $FeCl_3$ reaction and negative Benedict and ninhydrin reactions. Like the accompanying antibiotic, it is stable in neutral and alkaline solutions, unstable in acid solutions and ultraviolet light. It is active against gram-positive bacteria and 2–4 times more active against *Staphylococcus albus* and *Staph. aureus* than the preceding antibiotic.

Tsuruoka *et al.*, *Meiji Seika Kenkyu Nempo*, **13**, 21 (1973)

ANTIBIOTIC SF-701
$C_{18}H_{36}O_{11}N_7$
M.p. Indefinite

The culture filtrate of *Streptomyces griseochromogenes* yields this antibiotic which resembles streptothricin. It is normally obtained as the crystalline dihydrochloride, m.p. 210–213°C (*dec.*) with $[\alpha]_D^{24} - 68°$ (c 1·0, H_2O). The base antibiotic gives positive Fehling, Benedict, ninhydrin, Pauly and Elson-Morgan reactions and negative biuret, Sakaguchi, Molisch and $FeCl_3$ tests. It is a broad spectrum antibiotic, active against a range of gram-positive and gram-negative bacteria.

Tsuruoka *et al.*, *J. Antibiotics* (Japan), **21**, 237 (1968)

ANTIBIOTIC SF-767-A
$C_{23}H_{44}O_{15}N_4$
M.p. 190°C (*dec.*)

This antibiotic occurs in cultures of *Streptomyces microsporus*. It has a specific rotation of $[\alpha]_D^{25} + 67°$ (c 1·0, H_2O).

Shomura *et al.*, *Japanese Patent*, 7,017,157 (1970)

ANTIBIOTIC SF-733
$C_{17}H_{34}O_{10}N_4$
M.p. 192–195°C (*dec.*)

A glycosidic antibiotic, this compound has been isolated from cultures of *Streptomyces ribosidificus* and forms colourless needles when purified by recrystallization from CH_3OH. It is dextrorotatory with a specific rotation of $[\alpha]_D^{23} + 42°$ (c 1·0, H_2O). The structure has been deduced by chemical and spectroscopic methods and confirmed by synthesis. It is active against gram-positive bacteria and is comparatively non-toxic with LD_{50} in mice of 1000 mg/kg when administered intravenously.

Shomura *et al.*, *J. Antibiotics* (Japan), **23**, 155 (1970)
Akita *et al.*, *ibid.*, **23**, 173 (1970)
Synthesis
Ito *et al.*, *Agr. Biol. Chem.*, **34**, 980 (1970)
Ito *et al.*, *German Patent*, 2,104,129 (1971)

ANTIBIOTIC SF-773α
$C_{17}H_{34}O_{10}N_4$

Produced by a strain of *Streptomyces*, this antibiotic has the aminoglycosidic structure given above. It is active against a range of gram-positive bacteria. Oxidation of the hydroxymethyl group to the carboxylic acid almost completely destroys the antibacterial activity.

Tsuruoka et al., *Meiji Seika Kenkyu Nempo*, No. 11, 45 (1970)

ANTIBIOTIC SF-837 (*Mydecamycin*)
$C_{41}H_{67}O_{15}N$
M.p. 122–124°C and 155–156°C

Streptomyces mycarofaciens yields four closely related macrocyclic antibiotics which have been extensively investigated by Japanese workers. This compound is prepared by cultivating the organism on a medium consisting of peptone, glucose, soluble vegetable protein, beef extract, soybean oil, sodium chloride and calcium carbonate at pH 7·0 and 28°C for 60–70 hours. It forms a white powder having the lower melting point given above. When recrystallized from a mixture of C_6H_6 and cyclohexane, however, it forms colourless needles with the higher melting point. It has a specific rotation of $[\alpha]_D^{22} - 67°$ (c 1·0, EtOH). The diacetate forms colourless needles from CCl_4 with m.p. 123–124°C.

Antibiotic SF-837 is active *in vitro* against *Mycoplasma pneumoniae* and has a minimum inhibitory concentration against strains of staphylococci of 1·6 μg/ml. It is also highly active against a range of gram-positive bacteria and has a low toxicity. When examined *in vivo* it was as effective as kitasamycin (q.v.) for subcutaneous administration against staphylococcal infections in mice. Some two hours after oral administration to rabbits, the level of the antibiotic in the bile and urine increased to approximately 50 times that of the serum level. Clinical trials have proved promising, the antibiotic being effective in such diseases as acute enterogastritis, colitis and bacterial dysentry although it has no effect in cases of scarlet fever. Following oral or intravenous administration in rats, the antibiotic is rapidly absorbed and metabolized to 14-hydroxy-4″-depropionyl-SF-837 and 4″-depropionyl-SF-837, the former being the major metabolite in bile and the latter in the urine. Similar observations have been made in the cases of dogs and humans. The 3″-O-methylthiomethyl derivative and the corresponding deacetyl compound have been prepared and shown to be useful bactericides.

Niida et al., *J. Antibiotics* (Japan), **24**, 319 (1971)
Tsuruoka et al., *ibid.*, **24**, 452 (1971)
Inouye et al., *ibid.*, **24**, 460 (1971)
Inouye et al., *German Patent*, 2,316,705 (1972)
Fukaya, Nakamura, Kitamoto, *Chemotherapy* (Tokyo), **21**, 692 (1973)
Shomura, Umemura, *Chem. Pharm. Bull.*, **21**, 1824 (1973)

ANTIBIOTIC SF-837-A$_2$
$C_{42}H_{69}O_{15}N$
M.p. 125–128°C

A minor antibiotic obtained from cultures of *Streptomyces mycarofaciens*, this compound is also a white powder having a sharp melting point. It is laevorotatory with a specific rotation of $[\alpha]_D^{22} - 68°$ (c 1·0, EtOH) and gives an ultraviolet spectrum in EtOH having an absorption maximum at 232 nm. On hydrolysis it yields one mole each of propionic and butyric acids. The structure is very similar to that of antibiotic SF-837. The bacterial spectra both *in vitro* and *in vivo* are analogous to those of the preceding antibiotic.

Tsuruoka *et al.*, *J. Antibiotics* (Japan), **24**, 476 (1971)
Tsuruoka *et al.*, *ibid.*, **24**, 526 (1971)
Tsuruoka *et al.*, *Japanese Patent*, 7,203,158 (1972)

ANTIBIOTIC SF-837-A$_3$
$C_{41}H_{65}O_{15}N$
M.p. 122–125°C

A further minor component produced by *Streptomyces mycarofaciens*, antibiotic SF-837-A$_3$ is obtained as a white, amorphous powder. It has a specific rotation of $[\alpha]_D^{22}$ − 44° (c 1·0, EtOH) and is characterized as the acetate, m.p. 182–185°C. It differs in structure from antibiotic SF-837 in having two ketonic groups in the aglycone. The ultraviolet spectrum in EtOH has an absorption maximum at 280 nm. On hydrolysis it liberates two moles of propionic acid. Its biological activity is almost identical to those of the two preceding antibiotics.

Tsuruoka *et al.*, *J. Antibiotics* (Japan), **24**, 476 (1971)
Tsuruoka *et al.*, *ibid.*, **24**, 526 (1971)
Tsuruoka *et al.*, *Japanese Patent*, 7,203,158 (1972)

ANTIBIOTIC SF-837-A$_4$
$C_{42}H_{67}O_{15}N$
M.p. 120–122°C

Streptomyces mycarofaciens also elaborates this minor antibiotic which, like the preceding compounds, is a white amorphous powder. It is also laevo-rotatory having a specific rotation of $[\alpha]_D^{22}$ − 40° (c 1·0, EtOH). The ultra-violet spectrum in EtOH is identical to that of antibiotic SF-837-A$_3$ with a single absorption maximum at 280 nm. Hydrolysis gives one mole each of propionic and butyric acids. It has a similar biological activity and toxicity to that of the major antibiotic.

Tsuruoka *et al.*, *J. Antibiotics* (Japan), **24**, 476 (1971)
Tsuruoka *et al.*, *ibid.*, **24**, 526 (1971)
Tsuruoka *et al.*, *Japanese Patent*, 7,203,158 (1972)

ANTIBIOTIC SF-1130

This antibiotic has been obtained from cultures of *Streptomyces myxogenes* cultivated on media normally used for *Streptomyces* culture. The optimum fermentation temperature is 28°C and the duration is 2–5 days. The compound is isolated from the broth by adsorption on activated carbon at pH 2·0 followed by elution with 50 per cent aqueous $(CH_3)_2CO$ at pH 8·0, the crude material being purified by chromatography on a cellulose column. Antibiotic SF-1130 is active against a number of gram-negative bacteria.

Omoto *et al.*, *Japanese Patent*, 7,330,393 (1973)

ANTIBIOTIC SF-1195
$C_{38}H_{74}O_{11}$

A strain of *Streptomyces hygroscopicus*, SF-1195, freshly isolated from soil, yields this lactone antibiotic when cultivated on a medium containing glucose and Pharmamedia at 28°C for 3 days. The compound is isolated by extraction of the culture filtrate with AcOEt and the mycelium with CH_3OH and purified by crystallization from CH_3OH—AcOEt. It is active against most resistant strains of *Candida albicans*, *Piricularia oryzae* and *Staphylococcus aureus*. The LD_{50} in mice is approximately 100 mg/kg given orally.

Shomura *et al.*, *Japanese Patent*, 7,228,193 (1972)

ANTIBIOTIC SF-1223
$C_{32}H_{21}O_{11}N$ $(C_{30}H_{29}O_{12}N)$
M.p. Indefinite
An antibiotic produced by *Streptomyces hygroscopicus* strain SF-1223, isolated from soil, the compound is soluble in $CHCl_3$, slightly soluble in AcOEt and CH_3OH and insoluble in H_2O. It has a specific rotation of $[\alpha]_D^{23} - 507°$ (c 0·46, $CHCl_3$) and is active against a strain of *Staphylococcus aureus* resistant to erythromycin.

Kondo *et al.*, *Japanese Patent*, 7,301,194 (1973)

ANTIBIOTIC SF-1293
$C_{11}H_{22}O_6N_3P$
M.p. 159–161°C
This phosphorus-containing antibiotic is derived from *Streptomyces hygroscopicus*. Hydrolysis yields alanine and an unidentified phosphorus-containing amino acid, the latter acting as a precursor in the fermentation. Antibiotic SF-1293 inhibits numerous species including *Alternaria kikuchiana*, *A. mali*, *Botrytis cinerea*, *Glomerella cingulata*, *Sclerotinia sclerotiorum* and *Trichophyton asteroides*. *In vivo* studies show that mice tolerate 50 mg/kg (intravenous), 50 mg/kg (intraperitoneal) and 500 mg/kg (oral).

Kondo *et al.*, *Meiji Seika Kenkyu Nempo*, **13**, 34 (1973)

ANTIBIOTIC SF-1306A
$C_{16}H_{25}O_6N_7$
Dec. 170–178°C
When *Streptomyces stechinatus* was cultured on a medium containing soybean oil, millet jelly, soybean flour, soluble vegetable proteni and inorganic salts at pH 7·0 for 4 days at 28°C an antibiotic substance was produced designated antibiotic SF-1306. When adsorbed on Sephadex G-10 saturated with 0·2M-sodium chloride and eluted with the same solution, this is fractionated into two components, A and B. The former is obtained as a white powder, soluble in H_2O and AcOH, giving positive ninhydrin and Molisch tests and negative biuret, $FeCl_3$, Fehling and Sakaguchi reactions. It is laevorotatory with a specific rotation of $[\alpha]_D^{25} - 15·8°$ (H_2O) and gives an ultraviolet spectrum in H_2O with one absorption maximum at 258 nm. The antibiotic is active against plant moulds, especially *Piricularia oryzae* and is also effective against HeLa cells and infiuenza virus. It is more toxic than the accompanying compound, being lethal to mice when administered intravenously as the hydrochloride at a dose of 50 mg/kg.

Shomura *et al.*, *Japanese Patent*, 7,372,394 (1973)
Shomura *et al.*, *Meiji Seika Kenkyu Nempo*, **13**, 64 (1973)
Tsuruoka *et al.*, *Japanese Patent*, 7,380,795 (1973)

ANTIBIOTIC SF-1306B
$C_{18}H_{31}O_6N_7$
Dec. 158–162°C
This component of the antibiotic mixture produced by *Streptomyces echinatus* is separated from the preceding antibiotic by chromatography on Sephadex G-10 saturated with 0·2M-sodium chloride and elution with the same solution. It is a white powder, soluble in H_2O, giving a positive ninhydrin and Molisch test and negative anthrone, biuret, Fehling and $FeCl_3$ reactions. It is dextrorotatory with a specific rotation of $[\alpha]_D^{25} + 14·2°$ (H_2O) and gives an ultraviolet spectrum in H_2O with a single absorption maximum at 258 nm. The antibiotic is active against phytopathogenic fungi and *Candida* species. It is somewhat less toxic than the preceding compound, mice tolerating an intravenous injection of 150 mg/kg of the hydrochloride.

Shomura *et al.*, *Japanese Patent*, 7,372,394 (1973)
Shomura *et al.*, *Meiji Seika Kenkyu Nempo*, **13**, 64 (1973)
Tsuruoka *et al.*, *Japanese Patent*, 7,380,795 (1973)

ANTIBIOTIC SF-1346
$C_8H_{10}O_3N_2$
M.p. 260–261°C (*dec.*)
Streptomyces chiabaensis yields this antibiotic when cultivated on a medium containing soybean powder, millet jelly, soybean oil, soluble vegetable protein and inorganic salts, incubated at 28°C for 3 days. The culture filtrate is passed through a column of Dowex 50 Wx2, eluted with 1-N ammonium hydroxide, adsorbed on activated carbon, eluted with 10 per cent aqueous $(CH_3)_2CO$ and crystallized by concentration after maintaining at 5°C overnight. The antibiotic is soluble in H_2O and CH_3OH, slightly soluble in EtOH, and insoluble in $CHCl_3$, AcOEt, C_6H_6 and petroleum ether. It inhibits *Bacillus subtilis*, *Escherichia coli* and *Piricularia sasaki* and is also effective against rice blast disease.

Inoue *et al.*, *Japanese Patent*, 7,441,595 (1974)

ANTIBIOTIC SF-1623
$C_{15}H_{21}O_{10}N_3S_3$
M.p. Indefinite
Produced by aerobic culture of *Streptomyces chartreusis*, this antibiotic is

formed when sodium, potassium or ammonium thiosulphates are added to the usual fermentation medium for this genus. Purification is carried out by adsorption on an ion exchange resin followed by chromatography on Sephadex. It is usually isolated as the sodium salt which forms a white powder decomposing at 160–165°C, soluble in H_2O and giving a positive ninhydrin reaction. Both the antibiotic and its salts are active in inhibiting the growth of gram-negative bacteria.

Inoue et al., *German Patent*, 2,445,992 (1975)

ANTIBIOTIC SF-1768
B.p. Indefinite
One of a range of antibiotics isolated from cultures of *Streptoverticillium eurocidicus* strain SF 1768, this substance has been prepared by aerobic culture in a medium containing glucose, peptone, wheat germ and NaCl at 28°C for 23 hours at pH 7·0. Extraction of the culture filtrate with AcOEt, concentration of the extract under vacuum, gave a yellow syrup which was purified by dissolving in Me_2CO and subjecting to silica gel chromatography. Antibiotic SF-1768 is a colourless syrup which is soluble in H_2O, the lower alcohols, Me_2CO, AcOEt and $CHCl_3$, insoluble in hexane, C_6H_6, cyclohexane and petroleum ether. The antibiotic is active against both gram-positive and gram-negative bacteria.

Shomura et al., *Japanese Patent*, 76 82,792 (1976)

ANTIBIOTIC SF-1771
Isolated from the aerobic culture of *Streptomyces toyocaensis* strain SF-1771, this copper containing antibiotic forms an H_2O-soluble greenish-blue powder which is useful in cancer therapy. It is also active against gram-positive bacteria. The structure has not yet been fully elucidated.

Ohba et al., *German Patent*, 2,649,604 (1976)

ANTIBIOTIC SF-1771-B
This antibiotic has been prepared by the removal of the copper component from antibiotic SF-1771. It is a colourless, H_2O-soluble powder and has similar antibacterial properties to those of the preceding antibiotic but a lower toxicity.

Ohba et al., *German Patent*, 2,649,604 (1976)

ANTIBIOTIC SF-1774
$C_{10}H_{12}N_2O_5Na_2 \cdot 1 \cdot 5H_2O$
Decomp. 113–115°C
Streptomyces recifensis strain SF-1774 yields this antibiotic when cultured aerobically at 28°C for 24 hours in a liquid medium at pH 7·0. The culture filtrate is treated with activated carbon and an ion exchange resin and eluted with 0·5M NaCl, the eluate decoloured and concentrated to dryness. The residue is then extracted with MeOH and purified by chromatography on activated carbon and an ion exchange resin. The antibiotic is soluble in H_2O and MeOH, insoluble in Me_2CO and $CHCl_3$ and is unstable in acid solutions. It is active against gram-positive bacteria, particularly *Bacillus* and *Clostridium* species.

Shomura et al., *Japanese Patent*, 76 123,893 (1976)

ANTIBIOTIC SF-1854
Decomp. 220°C
This antibiotic is a white amorphous powder which decomposes without melting. It has been obtained by culturing *Micromonospora* strain SF-1854 at 28°C for 80 hours in a medium of wheat germ, starch, soybean meal, soybean oil and inorganic salts at pH 7·0. The antibiotic is adsorbed onto an ion-exchange resin, eluted with 0·5N HCl and purified as the salicylidene derivative. It is active against both gram-positive and gram-negative bacteria.

Shomura et al., *Japanese Patent*, 77 15,896 (1977)

ANTIBIOTIC SKCC-1377
An antibiotic produced by a *Streptomyces* species, this substance is obtained by extraction of the culture filtrate with C_6H_6, followed by concentration *in vacuo*, back extraction with 0·05N-HCl and lycophilization. When prepared in this manner it is a reddish-brown powder, soluble in H_2O, EtOH and $(CH_3)_2CO$, insoluble in C_6H_6 or Et_2O. The solution can withstand 10 minutes heating at 100°C with the pH adjusted to 3·5. Aqueous solutions are yellow at neutral or acid reaction and purple when alkaline. The antibiotic forms a picrate, m.p. 165–168°C (*dec.*) which gives an ultraviolet spectrum with absorption maxima at 245 and 255 nm. This antibiotic is active against gram-positive bacteria but inactive against fungi and *Escheri-*

chia coli. It is very toxic with LD_{50} in mice of only 5 mg/kg when given intraperitoneally.

Reilly, *Bact. Proc.*, 26 (1952)

ANTIBIOTIC SKF-59962
$C_{13}H_{12}O_4N_6S_3F_3Na$

A fluorinated cephalosporin antibiotic, this synthetic substance exhibits a high degree of antibacterial activity both *in vitro* and *in vivo*. It is effective against a wide spectrum of clinical isolates and is more active than either cephalothin and cefazolin (q.v.) when tested against gram-negative organisms *in vitro*. Its activity against gram-positive bacteria is comparable to that of cephalothin. When tested in mice infected with bacterial pathogens it proves more effective than cephalothin and comparable to cefazolin.

Actor *et al.*, *J. Antibiotics* (Japan), **28**, 471 (1975)

ANTIBIOTIC SL-1846
$C_{16}H_{24}O_3$
M.p. 89–92°C

This antitumour antibiotic is produced by preculturing *Pseudeurotium ovalis* NRRL 3194 and inoculating a medium containing glucose, peptone, Bacto-Yeast, malt extract and inorganic salts, fermenting at 27°C for 3 days with agitation and aeration. The antibiotic crystallizes as colourless plates from Et_2O-pentane and is laevorotatory with a specific rotation of $[\alpha]_D^{20} - 117°$ (c 0.4, $CHCl_3$). The ultraviolet spectrum in CH_3OH has a single absorption maximum at 284.5 nm. The compound is active against gram-positive and gram-negative bacteria and also inhibits mastocytoma P-815.

Sigg, Stoll, *French Patent*, 1,503,233 (1967)

ANTIBIOTIC SL-2052
$C_{23}H_{24}O_8$
M.p. 237–238°C

A crystalline antibiotic, this substance is produced by culturing the spores of *Myrothecium roridum* in a medium containing glucose, yeast extract, malt extract, peptone and inorganic salts at 27°C for 4 days with strong aeration. Antibiotic SL-2052 is useful in the treatment of various dermatomycoses in humans and animals. The LD_{50} in mice is 5 mg/kg given orally and 18 mg/kg administered intraperitoneally.

Sigg, Stoll, *French Patent*, 1,503,234 (1967)

ANTIBIOTIC SL-3238
$C_{27}H_{41}O_7N$
M.p. 160–161°C

Isolated from a culture of *Penicillium purpurogenum*, this antibiotic is obtained as colourless needles and is laevorotatory with a specific rotation of $[\alpha]_D^{20} - 102°$ (c 0.47, $CHCl_3$). It is active against gram-positive and gram-negative bacteria.

Bollinger, Sigg, Harri, *German Patent*, 2,005,976 (1970)

ANTIBIOTIC SL 7810 (*Echinocandin B*)
$C_{52}H_{81}N_7O_{16}$
M.p. 160–163°C

A complex macrocyclic antibiotic, this substance has been isolated from cultures of *Aspergillus rugulosus* NRRL 8039, grown in submerged culture. It is a white amorphous powder which is laevorotatory with a specific rotation of $[\alpha]_D^{20} - 48°$ (MeOH). The ultraviolet spectrum in MeOH has absorption maxima at 194 and 276 nm with a shoulder at 226 nm. Antibiotic SL 7810 has little, if any, activity against bacteria but is effective against a range of fungi.

Benz et al., *Helv. Chim. Acta*, **57**, 2459 (1974)
Structure
Keller-Juslen et al., *Tetrahedron Lett.*, 4147 (1976)

ANTIBIOTIC SL-21429

An antibiotic elaborated by *Chaetomium globosum* when cultivated on a medium containing maltose, peptone, yeast extract, bean flour and inorganic salts at 27°C for 10 days. The antibiotic is isolated by extraction of both the culture filtrate and mycelium with CH_2Cl_2 followed by chromatography on a silica gel column. The antibiotic exhibits immunosuppressive, antiulcerous and antiedemic activity in animals.

Closse, Thiele, *German Patent*, 2,200,377 (1972)

ANTIBIOTIC SOB-7

$C_{14}H_{27}O_7N_5$

Antibiotic SOB-7 is obtained by the aerobic fermentation of *Streptomyces lavendulae* ATCC 21,655 in an aqueous medium containing glucose, starch, soybean flour and inorganic salts at 27°C for 68 hours. It is normally obtained as the trihydrochloride or sulphate, both the antibiotic and its salts being active against gram-negative organisms and particularly against *Staphylococcus aureus*. It is comparatively non-toxic, the LD_{50} in mice when given intravenously being 500 mg/kg.

Ando et al., *Japanese Patent*, 7,220,395 (1972)
Ando et al., *German Patent*, 2,208,813 (1972)

ANTIBIOTIC SP-351

This antibiotic complex, consisting of at least four components, has been isolated from cultures of *Streptomyces phaeochromogenes* species 351. The complex is strongly active against gram-positive and gram-negative bacteria.

Yoshida et al., *Abg. Biol. Chem.*, **37**, 661 (1973)

ANTIBIOTIC SS-49

$C_{40}H_{66-68}O_{10-11}$

Streptomyces triangulata produces this antibiotic when grown in a common nutrient medium at 28°C for 2 days. It is isolated by extraction of the culture filtrate with AcOEt followed by chromatography on an alumina column and recrystallization from $CHCl_3$. The antibiotic is active against a range of fungi and yeasts but inactive against bacteria. It is highly toxic to mammals.

Ogawa et al., *Japanese Patent*, 7,228,194 (1972)

ANTIBIOTIC SS-56A

$C_{12}H_{24}O_8N_2$
M.p. 252–254°C (dec.)

One of a number of antibiotics derived from *Streptomyces eurocidicus*, this compound is laevorotatory with a specific rotation of $[\alpha]_D^{25} - 30°$ (c 0·62, H_2O). It forms colourless crystals when recrystallized from EtOH. It is active against gram-positive and gram-negative bacteria and some fungi.

Inouye et al., *J. Antibiotics* (Japan), **26**, 374 (1973)

ANTIBIOTIC SS-56B

$C_{12}H_{24}O_8N_2$
M.p. 229–231°C (dec.)

This antibiotic, obtained from cultures of *Streptomyces eurocidicus*, is an isomer of the preceding compound. It forms colourless crystals from EtOH and is also laevorotatory with a specific rotation of $[\alpha]_D^{25} - 11·5°$ (c 0·93, H_2O). It inhibits the growth of gram-positive and gram-negative bacteria and some fungi.

Inouye et al., *J. Antibiotics* (Japan), **26**, 374 (1973)

ANTIBIOTIC SS-56C

$C_{19}H_{35}O_{14}N_3$
M.p. 201–203°C (dec.)

Also derived from cultures of *Streptomyces eurocidicus*, this antibiotic forms a white amorphous powder. It is dextrorotatory with a specific rotation of

$[\alpha]_D^{25}$ + 12° (c 1·08, H$_2$O). The above aminoglycosidic structure has been established by chemical and spectroscopic methods.

Inouye et al., *J. Antibiotics* (Japan), **26**, 374 (1973)

ANTIBIOTIC SS-56D (*Antibiotic A-396-I*)
C$_{19}$H$_{35}$O$_{13}$N$_3$
M.p. 185–190°C (*dec.*)

This antibiotic which is elaborated by *Streptomyces eurocidicus*, has a structure very similar to that of the preceding compound. It is an amorphous white powder which decomposes at the melting point and is dextrorotatory with a specific rotation of $[\alpha]_D^{25}$ + 12·7° (c 1·02, H$_2$O).

Shoji et al., *J. Antibiotics* (Japan), **23**, 291 (1970)
Inouye et al., *ibid.*, **26**, 374 (1973)

ANTIBIOTIC SS-70-A
Decomp. 188–190°C (hydrochloride)
Streptomyces olivogriseus yields a mixture of two closely related copper-containing antibiotics when cultured on a fermentation medium containing a copper salt. The antibiotics have been isolated from the culture filtrate as their hydrochlorides and separated and purified by column chromatography on an ion-exchange resin. Chemical analysis has shown the antibiotic to contain nitrogen, sulphur and chlorine in addition to copper. It is a wide spectrum antibiotic active against both gram-positive and gram-negative bacteria.

Ohba et al., *Meiji Seika Kenkyu Nempo*, **16**, 29 (1976)

ANTIBIOTIC SS-70-B
Decomp. 188–190°C (hydrochloride)
A second constituent of the antibiotic mixture elaborated by *Streptomyces olivogriseus*, this antibiotic also contains nitrogen, sulphur, chlorine and copper in the molecule. It has been isolated as the hydrochloride which decomposes without melting. The antibiotic spectrum is virtually identical to that of the preceding antibiotic.

Ohba et al., *Meiji Seika Kenkyu Mempo*, **16**, 29 (1976)

ANTIBIOTIC SS-228Y
C$_{19}$H$_{14}$O$_6$
M.p. 256–266°C (*dec.*)

This *peri*-hydroxyquinone type antibiotic has been isolated from cultures of a species of *Chainia* found in shallow sea mud in Sagami Bay. It forms an orange or yellow-brown powder and is laevorotatory with a specific rotation of $[\alpha]_D$ − 85° (c 1·0, Me$_2$CO). The ultraviolet and visible spectrum in aqueous MeOH has absorption maxima at 218 and 440–460 nm with shoulders at 228 and 415 nm. The structure given above has been established from a study of the infrared, ultraviolet, NMR and mass spectra. Antibiotic SS-228Y is active against gram-positive bacteria and Ehlich carcinoma in mice. It inhibits dopamine-β-hydroxylase.

Okazaki, Kitahara, Okami, *J. Antibiotics* (Japan), **28**, 176 (1975)
Kitahara et al., *ibid.*, **28**, 280 (1975)

ANTIBIOTIC T
See Crotocin

ANTIBIOTIC T-1226
See Piperacillin

ANTIBIOTIC T-2636 A
See Bundlin B

ANTIBIOTIC T-2636 B
C$_{43}$H$_{72}$O$_{17}$
M.p. 205–207°C

This antibiotic is obtained from *Streptomyces rochei* var. *bolubilis*. It forms colourless crystals and has a specific rotation of $[\alpha]_D - 92.4°$ (c 1·0, EtOH).

Harada *et al.*, *Tetrahedron Lett.*, 2239 (1969)
Higeshide *et al.*, *J. Antibiotics* (Japan), **24**, 1 (1971)
Harada, Kishi, Mizuno, *ibid.*, **24**, 13 (1971)

ANTIBIOTIC T-2636 C
See Bundlin A

ANTIBIOTIC T-2636 D (*Lankacidinol A*)
$C_{27}H_{37}O_8N$
M.p. 190–191°C (dec.)

A further antibiotic isolated from *Streptomyces rochei* var. *bolubilis*, this macrocyclic compound is laevorotatory with a specific rotation of $[\alpha]_D - 226°$ (c 1·0, EtOH) and gives an ultraviolet spectrum in EtOH with an absorption maximum at 229 nm.

Harada *et al.*, *Tetrahedron Lett.*, 2239 (1969)
Higeshide *et al.*, *J. Antibiotics* (Japan), **24**, 1 (1971)
Harada, Kishi, Mizuno, *ibid.*, **24**, 13 (1971)

ANTIBIOTIC T-2636 E
$C_{26}H_{37}O_5N$
M.p. 228–230°C (dec.)

Streptomyces rochei var. *bolubilis* also elaborates this antibiotic which is obtained in the form of colourless needles when recrystallized from $(CH_3)_2CO$. It is strongly laevorotatory with a specific rotation of $[\alpha]_D^{25} - 320°$ (c 0·25, EtOH—$(CH_3)_2SO$).

Higashide *et al.*, *J. Antibiotics* (Japan), **24**, 1 (1971)
Harada, Kishi, Mizuno, *ibid.*, **24**, 13 (1971)

ANTIBIOTIC T-2636 F (*Lankacidinol F*)
$C_{25}H_{35}O_7N$
M.p. 178–179°C (dec.)

Isolated from cultures of *Streptomyces rochei* var. *bolubilis*, this antibiotic forms colourless needles and has a specific rotation of $[\alpha]_D - 210°$ (c 1·0, dimethylformamide). The ultraviolet spectrum in EtOH has a single absorption maximum at 228 nm. The 14-acetate is antibiotic T-2636 D and the 2′:8:14-triacetate has also been prepared as colourless needles with m.p. 211–215°C (dec.).

Harada *et al.*, *Tetrahedron Lett.*, 2230 (1969)
Higeshide *et al.*, *J. Antibiotics* (Japan), **24**, 1 (1971)
Harada, Kishi, Mizuno, *ibid.*, **24**, 13 (1971)
Fugono *et al.*, *ibid.*, **24**, 23 (1971)
Harada, Kishi, *Chem. Pharm. Bull.*, **22**, 99 (1974)

ANTIBIOTIC T-2636M
Japanese workers have isolated this antibiotic from cultures of *Streptomyces rochei* var. *bolubilis*. It forms a yellow crystalline powder and has a specific rotation of $[\alpha]_D^{24} - 210°$ (c 0·5, EtOH).

Higashide *et al.*, *J. Antibiotics* (Japan), **24**, 1 (1971)
Harada, Kishi, Mizuno, *ibid.*, **24**, 13 (1971)

ANTIBIOTIC T-7545
$C_{19-21}H_{33-37}O_{13-15}N$
M.p. Indefinite
An antibiotic isolated from cultures of *Streptomyces hygroscopicus* var. *limoneus* freshly obtained from soil, this compound is soluble in H_2O and has weakly basic properties. It is characterized as the crystalline hydrochloride and acetate. Antibiotic T-7545 is inactive *in vitro* but is effective against *Pellicularia sasaki* disease in rice at a level of 10–20 µg/ml.

Shibata *et al.*, *Japanese Patent*, 7,128,831 (1971)

ANTIBIOTIC T-24146
An antibiotic produced by the submerged culture of *Streptomyces viridochromogenes* strain T-24146 in common carbohydrate-containing media, cultivated at 28°C for 90 hours. The antibiotic is isolated by extracting the culture filtrate with AcOEt at pH 4·0 and evaporation of the solvent. It is active against gram-positive bacteria, particularly *Bacillus subtilis* and *Staphylococcus aureus* and is also effective against protozoa such as *Trichomonas vaginalis*, the minimum inhibition concentration against the latter being 0·062–0·125 µg/ml.

Hagegawa *et al.*, *German Patent*, 2,161,568 (1972)

ANTIBIOTIC T-41348
An antibiotic produced by *Streptomyces recifensis* strain T-41348, this substance is obtained by culturing the organism aerobically at 28°C for 36 hours on a medium containing glycerol, peptone, meat extract, NaCl and $FeCl_2$. The antibiotic is purified by extraction of the fermentation broth with an organic solvent followed by column chromatography.

Hasegawa *et al.*, *Japanese Patent*, 77 83,857 (1977)

ANTIBIOTIC T-42082
Streptomyces hygroscopicus T-42082 (FERM-P 2691) elaborates this antibiotic when cultured aerobically at 28°C for 140 hours in corn steep liquor, glucose, starch, soybean meal, peptone, NaCl and $CaCO_3$ The antibiotic is obtained by the addition of an equal volume of Me_2CO to the culture filtrate, stirring and filtering, concentrating the liquor to a syrup and chromatographing.

Imada *et al.*, *Japanese Patent*, 77 83,805 (1977)

ANTIBIOTIC Ta-146
Decomp. >150°C
This antibiotic forms a reddish-violet, optically inactive powder which is insoluble in H_2O but soluble in organics solvents. It has been obtained by culturing *Streptomyces* strain Ta-146 at 47°C for 24 hours at pH 7·0 in a medium comprising soybean meal, starch and inorganic salts, extracting the culture filtrate with BuOH at pH 3·0, concentrating the extract to dryness under vacuum, suspending the residue in C_6H_6 and chromatographing on silica gel. The antibiotic is effective against gram-positive bacteria, *Salmonella* and *Shigella*. It has LD_{50} in mice of 21·5 mg/kg when administered intraperitoneally.

Okazaki, Saito., *Japanese Patent*, 76 139,692 (1976)

ANTIBIOTIC TL-119
$C_{42}H_{56}N_6O_9$
Decomp. >250°C

A complex antibiotic isolated from cultures of *Bacillus subtilis*, this substance decomposes without melting and is laevorotatory with a specific rotation of $[\alpha]_D^{24} - 8·7°$ (c 0·482, Me_2SO). It is effective against bacteria and fungi and also acts as an enzyme inhibitor.

Shoji *et al.*, *J. Antibiotics* (Japan), **28**, 126 (1975)
Structure
Nakagawa, Nakazawa, Shoji, *J. Antibiotics* (Japan), **28**, 1004 (1975)

ANTIBIOTIC TS-106
M.p. Indefinite
Antibiotic TS-106 is produced by *Klebsiella* strain TS-106 grown in a medium containing glucose, sodium glutamate and inorganic salts and

cultured with shaking at 37°C for 3 days. The dried cells are extracted with aqueous phosphoric acid and precipitated with $(CH_3)_2CO$. The antibiotic is a lipopolysaccharide and is effective against gastric ulcer, hepatitis virus and Ehrlich ascites sarcoma. It has LD_{50} in mice of 215 mg/kg when given intravenously.

Tomioka et al., *Japanese Patent*, 7,118,597 (1971)

ANTIBIOTIC TS-0822

An antibacterial antibiotic produced by culturing *Streptomyces eurocidicus* var. *asterocidicus* at 27°C and pH 7·2 for 72 hours on a medium containing glucose, peptone and inorganic salts. The structure has not yet been fully established.

Ishida, Hokune, *Japanese Patent*, 75 126,893 (1975)

ANTIBIOTIC TS-885
$C_{17}H_{25}O_4N$
M.p. 135–140°C

A novel antibiotic produced by *Streptomyces pluricolorescens* var. *yamashitaensis*, the organism is cultured with shaking on a medium at pH 7·4 containing meat extract, peptone, starch, glycerol and inorganic salts at 27°C for 4 days. The antibiotic is isolated by extracting the filtrate at pH 5·0 with AcOEt and purified by silica gel chromatography eluting with AcOEt—C_6H_6 and by thin layer chromatography on silica, developing with AcOEt. The pure compound is a pale yellow oil which is dextrorotatory with a specific rotation of $[\alpha]_D^{27} + 105°$ and is soluble in $CHCl_3$, C_6H_6, $(CH_3)_2CO$, AcOEt, CH_3OH, EtOH, pyridine and dilute HCl but insoluble in Et_2O and H_2O. It gives positive Ehrlich and *m*-phenylenediamine tests and negative ninhydrin and Tollens reactions.

Antibiotic TS-885 has the structure 3-(5:7-dimethyl-2-hydroxy-4-oxo-6:8-decadienyl)glutarimide. It has only a slight activity against bacteria but is highly active against fungi and viruses, particularly poliovirus and tumours, inhibiting the growth of ascites tumours in mice. It also inhibits the growth of HeLa cells at a concentration of 1·2 µg/ml. It is relatively non-toxic, mice showing no abnormal symptoms when given 20 mg/kg each day for 10 days.

Ishida, Okada, Kamata, *Japanese Patent*, 7,447,596 (1974)
Ishida, Okada, Kamata, *German Patent*, 2,342,404 (1974)

ANTIBIOTIC U-11,921
$C_{19}H_{36}O_6N_2S$

This antibiotic, isolated from *Streptomyces lincolnensis*, is closely related to lincomycin (q.v.). It forms a crystalline hydrochloride as the monohydrate which has $[\alpha]_D^{25} + 143°$. The structure has been established by chemical and spectroscopic methods. It is active against gram-positive bacteria.

Argoudelis et al., *J. Amer. Chem. Soc.*, **96**, 5044 (1964)

ANTIBIOTIC U-11,973 (*N-Demethyllincomycin*)
$C_{17}H_{32}O_6N_2S$
M.p. Indefinite

A further antibiotic obtained from cultures of *Streptomyces lincolnensis*, this compound is characterized as the hydrochloride monohydrate which, like that of the preceding substance, is dextrorotatory with a specific rotation of $[\alpha]_D^{25} + 149°$ (c 0·9, H_2O). N-methylation yields lincomycin (q.v.). This antibiotic is active against a range of gram-positive and gram-negative organisms.

Argoudelis et al., *J. Amer. Chem. Soc.*, **86**, 5044 (1964)

ANTIBIOTIC U-12,241

A variant of *Streptomyces bellus*, *S. bellus* var. *cirolerosus*, elaborates this antibiotic which is active against a number of gram-positive bacteria *in vitro* and is highly cytotoxic to KB cells and L-120 cells grown in culture. It is also active *in vivo* against Walker carcinosarcoma 256. The LD_{50} for mice is 5·6 mg/kg given intraperitoneally and dogs tolerate a dose of 1·2 mg/kg given subcutaneously.

Bhuyan, Dietz, *Antimicrobial Agents & Chemotherapy*, 426 (1967)

ANTIBIOTIC U-12,898

See Bluensomycin

ANTIBIOTIC U-13,933 (*Asperlin*)

$C_{10}H_{12}O_5$
M.p. 71–73°C

Aspergillus nidulans produces this antibiotic which is of interest in that it contains a cyclopropane ring in the molecule. It forms colourless crystals and is dextrorotatory with a specific rotation of $[\alpha]_D^{25} + 345°$ (c 0·9, 95 per cent EtOH). The ultraviolet spectrum exhibits a single absorption maximum at 204 nm. The structure has been determined primarily from the NMR spectrum.

Argoudelis, Zieserl, *Tetrahedron Lett.*, 1969 (1966)
Tahabe et al., *J. Amer. Chem. Soc.*, **93**, 273 (1971)

ANTIBIOTIC U-20,943

$C_{18}H_{34}O_6N_2S$

One of several structurally similar antibiotics isolated from *Streptomyces lincolnensis*, this substance forms a hydrochloride as the crystalline monohydrate which is dextrorotatory with a specific rotation of $[\alpha]_D^{25} + 153°$. The structure has been established from chemical and spectroscopic evidence and comparison with those of similar antibiotics. It has an inhibitory activity against gram-positive bacteria.

Argoudelis et al., *J. Amer. Chem. Soc.*, **86**, 5044 (1964)

ANTIBIOTIC U-21,699

$C_{17}H_{32}O_6N_2S$

Also produced by *Streptomyces lincolnensis*, this antibiotic forms a crystalline hydrochloride as the hemihydrate. This salt is dextrorotatory with a specific rotation of $[\alpha]_D^{25} + 147°$. The structure is methylthio-antibiotic U-20,943. It has a similar activity against gram-positive bacteria.

Argoudelis et al., *J. Amer. Chem. Soc.*, **86**, 5044 (1964)

ANTIBIOTIC U-42,126

$C_5H_7O_3N_2Cl$

Streptomyces sviceus elaborates this simple antibiotic which forms colourless crystals from aqueous CH_3OH. The crystal structure has been determined by X-ray crystallographic analysis. The antibiotic is active only against fungi *in vitro*, but inhibits both *Bacillus subtilis* and *Escherichia coli* when cultivated on a synthetic medium. In mice infected with L-1210 and P-388 leukemias, it prolongs life by 40 per cent and 37 per cent respectively when given at a dose of 400 mg/kg.

Hanka, Dietz, *Antimicrobial Agents & Chemotherapy*, **3**, 425 (1973)

ANTIBIOTIC U-43,120
$C_{34}H_{44}N_2O_{18}S$

A complex antibiotic, this substance has been obtained by the aerobic culture of *Streptomyces paulus* NRRL 8115 in a medium of glucose, malt extract, corn steep liquor and peptone at 25°C for 5 days. It has been purified by filtering the culture broth followed by chromatography on silica gel. The antibiotic is active primarily against gram-positive bacteria.

Wiley, *J. Antibiotics* (Japan), **29**, 587 (1976)
Hanka, Wiley, *U.S. Patent*, 3,988,441 (1976)

ANTIBIOTIC U-43,795
$C_5H_7N_2O_4Cl$

A simple antitumour antibiotic, this compound has been isolated from cultures of *Streptomyces sviceus*. The structure given above has been elucidated from chemical and spectroscopic evidence.

Martin *et al.*, *J. Antibiotics* (Japan), **28**, 91 (1975)

ANTIBIOTIC U-50,147
This antibiotic has been obtained, together with antibiotic U-51,738 (q.v.) by culturing *Streptomyces lemensis* NRRL 8170 on a medium containing glucose monohydrate, Bacto-Yeast extract and Bactopeptone. A seed inoculum is then incubated on a fermentation medium comprising starch, cottonseed meal and glucose with agitation at 28°C for 5 days. The antibiotic has been separated and purified by filtration with diatomaceous earth and chromatography on ion-exchange resins. It is active against gram-positive bacteria.

Argoudelis, Johnson, *U.S. Patent*, 4,029,548 (1977)

ANTIBIOTIC U-50,228
An antibiotic elaborated by *Streptomyces platensis clarensis*, this substance is prepared by culturing the organism in a medium containing glucose, molasses, yeast extract, protease peptone and dextrin at 28°C for 5–12 days with shaking. The broth is filtered, passed through a column of activated carbon and eluted successively with 10 per cent, 25 per cent and 50 per cent Me_2CO in H_2O. The eluates are then lyophilized and subjected to countercurrent distribution chromatography in 1:1 $BuOH$–H_2O. Antibiotic U-50,228 has been characterized as the 1-methylpseudouridine.

Argoudelis, Mizsak, *U.S. Patent*, 3,988,314 (1976)

ANTIBIOTIC U-51,738
Produced with antibiotic U-50,147 (q.v.), this antibiotic has been separated from the latter by chromatographic methods. It is active against gram-positive bacteria.

Argoudelis, Johnson, *U.S. Patent*, 4,029,548 (1977)

ANTIBIOTIC vD-844
$C_7H_6O_2N_2S_2$
M.p. 181–182°C

An unclassified species of *Streptomyces* yields this antibiotic, isolated as yellow needles. The structure has been shown to be 4:5-dihydro-6-N-methylformylamino-5-oxo-1:2-dithiolo 4,3-b pyrrole. The crystal structure has been determined from X-ray crystallographic data.

von Daene *et al.*, *J. Antibiotics* (Japan), **22**, 233 (1969)
Crystal structure
Jensen, *J. Antibiotics* (Japan), **22**, 231 (1969)
Jensen, *Acta Cryst.*, **27B**, 392 (1971)

ANTIBIOTIC VI-7501
An antitumour antibiotic, this compound is produced by a number of *Actinomyces* and *Streptomyces* species, particularly *S. griseus*. Good yields have been obtained by culturing the latter on a medium of glucose, peptone, beef extract and NaCl at 28–29°C for 2 days. It is ineffective against bacteria

and yeasts but shows *in vitro* activity against AH-66, EAC, S-180 and Yoshada cells and has been found to protect mice against EAC and S-180 tumour cells *in vivo*. The LD_{50} in mice has been reported as 1.5×10^5 BDI units/kg when administered intraperitoneally.

Sumiyama *et al.*, *German Patent*, 2,639,410 (1977)
Tsukuni *et al.*, *Japanese Patent*, 77 83,501 (1977)

ANTIBIOTIC W7783
See Ambruticin

ANTIBIOTIC Wr-142
An antibiotic prepared from a *Streptomyces* species, this substance is a glycopeptide which inhibits DNA, RNA and protein synthesis in cells of *Bacillus subtilis*. Although the antibiotic inhibits the formation of 16S and 23S ribosomal RNA, it has no effect on the formation of low molecular weight RNA (4-5S). It would appear that the inhibitory effect of this antibiotic on protein and nucleic acid synthesis is responsible for the antitumour and antibacterial effect.

Szyba, Mordarski, *Acta Microbiol. Pol.*, **5A**, 81 (1973)

ANTIBIOTIC Wr-142-FPG
An antifungal antibiotic, this substance has been isolated from the culture broth and mycelia of *Streptomyces olivaceus*. It has a molecular weight of approximately 510. Antibiotic Wr-142-FPG is cytotoxic and has a higher pathogenic activity to yeasts than many commonly used antibiotics. It is toxic to mice having LD_{50} 5 mg/kg.

Mordarsku, Wieczorek, Szowazuk, *Arch. Immunol. Exp. Ther., Pol. Acad. Sci., Warsaw*, **25**, 273 (1977)

ANTIBIOTIC WS-4545
$C_{12}H_{18}O_7N_2$

ANTIBIOTIC X-206

Streptomyces sapporensis produces this antibiotic when cultivated aerobically in a common medium at 30°C for 2 days. The compound is extracted from the culture broth with CH_3CO and the solvent removed *in vacuo*. The antibiotic forms colourless crystals and is active against a number of gram-positive and gram-negative bacteria. When tested against antibiotic-resistant strains of *Escherichia coli* its activity was more than ten times greater than other known compounds.

A number of monoacylated derivatives have been prepared, including the acetyl, benzoyl, cinnamoyl, nicotinoyl, 2-thienoyl and cyclohexyl-carbonyl, which are more readily absorbed into the body on oral administration than the parent antibiotic.

Miyoshi *et al.*, *German Patent*, 2,150,593 (1972)
Kamyia, Maeno, *Belgian Patent*, 815,530 (1974)

ANTIBIOTIC WS-8096
$C_{22}H_{20}O_{10}$
M.p. Indefinite

This antibiotic is produced by both *Streptomyces candidus* var. *enterostaticus* and *S. viridochromogenes* strain M-127, both freshly isolated from soil. The culture filtrate is extracted with AcOEt and the extract chromatographed on an alumina column with $CHCl_3$—CH_3OH. The antibiotic is a neutral crystalline compound, soluble in H_2O and CH_3OH and giving a positive Fehling reaction. It is relatively non-toxic and possesses a synergistic action with both chloramphenicol and streptomycin.

Miyoshi *et al.*, *Japanese Patent*, 7,215,750 (1972)

ANTIBIOTIC X-206
$C_{45}H_{78}O_{13}$
M.p. 133–145°C

An antibiotic from *Streptomyces* species, this substance may be extracted both from the broth and the mycelium filtrate. From the former it is extracted with butyl acetate, followed by concentration *in vacuo* and back extraction with phosphate buffer at pH 8·9. From the mycelium it is extracted with EtOH—CH$_3$OH, concentrated *in vacuo*, extracted with butyl acetate followed by back extraction with phosphate buffer at pH 8·9. Further purification is then obtained by chromatography on an alumina column. The antibiotic is an organic acid which forms colourless crystals and is dextrorotatory with a specific rotation of $[\alpha]_D^{20} + 15°$ (CH$_3$OH). It is insoluble in H$_2$O or alkali but soluble in alcohols, (CH$_3$)$_2$CO, Et$_2$O, esters and petroleum ether. There is no characteristic absorption in the ultraviolet spectrum and the antibiotic is stable only in neutral solution.

While it is not active *in vivo* against either bacterial or protozoal infections, it is active *in vitro* against gram-positive bacteria and mycobacteria. It is highly toxic with LD$_{50}$ in mice of 11 mg/kg on subcutaneous administration.

Berger *et al.*, *J. Amer. Chem. Soc.*, **73**, 5295 (1951)
Crystal structure
  Blount, Westley, *Chem. Commun.*, 927 (1971)

ANTIBIOTIC X-464
See Polyetherin A

ANTIBIOTIC X-537A (*Lasalocid A*)
C$_{34}$H$_{54}$O$_8$
M.p. 110–114°C

An antibiotic produced by several *Streptomyces* species, this compound has a specific rotation of $[\alpha]_D^{25} - 7·55°$ (c 1·0, CH$_3$OH) and gives an ultraviolet spectrum in *iso*PrOH with absorption maxima at 248 and 318 nm. The sodium salt forms colourless crystals, m.p. 168–171°C; $[\alpha]_D^{25} - 30°$ (c 1·0, CH$_3$OH). The antibiotic has been shown to be identical with Lasalocid A obtained from cultures of *Streptomyces lasaliensis*. By the use of ^{13}C and ^{14}C labelled precursors in the substrate it has been demonstrated that the antibiotic is composed of five acetate, four propionate and three butyrate groups and that the ethyl group in the molecule arises from butyrate and 2-ethylmalonate.

Berger *et al.*, *J. Amer. Chem. Soc.*, **73**, 5295 (1951)
Westley *et al.*, *Chem. Commun.*, **71** (1970)
Johnston *et al.*, *J. Amer. Chem. Soc.*, **92**, 4428 (1970)
Johnston *et al.*, *Chem. Commun.*, 72 (1970)
Biosynthesis
  Westley *et al.*, *Chem. Commun.*, 1467 (1970)
  Westley *et al.*, *Chem. Commun.*, 161 (1972)
  Westley *et al.*, *J. Antibiotics* (Japan), **27**, 288 (1974)
Crystal structure
  Schmidt, Wang, Paul, *J. Amer. Chem. Soc.*, **96**, 6189 (1974)

ANTIBIOTIC X-5108 (*Goldinodox*)
C$_{44}$H$_{62}$O$_{12}$N$_2$
M.p. Indefinite

Antibiotic X-5108 has been obtained from *Streptomyces* X-5108, subculture 3191-2 (*S. goldiniensis*) by aerobic fermentation at 28°C and pH 6·8 on a medium containing carbon and nitrogen sources and inorganic salts. The filtered medium is extracted with butyl acetate and the isolated extract purified by chromatography on Sephadex LH-20. The antibiotic is insoluble in H$_2$O but soluble in the lower alcohols. It forms a sodium salt which is laevorotatory with a specific rotation of $[\alpha]_D^{25} - 82·8°$ (c 0·52, EtOH). Structurally, the antibiotic is the N-methyl derivative of mocimycin (q.v.). It exhibits a broad spectrum antimicrobial activity and enhances the growth rate of chicks when included in the feed at a concentration of 0·0001–0·01 parts by weight.

Maehr *et al.*, *Helv. Chim. Acta*, **55**, 3051 (1972)
Berger, *U.S. Patent*, 3,657,421 (1972)
Berger, *German Patent*, 2,140,322 (1972)
Maehr *et al.*, *J. Amer. Chem. Soc.*, **95**, 8449 (1973)
Maehr *et al.*, *Helv. Chim. Acta*, **57**, 212 (1974)
Maehr *et al.*, *J. Amer. Chem. Soc.*, **96**, 4034 (1974)

ANTIBIOTIC XB-94
$C_6H_8O_4$

A strain of *Streptomyces*, MCRL-0738 (FERM-P 1110), similar to *S. eurythermus*, yields this simple antibiotic when cultivated in a medium containing glucose, starch, glycerol, soybean flour and inorganic salts at 27°C and pH 7·0 for 6 days. The antibiotic is active against a wide range of gram-positive and gram-negative bacteria particularly against *Corynebacterium*, *Mycobacterium* and *Neisseria* species. No abnormal symptoms were observed in mice given 400 mg/kg intravenously.

Okuda, Awataguchi, *Japanese Patent*, 7,339,691 (1973)

ANTIBIOTIC XB-94-F$_2$
$C_8H_{10}O_5$
M.p. Indefinite

Streptomyces species MRCL-0738 (FERM-P1110) which has been identified as a mutant strain of *S. eurythermus* elaborates this antibiotic which is formed when the organism is cultured aerobically in a medium consisting of starch, glucose, glycerol, soybean flour, sodium chloride and calcium carbonate. The substance is isolated by adsorption on activated carbon and eluted with 20 per cent aqueous $(CH_3)_2CO$. It is further purified by column and paper chromatography when it forms a colourless gluten-like solid with no definite melting point. It is freely soluble in H_2O, moderately so in CH_3OH, EtOH, $CHCl_3$, $(CH_3)_2CO$, $(CH_3)_2SO$, pyridine and dimethylformamide. The structure has been established by chemical and spectroscopic methods. The antibiotic is active against gram-positive bacteria and is comparatively non-toxic, mice showing no abnormal symptoms when injected with 150 mg/kg intravenously.

Awaguchi, Okuda, *Japanese Patent*, 7,361,691 (1973)

ANTIBIOTIC XK-19-1-1
See Streptolysin

ANTIBIOTIC XK-19-1-2
M.p. Indefinite
One of a number of antibiotics produced by submerged culture of *Streptomyces verticillus* var. *tsukushiensis* on common media at 25–30°C and pH 7·0 for 3 days. Separation and purification of the components is carried out by repeated chromatography of the broth filtrate. This antibiotic is active against gram-positive and gram-negative bacteria.

Nara *et al.*, *Japanese Patent*, 7,330,399 (1973)

ANTIBIOTIC XK-19-2
M.p. >200°C (*dec.*)
A further antibiotic elaborated by *Streptomyces verticillus* var. *tsukushiensis*, this substance is separated from the accompanying compounds by repeated chromatography of the broth liquor. It forms a white amorphous powder and is active against gram-positive and gram-negative bacteria, acid-fast bacteria, dysentery bacilli and particularly against *Escherichia coli*, *Klebsiella pneumoniae* and *Salmonella* species.

Nara *et al.*, *Japanese Patent*, 7,330,399 (1973)
Takasawa *et al.*, *J. Antibiotics* (Japan), **26**, 471 (1973)

ANTIBIOTIC XK-33-F$_2$
M.p. Indefinite
Japanese workers have isolated this antibiotic by aerobically culturing *Streptomyces olivoreticuli* var. *cellulophilus* ATCC 21,632 on a medium containing glucose, soybean flour and calcium carbonate at 30°C for 3 days. This antibiotic is similar in many respects to the tuberactinomycins and viomycin.

Nara *et al.*, *German Patent*, 2,165,644 (1972)

ANTIBIOTIC XK-41
See Megalomycins

ANTIBIOTIC XK-46
Dec. 64–76°C
Isolated from cultures of a thermophilic *Streptomyces* species MK-46, this antibiotic is formed at an optimum incubation temperature of 46°C. It is obtained as deep red crystals which decompose without melting and is a colour indicator being red in acidic solutions and blue in alkalies. It is dextrorotatory with a specific rotation of $[\alpha]_D^{23} + 212°$. It is slightly soluble

in H_2O and freely soluble in organic solvents. Antibiotic XK-46 is active against gram-positive bacteria and also against *Proteus vulgaris*. It is a powerful inhibitor of tyrosine hydroxylase activity.

Nara *et al.*, *Japanese Patent*, 7,349,991 (1972)
Takasawa *et al.*, *J. Antibiotics* (Japan), **27**, 502 (1974)

ANTIBIOTIC XK-49-1-B-2

This antibiotic is produced by *Streptosporangium violaceochromogenes* ATGC 21807 cultured in an aqueous medium containing nutrients at 30°C with aeration. The compound is isolated by filtering the culture broth and chromatographing on an alumina column. Antibiotic XK-49-1-B-2 is active against both gram-positive and gram-negative bacteria and possesses antitumour activity against Ehrlich-Ascites tumour cells and sarcoma 180 *in vivo* in mice.

Nara *et al.*, *German Patent*, 2,344,780 (1974)

ANTIBIOTIC XK-62-2
See Sagamicin

ANTIBIOTIC XK-88-1
See Seldomycin Factor 1

ANTIBIOTIC XK-90
$C_9H_{10}N_2O_3$

Streptomyces species MK-90 yields this simple antibiotic which has the structure given above based upon chemical analysis and spectroscopic data. It is effective against gram-positive and gram-negative bacteria and also weakly active against *Mycobacterium tuberculosis* H37Rv with a minimum inhibitory concentration of 50–100 micrograms/millilitre. The acute toxicity in mice by intravenous injection is greater than 400 mg/kg.

Takasawa *et al.*, *J. Antibiotics* (Japan), **29**, 1015 (1976)
Structure
Takai *et al.*, *J. Antibiotics* (Japan), **29**, 1253 (1976)

ANTIBIOTIC Y-8495
Dec. 225–240°C

Bacillus bungoensis produces this antibiotic when cultured on a medium containing glucose, dried yeast and inorganic salts at pH 7·0 and 26–28°C for 4 days. The culture broth is extracted with BuOH and evaporated to dryness when the crude antibiotic is obtained as a brown powder. It may be purified further by dissolving in 2 per cent aqueous pyridine, adsorbing on CM-Sephadex C-25 and eluting with a mixture of 4 per cent pyridine and 2 per cent ammonium hydroxide when it forms a white powder which decomposes without melting. The substance has an elemental analysis of C 54·75, H 8·85 and N 16·30 per cent and a molecular weight of approximately 2000. It is soluble in pyridine, AcOH, mineral acids and $(CH_3)_2SO$, insoluble in CH_3OH, hexane, petroleum ether, $CHCl_3$, C_6H_6, AcOEt, $(CH_3)_2CO$ and H_2O. Dilute acids hydrolyse the antibiotic to give phenylalanine, leucine, α,γ-diaminobutyric acid and an unidentified oxyacid which is soluble in Et_2O. The compound is active against gram-positive and gram-negative bacteria and is relatively non-toxic with LD_{50} in rats of more than 1000 mg/kg on oral administration.

Yabuuchi *et al.*, *Japanese Patent*, 7,525,795 (1975)

ANTIBIOTIC YA-56X
M.p. 198–202°C (*dec.*)

Streptomyces humidus MCRL-0387 elaborates two antibiotics which have not been fully characterized. This substance has $[\alpha]_{589} + 20°$ and $[\alpha]_{330} + 90°$, is optically inactive at $[\alpha]_{296}$ and has $[\alpha]_{272} - 360°$ (c 0·05, H_2O). Acid hydrolysis furnishes a number of compounds, e.g. β-aminoalanine, L-*erythro*-β-hydroxyhistidine, β-amino-β-(4-amino-6-carboxy-5-methyl-2-pyrimidinyl)propionic acid, together with three unidentified aminoacids and also 2-acetylthiazole-4-carboxylic acid. The identification of the latter in the hydrolysate suggests the presence of 2-[2-(2-aminoethyl)-2-thiazolin-4-yl]thiazole-4-carboxylic acid in the molecule of the antibiotic. When the fungus is grown in the presence of 0·002 per cent copper sulphate and the culture filtrate treated with activated carbon, extracted and chromatographed, the copper chelate of the antibiotic hydrochloride is obtained, this being active against gram-positive and gram-negative bacteria and ascites sarcoma in mice. Removal of the copper has no effect upon the biological activity.

Okuda, Awataguchi, *Japanese Patent*, 7,202,557 (1972)
Ohashi, Abe, Ito, *Agr. Biol. Chem.*, **37**, 2277, 2283 (1973)

ANTIBIOTIC YA-56Y
M.p. 188–197°C (*dec.*)

A second antibiotic isolated from *Streptomyces humidus*, the hydrolysis products of this substance are identical with those of antibiotic YA-56X but with the addition of one more unidentified aminoacid. The biological activity of the compound is analogous to that of the preceding antibiotic.

Ito *et al.*, *J. Antibiotics* (Japan), **24**, 727 (1971)
Okuda, Awataguchi, *Japanese Patent*, 7,202,557 (1972)
Ohashi, Abe, Ito, *Agr. Biol. Chem.*, **37**, 2277, 2283 (1973)

ANTIBIOTIC YC-17 (*10-Deoxymethymycin*)
$C_{25}H_{43}O_6N$
M.p. 68–70°C

A macrocyclic antibiotic, this compound is elaborated by *Streptomyces venezuelae*. It is dextrorotatory with a specific rotation of $[\alpha]_D^{22} + 84°$ (c 1·0, $CHCl_3$), giving an ultraviolet spectrum in EtOH with absorption maxima at 225–226 and 285 nm.

Kinumaki, Suzuki, *J. Chem. Soc., Chem. Commun.*, 744 (1972)

ANTIBIOTIC YC-73
$C_4H_8O_2N_2S_2Cu$
M.p. 199°C (*dec.*)

This unique copper-containing antibiotic has been isolated from a culture of *Streptomyces* 4601 (ATCC 21,775, FERM-P1369) which was cultured by shaking in a medium containing glucose, soybean flour, yeast powder, meat extract, peptone and inorganic salts at pH 7·0 and 30°C for 4 days. The product was isolated by concentrating the culture filtrate under reduced pressure, adjusting the pH to 8·2, extracting with BuOH three times and washing with H_2O. The condensed extract was adsorbed on Amberlite IRC-50 and eluted with 50 per cent CH_3OH containing 2·88 per cent ammonium hydroxide. When pure, the antibiotic crystallizes from CH_3OH as dark green needles. It is soluble in $(CH_3)_2CO$, slightly soluble in H_2O, CH_3OH, EtOH and AcOEt. The solution in EtOH gives an ultraviolet spectrum with absorption maxima at 231, 253, 267, 320 and 365 nm.

Antibiotic YC-73 is active against a number of gram-positive and gram-negative bacteria and also against HeLa cells. The LD_{50} for mice is 4·5 mg/kg given intraperitoneally.

Egawa *et al.*, *J. Antibiotics* (Japan), **23**, 267 (1970)
Miyamura, Ogasawara, Otsuka, *Japanese Patent*, 7,387,087 (1973)

ANTIBIOTIC Y-G19ZD2
Decomp. 165–172°C

A 2-methoxycephalosporin, this antibiotic has been obtained by culturing *Streptomyces aganonensis* Y-G192 (FERM-P 2725) at 30°C for 24 hours in a liquid nutrient medium. The antibiotic is a white amphoteric powder which decomposes without melting. It is soluble in H_2O but insoluble in organic solvents and gives a positive ninhydrin reaction. It is primarily active against gram-negative bacteria.

Osono *et al.*, *Japanese Patent*, 77 70,087 (1977)
Osono *et al.*, *ibid.*, 77 83,701 (1977)

ANTIBIOTIC Y-G19ZD3
This antibiotic has been obtained by culturing *Streptomyces organonensis* Y-G19Z in a culture medium of starch, glycerol, corn steep liquor, gluten meal, soybean flour, casamino acid and $FeSO_4$ aerobically at 30°C for 90 hours. The culture filtrate is adjusted to pH 3·0, passed through an ion-exchange column, adjusted to pH 5·0 and treated with activated carbon. Final purification is carried out by column chromatography.

Osono *et al.*, *Japanese Patent*, 77 83,702 (1977)

ANTIBIOTIC YL-704
The culture broth of *Streptomyces platensis* subsp. *malvinus* MCRL 0388 yields a macrolide antibiotic complex designated YL-704. By sequential extractions with AcOEt and C_6H_6, followed by chromatography, it has been found possible to separate this complex into at least thirteen individual components, several of which have been characterized and their structures determined. In general, it is possible to divide these antibiotics into three broad groups, e.g. YL-704A_0–A_3 which have an ultraviolet spectrum with an absorption maximum at 232 nm such as is found in the leucomycins (q.v.); YL-704-W_1 and W_2 whose ultraviolet spectra have an absorption maximum at 280 nm like carbomycin B and YL-704-C_1–C_4 which show no characteristic absorption in the ultraviolet spectrum. These antibiotics possess an activity against bacteria but are primarily active against rickettsia. Details of the known antibiotics of this group are given below.

ANTIBIOTIC YL-704-A_0
$C_{44}H_{73}O_{15}N$
M.p. 116–118°C

A minor component of the antibiotic complex YL-704, the structure of this

Antibiotic YL-704-A₁

compound has been determined by chemical analysis, spectroscopic data and mass spectral examination of the acetate.

Furumai et al., *J. Antibiotics* (Japan), **27**, 95 (1974)
Kinumaki et al., *ibid.*, **27**, 102 (1974)
Kinumaki et al., *ibid.*, **27**, 117 (1974)

ANTIBIOTIC YL-704-A₁

$C_{43}H_{71}O_{15}N$
M.p. 122–123°C

A major constituent of YL-704 derived from cultures of *Streptomyces platensis* subsp. *malvinus*, this antibiotic forms colourless crystals and is laevorotatory with a specific rotation of $[\alpha]_D^{21} - 50·2°$ (c 1·0, CHCl₃). The compound is characterized as the crystalline diacetate, m.p. 114–115°C. It should be noted that this compound was originally known as antibiotic YL-704A. The structure has been established by chemical and spectroscopic methods.

Suzuki et al., *Tetrahedron Lett.*, 435 (1971)
Furumai et al., *J. Antibiotics* (Japan), **27**, 95 (1974)
Kinumaki et al., *ibid.*, **27**, 102, 117 (1974)

ANTIBIOTIC YL-704-A₂

$C_{43}H_{71}O_{15}N$
M.p. 193–194°C

A further antibiotic obtained by chromatography of the antibiotic complex from *Streptomyces platensis* subsp. *malvinus*, this substance is laevorotatory with a specific rotation of $[\alpha]_D^{22} - 49°$ (c 1·0, CHCl₃).

Furumai et al., *J. Antibiotics* (Japan), **27**, 95 (1974)
Kinumaki et al., *ibid.*, **27**, 102 (1974)

ANTIBIOTIC YL-704-A₃

$C_{42}H_{69}O_{15}N$
M.p. 121–122°C

This minor component of the antibiotic complex YL-704 is obtained in the form of colourless prisms. It is also laevorotatory with a specific rotation of $[\alpha]_D^{22} - 54°$ (c 1·0, CHCl₃). The above structure has been determined from chemical and spectroscopic evidence.

Furumai et al., *J. Antibiotics* (Japan), **27**, 95 (1974)
Kinumaki et al., *ibid.*, **27**, 102 (1974)

ANTIBIOTIC YL-704-B₁

$C_{41}H_{67}O_{15}N$
M.p. 131–133°C

Also isolated by chromatography of the antibiotic complex YL-704, this substance is laevorotatory with $[\alpha]_D^{21} - 42·1°$ (c 1·0, CHCl₃). It is characterized as the crystalline diacetate, m.p. 116–118°C.

Suzuki et al., *Tetrahedron Lett.*, 435 (1971)
Kinumaki et al., *J. Antibiotics* (Japan), **27**, 102, 107 (1974)

ANTIBIOTIC YL-704-B$_2$
C$_{41}$H$_{67}$O$_{15}$N
M.p. 185–186°C

A minor constituent of the antibiotic complex isolated from cultures of *Streptomyces platensis* subsp. *malvinus*, this compound form colourless needles and is laevorotatory with a specific rotation of $[\alpha]_D^{22} - 42°$ (c 1·0, CHCl$_3$).

Kinumaki *et al.*, *J. Antibiotics* (Japan), **27**, 102 (1974)

ANTIBIOTIC YL-704-B$_3$
C$_{40}$H$_{65}$O$_{15}$N
M.p. 136–137°C

Antibiotic YL-704-B$_3$ is obtained by chromatography of the antibiotic mixture YL-704 and purified by crystallization from EtOH when it forms colourless prisms. It is laevorotatory with a specific rotation of $[\alpha]_D^{22} - 55°$ (c 1·0, CHCl$_3$).

Kinumaki *et al.*, *J. Antibiotics* (Japan), **27**, 102, 117 (1974)

ANTIBIOTIC YL-704-C$_1$
C$_{41}$H$_{67}$O$_{16}$N

This antibiotic is present only in small quantities in YL-704 complex. The structure has been deduced from chemical analysis and spectroscopic examination.

Kinumaki *et al.*, *J. Antibiotics* (Japan), **27**, 117 (1974)

ANTIBIOTIC YL-704-C$_2$
C$_{41}$H$_{67}$O$_{15}$N

A minor component of YL-704 antibiotic complex from *Streptomyces platensis* subsp. *malvinus*, the structure of this compound closely resembles that of antibiotic YL-704-B$_3$ (q.v.). The above structure has been confirmed by NMR and mass spectrometry.

Suzuki *et al.*, *J. Antibiotics* (Japan), **24**, 904 (1971)
Kinumaki *et al.*, *ibid.*, **27**, 117 (1974)

ANTIBIOTIC YL-704-C$_3$
C$_{43}$H$_{71}$O$_{16}$N
M.p. 126–127°C

A crystalline antibiotic from YL-704 complex, this substance is one of a small number of these compounds, isolated from this source, which contains an epoxy ring in the molecule.

Kinumaki *et al.*, *J. Antibiotics* (Japan), **27**, 102, 117 (1974)

ANTIBIOTIC YL-704-C$_4$
C$_{42}$H$_{69}$O$_{16}$N
M.p. 130–132°C

Antibiotic YL-704-C$_4$ also contains an epoxy structure which has been established by chemical analysis and spectroscopic examination. It forms colourless needles from EtOH.

Kinumaki *et al.*, *J. Antibiotics* (Japan), **27**, 102, 117 (1974)

ANTIBIOTIC YL-704-W$_1$
C$_{43}$H$_{69}$O$_{15}$N

The structure of this component of the YL-704 antibiotic complex resembles those of the majority of this group but has two ketonic groups in the aglycone moiety.

Suzuki *et al.*, *J. Antibiotics* (Japan), **24**, 906 (1971)
Kinumaki *et al.*, *ibid.*, **27**, 102, 117 (1974)

ANTIBIOTIC YL-704-W$_2$
C$_{44}$H$_{71}$O$_{15}$N
M.p. 101–103°C

A further minor component of the complex of antibiotics isolated from cultures of *Streptomyces platensis* subsp. *malvinus*, the structure of this compound is closely related to that of the preceding antibiotic.

Kinumaki *et al.*, *J. Antibiotics* (Japan), **27**, 102, 117 (1974)

ANTIBIOTIC YO-7396

This antibiotic has been described by Japanese workers. It has been isolated from cultures of *Coleophoma* YO-7396 and is effective against a range of yeasts. It possesses little, or no, activity against bacteria.

Yamano et al., *Japanese Patent*, 77 83,804 (1977)

ANTIBIOTIC Y-U17W C

Streptomyces lavendulae strain Y-U17W yields an antibiotic complex when grown on a common nutrient medium. Three components have been separated and purified by column chromatography, antibiotics Y-U17W C-1, Y-U17W C-2 and Y-U17W C-3, the first of these being the major component. It forms a white amorphous powder which, on acid hydrolysis furnishes stroptolidine and β-lysine. It is active against a wide range of gram-negative bacteria at concentrations of 6·25–12·5 micrograms/millilitre and effective against *Staphylococcus aureus* at a concentration of between 3·15 and 12·5 micrograms/millilitre. An intravenous dose of 90 mg/kg given to mice showed no retardation of growth or any histological kidney changes and there was no delayed toxicity in mice following a single intravenous dose of 180 mg/kg.

Watanabe et al., *Yamanouchi Seiyaku Kenkyu Hokoku*, **2**, 164 (1974)

ANTIBIOTIC ZN-1636

$C_9H_{13}O_2N$
M.p. 186–187°C (dec.)

A simple antibiotic elaborated by a variant of *Streptomyces diastatochromogenes* when cultivated in a medium containing glucose, starch, cottonseed cake and inorganic salts at 28–29°C for 44 hours. The antibiotic has a specific rotation of $[\alpha]_D^{23} - 54°$ (c 1·0, H_2O), is freely soluble in H_2O but only slightly so in EtOH. It is fungistatic against both *Trichophyton interdigitale* and *Ustilago maydis*. It is relatively non-toxic, mice tolerating a dose of 0·5 g/kg given intravenously.

Ueda et al., *Japanese Patent*, 7,026,712 (1970)

ANTICAPSIN

$C_9H_{13}O_4N$
M. p. 240°C (dec.)

A crystalline antibiotic, anticapsin is produced by cultivating the spores of *Streptomyces griseoplanus* NRRL 3507 in a nutrient medium containing sucrose, soy grits, yeast, casein hydrolysate and antifoam at 34°C and pH 7·0 for 6 days. The culture filtrate is adjusted to pH 4·0, the activity adsorbed on activated carbon, eluted with CH_3OH and freeze-dried. Purification is carried out by chromatography on silica gel. Anticapsin forms white crystals stable at room temperature, soluble in H_2O and methylformamide, slight soluble in CH_3OH and insoluble in other organic solvents. It is active against *Salmonella gallinarum in vitro*, inhibits the formation of hyaluronic acid capsules in *Streptococcus* species and in many respects resembles bacilysin (q.v.) from which it may be obtained by acid cleavage.

Shah et al., *J. Antibiotics* (Japan), **23**, 613 (1970)
Lively, Shah, Whitney, *German Patent*, 1,962,239 (1971)

ANTIMYCIN A$_1$

$C_{28}H_{40}O_9N_2$
M.p. 149–150°C

Various species of *Streptomyces* produce this antibiotic, particularly *Streptomyces* NRRL 2288. The antibiotic is normally crystallized from a mixture of AcOEt and Skellysolve B. It is dextrorotatory with a specific rotation of $[\alpha]_D^{26} + 76°$ (c 1·0, $CHCl_3$) and has an ultraviolet spectrum in EtOH consisting of absorption maxima at 226 and 320 nm. Antimycin A$_1$ dissolves freely in $CHCl_3$, EtOH, $(CH_3)_2CO$ or Et_2O but is only slightly soluble in C_6H_6, CCl_4 and petroleum ether. It is virtually insoluble in H_2O, dilute HCl and aqueous solution of sodium carbonate and bicarbonate. When dissolved in aqueous sodium hydroxide it forms an opaque suspension which becomes clear on heating but then all activity is lost. It is weakly acid in reaction, gives positive Millon, Gibbs phenol and ferric chloride reactions, but negative Molisch, ninhydrin and Ehrlich reactions and does not react with either 2:4-dinitrophenylhydrazine or fuchsin aldehyde. While it is adsorbed by activated carbon it cannot be eluted therefrom and is not dialysable through cellophane.

Antimycin A$_1$ is normally assayed as an agar streak, paper disc with *Glomerella cingulata*. A large number of bacterial species have been tested but only *Ercina amylovora* and *Bacillus cereus* var. *mycoides* are inhibited by the antibiotic. A large number of fungi are, however, inhibited at low concentrations, typical inhibition concentrations (μg/ml) being: *Ascochyta* species (25); *Colletotrichum circinans* (1·6); *C. lindemuthianum* (12·5); *C. pisi* (1·6); *Glomerella cingulata* (0·8–62·5); *Nigrospora sphaerica* (0·2); *Pythium* species (250); *Stemphylium sarcinaeforme* (1·6); *Sclerotinia fructicola* (0·4–1·6) and *Venturia inaequalis* (0·4–0·8). As yet the antibiotic has only been employed on an experimental basis as an insecticide, fungicide and miticide.

Leben, Keitt, *Phytopath*, **37**, 14 (1947)
Leben, Keitt, *ibid.*, **38**, 16, 899 (1948)
Dunshee *et al.*, *J. Amer. Chem. Soc.*, **71**, 2436 (1949)
Tener *et al.*, *ibid.*, **75**, 1100, 3623 (1953)
Lockwood *et al.*, *Phytopath.*, **44**, 438 (1954)
Structure
van Tamelen *et al.*, *J. Amer. Chem. Soc.*, **83**, 1639 (1961)
Birch *et al.*, *J. Chem. Soc.*, 889 (1961)

ANTIMYCIN A$_{2b}$
C$_{26}$H$_{36}$O$_9$N$_2$?
M.p. 168°C
This antibiotic may be separated from the preceding compound by column chromatography. It forms colourless crystals when purified by crystallization from EtOH.

Liu, Strong, *J. Amer. Chem. Soc.*, **81**, 4387 (1959)

ANTIMYCIN A$_3$ (*Blastmycin*)
C$_{26}$H$_{36}$O$_9$N$_2$
M.p. 170·5–171·5°C

First isolated by Japanese workers from *Streptomyces blastmyceticus*, this antibiotic has been shown to be identical with blastmycin. The compound forms colourless needles when crystallized from a mixture of C$_6$H$_6$ and petroleum ether and is dextrorotatory with $[\alpha]_D^{25}$ + 64·3° (c 1·0, CHCl$_3$).

Watanabe *et al.*, *J. Antibiotics* (Japan), **10A**, 39 (1957)

Yonehara, Takeuchi, *ibid.*, **11A**, 122, 254 (1958)
Liu, Strong, *J. Amer. Chem. Soc.*, **81**, 4387 (1959)
Synthesis
Kinoshita, Wada, Umezawa, *J. Antibiotics* (Japan), **22**, 580 (1969)

ANTIMYCOIN (*Fungicidin RAW*)
This antibiotic, closely related to nystatin (q.v.), is obtained from the broth of a culture of *Streptomyces aureus* by extraction with BuOH, followed by concentration *in vacuo*, extraction of the residue with EtOH and precipitation with Et$_2$O. Antimycoin is soluble in EtOH and H$_2$O but insoluble in CHCl$_3$, (CH$_3$)$_2$CO and Et$_2$O. It is stable under slightly alkaline conditions and can withstand 100°C for 10 minutes at pH 7·0. The ultraviolet spectrum exhibits absorption maxima at 290, 305 and 316 nm.

The antibiotic is active against fungi but not against bacteria, mycobacteria or actinomycetes. It is moderately non-toxic with LD$_{50}$ in mice of 204 mg/kg when given intraperitoneally.

Raubitschek, Acker, Waksman, *Antibiotics & Chemotherapy*, **2**, 179 (1952)

ANTIPHLEI FACTOR
A complex substance produced by a *Streptomyces* species closely allied to *S. aureus*. It is obtained by concentration of the broth filtrate to dryness *in vacuo* followed by extraction with CH$_3$OH and precipitation with (CH$_3$)$_2$CO. The compound is thermostable and basic, forming a pale-yellow amorphous powder with no definite melting point.

It is active against *Mycobacterium phlei* and to a somewhat lesser degree against *M. smegmatis*, *M. avium* and the human type of *M. tuberculosis*. It possesses virtually no activity against either gram-positive or gram-negative bacteria. It has a low toxicity, an injection of 10–20 mg/kg of the hydrochloride both muscularly and intravenously into mice being well tolerated. No data has yet been released regarding its utilization in medicine.

Ouchi, *J. Antibiotics* (Japan), **3**, 517 (1950)

ANTISMEGMATIS FACTOR
A *Streptomyces* species resembling *S. lavendulae* elaborates this antibiotic which is obtained from the culture filtrate by freezing and then thawing slowly, the bottom layer of the liquid being separated and kept in the frozen state. It is thermostable at pH 7·0 and is most active at an alkaline reaction against *Mycobacterium phlei* and *M. smegmatis*. It shows negligible activity against a pathogenic strain of *M. bovis* or against bacteria and fungi. It is

comparatively non-toxic; a 2 ml culture filtrate containing 4000 *M. smegmatis* units is well tolerated by mice when given intraperitoneally.

Kelner, Morton, *Proc. Soc. Exptl. Biol. Med.*, **63**, 227 (1946)

APHIDICOLIN
$C_{20}H_{34}O_4$

This antiviral terpenoid antibiotic has been isolated from cultures of *Cephalosporium aphidicola* and *Nigrospora sphaerica*. The structure has been determined from chemical and spectroscopic data, particularly the infrared, NMR and mass spectrometry evidence. The antibiotic is a mitotic suppressant and is active against viruses containing DNA.

Borrow *et al.*, *British Patent*, 1,331,520 (1973)
Starratt, Loschiavo, *Can. J. Microbiol.*, **20**, 416 (1974)
Adams, Bu'lock, *J. Chem. Soc., Chem. Commun.*, 389 (1975)

APLASMOMYCIN
$C_{40}H_{60}O_{14}BNa \cdot H_2O$

A complex macrocyclic isolated from fermentation broth cultivated with a strain of *Streptomyces griseus* isolated from shallow sea sediment in Sagami Bay, this substance is produced in a selected medium designed to simulate a marine environment. It inhibits the growth of gram-positive bacteria including *Mycobacteria in vitro* and is active against Plasmodia berghei *in vivo*. The structure has been established from an X-ray crystallographic analysis of the silver salt.

Okami *et al.*, *J. Antibiotics* (Japan), **29**, 1019 (1976)
Nakamura *et al.*, *ibid.*, **30**, 714 (1977)

AQUACILLIN
See Procaine Penicillin G

AQUAMYCIN
See Cellocidin

AQUAYAMYCIN
$C_{25}H_{26}O_{10}$
M.p. 189–190°C (*dec.*)

An anthraquinone type antibiotic, this compound occurs in the cultures of *Streptomyces misawanensis*. It crystallizes as orange needles from butyl acetate which contain solvent of crystallization and have the above melting point. It is dextrorotatory having $[\alpha]_D^{20} + 160°$ (c 1·0, dioxan) and yields a triacetate which crystallizes from $CH_3OH-C_6H_6$ with m.p. 178–180°C. The structure has been established from chemical and spectroscopic data.

Sezaki *et al.*, *J. Antibiotics* (Japan), **21**, 91 (1968)
Sezaki *et al.*, *Tetrahedron*, **26**, 5171 (1970)

ARANCIAMYCIN
$C_{27}H_{28}O_{12}$
M.p. 240°C (*dec.*)

An antibiotic produced by *Streptomyces echinatus*, this substance crystallizes from CH_3OH and has a specific rotation of $[\alpha]_D + 149.5°$ (c 0·5, CH_3OH).

The ultraviolet spectrum in EtOH has absorption maxima at 241, 265 and 440 nm. It forms a crystalline tetraacetate, m.p. 128–130°C.

Keller-Schierlein et al., *Helv: Chim. Acta*, **53**, 779 (1970)

ARANOFLAVIN A
$C_{23}H_{33}O_6N$
M.p. Indefinite
Cultivation of *Arachniolus flavoluteus* in a medium containing potato starch for 3 days at 26°C yields two closely related antibiotics. The mixture is isolated from the cells by extraction with $(CH_3)_2CO$ and forms an oily liquid which is separated and purified by chromatography on a silica gel column. This antibiotic forms colourless crystals and is active against *Staphylococcus aureus* and *Trichomonas vaginalis in vitro* and also against *Pseudomonas aeruginosa* and Yoshida sarcoma in rats. It is comparatively toxic with LD_{50} of 4·6 mg/kg in mice given intraperitoneally.

Udagawa et al., *Japanese Patent*, 7,130,794 (1971)

ARANOFLAVIN B
$C_{26}H_{39}O_7N$
M.p. Indefinite
Also isolated from cultures of *Arachniolus flavoluteus*, this antibiotic forms colourless crystals from $(CH_3)_2CO$. Unlike the preceding compound it is active only against *Pseudomonas aeruginosa* and Yoshida sarcoma in rats. However, it is somewhat less toxic, the LD_{50} in mice being approximately 15 mg/kg.

Udegawa et al., *Japanese Patent*, 7,130,794 (1971)

ARAZOPEPTIN
M.p. Indefinite
A complex antibiotic, this compound is produced by cultivation of *Streptomyces candidus* var. *azaticus* under aerobic conditions on a medium at pH 7·0 containing starch, soybean flour and sodium chloride at 28°C for 30 hours. So far, the compound has not been obtained in the pure form. The antibiotic is effective against L-1210 leukemia in mice.

Hata et al., *Japanese Patent*, 7,450,193 (1974)

ARENOMYCIN B
M.p. Indefinite
A tetraene antibiotic, this compound occurs with aernomycin A (which has not been obtained in a pure form), in cultures of *Actinomyces tumemacerans* var. *griseoarenicolor*. The antibiotic has a pronounced activity against a range of fungi and yeasts but little effect against bacteria.

Tsyganov, Shenin, Solov'ev, *Antibiotiki*, **18**, 973 (1973)

ARGOMYCIN
$C_{25}H_{43}O_7N$
M.p. 164°C
Streptomyces griseolus elaborates this macrocyclic antibiotic which forms colourless crystals from EtOH. It has a specific rotation of $[\alpha]_D^{25} + 8·2°$ (c 1·0. EtOH). It is active against a range of gram-positive bacteria.

Hata et al., *J. Antibiotics* (Japan), **8A**, 9 (1955)

ARISTEROMYCIN
$C_{11}H_{15}O_3N_5$
M.p. 213–215°C

This antibiotic derived from *Streptomyces citricolor* forms colourless prisms from EtOH and is laevorotatory with $[\alpha]_D - 52·5°$. The substance forms a hydrobromide as colourless prisms, m.p. 229°C (*dec.*). In aqueous solution, the antibiotic gives an ultraviolet spectrum consisting of a single absorption maximum at 262 nm. The (±)-form has been synthesized and forms colourless crystals from H_2O, m.p. 238–242°C (*dec.*). The antibiotic inhibits *Piricularia oryzae* and *Xanthomonas oryzae* at a minimum inhibition concentration of 5 µg/ml both *in vitro* and *in vivo*.

Kusaka et al., *J. Antibiotics* (Japan), **21A**, 255 (1967)
Kishi et al., *Chem. Pharm. Bull.*, **20**, 940 (1972)
Crystal structure
Kishi et al., *Chem. Commun.*, 852 (1967)
Synthesis
Shealy, Clayton, *J. Amer. Chem. Soc.*, **88**, 3885 (1966)

ARMENTOMYCIN

$C_4H_7NO_2Cl_2$
M.p. 153°C (dec.)

$$Cl_2-CH-CH_2-\underset{NH_2}{CH}-COOH$$

A simple aminoacid, armentomycin is elaborated by *Streptomyces armentosus*. It forms colourless crystals and is dextrorotatory with a specific rotation of $[\alpha]_D^{25} + 26 \cdot 2°$ (c 0·74, HCl, pH = 1·0). The structure has been elucidated from chemical and spectroscopic evidence. Armentomycin is active against a number of gram-positive bacteria.

Argoudelis *et al.*, *Biochem.*, **6**, 165 (1967)
Structure
Urabe *et al.*, *Tetrahedron Lett.*, 997 (1975)

ASCOCHLORIN (*Illicicolin, LL-Z1272*)

$C_{23}H_{29}O_4Cl$
M.p. 153–154°C (dec.)

Asochyta viciae yields this antibiotic which exists in two tautomeric forms. The α-form crystallizes as colourless needles with the melting point given above. In CH_3OH it gives an ultraviolet spectrum with absorption maxima at 240, 290 and 346 nm. It inhibits plaque formation by herpes simplex virus and Newcastle disease virus without forming any cytotoxic zones in the host chick embryo fibroblast cells at 6·0–50 μg/ml in the agar-diffusion plaque inhibition assay, thereby being effective against both DNA and RNA viruses. In the tube-culture method, however, it shows no antiviral activity. It is also active against *Candida albicans* and has LD_{50} of 20 mg/kg in mice given intraperitoneally. When given intraperitoneally to mice at 100 μg/kg for 5 days it affords some protection against Ehrlich carcinoma in mice. The β-form of the antibiotic is a colourless oil that cannot be crystallized.

Tamura *et al.*, *J. Antibiotics* (Japan), **21**, 539 (1968)
Structure
Nawata *et al.*, *J. Antibiotics* (Japan), **22**, 511 (1969)
Crystal structure
Nawata, Iitaka, *Bull. Chem. Soc., Japan*, **44**, 2652 (1971)

ASCOFURANONE

$C_{23}H_{29}O_5Cl$
M.p. 84°C

A second antibiotic elaborated by *Ascochyta viciae* (FERM-P 129), this compound cyrstallizes from a mixture of $(CH_3)_2CO$ and hexane as colourless needles. It is laevorotatory with a specific rotation of $[\alpha]_D^5 - 50°$ (c 1·0, CH_3OH) and the ultraviolet spectrum in EtOH has absorption maxima at 228, 295 and 350 nm. The compound is soluble in C_6H_6, AcOEt, $CHCl_3$, $(CH_3)_2CO$, CH_3OH, EtOH and hexane but insoluble in H_2O. Ascofuranone is inactive against bacteria, fungi or yeasts but is active against viruses and certain tumours.

Sasaki *et al.*, *Tetrahedron Lett.*, 2541 (1972)
Hosokawa *et al.*, *Japanese Patent*, 7,391,278 (1973)

ASIATICOSIDE

$C_{54}H_{88}O_{23}$
M.p. 230–233°C (dec.)

A glycosidic antibiotic, this substance occurs in the Madagascar varieties of *Centella asiatica* (*Hydrocotyle asiatica*) and was isolated and named by Bontemps. It is noteworthy that the Ceylon varieties of this plant do not contain asiaticoside but yield centoic acid and centelloside. Asiaticoside forms colourless prisms when recrystallized from aqueous EtOH and is laevorotatory with $[\alpha]_D - 14°$ (EtOH). It is insoluble in H_2O, slightly soluble in EtOH and freely so in pyridine. Hydrolysis first yields D-glucose and an amorphous glucone which may be further hydrolysed to give L-rhamnose and asiatic acid, $C_{30}H_{48}O_5$, the structure of which has been shown to be 2β,3β,23-trihydroxyurs-12-en-28-oic acid. Four sugar molecules are present in asiaticoside but their mode of linkage is not yet known with certainty. Most bacteriological examination has been carried out with oxyasiaticoside which is a water-soluble derivative of the parent antibiotic. *In vitro*, this material inhibits *Mycobacterium* tuberculosis at a concentration of 0·015 mg/ml. Experiments with rats, rabbits and guinea pigs *in vivo* have shown that, when treated with an experimental *M. tuberculosis* infection, 0·5 ml of a 4 per cent solution of oxyasiaticoside given subcutaneously twice a day for 68 days resulted in approximately one third as many tubercular lesions as were present in the control animals. The toxic level of oxyasiaticoside is said to be appreciably less than the tuberculosis therapy level.

Boiteau, Dureuil, Rakoto-Ratsimamanga, *Compt. rend. acad. sci.*, **228**, 1165 (1949)
Boiteau *et al.*, *Bull. soc. chim.*, **31**, 46 (1949)
Boiteau *et al.*, *Nature*, **163**, 258 (1949)
Bhattacharyya, Lythgoe, *Ibid.*, **163**, 259 (1949)

ASPERGILLIC ACID (*Aspergillin*)

$C_{12}H_{20}O_2N_2$
M.p. 97·9°C

Aspergillic acid has been isolated from cultures of *Aspergillus flavus* and has been studied by several observers. When grown on a tryptone medium, this antibiotic is produced as the major component in surface culture whereas in submerged culture on Czapek-Dox medium, more hydroxyaspergillic acid and penicillin-like antibiotics are formed. The presence of sugars in the medium also increases the amount of hydroxyaspergillic acid formed and since this is extremely difficult to separate from aspergillic acid, it has been proposed that sugar-free media should be used for the preparation of pure aspergillic acid. Crude aspergillic acid is obtained as a pale yellow, waxy amorphous solid which may be dissolved in boiling hexane, filtered, concentrated, and then precipitated. The precipitate is then dissolved in CH_3OH or $(CH_3)_2CO$, treated with activated carbon and recrystallized from aqueous EtOH when it forms pale yellow rods or plates, soluble in hot H_2O, C_6H_6, $CHCl_3$, CCl_4, pyridine, EtOH, Et_2O and $(CH_3)_2CO$, insoluble in cold H_2O, dilute acids and petroleum ether. It is dextrorotatory having $[\alpha]_D^{24} + 13\cdot4°$ (c 0·85, EtOH) and $+18\cdot5°$ (c 1·05, 1N-NaOH). The ultraviolet spectrum has absorption maxima at 230–250 and 300–350 nm, the positions varying with the pH and the solvent used. Aspergillic acid yields several salts and derivatives including the hydrochloride, m.p. 182°C (*dec.*); the methiodide which crystallizes with CH_3I, m.p. 169°C; the 3:5-dinitrobenzoyl derivative existing in two modifications with m.p. 123°C and 166–169°C; the silver salt decomposing at 190°C; the copper salt as green rectangular leaflets, m.p. 198–199°C and the phenylhydrazine salt, m.p. 99·5°C. It gives negative Molisch, Millon, Fehling, biuret and ninhydrin tests and a vivid red colour with $FeCl_3$ solution. Of the derivatives investigated, bromoaspergillic acid has an antibiotic activity similar to that of aspergillic acid and deoxyaspergillic acid, while antibiotically inactive, inhibits the sore germination of *Aspergillus flavus* at a concentration of 3 mg/ml.

This antibiotic may be assayed by several methods, e.g. the cylinder plate method with *Mycobacterium tuberculosis*, serial dilution using *Pasteurella multocida*, *Staphylococcus aureus* and *Streptococcus pyogenes*, antiluminescent activity against *Photobacterium fischeri* and by the ultraviolet absorption spectrum. Since, as already stated, aspergillic acid is often contaminated by varying amounts of hydroaspergillic acid and penicillin-type antibiotics produced by *Aspergillus flavus*, the bacterial assays will be influenced by the presence of these latter compounds. They do not, however, appear in the ultraviolet spectrum in the region between 300 and 350 nm and if a precise assay is required, the ultraviolet assay must be used in conjunction with the bioassay.

Aspergillic acid is active against a number of bacteria *in vitro*, typical inhibition concentrations (μg/ml) being: *Aerobacter aerogenes* (30); *Clostridium bifermentans* (60); *C. histolyticum* (60); *C. novyi* (20); *C. perfringens* (40); *C. septicum* (40); *C. sporogenes* (60); *Diplococcus pneumoniae* (4); *Escherichia coli* (30); *Klebsiella pneumoniae* (8); *Salmonella enteriditis* (30); *Staphylococcus aureus* (10) and *Streptococcus pyogenes* (2). Several factors affect the activity of this antibiotic. It is reduced by iron and also defibrinated rabbit blood but increased by various metals, e.g. arsenic, bismuth, cobalt, nickel and zinc with bismuth being the most effective. When administered intraperitoneally to mice, aspergillic acid afforded no protection against pneumococcus, *Pseudomonas aeruginosa*, *Staphylococcus aureus* or hemolytic streptococcus. There is some evidence, however, that it affords protection against gas gangrene and gonorrhea. The LD_{50} in mice has been given as 3 mg/20 g and 40 mg/kg (intraperitoneally) and 5 mg/20 g (orally).

White, *Science*, **92**, 127 (1940)
Glister, *Nature*, **148**, 470 (1941)
Rake, McKee, Jones, *Proc. Soc. Exptl. Biol. Med.*, **51**, 273 (1942)

White, Hill, *J. Bact.*, **45**, 433 (1943)
Bush, Goth, *Fed. Proc.*, **2**, 75 (1943)
Menzel, Wintersteiner, Rake, *J. Bact.*, **46**, 109 (1943)
McKee, MacPhillamy, *Proc. Soc. Exptl. Biol. Med.*, **53**, 247 (1943)
Jones, Rake, Hamre, *J. Bact.*, **45**, 461 (1943)
Menzel, Wintersteiner, Hoogerheide, *J. Biol. Chem.*, **152**, 419 (1944)
Dutcher, Wintersteiner, *ibid.*, **155**, 359 (1944)
Goth, *J. Lab. Clin. Med.*, **30**, 899 (1945)
Dutcher, Wintersteiner, *Fed. Proc.*, **4**, 88 (1945)
Bush, Dickison, Ward, Avery, *J. Pharm. Exp. Therapy*, **85**, 237 (1945)
Salvin, *J. Bact.*, **52**, 614 (1946)
Goth, *Fed. Proc.*, **5**, 180 (1946)
Woodward, *J. Bact.*, **54**, 375 (1947)
Tobie, Alverson, *ibid.*, **54**, 543 (1947)
Dutcher *et al.*, *J. Biol. Chem.*, **171**, 321, 341 (1947)
Dunn *et al.*, *J. Chem. Soc., Suppl.*, 126 (1949)
Dunn, Newbold, Spring, *ibid.*, 131 (1949)
Newbold, Sharp, Spring, *J. Chem. Soc.*, 2679 (1951)
Newbold, Sharp, Spring, *ibid.*, 4870 (1952)

ASPERGILLIN

First used to describe a black pigment found in the spores of *Aspergillus niger*, the name aspergillin has also been given to a number of antibiotics which have subsequently been shown to be aspergillic acid, gliotoxin, flavacin and fumigacin. The name is now no longer in use.

Bush, Goth, *Fed. Proc.*, **2**, 75 (1943)
Soltys, *Nature*, **154**, 550 (1944)
Stanley, Mills, *Aust. J. Science*, **6**, 141 (1944)
Krassilnikov, Koreniako, *Microbiologia* (USSR), **14**, 347 (1945)
Bush *et al.*, *Fed. Proc.*, **4**, 113 (1945)
Tobie, *Nature*, **158**, 709 (1946)
Stanley, Mills, *Aust. J. Exp. Biol. Med. Sci.*, **24**, 133 (1946)

ASPERGIN
$C_{19}H_{26}O_3$
M.p. 90·5–91·5°C

A benzenoid antibiotic, aspergin is isolated from cultures of an unidentified *Aspergillus* strain. When purified it forms a yellow powder which is insoluble in H_2O and optically inactive. The structure has been deduced from chemical and spectroscopic data, particularly the infrared, NMR and mass spectra. It is active against gram-positive bacteria.

Sokolov *et al.*, *Antibiotiki*, **16**, 504 (1971)
Kul'bakh *et al.*, *Soviet Patent*, 359,961 (1973)

ASPERLIN
See Antibiotic U-13,933

ASPICULAMYCIN
$C_{19}H_{30}O_{10}N_8$
Decomp. ~250°C

Streptomyces toyocaensis var. *aspiculamyceticus* No. 1040 elaborates this cytosine nucleoside antibiotic when cultivated in an agitated medium containing glucose, starch, corn steep liquor, meat extract and Pharmamedia at pH 7·4 at 27°C for 2 days. Aspiculamycin forms colourless needles from aqueous $(CH_3)_2CO$. The antibiotic is active against gram-positive and gram-negative bacteria, mycoplasms and pinworms in mice.

Arai *et al.*, *Ger. Patent*, 2,238,259 (1973)
Arai *et al.*, *J. Antibiotics* (Japan), **27**, 329 (1974)
Haneishi, Terahara, Arai, *ibid.*, **27**, 334 (1974)

ASTEROMYCIN
See Gougerotin

ASUKAMYCIN
$C_{29}H_{22}N_2O_9$

Streptomyces nodosus subsp. *asukaensis* elaborates this antibiotic which has been obtained by extraction of the fermentation broth with organic solvents and purified by column chromatography. It possesses antibacterial, antifungal and anticoccidial properties and is relatively non-toxic with no effect on mice when given 450 mg/kg *per os*. The acute LD_{50} in mice has been reported as 48·5 mg/kg given intraperitoneally.

Nakagawa, Shimada, Iwai., *J. Antibiotics* (Japan), **29**, 876 (1976)

ATHLESTATIN
$C_{32}H_{53}O_{12}N_5$
M.p. 160–165°C (*dec.*)

This antibiotic is obtained from the mycelium of *Aspergillus niger* strain F-172 by extraction with $(CH_3)_2CO$, concentration *in vacuo* to a reduced volume, precipitation at pH 2·0, dissolving in CH_3OH—$CHCl_3$, concentrating to a syrup, adsorbing on an alumina column, eluting with AcOEt, concentration *in vacuo* and addition of Et_2O. Athlestatin forms a yellow powder and is laevorotatory with a specific rotation of $[\alpha]_D^{20} - 64°$ (c 0·5, CH_3OH). The ultraviolet spectrum in CH_3OH has two absorption maxima at 225 and 278 nm. It is soluble in the lower alcohols, pyridine, $(CH_3)_2CO$ and methyl ethyl ketone, slightly soluble in AcOEt and $CHCl_3$, insoluble in C_6H_6, Et_2O, hexane and H_2O. It is stable in neutral and acid solutions, unstable towards alkalies. Although having little activity towards bacteria, it is active against fungi and yeasts. It is relatively non-toxic, mice tolerating a dose of 300 mg/kg given intraperitoneally.

Miyairi *et al.*, *Yakugaku Kenkyu*, **39**, 165 (1968)

AURANTIOGLIOCLADIN
$C_{10}H_{12}O_4$
M.p. 62·5°C

A simple antibiotic produced by a species of *Gliocladium*, this compound is obtained as bright orange plates when purified by recrystallization from petroleum ether. When dissolved in concentrated H_2SO_4 it gives a vivid violet colour. Reduction with Zn and HCl yields 2:3-dimethoxy-5:6-dimethylquinol, confirming the structure of the antibiotic as 2:3-dimethoxy-5:6-dimethyl-*p*-benzoquinone. The mono-2:4-dinitrophenylhydrazone crystallizes as red needles from AcOEt, m.p. 228–229°C (*dec.*). A higher m.p. of 243–244°C is obtained on a block.

Brian *et al.*, *Experientia*, **7**, 266 (1951)
Vischer, *J. Chem. Soc.*, 815 (1953)
Baker, McOMie, Miles, *ibid.*, 820 (1953)

AUREOLIC ACID (*Mithramycin, Antibiotic LA-7017*)
$C_{52}H_{76}O_{24}$
M.p. 180–183°C

A strain of *Streptomyces* yields this antibiotic which crystallizes well from $(CH_3)_2CO$. It is laevorotatory having $[\alpha]_D^{20} - 51°$ (c 0·4, EtOH). The ultraviolet spectrum in ethanol has absorption maxima at 229, 280, 317, 330 and 417 nm. Hydrolysis with dilute acids furnishes chromomycinone, one mole each of D-mycarose and D-oliose and three moles of D-olivose.

Grundy *et al.*, *Antibiotics & Chemotherapy*, **3**, 1215 (1953)
Phillips, Schenck, *ibid.*, **3**, 1218 (1953)
Sensi, Greco, Pagani, *ibid.*, **8**, 241 (1958)
Rao, Cullen, Sobin, *ibid.*, **12**, 182 (1962)
Berlin *et al.*, *Nature*, **218**, 193 (1968)
Structure
Bakhaeva *et al.*, *Tetrahedron Lett.*, 3595 (1968)

AUREOMYCIN (Biomycin, Chlorotetracycline)
$C_{22}H_{23}O_8N_2Cl$
M.p. 168–169°C

A broad-spectrum antibiotic elaborated by *Streptomyces aureofaciens*, this compound forms colourless small crystals, acicular to bladed in habit, from EtOH and is laevorotatory having a specific rotation of $[\alpha]_D^{23} - 275°$ (c 1·0, CH_3OH). It is readily soluble in dioxan and cellosolve, sparingly so in CH_3OH, EtOH, butanol, AcOEt, $(CH_3)_2CO$ and C_6H_6 and almost insoluble in H_2O, Et_2O and petroleum ether. The hydrochloride forms clear lemon-yellow rhomboid crystals which decompose above 210°C and has $[\alpha]_D^{23} - 24·0°$ (c 1·0, H_2O). In 0·1 N-NaOH the ultraviolet spectrum has absorption maxima at 255, 285 and 345 nm and in 0·1M phosphoric acid, at 226, 264 and 365 nm. The ultraviolet inflections vary according to pH and are not sharply defined. The antibiotic gives a greenish-brown colour with alcoholic $FeCl_3$ when viewed by reflected light, the colour being red by transmitted light. It is unstable on heating in strong mineral acids and alkalies, stable at pH 2·5 but unstable above pH 7·0, particularly in culture media. The latter characteristic, together with its instability at 37°C, makes it difficult to assay aureomycin. Methods which have been used include turbidimetric means using *Staphylococcus aureus*, the cylinder plate method with *Bacillus subtilis*, and serial dilution in blood serum with *B. subtilis* and *B. cereus* var. *mycoides*. In all of these methods it has been found that the turbidimetric assays are lower and more consistent than the plate assays.

In vitro studies with aureomycin show that its mode of action is bacteriostatic and typical complete inhibition concentrations (μg/ml) are: *Aerobacter aerogenes* (12·5–50); *Alkaligenes* species (6·0); *Bacillus megatherium* (3·1); *B. subtilis* (0·78–12·5); *Diplococcus pneumoniae* (0·1–1·0); *Escherichia coli* (3·1–100); *E. intermedia* (50); *Neisseria gonorrheas* (0·25–1·0); *N. meningitidis* (0·5); *Proteus morganii* (4·0); *Pr. vulgaris* (50–250); *Pseudomonas aeruginosa* (100–250); *Salmonella choleras-suis* (6·3); *S. derby* (50); *S. manhattan* (50); *S. pullorum* (12); *S. typhimurium* (50); *S. typhosa* (3·1–50); *Sarcina lutea* (3·0–50); *Serratia marcescens* (100–200); *Staphylococcus albus* (1·0–2·0); *Staph. aureus* (1·0–50); *Staph. citreus* (12). Aureomycin possesses no activity against viruses or rickettsia *in vitro* but is effective *in vivo*. The activity is decreased with an increase in pH above 6·1 and by various other factors including antagonism by blood and serum and anaerobiosis. Several workers have shown that there is increased resistance to the antibiotic after a number of transfers on media with an increasing concentration of aureomycin.

The antibiotic spectrum *in vivo* differs appreciably from that *in vitro*. Price and his colleagues have investigated the effect of the antibiotic against experimental bacterial infections in mice, the dose being injected intraperitoneally. A dose of 0·5 mg gave 100 per cent protection against *Escherichia coli* and *Salmonella typhosa* but only 10 per cent protection against *S. typhimurium*. A lower dose of 0·05 mg gave 85 per cent protection against *Proteus vulgaris* and 65 per cent protection against *Streptococcus hemolyticus* under the same conditions. The smaller dose gave no protection against *Klebsiella pneumoniae*. In general single doses are less effective than the same amount of antibiotic administered over two or three days. Protection against *Brucella* infections is enhanced when given in combination with streptomycin or sulfadiazine. *In vivo*, aureomycin is effective against both virus and rickettsial infections. 1·0 mg gives complete protection against psittacosis virus in 7-day chick embryos, while Wong and Cox have demonstrated that protection is afforded against the rickettsia of rickettsialpox, Q. fever, epidemic typhus, murine typhus, scrub typhus, South African tickbite fever, Queensland tick typhus, Rocky Mountain spotted fever and boutonneuse fever. The antibiotic is also effective against the viruses of the psittacosis-lymphogranuloma group.

Several clinical trials have been carried out with this antibiotic. Oral administration is effective in cases of amebiasis, brucellosis, epidemic typhus, Rocky Mountain spotted fever, Q fever, *Staphylococcus aureus* infections and urinary infections with bacteria of the coli-aerogenes group. When given intramuscularly it is also active against granuloma inguinale and lymphogranuloma venereum. It is, however, ineffective against *Escherichia coli*, *Proteus*, *Pseudomonas*, measles and typhoid when given orally. In the case of ocular infections the antibiotic gives excellent response against *Diplococcus pneumoniae*, *Escherichia coli*, *Moraxella lacunata*, *Staphylococcus aureus* and the herpes virus.

Aureomycin is relatively non-toxic in animals. When administered intravenously, the LD_{50} has been given as 118 mg/kg in rats and 50–134 mg/kg in mice while 50 mg/kg is tolerated in guinea pigs, cats, dogs and rabbits, although 150 mg/kg proved fatal in dogs. Given orally, 3 g/kg was tolerated by rats and 1500 mg/kg by mice. Side effects observed in humans include inflammation, severe pain, nausea, vomiting, loss of appetite and secondary anemia. In ointments, the free antibiotic irritates the eye and although the borate is non-irritating, it rapidly loses its activity. When administered intravenously in humans, the antibiotic appeared in both the blood and the spinal fluids while when given orally, a high percentage is excreted in the urine. The uses of the antibiotic are in the treatment of rickettsial Q-fever endocarditis, pneumonia, sinusitis and undulant fever. The main use of this antibiotic varies in tropical and non-tropical countries.

    Duggar, *Ann. N.Y. Acad. Sci.*, **51**, 177 (1948)
    Duggar, *U.S. Patent*, 2,482,055 (1949)
    Broschard, *Science*, **109**, 199 (1949)
  Treatment of bacterial infections
    Price, Randall, Welch, *Ann. N.Y. Acad. Sci.*, **51**, 211 (1948)
    Chandler, Bliss, *ibid.*, **51**, 221 (1948)
    Little, *ibid.*, **51**, 246 (1948)
    Bryer et al., *ibid.*, **51**, 254 (1948)
    Paine, Collins, Finland, *ibid.*, **51**, 228 (1948)
    Spink et al., *J.A.M.A.*, **138**, 1145 (1948)
    Beigelman, *Proc. Soc. Exptl. Biol. Med.*, **92**, 89 (1949)
    Perry, *ibid.*, **92**, 45 (1949)
    Brande, Hall, Spink, *J.A.M.A.*, **141**, 831 (1949)
    Magoffin, Anderson, Spink, *J. Immunol.*, **62**, 125 (1949)
    Rodriguez et al., *J.A.M.A.*, **141**, 771 (1949)
    Larson, *J. Immunol.*, **62**, 425 (1949)
    Wilhelm, *J.A.M.A.*, **141**, 837 (1949)
    Bryer et al., *Bull. John Hopkins Hosp.*, **84**, 444 (1949)
    Heilman, *Proc. Staff Meet. Mayo Clin.*, **24**, 133 (1949)
    Hersell, Barber, *ibid.*, **24**, 138 (1949)
  Treatment of virus and rickettsial infections
    Wong, Cox, *Ann. N.Y. Acad. Sci.*, **51**, 290 (1948)
    Anigstein, Whitmey, Beninson, *ibid.*, **51**, 306 (1948)
    Wright et al., *ibid.*, **51**, 318 (1948)
    Lennette, Meiklejohn, Thelen, *ibid.*, **51**, 331 (1948)
    McVay, Laird, Sprunt, *Science*, **109**, 590 (1949)
  Treatment of ocular infections
    Braley, Sanders, *Ann. N.Y. Acad. Sci.*, **51**, 280 (1948)
  Clinical studies
    Dornbush, Pelcak, *Ann. N.Y. Acad. Sci.*, **51**, 218 (1948)
    Collins, Paine, Finland, *ibid.*, **51**, 231 (1948)
    Dowling et al., *ibid.*, **51**, 241 (1948)
    Schoenbach, Bryer, Long, *ibid.*, **51**, 267 (1948)
    Brainerd et al., *Proc. Soc. Exptl. Biol. Med.*, **70**, 318 (1949)

    Schneierson, Toharsky, *J. Bact.*, **57**, 483 (1949)
Structure
    Stephens et al., *J. Amer. Chem. Soc.*, **74**, 4976 (1952)
    Waller et al., *ibid.*, **74**, 4978 (1952)
    Woodward et al., *ibid.*, **75**, 5455 (1953)
    Woodward et al., *ibid.*, **76**, 3568 (1954)
    Woodward et al., *ibid.*, **78**, 4155 (1956)
    Petty, *U.S. Patent*, 2,709,672 (1955)

AUREOTHRICIN
See Thiolutin

AVENACIOLIDE
$C_{15}H_{22}O_4$
M.p. 49–50°C and 54–56°C

This antifungal antibiotic is produced by both *Aspergillus avenaceus* G. Smith and *A. fischeri* var. *glaber*. It is best crystallized from a mixture of Et_2O and light petroleum when it forms colourless crystals having the double melting point given above. It has a specific rotation of $[\alpha]_D^{26 \cdot 5}$ − 41·6° (c 1·2, EtOH) and gives an ultraviolet spectrum with a single absorption maximum at 210 nm. The stereochemistry has been deduced primarily from the NMR spectrum.

    Brookes, Kidd, Turner, *J. Chem. Soc.*, 5385 (1963)
    Ellis et al., *Nature*, **203**, 1382 (1964)
NMR spectrum
    Brookes et al., *Austral. J. Chem.*, **18**, 373 (1965)

AVENACEIN
$C_{25}H_{44}O_7N_2$
M.p. 139°C

This antibiotic has been isolated from cultures of *Fusarium avenaceum* and forms colourless tetrahedra when crystallized from aqueous CH_3OH. It has a specific rotation of $[\alpha]_D^{19}$ − 101° ± 2° (c 1·0, EtOH). Hydrolysis with dilute HCl yields N-methyl-D-valine hydrochloride and D-α-hydroxyvaleric acid.

Cook, Cox, Farmer, *J. Chem. Soc.*, 1022 (1949)

AVILAMYCIN
$C_{63}H_{94}O_{35}Cl_2$
M.p. 188–189°C
An antibiotic related to curamycin, this complex substance is elaborated by *Streptomyces viridochromogenes*. The antibiotic forms colourless crystals and has specific rotations of $[\alpha]_D - 7\cdot7°$ (CHCl$_3$) and $[\alpha]_D + 0\cdot8°$ (EtOH). It gives a pentaacetate, m.p. 175–176°C and acid hydrolysis yields curacin, m.p. 144–145°C, 2-deoxy-D-rhamnose, Curaminose, D-coracose, m.p. 112–114°C, L-lyxose, m.p. 95–96°C and 3:5-diacetoxy-1:4-caprolactone, m.p. 102°C. Avilamycin possesses a high activity against gram-positive bacteria *in vitro* and also shows some activity *in vivo*.

Buzzetti *et al., Experimentia*, **24**, 320 (1968)

AVOPARICIN (*Antibiotic LL-AV290*)
M.p. Indefinite
This antibiotic isolated from cultures of *Streptomyces candidus* forms a white amorphous solid with no definite melting point. It is laevorotatory with a specific rotation of $[\alpha]_D^{25} - 95°$ (c 0·78, H$_2$O) and is active against a range of gram-positive bacteria.

Kunstmann *et al., Antimicrobial Agents & Chemotherapy*, 242 (1968)
Partial structure
Hlavka *et al., Tetrahedron Lett.*, 175 (1974)

AXENOMYCIN A
M.p. 127–142°C
This antibiotic has been reported from cultures of *Streptomyces lisandri*. It forms a powder which melts over a wide range of temperature. The structure has not yet been determined.

Cotta *et al., German Patent*, 1,929,107 (1970)
Bianchi *et al., Arch. Microbiol.*, **98**, 289 (1974)

AXENOMYCIN B
$C_{29}H_{38}O_{10}$
M.p. 122–140°C
A further antibiotic produced by *Streptomyces lisandri*, this compound also has a wide melting range. It has no activity against bacteria but possesses marked antifungal, antiprotozoal and anthelmintic properties. The structure has been determined by chemical and spectroscopic methods.

Cotta *et al., German Patent*, 1,929,107 (1970)
Bianchi *et al., Arch. Microbiol.*, **98**, 289 (1974)

AXENOMYCIN D
Streptomyces lisandri also yields this antibiotic when grown aerobically on a medium containing more than 10 per cent of assimilable carbon sources but no phosphates. It is extracted from the culture filtrate with BuOH and separated and purified by chromatography on a silica gel column. It has antifungal, antiprotozoal and anthelmintic activity and is particularly active against *Hymenolepis nana*. The LD$_{50}$ in mice is 200 mg/kg when given orally.

Bianchi *et al., Arch. Microbiol.*, **98**, 289 (1974)

AYFIVIN
M.p. Indefinite
An antibiotic of the polypeptide group, this substance is elaborated by *Bacillus licheniformis* and is isolated by adsorbing the activity of the culture filtrate on activated carbon and eluting with aqueous acid BuOH. The eluate is saturated with sodium chloride, further extracted with BuOH, shaken with H$_2$O at pH 2·0 and the aqueous fraction adjusted to pH 5·0. After precipitation of the crude antibiotic with picric acid, the residue is reacted with ethanolic HCl and the hydrochloride purified by counter-current distribution. Ayfivin contains the aminoacids, aspartic acid, cystine, glutamic acid, histidine, leucine, lysine, ornithine, phenylalanine and possibly *iso*leucine. It is soluble in H$_2$O and EtOH, sparingly so in (CH$_3$)$_2$CO and insoluble in Et$_2$O. It gives no typical absorption maxima in the ultraviolet and is a weak base, stable at pH 2·0 to 10·0 but rapidly deactivated by

alkali or acid at 100°C. It gives negative Adamkiewicz and Sakaguchi reactions and although not inactivated by pepsin or trypsin, is rapidly inactivated by copper.

The antibiotic is normally assayed by the cylinder plate method using *Mycobacterium phlei* or *Corynebacterium xerosis* as the test organism. Sharp and his coworkers have used an arbitrary unit of activity, the purified ayfivin hydrochloride being 40 units/mg. Typical inhibition concentrations (units/ml) have been determined by Arriagada and his colleagues and are as follows: *Corynebacterium xerosis* (0·008); *C. diphtheriae* (0·063–>1·0); *Diplococcus pneumoniae* (0·031–0·5); *Mycobacterium tuberculosis bovis* (>2·0); *Myco. tuberculosis hominis* (0·5–72); *Myco. tuberculosis* BCG (0·5); *Micrococcus lysodeikticus* (0·031); *M. tetragenus* (1·0); *Neisseria gonorrheae* (0·25); *N. intracellularis* (0·5–>1·0); *Staphylococcus albus* (1·0); *Staph. aureus* (0·125–>1·0). The antibiotic inhibits *Bacillus anthracis*, *Clostridium edematiens*, *Cl. novyi*, *Cl. septicus*, *Cl. welchii*, *Escherichia coli*, *Mycobacterium phlei*, *Pasteurella pestis*, *Salmonella enteritidis*, *S. typhi*, *Pseudomonas aeruginosa* and *Vibrio comma* at concentrations greater than 1·0 unit/ml. No resistance to the antibiotic has been reported with *Staphylococcus aureus* although some develops with *Mycobacterium tuberculosis*.

The antibiotic spectrum *in vivo* has been investigated by Arriagada and his coworkers who have demonstrated that 150 units given intravenously to mice over a period of 2 days gave complete protection against *Staphylococcus aureus* and *Streptococcus pyogenes*, but only partial protection against the former unless the treatment was continued for more than 7 days. The antibiotic has been detected in the urine of mice after subcutaneous injection but not following oral administration.

Arriagada *et al.*, *Brit. J. Exptl. Path.*, **30**, 425 (1949)
Hills, Belton, Blatchley, *ibid.*, **30**, 427 (1949)
Sharp *et al.*, *ibid.*, **30**, 444 (1949)
Arriagada *et al.*, *ibid.*, **30**, 458 (1949)

AZALOMYCIN B
$C_{14}H_{24}O_5$
M.p. 185–187°C (*dec.*)
Produced by *Streptomyces hygroscopicus*, this antibiotic forms colourless needles from CH_3OH. It is laevorotatory with a specific rotation of $[\alpha]_D^{25} - 48°$ (c 1·0, CH_3OH) and gives an ultraviolet spectrum in CH_3OH with a single absorption maximum at 252·5 nm. It is active against a number of gram-positive bacteria.

Arai, *J. Antibiotics* (Japan), **13A**, 51 (1960)

AZALOMYCIN F
$C_{30}H_{50}O_{10}N_2$
This antibiotic complex is produced by *Streptomyces hygroscopicus* and has been separated by countercurrent distribution into five components of which the three major constituents have been isolated. These are described below. The complex inhibits the growth of *Bacillus subtilis* PCI 219 in synthetic and natural media, even 5 µg/ml bringing about a rapid release of the cell constituents into the surrounding medium. It also has some activity against fungi, including *Candida albicans*, but does not inhibit the growth of *Escherichia coli* NIHJ even at concentrations as high as 200 µg/ml.

Tresner, Backus, *Appl. Microbiol.*, **4**, 243 (1956)
Arai, *J. Antibiotics* (Japan), **13A**, 51 (1960)
Sugawara, *ibid.*, **21**, 83 (1968)

AZALOMYCIN F_3
M.p. 132–133°C
One of the major components of azalomycin F, this antibiotic forms colourless crystals and has a specific rotation of $[\alpha]_D^{27} + 35°$ (c 1·0, aqueous CH_3OH).

Arai, *Arzneimittel-Forsch.*, **18**, 1396 (1968)
Arai, Hamano, *J. Antibiotics* (Japan), **23**, 107 (1970)

AZALOMYCIN F_4
M.p. 131–132°C
A further major constituent of azalomycin F, this compound crystallizes from CH_3OH as colourless needles and has a specific rotation of $[\alpha]_D^{27} + 39°$ (c 1·0, aqueous CH_3OH).

Arai, *Arzneimittel-Forsch.*, **18**, 1396 (1968)
Arai, Hamano, *J. Antibiotics* (Japan), **23**, 107 (1970)

AZALOMYCIN F_5
M.p. 125–126°C
A third major component of the antibiotic complex, azalomycin F, this antibiotic is also dextrorotatory with a specific rotation of $[\alpha]_D^{27} + 44°$ (c 1·0, aqueous CH_3OH).

Arai, *Arzneimittel-Forsch.*, **18**, 1396 (1968)
Arai, Hamano, *J. Antibiotics* (Japan), **23**, 107 (1970)

AZIRINOMYCIN
$C_4H_5O_2N$

A simple azirine antibiotic isolated from cultures of *Streptomyces aureus*, this substance is unstable, particularly in solution. The structure has been determined as 3-methyl-2-(2*H*)-azirinecarboxylic acid. Both it and the methyl ester are broad-spectrum antibiotics, active against gram-positive and gram-negative bacteria. They are, however, highly toxic to mice and give no protection against lethal bacterial infections.

Stapley *et al.*, *J. Antibiotics* (Japan), **24**, 42 (1971)
Miller, Tristam, Wolf, *ibid.*, **24**, 48 (1971)

AZLOCILLIN
$C_{20}H_{23}N_5O_6S$

A semi-synthetic antibiotic, azlocillin has been shown to be active against gram-positive bacteria such as *Pseudomonas aeruginosa*, *Escherichia coli*, indole-positive and indole-negative *Proteus* species and gram-positive cocci with the exception of penicillin G-resistant *Staphylococcus aureus*. When larger inocula were used it did not inhibit gram-negative bacteria. Experiments have shown it to be more active than carbenicillin or ticarcillin.

Wirth *et al.*, *Infection* (Munich), **4**, 25 (1976)
Stewart, Bodey, *Antimicrobial Agents & Chemotherapy*, **11**, 865 (1977)

AZOMULTIN
$C_{13}H_{22}O_4N_6$
M.p. Indefinite

Streptomyces noborieoensis var. *azomultinus* elaborates this antibiotic which has been obtained as the crystalline hydrochloride, m.p. 209–210°C; $[\alpha]_D^{25}$ + 12·5° (c 1·0, H_2O). The salt gives an ultraviolet spectrum with two absorption maxima at 240 and 325 nm. It is active against gram-positive bacteria.

Misato, Shirato, *Japanese Patent*, 7,006,073 (1970)

AZOMYCIN
$C_3H_3O_2N_3$
M.p. 287–288°C (*dec.*)

This substance is elaborated by several *Nocardia* species and forms pale yellow crystals from EtOH. The ultraviolet spectrum in 0·1 *N*-NaOH has a single absorption maximum at 374 nm. The structure, as 2-nitroimidazole, has been confirmed by synthesis. The inhibitory action of the antibiotic on bacterial synthesis is most rapid for DNA and from experimental work carried out with *Escherichia coli*, it appears that it blocks ribonucleotide reductase but not the polymerization step in the synthesis of DNA or the RNA polymerase reaction. Accordingly, it does not seem to interact with the DNA template.

Nakamura, Umezawa, *J. Antibiotics* (Japan), **8A**, 66 (1955)
Saeki *et al.*, *ibid.*, **27**, 225 (1974)
Synthesis
Beaman *et al.*, *J. Amer. Chem. Soc.*, **87**, 389 (1965)

AZOTOMYCIN (*Antibiotic 1719*)

This antineoplastic antibiotic is produced by *Streptomyces* species. Its cumulative effect in mice has been compared with those of bruneomycin, rubomycin and sibiromycin. When administered intravenously to mice in four 24-hourly doses of 0·36 mg/kg it exhibits a far higher cumulative action than the above-mentioned antibiotics, but this effect is not found when the doses are given at 72-hourly intervals. The Russian workers have suggested that this cumulative effect of the antibiotic may be related to its known inhibitory effects on *de novo* synthesis of purines.

Gol'dberg, Filippos'yants, Stepanova, *Antibiotiki*, **18**, 701 (1973)

B

BACILIPIN A

This antibiotic is obtained from *Bacillus subtilis*, fermentation being carried out on Czapek-Dox medium containing neutral corn steep liquor and glucose as submerged growth in aerated vessels. The bacilipin is isolated by extracting the culture filtrate with amyl acetate at pH 5·0 and purified by adsorbing on alumina at pH 9·0, the activity being eluted with a phosphate buffer saturated with $(CH_3)_2CO$ and then extracted into Et_2O. Countercurrent distribution between the Et_2O and buffer separates the antibiotic into bacilipin A and B. Bacilipin A is soluble in $CHCl_3$, C_6H_6, Et_2O and amyl acetate, slightly soluble in H_2O and insoluble in petroleum ether. It forms salts, e.g. the barium salt, which are all soluble in H_2O and EtOH. The antibiotic is an organic acid which is unstable, is not digested by trypsin and gives negative reactions with Molisch reagent, ammoniacal silver nitrate and 2:4-dinitrophenylhydrazine. It is unsaturated and may be hydrogenated catalytically. The activity is readily lost on drying. The salts, however, are comparatively stable over the pH range from 2·0 to 10·0.

The antibiotic is normally assayed by the cylinder plate method using *Mycobacterium phlei* and *Staphylococcus aureus* as test organisms. It is active *in vitro* against *Corynebacterium diphtheriae gravis*, *Bacillus anthracis*, *Mycobacterium phlei*, *Salmonella enteriditis*, *S. typhi*, *Escherichia coli* and *Staphylococcus aureus*. The antibiotic is a bacteriostatic and is not affected by serum.

Newton, *Brit. J. Exper. Path.*, **30**, 306 (1949)

BACILIPIN B

This component of bacilipin is separated from the preceding antibiotic by countercurrent distribution and is also an organic acid forming stable salts. The antibiotic spectrum *in vitro* is similar to that given for bacilipin A (q.v.).

—Newton, *Brit. J. Exper. Path.*, **30**, 306 (1949)

BACILLIN

This antibiotic has been isolated from a soil isolate of *Bacillus subtilis* by Foster and Woodruff by surface growth on a medium containing alanine salts, glucose and 20 ppm of manganese sulphate tetrahydrate. The yield is 48 *Escherichia coli* units/ml. The antibiotic may be isolated from the culture filtrate either by adsorbing the activity on a cationic resin and eluting with aqueous pyridine or adsorbing on activated carbon, eluting with 90 per cent EtOH and evaporating the eluate to dryness *in vacuo*. The antibiotic is insoluble in all common organic solvents, is thermostable but rapidly inactivated by hydrogen sulphide.

The assay is usually done by serial dilution by agar streak or by the cylinder plate method with *Escherichia coli* as the test organism. Typical inhibition dilutions *in vitro* have been determined by Foster and Woodruff, e.g. *Diplococcus pneumoniae* I (480); *D. pneumoniae* II (120); *Escherichia coli* (160–240); *Micrococcus conglomeratus* (160); *Pasteurella* species (320); *Salmonella paratyphi* (1280); *S. schottmuelleri* (80); *Staphylococcus albus* (320) and *Staph. aureus* (320). The activity *in vitro* is decreased by antibacillin, brain heart media and rabbit blood. Bacillin is not active *in vivo* giving no protection in mice against either *Diplococcus pneumoniae* or *Staphylococcus aureus*. It is relatively toxic, the highest tolerated dose in mice being 20 mg when given intraperitoneally.

Foster, Woodruff, *J. Bact.*, **51**, 363 (1946)
Woodruff, Foster, *ibid.*, **51**, 371 (1946)
Rudert, Foter, *ibid.*, **54**, 793 (1947)

BACILLOMYCIN A (*Bacillomycin R, Fungosin*)

M.p. Indefinite

An antibiotic produced by *Bacillus subtilis*, this substance is an acidic polypeptide which, on acid hydrolysis furnishes aspartic acid, glutaric acid, serine, threonine and tyrosine.

Landy, Rosenman, Warren, *J. Bact.*, **54**, 24 (1947)
Tint, Reiss, *J. Biol. Chem.*, **190**, 133 (1951)
Turner, *Arch. Biochem. Biophys.*, **60**, 364 (1956)

BACILLOMYCIN B

M.p. Indefinite

Bacillus subtilis strain AF 1 furnishes this antibiotic polypeptide. The substance has an *iso*electric point at pH 4·3–4·5 and is non-dialyzable through cellophane. In the dry form it is quite stable and also in solution between pH 3·0 and 9·0. It is not destroyed by either pepsin or trypsin. Bacillomycin B dissolves freely in CH_3OH, EtOH, BuOH, $(CH_3)_2CO$ and dilute alkalies, sparingly soluble in H_2O and insoluble in Et_2O and C_6H_6. It is precipitated by ammonium sulphate, indicative of its peptide character. Acid hydrolysis gives aspartic acid, glutamic acid, leucine, proline and tyrosine. With concentrated H_2SO_4 it furnishes a red-brown colour.

The antibiotic is assayed by the cylinder plate method on Sabouraud's maltose agar using a spore suspension of *Trichophyton mentagrophytes* incubated for 72 hours at 30°C. It has only a negligible activity against bacteria *in vitro* but possesses a high fungistatic activity, typical inhibition concentrations (mg/ml) being: *Blastomyces dermatitidis* (mycelial) (0·010); (yeast) (0·0025); *Candida albicans* (0·05); *Coccidiodes immitis* (0·025); *Epidermophyton floccosum* (0·025); *Histoplasma capsulatum* (0·025); *Microsporon audouini* (0·025); *M. gypseum* (0·025); *Monosporium apiospermum* (0·025); *Nocardia asteroides* (>0·5); *Phialophora verrucosa* (>0·5); *Sporotrichum schenkii* (0·05); *Torula histolytica* (0·05); *Trichophyton mentagrophytes* (0·025); *T. rubrum* (0·025) and *T. schoenleini* (0·026). No details are available concerning its toxicity.

Landy et al., *Proc. Soc. Exptl. Biol. Med.*, **67**, 539 (1948)
Tint, Reiss, *J. Biol. Med.*, **190**, 133 (1951)
Shibazaki, Terui, *J. Fermentation Technol.*, **31**, 339 (1953)
Turner, Schmerzler, *Biochim. Biophys. Acta*, **13**, 553 (1954)

BACILLOMYCIN C
M.p. Indefinite
A further polypeptide antibiotic isolated from *Bacillus subtilis* strain AF 2, this compound is freely soluble in CH_3OH, EtOH, BuOH, $(CH_3)_2CO$, AcOEt, but insoluble in H_2O, Et_2O, $CHCl_3$, CCl_4 and light petroleum. It gives a red colour with concentrated H_2SO_4 and on acid hydrolysis yields aspartic acid, glutamic acid, leucine, tyrosine and valine.

Shibazaki, Terui, *J. Fermentation Technol.*, **32**, 115 (1954)

BACILLOMYCIN R
See Bacillomycin A

BACILLOSPORIN
See Polymixin

BACILYSIN
$C_{12}H_{18}O_5N_2$
M.p. Indefinite

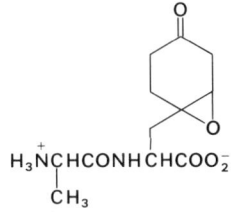

This antibiotic is elaborated by a strain of *Bacillus subtilis* (N.C.T.C. 7197) and forms a white amorphous powder with no definite melting point. It is produced by exactly the same method as bacilipins A and B (q.v.) but by varying the aeration rate. The culture filtrate is clarified at pH 3·0, then adjusted to pH 2·0, the activity adsorbed on activated carbon and eluted with an EtOH-phosphate buffer. Purification is carried out by adsorbing the activity on an alumina column at pH 5·0, eluting with 25 per cent EtOH, distilling the eluate *in vacuo* and freeze-drying the residue. Bacilysin is soluble in CH_3OH and H_2O but insoluble in organic solvents in the absence of moisture. It is dextrorotatory having a specific rotation of $[\alpha]_D^{20} + 103°$ (c 0·643, H_2O) and has pK_a 3·0 and 8·2. It is thermostable, stable in solution in the pH range between 1·4 and 12·0 and is not precipitated by ammonium sulphate, picric, phosphotungstic or trichloroacetic acids. It gives a negative Molisch reaction and a positive Pauly and ninhydrin reaction. It is inactivated by hydrogen sulphide, trypsin and tissue enzymes. Acid hydrolysis yields ammonia, alanine and tyrosine although it is noteworthy that the parent substance does not contain a tyrosyl residue in its structure. The earlier claim that sulphur is present in the molecule has been shown to be incorrect.

Bacilysin is assayed by the cylinder plate method with *Mycobacterium phlei* or *Staphylococcus aureus*. *In vitro* it is active against *Corynebacterium xerosis* and *Staphylococcus aureus* but less so against *Escherichia coli* and *Mycobacterium phlei*. Some resistant colonies are found inside the zone of the assay plate.

Newton, *Brit. J. Exper. Path.*, **30**, 306 (1949)
Rogers, Lomakina, Abraham, *Biochem. J.*, **97**, 573, 579 (1965)
Biosynthesis
Roscoe, Abraham, *Biochem. J.*, **99**, 793 (1966)

BACIMETHRIN
$C_6H_9O_2N_3$
M.p. 174°C
This simple pyrimidine antibiotic has been isolated from cultures of

Bacillus megatherium. It forms colourless crystals from CH_3OH and has the structure 4-amino-5-hydroxymethyl-2-β methoxypyrimidine.

Tanaka et al., *J. Antibiotics* (Japan), **14A**, 161 (1961)

BACIPHELACIN
$C_{22}H_{34}N_2O_6$
M.p. Indefinite

Bacillus thiaminolyticus yields this antibiotic which has been obtained as a white powder having no definite melting point. The structure given above has been determined from chemical analysis and a study of the infrared, NMR and mass spectra. Beciphelacin possesses antibacterial and antileukemic activity.

Okazaki et al., *J. Antibiotics* (Japan), **28**, 717 (1975)

BACITRACIN

This antibiotic substance has been isolated from both *Bacillus licheniformis* and *B. subtilis* and was originally considered to be a single compound. It has now been demonstrated that it consists of several components, the major constituents being bacitracins A, B and C. Other components have also been obtained in smaller amounts and are described below. Much of the bacteriological work has been carried out with the mixture of bacitracins obtained as an amorphous white powder which is highly hygroscopic. This material is soluble in CH_3OH, EtOH, *iso*PrOH, BuOH and cyclohexanol, slightly soluble in cyclohexanone and insoluble in $CHCl_3$, C_6H_6, $(CH_3)_2CO$, Et_2O and AcOEt. It readily diffuses through a nitrocellulose membrane. Bacitracin is stable in neutral and slightly acid solutions at 0–5°C and is precipitated by benzoic, furoic, salicylic, tannic and trichloroacetic acids, the salts of heavy metals and also by high concentrations of CH_3CO, sodium chloride, molybdic acid and Reinecke's salt. It gives a negative Sakaguchi and biuret reaction and is not digested by either pepsin or trypsin.

Several methods of assay have been employed, e.g. cylinder plate and turbidimetric with *Staphylococcus aureus*, serial dilution with *Streptococcus hemolyticus* and the cylinder plate method with *S. hemolyticus* for the determination of the antibiotic in saliva, serum and urine. Craig and his colleagues obtained a maximum activity of 66 units/mg for their material. Bacitracin is active *in vitro* against a number of pathogenic bacteria, typical inhibition concentrations (units/ml) being: *Bacillus anthracis* (4·0–12·5); *Clostridium histolyticum* (0·025–0·004); *Cl. novyi* (0·01); *Cl. speticum* (0·01–0·002); *Cl. sordellii* (0·01–0·005); *Cl. tetani* 0·01–0·006); *Cl. welchii* (0·025–0·002); *Corynebacterium diphtheriae* (0·015–0·004); *C. xerosis* (0·005–0·003); aerobic *Micrococci* (5·0–0·008); *Neisseria gonorrheae* (0·006); *N. meningitidis* (0·01); *Streptococcus hemolyticus* (ABDFG) (0·025–0·005); *St. hemolyticus* (D) (3·0–0·008) and *St. non-hemolyticus* (3·0–0·025). It is also active against *Actinomyces israeli* at a concentration of 0·075–0·005 units/ml. Meleney and Johnson have shown that at a concentration of 50 units/ml the following bacteria and fungi were not inhibited: *Aerobacter aerogenes*, *A. cloacae*, *Bacillus alkaligenes*, *B. subtilis*, *Cryptococcus hominis*, *Escherichia coli*, *Monilia albicans*, *Nocardia asteroides*, *Proteus*, *Pseudomonas aeruginosa*, *Shigella alkalescens* and *Salmonella typhosa*. Bachman has also shown that bacitracin is synergistic with penicillin against a number of strains of α- and β-hemolytic streptococci.

A number of workers have examined the effect of bacitracin upon experimental infections in animals. Meleney and Teng have shown that 4000–10,000 units given intramuscularly 3 hours after infection of dogs with staphylococcal meningitis gave complete protection while Bond and his colleagues showed that in the same animals a dose of 2000–10,000 mg/kg/day, administered orally, substantially reduced spore-forming anaerobes and fecal streptococci. Johnson, Anker and Meleney found that in guinea pigs infected with *Clostridium septicum* or *Cl. welchii*, 50–100 units administered subcutaneously every 3 hours for 36 hours gave a survival rate of 80 per cent and in mice infected with hemolytic streptococcus, 1–2 units administered intraperitoneally gave an 80 per cent survival rate.

Numerous clinical tests have been carried out with bacitracin, particularly in the form of an ointment giving a favourable response in a large number of cases resistant to penicillin, streptomycin and sulphonamides. It has also proved useful in the treatment of eye infections either in the form of a fine powder or in saline solution. In concentrations of 100 units/ml or greater, it is very effective against mastoid infections but somewhat less so against chronic suppurative mastoiditis and external otitis. Bacitracin is unabsorbed when given orally and is too nephrotoxic for parenteral administration.

Bacitracin has also found a use in veterinary medicine being effective against bovine mastitis caused by *Streptococcus agalactiae*.

The toxicity in mice has been determined by Scudi and Antopol, the LD_{50} being 360 mg/kg (intravenous), 1300–2500 mg/kg (subcutaneous), 200–650 mg/kg (intraperitoneal) and 3750 mg/kg (oral). Repeated sublethal doses gave no chronic toxicity in rats or mice. When applied topically, sensitivity reactions to the antibiotic are rare even following prolonged therapy. Following administration of bacitracin, only negligible concentrations are found in the blood and spinal fluids. Upon intravenous injection, bacitracin is found in all of the organs, body fluids and tissues although concentrations are extremely low in the brain and cerebrospinal fluid.

Johnson, Anker, Meleney, *Science*, **102**, 376 (1945)
Darker et al., *J. Amer. Pharm. Assoc.*, **37**, 156 (1948)
Anker et al., *J. Bact.*, **55**, 249 (1949)
Craig, Gregory, Barry, *J. Clin. Invest.*, **28**, 1014 (1949)
Meleney, Johnson, *Amer. J. Med.*, **7**, 794 (1949)
Bacteriological studies
Benson, *J. Amer. Vet. Med. Assoc.*, **111**, 160 (1947)
Meleney, Johnson, *J. Amer. Med. Assoc.*, **133**, 675 (1947)
Scudi, Antopol, *Proc. Soc. Exper. Biol. Med.*, **64**, 503 (1947)
Scudi, Clift, Kreuger, *ibid.*, **65**, 9 (1947)
Scudi, Coret, Antopol, *ibid.*, **66**, 558 (1947)
Eagle, Fleischmann, *J. Bact.*, **55**, 341 (1948)
Eagle, Musselman, Fleischman, *ibid.*, **55**, 347 (1948)
Evans, *ibid.*, **56**, 507 (1948)
Bond et al., *Proc. Soc. Exper. Biol. Med.*, **68**, 395 (1948)
Eagle, Fleischman, *ibid.*, **68**, 415 (1948)
Benson, *J. Amer. Vet. Med. Assoc.*, **112**, 160 (1948)
Miller, Slatkin, Johnson, *J. Invest. Dermatol.*, **10**, 179 (1948)
Bellows, Farmer, *Amer. J. Ophthalmol.*, **31**, 1070 (1948)
Sandusky, Keeble, *Ann. Surg.*, **130**, 674 (1949)
Meleney, Teng, *J. Clin. Invest.*, **28**, 1054 (1949)
Coyle, Collins, Nungester, *Arch. Otalaryng.*, **50**, 284 (1949)

Synergism with penicillin
Eagle, Fleischman, *Proc. Soc. Exper. Biol. Med.*, **68**, 415 (1948)

BACITRACIN A
$C_{66}H_{103}O_{16}N_{17}S$
M.p. Indefinite

This component of bacitracin (q.v.) is a complex polypeptide, separated by countercurrent distribution methods. It has been shown to possess the structure given above which is based primarily upon a study of the hydrolysis products. It forms a white, amorphous powder which is slightly dextrorotatory with $[\alpha]_D^{23} + 5°$ (c 0·1, 0·02 N-HCl). Together with bacitracin C it is the most active of the constituents of the original mixture.

Lockhart, Abraham, Newton, *Biochem. J.*, **61**, 534 (1955)
Weisiger, Hausmann, Craig, *J. Amer. Chem. Soc.*, **77**, 731, 3123 (1955)
Wrinch, *Nature*, **179**, 536 (1957)

BACITRACIN B
M.p. Indefinite
A further major component of bacitracin, obtained from *Bacillus licheniformis* and *B. subtilis*, this polypeptide antibiotic has only about a third of

the biological activity of bacitracins A and C. The structure is not yet completely known.

>   Sharp et al., *Brit. J. Exptl. Path.*, **30**, 444 (1949)
>   Newton, Abraham, *Biochem. J.*, **47**, 257 (1950)
>   Lockhart, Abraham, *ibid.*, **58**, 633 (1954)
>   Hausmann, Weisiger, Craig, *J. Amer. Chem. Soc.*, **77**, 721, 723, 3123 (1955)
>   Hausmann, Weisiger, Craig, *ibid.*, **76**, 2839 (1954)

BACITRACIN C
M.p. Indefinite
The third major component of bacitracin, this antibiotic is also a polypeptide and forms a white amorphous powder with no definite melting point. The biological activity is similar to that of bacitracin A (q.v.).

>   Sharp et al., *Brit. J. Exptl. Path.*, **30**, 444 (1949)
>   Newton, Abraham, *Biochem. J.*, **47**, 257 (1949)
>   Lockhart, Abraham, *ibid.*, **58**, 633 (1950)
>   Hausmann, Weisiger, Craig, *J. Amer. Chem. Soc.*, **76**, 2839 (1954)
>   Hausmann, Weisiger, Craig, *ibid.*, **77**, 721, 723, 3123 (1955)

BACITRACIN D
A minor constituent of bacitracin, this antibiotic substance has not yet been fully characterized.

>   Sharp et al., *Brit. J. Exptl. Path.*, **30**, 444 (1949)
>   Newton, Abraham, *Biochem. J.*, **47**, 257 (1950)
>   Lockhart, Abraham, *ibid.*, **58**, 633 (1954)
>   Hausmann, Weisiger, Craig, *J. Amer. Chem. Soc.*, **76**, 2839 (1954)
>   Hausmann, Weisiger, Craig, *ibid.*, **77**, 721, 723, 3123 (1955)

BACITRACIN E
Also present in bacitracin, isolated from *Bacillus licheniformis* and *B. subtilis*, this antibiotic is a polypeptide like the remaining components of the mixture.

>   Sharp et al., *Brit. J. Exptl. Path.*, **30**, 444 (1949)
>   Newton, Abraham, *Biochem. J.*, **47**, 257 (1950)
>   Lockhart, Abraham, *ibid.*, **58**, 633 (1954)
>   Hausmann, Weisiger, Craig, *J. Amer. Chem. Soc.*, **76**, 2839 (1954)
>   Hausmann, Weisiger, Craig, *ibid.*, **77**, 721, 723, 3123 (1955)

BACITRACIN F_1
M.p. Indefinite
This minor component of bacitracin has been distinguished by column chromatography but has not been extensively studied.

>   Sharp et al., *J. Brit. Exptl. Path.*, **30**, 444 (1949)
>   Newton, Abraham, *Biochem. J.*, **47**, 257 (1950)
>   Lockhart, Abraham, *ibid.*, **58**, 633 (1954)
>   Hausmann, Weisiger, Craig, *J. Amer. Chem. Soc.*, **76**, 2839 (1954)
>   Hausmann, Weisiger, Craig, *ibid.*, **77**, 721, 723, 3123 (1955)

BACITRACIN F_2
M.p. Indefinite
A polypeptide antibiotic found in bacitracin (q.v.), this substance is present only in small quantities and has not yet been fully characterized.

>   Sharp et al., *Brit. J. Exptl. Path.*, **30**, 444 (1949)
>   Newton, Abraham, *Biochem. J.*, **47**, 257 (1950)
>   Lockhart, Abraham, *ibid.*, **58**, 633 (1954)
>   Hausmann, Weisiger, Craig, *J. Amer. Chem. Soc.*, **76**, 2839 (1954)
>   Hausmann, Weisiger, Craig, *ibid.*, **77**, 721, 723, 3123 (1955)

BACITRACIN F_3
An antibiotic obtained from bacitracin (q.v.), little is yet known concerning its chemical or physical characteristics.

>   Sharp et al., *Brit. J. Exptl. Path.*, **30**, 444 (1949)
>   Newton, Abraham, *Biochem. J.*, **47**, 257 (1950)
>   Lockhart, Abraham, *ibid.*, **58**, 633 (1954)
>   Hausmann, Weisiger, Craig, *J. Amer. Chem. Soc.*, **76**, 2839 (1954)
>   Hausmann, Weisiger, Craig, *ibid.*, **77**, 721, 723, 3123 (1955)

BACITRACIN G
This minor component of bacitracin has also been distinguished in the mixture by column chromatography. No details are yet available regarding its chemical, physical and biological properties.

>   Sharp et al., *Brit. J. Exptl. Path.*, **30**, 444 (1949)
>   Newton, Abraham, *Biochem. J.*, **47**, 257 (1950)
>   Lockhart, Abraham, *ibid.*, **58**, 633 (1954)
>   Hausmann, Weisiger, Craig, *J. Amer. Chem. Soc.*, **76**, 2839 (1954)
>   Hausmann, Weisiger, Craig, *ibid.*, **77**, 721, 723, 3123 (1955)

BAKUCHIOL
$C_{18}H_{24}O$
A plant antibiotic substance, bakuchiol has been isolated from *Psoralea*

drupacea Bge. Bakuchiol is not effective against gram-negative bacteria, saprophytes or phytopathogenic fungi. It does, however, inhibit gram-positive bacteria, particularly a number of antibiotic-resistant staphylococci at a concentration of 1–5 micrograms/millilitre and also certain dermatophytes at 2–20 micrograms/millilitre. The structure has been established from chemical and spectroscopic examination.

Bondarenko *et al.*, *Tr. S'ezda Mikrobiol. Ukr.* 4th, 208 (1975)

BAMICETIN
$C_{28}H_{40}O_9N_6$
M.p. 240°C (*dec.*)

A peptide antibiotic, bamicetin is produced by *Streptomyces plicatus* and forms colourless crystals from CH_3OH. It is dextrorotatory having a specific rotation of $[\alpha]_D^{26}$ + 123° (c 0·5, 0·1 *N*-HCl). The partial structure given above is based upon chemical and spectroscopic evidence.

Haskell *et al.*, *J. Amer. Chem. Soc.*, **80**, 743 (1958)

BAUMYCIN A$_1$
$C_{34}H_{43}NO_{13}$

An antibiotic complex has recently been isolated from cultures of an unclassified *Streptomyces* species and separated into six components by column and thin layer chromatography. These antibiotics are structurally related to daunomycin and all have antitumour activity.

Komiyama *et al.*, *J. Antibiotics* (Japan), **30**, 619 (1977)
Structure
Takahasi *et al.*, *J. Antibiotics* (Japan), **30**, 622 (1977)

BAUMYCIN A$_2$
$C_{34}H_{43}NO_{13}$

Baumycin B₁

A stereoisomer of baumycin A₁, this antibiotic also occurs in the baumycin complex isolated from cultures of an unclassified species of *Streptomyces*. The structure has been elucidated from chemical and spectroscopic data.

Komiyama *et al.*, *J. Antibiotics* (Japan), **30**, 619 (1977)
Structure
Takahashi *et al.*, *J. Antibiotics* (Japan), **30**, 622 (1977)

BAUMYCIN B₁
$C_{34}H_{41}NO_{14}$

A further antitumour antibiotic related to daunomycin isolated from the culture broth of an unclassified *Streptomyces* species, this substance has been shown to be the acid corresponding to the preceding antibiotics.

Komiyama *et al.*, *J. Antibiotics* (Japan), **30**, 619 (1977)
Structure
Takahashi *et al.*, *J. Antibiotics* (Japan), **30**, 622 (1977)

BAUMYCIN B₂
$C_{34}H_{41}NO_{14}$

This antibiotic isolated from the baumycin complex by column and thin layer chromatography is a stereoisomer of baumycin B₁, the structure having been established from chemical analysis, spectroscopic data and comparison with the preceding antibiotics. It possesses antitumour activity.

Komiyama *et al.*, *J. Antibiotics* (Japan), **30**, 619 (1977)
Structure
Takahashi *et al.*, *J. Antibiotics* (Japan), **30**, 622 (1977)

BAUMYCIN C₁
$C_{28}H_{29}NO_{11}$

Baumycin C₂

A fifth component of the baumycin antibiotic complex, this substance has the simpler structure given above based upon chemical and spectroscopic evidence.

Komiyama et al., *J. Antibiotics* (Japan), **30**, 619 (1977)
Structure
Takahashi et al., *J. Antibiotics* (Japan), **30**, 622 (1977)

BAUMYCIN C₂
$C_{28}H_{31}NO_{11}$

The secondary alcohol corresponding to baumycin C_1, this antibiotic has also been isolated from the culture broth of an unclassified species of *Streptomyces* and has the above structures based upon chemical analysis and a study of the infrared, NMR and mass spectra. It has antitumour activity.

Komiyama et al., *J. Antibiotics* (Japan), **30**, 619 (1977)
Structure
Takahashi et al., *J. Antibiotics* (Japan), **30**, 622 (1977)

BEAUVERICIN
$C_{45}H_{57}O_9N_3$
M.p. 93–4°C (147–148°C)

A depsipeptide antibiotic from *Streptomyces* species, this compound has also been synthesized, the synthetic material having the higher of the two melting points given above. Beauvericin is markedly active against a wide range of bacteria, particularly *Escherichia coli*, *Sarcina lutea* and *Staphylococcus aureus* and also against *Candida albicans*.

Ovchinnikov, Ivanov, Mikhaleva, *Tetrahedron Lett.*, 159 (1971)

BELFACILLIN
See Methicillin

4-N-BENZYLDEMETHYLRIFAMPICIN
$C_{49}H_{62}O_{12}N_4$

A semi-synthetic antibiotic, this compound increases the number of survivors among mice injected with Rauscher leukaemia virus when given subcutaneously shortly after the injection but does not prolong the survival time.

Okunewick, Phillips, Erhard, *Int. J. Cancer*, **11**, 460 (1973)

2-BENZYL-1:4-DIMETHYL-5-HYDROXYMETHYL-2:5-EPIDITHIA-3:6-DIKETOPIPERAZINE
$C_{14}H_{16}O_3N_2S_2$

An antibiotic metabolite isolated from an unidentified fungus, this compound is a potent antibacterial against gram-positive bacteria and is also effective against a range of fungi.

De Vault, Rosenbrook, *J. Antibiotics* (Japan), **26**, 532 (1973)

2-BENZYL-1:4-DIMETHYL-5-HYDROXYMETHYL-2:5-EPITRITHIA-3:6-DIKETOPIPERAZINE
$C_{14}H_{16}O_3N_2S_3$

The trithia analogue of the preceding antibiotic has also been isolated from the same fungus. Its antibiotic activity is virtually identical.

De Vault, Rosenbrook, *J. Antibiotics* (Japan), **26**, 532 (1973)

BENZYLPENICILLIN (*Parasiticin, Penicillin G, Penicillin II*)
$C_{16}H_{18}O_4N_2S$
M.p. Indefinite

Several strains of *Aspergillus* and *Penicillium*, particularly *P. notatum*, yield this potent antibiotic when cultivated on suitable media. The parent acid, 6-phenylacetamidapenicillanic acid, is an amorphous white powder having no definite melting point. It is dextrorotatory with a specific rotation of $[\alpha]_D + 282°$ (c 1·0, EtOH) and is normally isolated as the potassium or sodium salt, the latter forming colourless needles with m.p. 215°C (*dec.*) when crystallized from equeous BuOH or MeOH–AcOEt. The sodium salt is dextrorotatory having a specific rotation of $[\alpha]_D^{24·8} + 301°$ (c 1·0, H$_2$O) and gives an ultraviolet spectrum in ethanolic solution with absorption maxima at 252, 257·5 and 264 nm. Both salts are freely soluble in H$_2$O, moderately soluble in the lower alcohols and virtually insoluble in Et$_2$O, CHCl$_3$ and liquid paraffin.

Benzylpenicillin is inactivated by oxidizing and reducing agents, glycerol and alcohols in the cold although it is possible that under these conditions, the presence of impurities may be responsible for the deactivation. When highly purified, the parent acid is stated to be quite stable. In the cold, dilute acids furnish benzylpenicillic acid and penicillamine. How alkalis yield γ-phenyllevulinic acid and when heated with alcohols it gives a series of alkylbenzylpenicilloates. In cold alkaline solution it is rapidly inactivated by cysteine and other aminothiol compounds. Dehydrogenation with selenium furnishes phenylacetamide.

Benzylpenicillin possesses bacteriostatic and bactericidal activity, depending on concentration, against the majority of gram-positive bacteria and gram-negative cocci and also against some actinomycetes and spirochaetes. The antibiotic is believed to act by interfering with the utilization of certain substances required for the synthesis of the bacterial cell wall and accordingly exerts its effect against bacteria during cell division. This action is inhibited by the enzyme penicillinase which is produced during the growth of certain microorganisms. It is not, however, inactivated by pus, serum or the products forms by autolysis of tissue.

The parent acid has an antibiotic activity of 1250 penicillin units and the sodium salt 2100 units. A large number of organisms are normally sensitive to the antibiotic including *Actinomyces israelii*, *Bacillus anthracis*, *Clostridium* species, *Corynebacterium diphtheriae*, *Erysipelothrix rhusiopathiae*, *Haemophilus influenzae*, *Leptospira* species, *Listeria monocytogenes*, *Neisseria* species, *Spirillum minus* and *Treponema* species at minimum inhibitory concentrations between 0·006 and 2·0 micrograms/millilitre.

Among the pathogenic microorganisms which are naturally insensitive to the antibiotic are *Brucella*, the *Escherichia coli* group, *Klebsiella*, *Mycobacterium*, *Pasturella*, *Proteus* (with the exception of certain strains of *P. mirabilis*), *Pseudomonas*, *Vibrio*, fungi, rickettsia, mycoplasmas and viruses. The susceptibility of individual species to the antibiotic varies widely, however, and in many cases resistant strains of normally sensitive organisms have been encountered.

In common with most of the penicillin antibiotics, benzylpenicillin produces toxic symptoms in allergic patients. When administered to hypersensitive patients, anaphylactic shock with collapse and sometimes death may occur within minutes. A generalized sensitivity reaction can occur, usually within 1–3 weeks with fever, joint pains, urticaria, erythema multiforme, angioneurotic oedema and exfoliative dermatitis, while an accelerated form of urticaria has been known to develop within hours.

Doses of more than 6 grams given intravenously have been associated with haemolytic anemia in patients with circulating IgG antibody and convulsions and other signs of toxicity to the central nervous system can occur with very high doses of benzylpenicillin.

Weihrauch and his colleagues have compared the neurotoxic effect of this antibiotic in the rabbit with ampicillin (q.v.), showing that ampicillin has no such effects on the central nervous system. Single spikes are found on the electroencephalogram with blood levels of 1000–1500 units/ml followed by spike-wave paroxysms. With blood levels higher than this, generalized spike-waves then developed leading to generalized convulsions. Neurotoxic concentrations of the antibiotic appear in the brain with 15–33 minutes and even when the blood levels return to zero, the pathological encephalogram changes persist for more than 2 hours.

Russian workers have demonstrated that where female rabbits are immunized with benzylpenicillin before or during gestation, antibodies of the IgG and IgM type appear in the progeny.

Medical Research Committee, Washington and Medical Research Council, London, *Science*, **102**, 626 (1945)
du Vigneaud *et al.*, *ibid.*, **104**, 431 (1946)
Arnstein, Cook, *Brit. J. Exptl. Path.*, **28**, 94 (1947)
Sato, Barry, Craig, *J. Biol. Chem.*, **174**, 217 (1948)
Behrens *et al.*, *ibid.*, **175**, 751 (1948)
Carpenter, *J. Amer. Chem. Soc.*, **70**, 2964 (1948)
Cooper, Binkley, *ibid.*, **70**, 2964 (1948)
Salivar, Hedger, Brown, *ibid.*, **70**, 1287 (1948)
du Vigneaus *et al.*, *J. Biol. Chem.*, **175**, 721 (1948)
du Vigneaud *et al.*, *ibid.*, **176**, 893, 915 (1948)
Hockenbull, Ramachandran, Walker, *Arch. Biochem.*, **23**, 160 (1949)
Peck, Folkers, *The Chemistry of Penicillin*, Princeton Univ. Press, **52**, 144 (1949)
Wintersteiner, *ibid.*, 81 (1949)
Johnson, Woodward, Robinson, *ibid.*, 440 (1949)
Behrens, *ibid.*, 657 (1949)
du Vigneaud, Wood, Wright, *ibid.*, 892 (1949)
Süs, *Annalen*, **571**, 201 (1951)
Batchelor, Chain, Robinson, *Proc. Roy. Soc.*, **154B**, 478 (1961)
Sheehan, Henery-Logan, *J. Amer. Chem. Soc.*, **84**, 2983 (1962)
Keusch, O'Connell, *Amer. J. med. Sci.*, **251**, 428 (1966)
Sabath *et al.*, *Antimicrobial Agents & Chemotherapy*, 53 (1970)
Kiktenko *et al.*, *Antibiotiki*, **18**, 1085 (1973)
Paroli, Samueli, Valeri, *Fegato*, **19**, 293 (1973)
Weihrauch *et al.*, *Arzneim-Forsch.*, **24**, 317 (1974)
Kovalenko, Solov'ev, Borodin, *Antibiotiki*, **20**, 266 (1975)
Bacterial resistance
Okubadejo *et al.*, *Brit. med. J.*, 212 (ii/1973)
Hansman, *Med. J. Aust.*, 353 (ii/1974)
Ross *et al.*, *J. Amer. med. Assoc.*, **229**, 1075 (1974)
Thin, *Brit. J. vener. Dis.*, **50**, 57 (1974)
Incompatibility
Woodward, *J. Pharm. Pharmacol.*, **4**, 1009 (1952)
Schwartz, Buckwalter, *J. Pharm. Sci.*, **51**, 1119 (1962)
Thoma *et al.*, *Acta Pharm. Hung.*, **35**, 1 (1965)
Patel, Phillips, *Amer. J. Hosp. Pharm.*, **23**, 409 (1966)
Lynn, *J. Hosp. Pharm.*, **28**, 71 (1970)
Toxic effects
Bertelsen, Dalgaard, *Bull. Hyg. Lond.*, **40**, 1013 (1965)
Levin, *N. Engl. J. Med.*, **275**, 1115 (1966)
Batchelor *et al.*, *Lancet*, 1175 (i/1967)
Idsoe *et al.*, *Bull. World Health Org.*, **38**, 159 (1968)
Wicher *et al.*, *J. Amer. med. Assoc.*, **208**, 143 (1969)
Copeman, *Brit. J. Hops. Med.*, **7**, 339 (1972)
Pevny, *J. Amer. med. Assoc.*, **226**, 583 (1973)

BERNINAMYCIN
M.p. Indefinite

A polypeptide antibiotic isolated from cultures of *Streptomyces bernensis*, this antibiotic forms a white amorphous powder with no definite melting point. The organism is grown under submerged aerobic conditions in a medium containing unpurified ingredients at 20–32°C for 10 days. The antibiotic substance is isolated by filtration of the medium followed by liquid:liquid extraction from the broth with methyl ethyl ketone. Further purification is carried out by chromatography on silica gel, eluting with $CH_3OH-CH_2Cl_2$. Berninamycin inhibits the growth of a number of gram-positive bacteria and its use has been proposed to inhibit the growth of *Bacillus subtilis* in yeast.

Bergy, Coats, Reusser, *U.S. Patent*, 3,689,639 (1972)

BEROMYCIN
$C_{27}H_{29}O_{10}N$

Streptomyces griseoruber var. *beromycini* produces this antibiotic which is of the anthrocycline group. Optimum results are obtained by a selection of organisms from tropical soils fermented upon one of two media based upon soybean flour and glucose respectively and incubated at 28°C for 5 days. The final yield obtained in this manner is between 500 and 1200 μg/ml of the antibiotic. The antibiotic is amphoteric giving H_2O-soluble salts with alkalies. It is active against a number of experimental tumours in mice.

Gauze et al., *Antibiotiki*, **17**, 8 (1972)
Kudinova et al., *ibid.*, **17**, 689 (1972)
Shapovalova, *ibid.*, **19**, 260 (1974)

BICYCLOMYCIN
$C_{12}H_{18}O_7N_2$
M.p. 187–189°C and 188–191°C

This bicyclic antibiotic is obtained from cultures of *Streptomyces sapporonensis* and exists in two crystal forms having the melting points given above. It is dextrorotatory with a specific rotation of $[\alpha]_D^{23}$ + 63·5° (c 1·0, CH_3OH). Determinations made by NMR and X-ray crystallographic analysis have established the structure as 8:10-diaza-6-hydroxy-5-methylene-1-(2'-methyl-1':2':3'-trihydroxypropyl)-2-oxabicyclo[4,2,2]decan-7:9-dione.

Bicyclomycin is active primarily against gram-negative bacteria, e.g. *Citrobacter*, *Enterobacter cloacae*, *Escherichia coli*, *Klebsiella*, *Neisseria*, *Salmonella* and *Shigella* but inactive against *Proteus* spp., *Pseudomonas aeruginosa* and gram-positive organisms. It is not deactivated by rat tissue homogenates or by cultures of sensitive or resistant organisms and is highly effective in curing mice infected with *Escherichia coli* strains which prove resistant to common antibiotics. The binding of the antibiotic with serum proteins is extremely low. Bicyclomycin shows no cross resistance with other common antibiotics. On administration *in vivo*, the peak blood level following a dose of 50 mg/kg given intramuscularly to mice, rats, rabbits and dogs is quite high and more than 70 per cent of the dose is recovered from the first 24-hour sample of urine. The antibiotic is distributed among various organs and tissues with the maximum concentration being found in the kidneys. When administered to humans, only 2·9 per cent of the given dose is found in the urine, compared with 24 per cent found in the urine of rats. The toxicity *in vivo* is low, doses of 500–1000 mg being tolerated by human volunteers.

Several acyl derivatives of this antibiotic have been prepared and administered orally to rats when it is found that their recovery after urinary excretion increases with the increasing lipophilicity of the derivatives. The monoacyl derivatives are readily hydrolysed by esterases whereas the diacyl derivatives are unattacked.

Kamiya et al., *J. Antibiotics* (Japan), **25**, 576 (1972)
Miyoshi et al., *ibid.*, **25**, 569 (1972)
Nishida et al., *ibid.*, **25**, 582, 594 (1972)

BIFLORINE
$C_{20}H_{20}O_3$
M.p. 97°C

This antibiotic, isolated from the roots of *Capraria biflora*, must not be confused with the alkaloid of the same name. Biflorine forms colourless crystals from $(CH_3)_2CO$ and is soluble in most common organic solvents forming deep violet solutions. It is active against gram-positive bacteria.

de Lima et al., *Rev. quim. ind.*, (Rio de Janeiro), **22**, 14 (1953)
Comin et al., *Helv. Chim. Acta*, **46**, 409 (1963)

BIFORMIN
Polyporus biformis yields both the neutral and the acid form of this antibiotic, the latter being designated biforminic acid (q.v.). Biformin is isolated from the fermented liquor by extraction with $CHCl_3$ followed by evaporation with the addition of H_2O to form a brown aqueous concentrate which yields a solution of the product on filtration. It may be purified by precipitation with acidified silver nitrate, the metallic silver removed from the precipitate by acidified potassium iodide, the filtrate neutralized, extracted with Et_2O, evaporated to an aqueous concentrate and filtered. Biformin is soluble in EtOH, $CHCl_3$, Et_2O and H_2O. It is stable in dilute solution but not in concentrated solutions, gives no colour reaction with $FeCl_3$ or potassium cyanide and is not affected by boiling in dilute acid or alkali.

The antibiotic is active against a number of bacteria *in vitro*, typical inhibition concentrations (μg/ml) being: *Bacillus mycoides* (5·0–13); *B. subtilis* (0·04); *Escherichia coli* (1·6); *Klebsiella pneumoniae* (0·6–1·6); *Pseudomonas aeruginosa* (32–50); *Mycobacterium phlei* (0·6–1·5); *M. smegmatis* (3·0–3·5); *M. tuberculosis* (0·56) and *Staphylococcus aureus* (0·3–0·8). No resistance to the antibiotic is developed by *Staph. aureus* and serum has little effect upon the activity with the same organism.

Biformin shows no activity *in vivo* against *Mycobacterium tuberculosis* and *Staphylococcus aureus* in mice. The LD_{50} in mice in 77 mg/kg (subcutaneous), 18·8 mg/kg (intravenous) and 37·5 mg/kg (intraperitoneal). In humans it produces severe dermatitis upon contact with the skin.

Robbins et al., Proc. Nat. Acad. Sci., **33**, 176 (1947)

BIFORMINIC ACID

This form of the antibiotic is produced in approximately 10 per cent yield from cultures of *Polyporus biformis* together with biformin. It is isolated by re-extracting with $CHCl_3$ at pH 2·0 following the isolation of biformin. It gives the same chemical reactions as biformin with the exception that impure biforminic acid forms a brown colour with $FeCl_3$. The antibiotic spectrum *in vitro* differs somewhat from that of biformin as may be seen from the inhibition concentrations (µg/ml): *Bacillus mycoides* (3·4); *B. subtilis* (0·2); *Escherichia coli* (3·4); *Klebsiella pneumoniae* (6·8); *Mycobacterium phlei* (0·8); *M. smegmatis* (6·8); *Pseudomonas aeruginosa* (220) and *Staphylococcus aureus* (0·7).

Robbins et al., Proc. Nat. Acad. Sci., **33**, 176 (1947)

BIHOROMYCIN
$C_{41}H_{76}O_{13}$

A crystalline antibiotic isolated from cultures of *Streptomyces filipinensis* var. *bihoroensis* freshly isolated from soil and incubated at 28°C for 3 days. The substance is obtained by adjusting the pH of the culture filtrate to 2·0 and extracting the precipitate with CH_3OH. Chromatography of the extract gives pure bihoromycin as colourless needles. The antibiotic inhibits the growth of tobacco mosaic virus on the leaf disc and is also active against *Piricularia oryzae* and *Staphylococcus aureus*.

Koaze et al., Japanese Patent, 7,218,636 (1972)

BIKAVERIN (*Lycopersin*)

This antibiotic is produced by *Fusarium oxysporum* grown on a medium containing glucose and ammonium tartrate. The glucose may be replaced by other carbohydrates and although the production of the antibiotic differs in this case, it has been shown that the source of carbon in the medium is not as critical as the initial ratio of carbon to nitrogen. The yield of bikaverin increases with increasing nitrogen content up to 0·7 g/l but, thereafter, unutilized ammonium tartrate remained and none of the antibiotic pigment is formed. It appears that bikaverin is only synthesized during unbalanced growth in acidic media when the source of nitrogen is depleted and an excess carbon source is still present. From the infrared spectrum it has been concluded that bikaverin is identical with lycopersin.

Brewer et al., J. Antibiotics (Japan), **26**, 778 (1973)

BIOCERIN

An antibiotic derived from *Bacillus cereus*, biocerin is obtained from the culture filtrate by extraction with Et_2O, the ethereal extract yielding a yellow-brown oily residue. This substance dissolves readily in $(CH_3)_2CO$, $CHCl_3$, Et_2O and 95 per cent EtOH, but is insoluble in H_2O.

Johnson and his colleagues have determined the inhibition concentrations of a crude biocerin (µg/ml) as follows: *Aerobacter aerogenes* (0·5–1·0); *Bacillus anthracis* (0·5–1·0); *B. subtilis* (0·5–1·0); *Brucellus suis* (0·5–1·0); *Corynebacterium diphtheriae* (0·5–1·0); *Escherichia coli* (0·5–1·0); *Neisseria catarrhalis* (0·5–1·0); *Salmonella paratyphi* (0·1–1·0); *S. paratyphi* B (0·5–1·0); *S. typhosa* (0·5–1·0); *Sarcina lutea* (0·5–1·0) and *Staphylococcus aureus* (0·05–0·025).

The antibiotic appears to be comparatively non-toxic since 20 mg of the crude material in mineral oil produced no fatalities or toxic symptoms when injected intraperitoneally into mice.

Goodlow, Johnson, Shafer, J. Bact., **54**, 268 (1947)
Johnson et al., ibid., **57**, 63 (1949)

BIOMYCIN (*Aureomycin*)
$C_{22}H_{23}O_8N_2Cl$

An anthraquinoid type antibiotic, biomycin is obtained from cultures of *Streptomyces aureofaciens*. The antibiotic spectrum *in vitro* shows it to be a more powerful bacteriostatic and bactericidal agent than either neomycin or streptomycin (q.v.). The structure has been established on the basis of chemical and spectroscopic evidence and is identical with that of aureomycin (q.v.).

Len'kova, *Nauch. Tr. Nauch.-Issled. Vet. Inst. Minsk*, **8**, 57 (1970)

BIOMYCIN LS-B 16

To obtain this antibiotic, the spores of *Streptomyces aureofaciens* LS-536 are suspended in H_2O and irradiated twice by X-rays and then exposed to ultraviolet light. High productivity colonies are then separated and their spores irradiated as before followed by a separation of live colonies according to their antibiotic activity. These are then cultured on a normal nutrient medium. The antibiotic has bactericidal activity against a number of gram-positive and gram-negative bacteria.

Gol'dat, *Soviet Patent*, 120,783 (1967)

3:6-BIS-(5-CHLORO-2-PIPERIDYL)-2:5-PIPERAZINEDIONE
(*Compound 593A*)
$C_{14}H_{22}O_2N_4Cl_2$

This compound, isolated from cultures of *Streptomyces griseoluteus*, has shown some promise as an antitumour agent. The structure has been elucidated by chemical and spectroscopic methods.

Gitterman *et al.*, *J. Antibiotics* (Japan), **23**, 305 (1970)
Structure
Arison, Beck, *Tetrahedron*, **29**, 2743 (1973)

BISNORPENICILLIN V
$C_{14}H_{14}O_5N_2S$

A synthetic penicillin-type antibiotic, this compound has been prepared from *tert*-butyl-(3-carboxy-5-thiazolidino)phthalimidoacetate and isolated as the potassium salt. When tested *in vitro* and *in vivo*, the activity of the antibiotic was substantially lower than that of penicillin V.

Hoogmartens, Claes, Vanderhaeghe, *J. Med. Chem.*, **17**, 389 (1974)

BLASTICIDIN A
$C_{46-52}H_{81-82}N_{4-7}$
M.p. 197–201°C

This antibiotic has been described by Japanese workers. So far, few details are available concerning the method of extraction or the species from which it has been isolated.

Fukunaga *et al.*, *Bull. Agr. Chem. Soc.* (Japan), **19**, 181 (1955)

BLASTICIDIN C
M.p. Indefinite
Also isolated by Japanese workers from *Streptomyces griseochromogenes*, this antibiotic forms a red-brown amorphous powder having no definite melting point.

Fukunaga *et al.*, *Bull. Agr. Chem. Soc.* (Japan), **19**, 181 (1955)

BLASTICIDIN S
$C_{17}H_{26}O_5N_8$
M.p. 252–253°C (*dec.*)

A basic antibiotic, blasticidin S has been obtained from *Streptomyces globifer* and *S. griseochromogenes* by fermentation in a medium at pH 7·0 containing glucose, soybean flour, peptone and calcium carbonate. The substance was originally assigned the empirical formula $C_{14}H_{20}O_5N_6$, later altered to that given above. It has a specific rotation of $[\alpha]_D^{11} + 108\cdot4°$ (c 1·0, H_2O). The ultraviolet spectrum in 0·1 *N*-HCl has an absorption maximum at 274 nm which is shifted to 266 nm in 0·1 *N*-NaOH solution. When hydrolysed the antibiotic yields cytosinine. The monohydrochloride has m.p. 229°C (*dec.*), the dihydrochloride, m.p. 195°C (*dec.*) and the methyl ester forms a crystalline trihydrochloride, m.p. 206–208·5°C (*dec.*).

Takeuchi *et al.*, *J. Antibiotics* (Japan), **11A**, 1 (1958)
Yonehara *et al.*, *ibid.*, **16A**, 195 (1963)
Yamamoto *et al.*, *Japanese Patent*, 7,137,240 (1971)
Revised structure
Otake *et al.*, *Tetrahedron Lett.*, 1411 (1965)
Fox, Watanabe, *ibid.*, 897 (1966)
Absolute configuration
Yonehara, Otake, *Tetrahedron Lett.*, 3785 (1966)
Biosynthesis
Srto *et al.*, *Tetrahedron Lett.*, 3793 (1966)

BLASTMYCIN

See Antimycin A_3

BLEOMYCIN

$C_{50}H_{72}O_{21}N_{14}S_2$
M.p. Indefinite

BLUENSOMYCIN

A complex aminoglycosidic antibiotic elaborated by *Streptomyces verticillus*, the complete structure of this substance has been determined by hydrolysis studies, NMR spectroscopy and partial synthesis. The antibiotic is active *in vivo* experiments with mice against Ehrlich carcinoma, arresting development of the tumour at the end of the S-phase and in the $(C_2 + M)$-phase of the cell cycle. The arrest of cell division at the end of the cell cycle increases inactivation of such tumour cells by radiotherapy. When tested against C3H mammary adenocarcinoma cells in mice, it appears that about 10 per cent of the tumour cells are drug-resistant and the growth is inhibited more effectively by small administrations of bleomycin than by a single administration of the same total dose.

A number of new bleomycins have been produced biosynthetically by the addition of various amines to the culture broth, each particular amine suppressing the production of the other natural bleomycins. These compounds include bleomycins A_2, A'_2-a, A'_2-b, A'_2-c, A_5, B_2 and B_4. Of these, bleomycin B_2 has been found to cause scission of virus SV40 DNA, the effect increasing with an increase in the concentration of the antibiotic until at 2 µg/ml virtually all of the DNA molecules had undergone scission. Additional DNA inhibits this reaction but RNA has no effect. The reaction is stimulated about 20-fold in the presence of 2-mercaptoethanol. Toxicological studies have been carried out on the effect of bleomycin ointment on the skin of rabbits and also given orally to mice, rats and dogs. In every case, there was no observable effect on the behaviour or anatomy of the animals.

Takita *et al.*, *Progr. Antimicrob. Anticancer Chemother.*, *Proc. Int. Congr. Chemother.*, 6th, **2**, 1031 (1969)
Suzuki *et al.*, *J. Antibiotics* (Japan), **23**, 473 (1970)
Takita *et al.*, *ibid.*, **25**, 755 (1972)
Umezawa *et al.*, *German Patent*, 2,307,986 (1973)
Nakayama *et al.*, *J. Antibiotics* (Japan), **26**, 400 (1973)
Umezawa *et al.*, *ibid.*, **26**, 521 (1973)
Urano *et al.*, *Cancer Res.*, **33**, 2849 (1973)
Schumann, Goehde, *Strahlentherapie*, **147**, 298 (1974)
Fujii *et al.*, *J. Antibiotics* (Japan), **27**, 73 (1974)
Tanaka *et al.*, *ibid.*, **28**, 3 (1975)
Promchainant, *Mutat. Res.*, **28**, 107 (1975)

BLUENSOMYCIN (*Antibiotic U-12,898*)

$C_{21}H_{39}O_{14}N_5$
M.p. Indefinite

A glycosidic antibiotic, bluensomycin is usually obtained as the crystalline hydrochloride, m.p. 190–194°C (*dec.*). This salt is only slightly dextrorotatory with $[\alpha]_D^{24}$ + 0.5° ± 0.5° (c 1.0, H_2O). The antibiotic yields *scyllo*-imosamine when hydrolysed with barium hydroxide. It forms a dihydrochloride which, on treatment with methanolic HCl furnishes bluensidine, the structure of the latter having been established as 1-deoxy-1-guianidine-3-O-carbamoyl-*scyllo*-inositol. Bluensomycin is active against a range of bacteria and fungi.

Bergy *et al.*, *2nd Interscience Conf. on Antimicrobial Agents and Chemotherapy* (1962)
Bannister, Argoudelis, *J. Amer. Chem. Soc.*, **85**, 119, 235 (1963)
Barlow, Anderson, *J. Antibiotics* (Japan), **25**, 281 (1972)

BONGKREKIC ACID
$C_{28}H_{38}O_7$
M.p. Indefinite

A toxin elaborated by *Pseudomonas cocovenenans* grown on a medium containing copra, this antibiotic is obtained as a resin which possesses no definite melting point and cannot be crystallized. It has a specific rotation of $[\alpha]_D^{22}$ + 165° (c 2.0, $NaHCO_3$.aq.).

Nugteren, Berends, *Rec. Trav. Chim.*, **76**, 13 (1957)
Structure
Lijmbach, Cox, Berends, *Tetrahedron*, **26**, 5993 (1970)
Lijmbach, Cox, Berends, *ibid.*, **27**, 1839 (1971)
de Bruun *et al.*, *ibid.*, **29**, 1541 (1973)
Absolute configuration
Zylber, Gaudemer, Gaudemer, *Experientia*, **29**, 387, 648 (1973)

BONOMYCIN
See Sencycline

BOROMYCIN
$C_{45}H_{74}O_{15}NB$
M.p. 223–228°C (*dec.*)

This complex boron-containing antibiotic has been obtained from cultures of *Streptomyces antibioticus*. It crystallizes from EtOH and is dextrorotatory with a specific rotation of $[\alpha]_D$ + 63.5° (c 0.55, $CHCl_3$). The structure has been elucidated from chemical and spectroscopic evidence.

Hutter *et al.*, *Helv. Chim. Acta*, **50**, 1533 (1967)
Structure
Dunitz *et al.*, *Helv. Chim. Acta*, **54**, 1709 (1971)

BORRELIDIN
$C_{28}H_{43}O_6N$
M.p. 145–146°C

Elaborated by a strain of *Streptomyces rochei* (C2989), borrelidin possesses anti-viral activity. The mould is fermented by both surface and submerged growth on a medium containing glucose, phosphate and soybean meal and isolated by extraction of the liquor with butyl acetate, the residue formed on evaporation of the solvent being redissolved in a suitable solvent, treated with bentonite and extracted with alkali from Et_2O. The antibiotic is then purified by recrystallization from C_6H_6. It forms colourless crystals and is laevorotatory with a specific rotation of $[\alpha]_D^{27} - 28°$ (EtOH), the ultraviolet spectrum showing a single absorption maximum at 256 nm.

Borrelidin, being an organic acid, forms a crystalline methyl ester, m.p. 155·5–156·5°C which may be further characterized as the acetate, m.p. 190–192°C. Chemical and spectroscopic investigations have shown it to possess the macrocyclic structure given above.

It is highly active *in vivo* against *Borrelia*. When given subcutaneously to mice, the curative doses, determined by Buck, Farr and Schnitzer are: *Borrelia novyi* 3·25 mg/kg; *B. obermeieri* 3·6 mg/kg and the Tick strain 0·815 mg/kg. Several workers have shown a synergistic effect with penicillin G, the activity being enhanced by small doses of borrelidin against β-hemolytic streptococcus and meningococcus endotoxin in mice and syphilis in rabbits. There is, however, no such effect observed against *Diplococcus pneumoniae*, *Eberella typhi* or *Salmonella schottmuelleri*. Borrelidin is relatively toxic. The LD_{50} in mice is 39·0 mg/kg (intravenous) and 74–7 mg/kg (subcutaneous). It has an irritating effect upon the skin of humans and the tissues of animals.

Berger, Goldberg, *J. Clin. Invest.*, **28**, 1046 (1949)
Jampolsky, Goldberg, *ibid.*, **28**, 1046 (1949)
Grunberg, Eldridge, Soo-Hoo, *ibid.*, **28**, 1046 (1949)
Schnitzer, Buck, Farr, *ibid.*, **28**, 1047 (1949)
Buck, Farr, Schnitzer, *Trans. N.Y. Acad. Sci.*, Ser II, **11**, No. 6207 (1949)
Grunberg et al., *ibid.*, No. 6210 (1949)
Lumb et al., *Nature*, **206**, 263 (1965)
Anderton, Rickards, *ibid.*, **206**, 269 (1965)
Structure
Keller-Schlierlein, *Experientia*, **22**, 355 (1966)

BOSEIMYCIN
$C_{24}H_{46}O_8N_9$
M.p. Indefinite

A streptothricin type antibiotic, elaborated by *Streptomyces* species Ac6569 grown in a medium containing yeast extract, soya peptone and inorganic salts at pH 7·2, this compound is isolated as the tetrahydrochloride, a yellow amorphous powder, m.p. 216–218°C (*dec.*). The antibiotic is soluble in H_2O, stable at room temperature, gives positive ninhydron, Sakaguchi and Elson-Morgan tests and negative Fehling, Tollen and maltol reactions. The compound is assayed with *Staphylococcus aureus* as the test organism and the following minimum inhibition concentrations have been determined by Sinha and Nandy; given as (µg/ml): *Aerobacter aerogenes* (3·0); *Bacillus anthracis* (8·0); *B. megaterium* (2·5); *B. subtilis* (3·0); *Candida albicans* (2·0); *Pseudomonas aeruginosa* (4·0); *Proteus vulgaris* (12); *Salmonella typhosa* (6·0); *Staphylococcus albus* (0·5); *Staph. aureus*, sensitive (3.0) and *Staph. aureus* resistant (5·0). Boseimycin is non-toxic to mice at a dose of 25 mg/kg given intravenously.

Sinha, Nandy, *Experientia*, **24**, 795 (1968)
Sinha, *J. Antibiotics* (Japan), **23**, 360 (1970)

BOSTRYCIN
$C_{16}H_{16}O_7$
M.p. 222–224°C

An anthraquinoid antibiotic produced by *Bostrychonema alpestre*, bostrycin forms bright red crystals when recrystallized from aqueous pyridine. The ultraviolet and visible spectra in EtOH consist of absorption maxima at 228, 303, 472, 505 and 542 nm. Five hydroxyl groups are present in the molecule but, when acetylated, the antibiotic forms the crystalline triacetate, m.p. 255·5–260·5°C. The compound is active against gram-positive bacteria and also possesses antitumour properties.

    Noda et al., Tetrahedron Lett., 6087 (1968)
Crystal structure
    Takenake et al., Tetrahedron Lett., 6091 (1968)
    Noda et al., Tetrahedron, **26**, 1339 (1970)

BOTRIC ACID
$C_{25}H_{32}O_4$
M.p. 214–216°C (dec.)

A new antibiotic, botric acid is elaborated by *Botrytis*. It is produced by submerged culture in a medium containing glucose, peptone, corn steep liquor and inorganic salts at pH 6·4 and 27–28°C for 66 hours. The wet cells are extracted twice with $(CH_3)_2CO$, the extracts combined and concentrated and then diluted with H_2O. The antibiotic is then extracted with BuOAc and precipitated with CH_3OH at 5°C. Botric acid forms yellow plates and is laevorotatory with a specific rotation of $[\alpha]_D^{24} - 294°$ (c 0·1, $CHCl_3$). The antibiotic is weakly acidic and soluble in $CHCl_3$, $(CH_3)_2CO$, AcOEt, dimethylformamide, $(CH_3)_2SO$ and alkaline H_2O, slightly soluble in the lower alcohols, hexane and petroleum ether and insoluble in H_2O. Botric acid is virtually inactive against bacteria but effective against *Candida*. The LD_{50} in mice is 250 mg/kg (intraperitoneally) and 125 mg/kg (intravenously).

    Mizuno, Miyazawa, Takada, *J. Antibiotics* (Japan), **27**, 552 (1974)
    Mizuno, Takada, Miyazawa, *Japanese Patent*, 7,436,891 (1974)

BOTRYDIAL
$C_{17}H_{26}O_5$
M.p. 108–110°C

Botrytis cinerea furnishes this antibiotic when grown by submerged culture in a common nutrient medium at 27–28°C for 3 days. The compound is dextrorotatory with a specific rotation of $[\alpha]_D^{20} + 34°$ (c 1·4, $CHCl_3$). It is active against *Candida* but only weakly so against bacteria.

    Fehlhaber et al., *Chem. Ber.*, **107**, 1720 (1974)

BOTRYODIPLODIN
$C_7H_{12}O_3$
M.p. 42°C

This simple antibiotic is elaborated by *Botryodiplodia theobromae* Pat. It forms colourless crystals having a low melting point. The structure, which has been confirmed by synthesis, is 4-acetyl-2-hydroxyl-3-methyltetrahydrofuran. It shows some activity against gram-positive bacteria.

    Sen Gupta, Chandran, Divekar, *Ind. J. Exp. Biol.*, **4**, 152 (1966)
Structure
    Arsenault, Althaus, Divekar, *Chem. Commun.*, 1414 (1969)
Synthesis
    McCurry, Abe, *J. Amer. Chem. Soc.*, **95**, 5824 (1973)
    McCurry, Abe., *Tetrahedron Lett.*, 4103 (1973)

BOTTROMYCIN
$C_{38}H_{57-61}O_{7-8}N_7S$
M.p. Indefinite

An amorphous polypeptide antibiotic complex, bottromycin is produced by *Streptomyces bottropensis*, *S. canadensis* and various strains of *Kitasatoa purpurea*, KA-279, KA-280, KA-281 and KA-282. The complex has been separated into five components, the major constituents being bottromycins A, A_2, B and C. The complex and the individual components are active against *Mycoplasma* species, particularly *M. gallisepticum* and *M. mycoides*. The minimum inhibition concentration of bottromycin A against *M. gallisepticum* is 0·001–0·01 µg/ml.

    Waisvisz et al., *J. Amer. Chem. Soc.*, **79**, 4520, 4522, 4524 (1957)
    Miller et al., *Antimicrobial Agents & Chemotherapy*, 407 (1968)
    Tanaka et al., *J. Antibiotics* (Japan), **21**, 75 (1968)
    Umezawa et al., *Japanese Patent*, 10,998 (1968)
    Hata et al., *Japanese Patent*, 7,210,036 (1972)

BOUVARDIN
$C_{40}H_{48}N_6O_{10}$
M.p. 254–255°C

A plant antibiotic, bouvardin has been isolated from the MeOH extract of the flowers, leaves and stems of *Bouvardia ternifolia*. It forms colourless needles when crystallized from MeOH–CH$_2$Cl$_2$ containing MeOH of crystallization. It is laevorotatory having a specific rotation of $[\alpha]_D^{25} - 181°$ (c 1·0, CHCl$_3$) and forms orthorhombic crystals with space group P2$_1$2$_1$2$_1$ and a = 9·009, b = 12·623 and c = 42·970 Å with Z = 4. Bouvardin exhibits an inhibitory action towards P388 lymphocytic leukemia and B16 melanotic melanoma.

Jolad et al., J. Amer. Chem. Soc., **99**, 8040 (1977)

BRAMYCIN
M.p. 166–166·5°C
An antibiotic isolated from cultures of *Streptomyces diastatochromogenes* var. *bracus*, this substance forms crystals from EtOH and has a specific rotation of $[\alpha]_D^{25} - 2·5°$ (c 0·2, CH$_3$OH). It is active against gram-positive and some gram-negative bacteria.

Sakagami, *Japanese Patent*, 7,002,077 (1970)

BREDININ
C$_9$H$_{13}$O$_6$N$_3$
M.p. >200°C (*dec.*)
A simple antibiotic, bredinin has been isolated from cultures of *Eupenicillum brefeldianum* M-2166 (FERM-P 1104). The culture supernatant is adsorbed on a strong basic anion exchanged resin, eluted with 2 per cent aqueous AcOH and precipitated with CH$_3$OH and (CH$_3$)$_2$CO. Further purification is carried out by silica gel and Sephadex A-25 column chromatography and recrystallization from CH$_3$OH. It is laevorotatory with $[\alpha]_D^{28} - 35°$ (c 0·8, H$_2$O) and gives an ultraviolet spectrum with absorption maxima at 245 and 279 nm. The antibiotic is soluble in H$_2$O, slightly so in CH$_3$OH and EtOH and insoluble in other organic solvents. It exhibits pronounced antitumour and antiviral properties and inhibits *Candida albicans*. It produced no toxic symptoms in mice when given intravenously at 250 mg/kg.

Mizuno et al., *J. Antibiotics* (Japan), **27**, 775 (1974)
Production
Mizuno et al., *Japanese Patent*, 7,356,894 (1973)

BREFELDIN A
C$_{16}$H$_{24}$O$_4$
M.p. Indefinite

Phyllosticta medicaginis CBS 47,963 produces this bicyclic antibiotic when grown on a medium containing peptone, yeast extract and inorganic salts at 25°C for 3 days. It is extracted from the culture filtrate with AcOEt. The compound is characterized as the acetate, m.p. 129–139°C. Brefeldin A is only weakly active against bacteria but is effective against a number of fungi, particularly *Candida albicans*.

Taniguchi et al., *J. Fac. Agr., Kyushu Univ.*, **17**, 129 (1973)
Howard, Johnstone, Entwistle, *German Patent*, 2,325,330 (1973)
Hayashi, Takatsuki, Tamura, *J. Antibiotics* (Japan), **27**, 65 (1974)

BREVIMYCINS
M.p. Indefinite

Brevibacterium ammoniagenes yields an antibiotic mixture consisting of brevimycins A and B when cultured aerobically and with stirring on a common nutrient medium. The mixture is separated by extraction of the broth with an organic solvent and purified by paper chromatography. Brevimycin B is active against a range of gram-positive and gram-negative bacteria.

Murdia *et al.*, *Hakko Kogaku Zasshi.*, **52**, 598 (1974)

BREVISTIN
$C_{63}H_{91}N_{15}O_{18}$

Cultures of *Bacillus brevis* 342-14 contain this antibiotic which is an acyl peptide having the approximate empirical formula given above. It has been shown, from hydrolysis experiments, to contain aspartic acid, isoleucine, glycine, valine, threonine, tryptophan, phenylalanine and 2,4-diaminobutyric acid in the molecule. The hydrochloride is soluble in MeOH. Brevistin is effective against gram-positive bacteria *in vitro* and *in vivo*. It possesses a low toxicity in mice.

Shoji *et al.*, *J. Antibiotics* (Japan), **29**, 375 (1976)
Shoji, Kato., *ibid.*, **29**, 380 (1976)

BROMONITRIN A
$C_{10}H_4O_2N_2Br_4$

Pseudomonas pyrrolnitrica furnishes a mixture of three bromine-containing antibiotics when grown on a common medium in the presence of 0·3–0·5 per cent of potassium or ammonium bromide. Separation and purification are carried out by chromatography on a silica gel column. The antibiotic is active against *Penicillium chrysogenum* and *Trichophyton interdigitale*.

Ajisaka *et al.*, *Japanese Patent*, 7,214,916 (1972)

BROMONITRIN B
$C_{10}H_3O_2N_2Br_5$

Also elaborated by *Pseudomonas pyrrolnitrica* grown in a medium containing potassium or ammonium bromide, this antibiotic has a similar inhibitory activity against *Penicillium chrysogenum* and *Trichophyton interdigitale*.

Ajisaka *et al.*, *Japanese Patent*, 7,214,916 (1972)

BROMONITRIN C
$C_{10}HO_2N_2Br_7$

A further brominated antibiotic, this compound has been isolated from the mixture produced by *Pseudomonas pyrrolnitrica* grown on a medium containing inorganic bromides. It is active against *Penicillium chrysogenum* and *Trichophyton interdigitale*.

Ajisaka *et al.*, *Japanese Patent*, 7,214,916 (1972)

BRUNEOMYCIN
$C_{25}H_{22}O_8N_4$

A quinolone type antibiotic, bruneomycin is obtained from cultures of various *Streptomyces* species and has the structure given above which is based upon chemical and spectroscopic evidence. Bruneomycin is mainly active against tumours although it shows some activity against *Staphylococcus aureus* and hemolytic *Streptococcus*. The antibiotic is toxic with lethal doses of 0·15 and 0·52 mg/kg when given intraperitoneally to mice and rats respectively. In mice, the maximum tolerated dose decreases the numbers of antibody-forming cells and erythropoietic stem cell colonies. It also exhibits a transient hypertensive effect and has marked antidiuretic activity. Resistant tumour cells appear in mice transplanted with Fisher lymphadenosis following ten passages on single use of the drug.

Kats et al., *Antibiotiki*, **16**, 60 (1971)
Revina, Sal'nik, *Vop. Radiobiol. Biol. Deistviya Tsitostaticheskikh*, **3**, 276 (1971)
Todorov, Vulkov, *Farmatsiya* (Sofia), **23**, 69 (1973)
Pasqual, Rivera, *Farmakol. Toksikol.* (Moscow), **37**, 197 (1974)
Averbukh, *Antibiotiki*, **20**, 307 (1975)

BULGERIN
$C_{17}H_{24}O_{10}N_4$
M.p. Indefinite

Streptomyces aburaviensis var. *tuftformis* produces this antibiotic which has a specific rotation of $[\alpha]_D + 24°$ (H_2O). The ultraviolet spectrum in 0·05 N-HCl has an absorption maximum at 289 nm and a shoulder at 230 nm.

Shoki et al., *J. Antibiotics* (Japan), **23**, 295 (1970)

BUNDLIN A (*Antibiotic T-2636C*)
$C_{25}H_{33}O_7N$
M.p. 205–207°C (*dec.*)

Obtained from cultures of *Streptomyces rochei* var. *bolubilis*, bundlin A crystallizes as colourless needles. It is laevorotatory with a specific rotation of $[\alpha]_D - 240°$ (c 1·0, EtOH). The ultraviolet spectrum in ethanol has an absorption maximum at 227 nm. The 8-acetate is crystalline with m.p. 203–204°C (*dec.*) and the 8:14-diacetate, also colourless crystals, melts at 136–140°C (*dec.*). The 14-acetate is bundlin B (q.v.).

Harada et al., *Tetrahedron Lett.*, 2239 (1969)
Uramoto et al., *ibid.*, 2249 (1969)
Higashide et al., *J. Antibiotics* (Japan), **23**, 1 (1971)
Harada, Kishi, Mizumo, *ibid.*, **23**, 13 (1971)
Crystal structure
Uramoto et al., *Acta Cryst.*, **27B**, 236 (1971)
Uramoto et al., *Agr. Biol. Chem.*, **35**, 27 (1971)

BUNDLIN B
$C_{27}H_{35}O_8N$
M.p. 213–215°C (*dec.*)

Also isolated from cultures of *Streptomyces rochei* var. *bolubilis*, this antibiotic is the 14-acetate of the preceding compound. It forms colourless needles and has a specific rotation of $[\alpha]_D - 235°$ (c 1·0, EtOH). The ultraviolet spectrum in EtOH is identical with that of bundlin A with a single absorption maximum at 227 nm.

Harada et al., *Tetrahedron Lett.*, 2239 (1969)
Uramoto et al., *ibid.*, 2249 (1969)
Absolute configuration
Kamiya et al., *Tetrahedron Lett.*, 2245 (1969)
Higashide et al., *J. Antibiotics* (Japan), **24**, 1 (1971)
Harada et al., *ibid.*, **24**, 13 (1971)
Crystal structure
Uramoto et al., *Agr. Biol. Chem.*, **35**, 27 (1971)

BUTIROSIN A
$C_{21}H_{41}O_{12}N_5$

Bacillus circulans produces two similar antibiotics when cultivated by submerged techniques in a medium containing glycerol, meat peptone, soybean flour and inorganic salts at 27–28°C. The structure of the antibiotic butirosin

A has been established by mass spectrometry of poly-N-acetyl-poly-O-trimethylsilylbutirosin A. The antibiotic is assayed by the paper disc method using *Escherichia coli* as the test organism. It is active against a number of gram-positive and gram-negative organisms, particularly *Pseudomonas aeruginosa*. Resistant strains of *Escherichia* and *Pseudomonas* inactivate the antibiotic due to 3'-O-phosphorylation, the resulting 3'-O-phosphorylbutirosin A having been isolated and identified by thin-layer and paper chromatography.

Woo, *Tetrahedron Lett.*, 2621 (1971)
Howells *et al.*, *Antimicrobial Agents & Chemotherapy*, **2**, 79 (1972)
Sugawara *et al.*, *Sankyo Kenkyusho Nempo*, **25**, 56 (1973)

BUTIROSIN B
$C_{21}H_{41}O_{12}N_5$
M.p. Indefinite
This antibiotic which is stereoisomeric with the preceding compound, is isolated from the complex produced by cultivation of *Bacillus circulans* on a medium of glycerol, meat peptone, soybean flour and inorganic salts under submerged conditions. The structure has been determined in the same manner as for butirosin A. It also possesses a similar antibiotic spectrum.

Woo, *Tetrahedron Lett.*, 2621 (1971)
Howells *et al.*, *Antimicrobial Agents & Chemotherapy*, **2**, 79 (1972)
Sugawara *et al.*, *Sankyo Kenkyusho Nempo*, **25**, 56 (1973)

BUTYLCYCLOHEPTYLPRODIGININE
$C_{25}H_{33}N_3O$

An unclassified *Streptomyces* species elaborates this antibiotic pigment which has antimalarial activity. It is produced with the undecyl derivative (q.v.) from which it is separated by column chromatography. The structure has been elucidated from chemical and spectroscopic evidence.

Gerber, *J. Antibiotics* (Japan), **28**, 194 (1975)

CAERULOMYCIN
$C_{12}H_{11}O_2N_3$
M.p. 174–175°C

A bipyridyl antibiotic, this compound is produced by *Streptomyces caeruleus* and is obtained in the form of colourless needles when crystallised from EtOH. It gives a deep red colour with $FeCl_3$ solution. Caerulomycin is characterized as the acetate, colourless needles with m.p. 102°C and the methyl ether, colourless crystals, m.p. 90°C. It has been synthesized from 4-methoxy-2:2'-bipyridyl-1-oxide. Although only slightly active against bacteria, the antibiotic has powerful antifungal properties and is a potent plant-wilt toxin.

Funk, Divekar, *Can. J. Microbiol.*, **5**, 317 (1959)
Structure
Divekar, Read, Vining, *Can. J. Chem.*, **45**, 1215 (1967)
Synthesis
Ranganathan, Singh, Divekar, *Can. J. Chem.*, **47**, 165 (1969)

CAIROMYCIN B
$C_{10}H_{15}N_3O_3$
M.p. 120–121°C

A *Streptomyces* strain As-C-19 isolated from soil in Cairo yields this macrocyclic antibiotic which forms colourless crystals from EtOH. It is freely soluble in $CHCl_3$, AcOEt and Me_2CO, slightly soluble in the lower alcohols and insoluble in H_2O and petroleum ether. On acid hydrolysis it yields aspartic acid and lysine. Cairomycin B is active against gram-positive bacteria but has a high toxicity in experimental animals. The LD_{50} in mice is 12·5 mg/kg administered intraperitoneally.

Shimi, Abedalla, Fathy, *Antimicrob. Agents Chemother.*, **11**, 883 (1977)

CALDARIOMYCIN
$C_5H_8O_2Cl_2$
M.p. 121°C

This substance is elaborated by *Caldariomyces fumago* and forms colourless needles from $CHCl_3$. It is freely soluble in EtOH, CH_3OH, Et_2O and H_2O and moderately soluble in petroleum ether. It has $[\alpha]_{5461}^{20}$ + 59·2° (c 1·0, H_2O) and gives a red-brown colour with concentrated H_2SO_4 having a green fluorescence. It reduces Fehling's solution in the cold and has the structure given above which is based upon chemical and spectroscopic data. It is active against a number of gram-positive bacteria.

Clutterbuck *et al.*, *Biochem. J.*, **34**, 664 (1940)
Beckwith, Hager, *J. Org. Chem.*, **26**, 5206 (1961)

CALVATIC ACID
$C_7H_5O_3N_3$

This novel antibiotic is produced by fermentation of a medium containing glucose, peptone, yeast extract and inorganic salts by *Calvatia craniformis* at 28°C for 10 days. The culture filtrate is then extracted with BuOH at pH 2·0, concentrated to dryness, the solid dissolved in CH_3OH, the impurities precipitated with AcOEt and the antibiotic purified by silica gel chromatography. Calvatic acid is soluble in the lower alcohols, $(CH_3)_2CO$ and $(CH_3)_2SO$, insoluble in AcOEt, C_6H_6, Et_2O and hexane. It is effective against gram-positive bacteria and also possesses antitumour properties. The LD_{50} in mice is about 100 mg/kg given intraperitoneally. The methyl ester has been prepared by the action of CH_2N_2 and found to be more effective than the free acid.

Umezawa et al., *Japanese Patent*, 7,552,290 (1975)

CANDICIDIN A
M.p. Indefinite

Several species of *Streptomyces*, and in particular *S. griseus*, produce an antibiotic, candicidin, which may be separated into two components by extraction with EtOH. Candicidin A is soluble in H_2O, EtOH and ethylene glycol but insoluble in $(CH_3)_2CO$ or petroleum ether. It has, however, the same R_f value by paper chromatography as candicidin B (q.v.) and gives an identical ultraviolet spectrum with absorption maxima at 360–361, 380–381 and 405 nm. It is very unstable in acid media.

The antibiotic is active against yeasts and also against certain protozoa and filamentous fungi. It possesses a powerful fungicidal action against *Candida albicans* and is active in mice against both *C. albicans* and *Bacillus dermatitidis*. It exhibits its maximum activity at a pH between 7·0 and 8·0. In mice, the subcutaneous LD_{50} is approximately 200 mg/kg and the intraperitoneal about 50 mg/kg.

Lechavalier et al., *Mycologia*, **45**, 155 (1953)
Kligman, Lewis, *Proc. Soc. Exptl. Biol. Med.*, **82**, 399 (1953)

CANDICIDIN B
M.p. Indefinite

Also produced by species of *Streptomyces*, especially *S. griseus*, this fraction of the original antibiotic is left after extraction with EtOH. It is only slightly soluble in ethylene glycol and BuOH and insoluble in H_2O, EtOH, $(CH_3)_2CO$ and petroleum ether. Both the biological activity and toxicity are the same as for candicidin A.

Lechevalier et al., *Mycologia*, **45**, 155 (1953)
Kligman, Lewis, *Proc. Soc. Exptl. Biol. Med.*, **82**, 399 (1953)

CANDIDIN
$C_{47}H_{71}O_{17}N$
M.p. Indefinite

A macrocyclic antifungal antibiotic, this substance has been obtained from *Streptomyces viridoflavus*. The structure given above is based upon chemical analysis and spectroscopic techniques, especially infrared, ultraviolet, NMR and mass spectra.

Taber, Vining, Waksman, *Antibiotics & Chemotherapy*, **4**, 455 (1953)
Borowski et al., *Tetrahedron Lett.*, 1987 (1971)

CANDIDULIN
$C_{11}H_{15}O_3N$
M.p. 88–89°C

Candidulin is produced by *Aspergillus candidus*, fermentation usually being by surface growth on a medium containing glucose, potassium phosphate and sodium nitrate. The yield obtained is 64 *Mycobacterium ranae* units/ml. No antibiotic is formed in the presence of corn steep liquor, soybean flour or yeast extract. The antibiotic is isolated by extraction of the filtrate with $CHCl_3$ or Et_2O, washing the extract with H_2O, drying and then evaporating to dryness *in vacuo*. Purification is by taking up the residue in hot *n*-hexane, cooling and crystallizing. Candidulin forms long whitish needles which are soluble in CH_3OH, EtOH, Et_2O and $(CH_3)_2CO$, less soluble in CCl_4, C_6H_6, *n*-hexane and H_2O. It is dextrorotatory with a specific rotation of $[\alpha]_D^{24} + 15° \pm 2°$ (c 1·0, $CHCl_3$) and gives no characteristic absorptions in the ultraviolet spectrum. Candidulin is thermostable but alkali-labile and does not react with ninhydrin, ferric chloride or 2:4-dinitrophenylhydrazine.

The antibiotic is normally assayed by the agar streak method using *Mycobacterium ranae* as the test organism. It is active against both bacteria and fungi and has the following typical inhibition concentrations (μg/ml): *Aspergillus fumigatus* (80); *Bacillus polymyxa* (160); *B. subtilis* (10); *Brucella abortus* (20); *Escherichia coli* (160); *Klebsiella pneumoniae* (10); *Mycobacterium ranae* (2·5); *Myco. smegmatis* (2·5); *Penicillium puberulum* (40);

Pseudomonas aeruginosa (640); *Sarcina lutea* (320); *Staphylococcus aureus* (320); *Streptococcus hemolyticus* (160) and *Streptomyces griseus* (320).

In vivo experiments have demonstrated that the antibiotic affords no protection in mice against *Mycobacterium tuberculosis*. The LD_{50} in mice is approximately 250 mg/kg when given subcutaneously.

Stanley, Anenenko, *J. Clin. Invest.*, **28**, 1047 (1949)
Stanley, Anenenko, *Arch. Biochem.*, **23**, 256 (1949)

CANESCIN
$C_{15}H_{14}O_7$
M.p. 200–202°C

Both *Penicillium canescens* and *Aspergillus malignus* produce this antibiotic which forms colourless crystals when purified by recrystallization from CH_3OH. It is slightly dextrorotatory with a specific rotation of $[\alpha]_D^{23}$ + 17·8° and the ultraviolet spectrum in EtOH has absorption maxima at 247, 278, 290 and 327 nm.

Brian *et al.*, *Trans. Brit. Mycol. Soc.*, **36**, 243 (1953)
Birch *et al.*, *Tetrahedron Lett.*, 29 (1965)

CAPREOMYCIN IA
$C_{25}H_{44}O_8N_{14}$

The antibiotic produced by *Streptomyces capreolus* and earlier given the tentative empirical formula $C_{25-27}H_{50-53}O_{9-10}N_{13-14}Cl_4$ has recently been shown to consist of two components, neither of which contain chlorine. Hydrolysis of capromycin IA furnishes serine, alanine, α-lysine, 2:3-diaminopropionic acid and capreomycidine.

Herr, Sutton, Stark, *Trans. 21st Res. Conf. Pulmonary Diseases*, 367 (1962)
Herr, *Antimicrobial Agents & Chemotherapy*, 201 (1962)
Stark *et al.*, *ibid.*, 596 (1962)
Bycroft *et al.*, *Nature*, **231**, 301 (1971)

CAPREOMYCIN IB
$C_{25}H_{44}O_7N_{14}$

This antibiotic from *Streptomyces capreolus* has a structure virtually identical with that of the preceding compound. The hydrolysis products are the same as for capreomycin IA.

Herr, *Antimicrobial Agents & Chemotherapy*, 201 (1962)
Stark *et al.*, *ibid.*, 596 (1962)
Bycroft *et al.*, *Nature*, **231**, 301 (1971)

CAPREOMYCIN II
M.p. Indefinite

A further antibiotic elaborated by *Streptomyces capreolus*, this substance is slightly dextrorotatory with a specific rotation of $[\alpha]_D$ + 2·5° (c 1·0, H_2O). Hydrolysis yields alanine, serine, 2:3-diaminopropionic acid and capreomycidine.

Herr, *Antimicrobial Agents & Chemotherapy*, 201 (1962)

CARBENICILLIN (Pyopen[R])

$C_{17}H_{18}O_6N_2S$
M.p. Indefinite

This semi-synthetic antibiotic has the structure α-carboxybenzyl-penicillin. It is highly active against a range of gram-positive and gram-negative bacteria, being generally more active than ampicillin (q.v.) against strains of *Staphylococcus aureus in vitro* and experimental *S. aureus* infections in mice. It is also somewhat more stable than ampicillin to hydrolysis by β-lactamase. With the exception of a small number of strains of *Bacteroides fragilis* and *B. melaninogenicus*, it is active against all anaerobic bacteria examined at concentrations readily achieved in the blood. The minimum inhibition concentrations for 13 strains of *Pseudomonas aeruginosa* were 50–200 μg/ml and for 11 strains of *Proteus* between 0·4–3·1 μg/ml. The general toxicity is low and doses of 200–300 mg daily for children and 12 g for adults have been recommended for *Escherichia coli* and *Proteus* infections and larger doses for the treatment of *Pseudomonas aeruginosa* infections. It is, however, possible to develop a high degree of *in vitro* resistance in strains of *Klebsiella pneumoniae*, *Proteus mirabilis* and *Pseudomonas aeruginosa*. Comparatively higher blood concentrations are reached using the indanyl sodium salt of the antibiotic, this being readily hydrolysed by tissue esterases to the parent antibiotic.

Acred *et al.*, *Nature*, **215**, 25 (1967)
Simon *et al.*, *Arzneimittel-Forsch.*, **21**, 78 (1971)
Bononi, Renzini, *Advan. Antimicrob. Antineoplastic Chemother.*, *Proc. Int. Congr. Chemother.*, 7th, **1**, 711 (1971)
Ceccarelli *et al.*, *Aggiorn. Pediat.*, **23**, 123 (1972)
Blazevic, Matsen, *Antimicrobial Agents & Chemotherapy*, **5**, 462 (1972)
Perrotta, Shioppacassi, Curcio, *Bull. Chim. Farm.*, **113**, 37 (1974)
Brown *et al.*, *N. Engl. J. Med.*, **291**, 265 (1974)
Brogard *et al.*, *J. Int. Med. Res.*, **2**, 142 (1974)
Athar, *Hindustan Antibiot. Bull.*, **13**, 1 (1974)
Kawai *et al.*, *Nippon Kakuka Gakkai Zasshi*, **23**, 666 (1974)
Noguchi *et al.*, *Chemotherapy*, **23**, 572 (1975)
Otsuki, Ishiko, *ibid.*, **23**, 583 (1975)
Kimura *et al.*, *ibid.*, **23**, 591 (1975)

CARBOMYCIN (*Magnamycin*)

$C_{40}H_{67}O_{16}N$
M.p. 210–214°C (*dec.*)

A macrocyclic antibiotic isolated from *Streptomyces halstedii*, carbomycin crystallizes from aqueous CH_3OH in colourless needles-shaped crystals and decomposes somewhat at 200°C. The antibiotic is laevorotatory with specific rotations of $[\alpha]_D^{25} - 58·6°$ (c 1·0, $CHCl_3$) and $-54°$ (c 1·0, CH_3OH). The ultraviolet spectrum in EtOH consists of a single absorption maximum at 240 nm. The free antibiotic is only slightly soluble in H_2O although the acid salts such as the sulphate and hydrochloride are H_2O-soluble. A number of salts and derivatives have been prepared including the hydrochloride, m.p. 158–160°C (*dec.*); sulphate, m.p. 163–164°C (*dec.*); oxime, m.p. 198–199°C; thiosemicarbazone, m.p. 172–173°C; diacetate, m.p. 150°C $[\alpha]_D^{25} - 81°$ (c 1·0, $CHCl_3$); pentaacetate, m.p. 134–135°C; dibenzoate, m.p. 164–166°C and the dipropionate, m.p. 197–198°C. Catalytic reduction with palladium yields the tetrahydro derivative, m.p. 121–122°C. $[\alpha]_D^{25} - 53°$ (c 0·5, EtOH). Treatment with ethanolic HCl furnishes mycaminose and 4-*isovaleryl*-C-methylmycaroside.

Carbomycin is active against gram-positive bacteria, rickettsiae and large viruses. It has no activity against gram-negative bacteria with the exception of *Hemophilus* and *Neisseria* and little activity against *Mycobacteria*. The development of resistance is slow and there appears to be no cross resistance with other common antibiotics. It has been demonstrated to possess a growth-promoting action on chicks. It is comparatively non-toxic with an LD_{50} of 550 mg/kg on intravenous injection in mice. So far, it has found some utilization in the treatment of infections caused by gram-positive bacteria and rickettsiae.

Tanner *et al.*, *Antibiotics & Chemotherapy*, **2**, 441 (1952)
Wagner *et al.*, *J. Amer. Chem. Soc.*, **75**, 4684 (1953)
Regna *et al.*, *ibid.*, **75**, 4625 (1953)
Pagano *et al.*, *Antibiotics & Chemotherapy*, **3**, 899, 910 (1953)

Woodward, *Festschrift Arthur Stoll*, Birkhauser, 524 (1957)
Tanner, Lees, Routein, *U.S. Patent*, 2,796,379 (1957)
Gilner, Srinivasan, *Biochem. Biophys. Res. Commun.*, **8**, 299 (1962)
Revised structure
Kuehne, Benson, *J. Amer. Chem. Soc.*, **87**, 4660 (1965)
Woodward, Weiler, Dutta, *ibid.*, **87**, 4662 (1965)
Configuration
Hofheinz, Grisebach, *Chem. Ber.*, **96**, 2867 (1963)

CARBOMYCIN B
$C_{42}H_{67}O_{15}N$
M.p. 141–144°C (*dec.*)

Streptomyces halstedii also produces this antibiotic closely related in structure to the preceding compound. It forms colourless crystals from $(CH_3)_2CO$ and is characterized as the hydrochloride, m.p. 164–166°C (*dec.*) with $[\alpha]_D^{25} - 35°$ (c 2·0, $CHCl_3$).

Hochstein, Murai, *J. Amer. Chem. Soc.*, **76**, 5080 (1954)
Woodward, *Angew. Chem.*, **69**, 50 (1957)

3-CARBOXY-2-QUINOXALINYLPENICILLIC ACID
$C_{18}H_{16}O_6N_4S$

One of the large number of known penicillins, this antibiotic is of particular value in medicine since it is active against penicillinase-producing bacteria.

It gives a deep red colour with solutions of cuprous salts and a violet colour with ferrous sulphate. The sodium salt (quinacillin) furnishes cream-yellow needles from H_2O, melts at 260°C and decomposes at 261–262°C. It has $[\alpha]_D^{23} + 183·5°$ (H_2O). The parent antibiotic forms a bis-triethyl-ammonium salt which crystallizes as the monohydrate, m.p. 135–137°C (*dec.*) and has $[\alpha]_D^{20} + 142°$ (c 0·376, H_2O). The antibiotic is active against a wide range of gram-positive and gram-negative bacteria.

Richards, Housley, Spooner, *Nature*, **199**, 354 (1963)

α-CARBOXY-3-THIENYLMETHYLPENICILLIN
$C_{15}H_{16}O_6N_2S_2$

A semi-synthetic penicillin, this antibiotic is more active than carbenicillin against *Pseudomonas aeruginosa* and is also effective against *Enterobacter* and indole-positive *Proteus* species, together with *Hemophilus influenzae*, *Neisseria gonorrhoeae*, *N. meningitidis* and *Proteus mirabilis*. Isolates of *Klebsiella* are routinely resistant to the antibiotic.

Neu, Winshell, *Antimicrobial Agents & Chemotherapy*, 385 (1970)
Sutherland, Burnett, Rolinson, *ibid.*, 390 (1970)
Bodey, Deerhake, *Appl. Microbiol.*, **21**, 61 (1971)
Neu, Winshell, *ibid.*, **21**, 66 (1971)

CARCINOCIDIN
A highly complex antibiotic of the polypeptide group, carcinocidin is produced by *Streptomyces kitazawaensis*. The structure is not yet known, but on acid hydrolysis it furnishes cystine, glutamic acid, glycine and lysine. Molecular weight determinations indicate a value greater than 6000. The antibiotic possesses marked antitumour properties.

Okamoto *et al.*, *Japanese Patent*, 6894 (1959)

CARCINOMYCIN
M.p. Indefinite
Streptomyces carcinomycinus elaborates this polypeptide antibiotic which is obtained as a dark green amorphous powder with no definite melting point.

It is active against a number of experimental tumours. Little is known of its chemical constitution.

Hosotani, Soeda, *Japanese Patent*, 6893 (1959)

CARFECILLIN
$C_{23}H_{22}N_2O_6S$

A semi-synthetic antibiotic, carfecillin is the α-phenyl ester of carbenicillin (q.v.). It has a comparable activity against gram-negative bacilli as carbenicillin but is more active than this antibiotic against gram-positive cocci and penicillin-sensitive strains of staphylococci and β-hemolytic streptococci. It is significantly more effective than carbenicillin against enterococci and pneumococci.

Basker, Sutherland, *Chemother. Proc. Int. Congr. Chemother.*, 9th, **5**, 51 (1975)

CARMINOMYCIN 1
$C_{26}H_{27}O_{10}N$
M.p. Indefinite

An anthraquinoid antibiotic, this compound is the major component of an antibiotic complex produced by *Actinomadura carminata* grown on a nutrient medium to which streptomycin has been added. The antibiotic yields a crystalline hydrochloride as bright red needles with a specific rotation of $[\alpha]_D^{20}$ + 289°. Carminomycin 1 has antineoplastic properties, significantly decreasing the growth of bronchogenic cancer, transplantable prestomach cancer, lymphatic leukosis L-1210 and lymphosarcoma in mice with 2–4 intravenous injections of between 1·3 and 2·25 mg. The inhibitory effects on sarcoma 180 and lymphadenosis are less pronounced and carminomycin 1 is ineffective against Ehrlich ascites carcinoma.

Gauze et al., *Antibiotiki*, **18**, 675 (1973)
Shorin et al., *ibid.*, **18**, 681 (1973)
Brazhnikova et al., *J. Antibiotics* (Japan), **27**, 254 (1974)
Gauze et al., *Cancer Chemother. Rep.*, Part 1, **58**, 255 (1974)

CASSIC ACID
M.p. 330°C (*dec.* and *subl.*)

For many decades it has been known by the natives of Costa Rica that the leaves of *Cassia reticulata* Wild may be used orally in the treatment of chronic gonorrhea, but it was not until 1947 that the active agent was described by Robbins, Kavanagh and Thayer. Cassic acid is isolated by washing the leaves with boiling H_2O, then boiling the washed leaves with H_2O and dilute sodium carbonate, the cooled extract being acidified with HCl to pH 3·2, extracted with methyl *iso*butyl ketone and the organic layer concentrated *in vacuo* to an oily material. The crude compound thus obtained may be purified by dissolving in $(CH_3)_2CO$, adding H_2O and removing the active material with Et_2O. On extracting the ethereal solution with sodium bicarbonate, acidifying the bicarbonate fraction, crystalline cassic acid is precipitated. Cassic acid forms light yellow needles which are slightly soluble in EtOH, $CHCl_3$, Et_2O, H_2O and methyl *iso*butyl ketone and virtually insoluble in petroleum ether. It gives a yellow colour with dilute acids, changing to red under alkaline conditions.

Cassic acid is normally assayed by serial dilution using *Escherichia coli* and *Staphylococcus aureus* as test organisms. When used as the crystalline sodium salt, it has the following inhibition concentrations (μg/ml): *Bacillus mycoides* (4·0); *B. subtilis* (8·0); *Escherichia coli* (>250); *Mycobacterium phlei* (8·0); *Myco. smegmatis* (32); *Neisseria gonorrheae* (8·0) and *Staphylococcus aureus* (8·0). Cassic acid has a low toxicity in rabbits and mice when administered orally. Some is excreted in the urine.

Robbins, Kavanagh, Thayer, *Bull. Torrey Bot. Club*, **74**, 287 (1947)

CATENULIN (*Paromomycin*)
An antibiotic obtained from an unclassified *Streptomyces* species, this compound is closely related to neomycin B. It may, however, be distin-

guished from both neomycin A and B and the streptomycins by paper chromatography. Catenulin is extracted from the broth by adsorption on activated carbon followed by elution. It is normally crystallized as the helianthate or the p-(p'-hydroxyphenylazo)-benzene sulphonate from hot H_2O. The sulphate is optically active with a specific rotation of $[\alpha]_D^{25}$ + 51·9° (c 1·0, H_2) and gives no typical ultraviolet spectrum although the infrared spectrum is typical of a polypeptide. Catenulin is stable in acid solution and upon prolonged hydrolysis yields a substance tentatively identified as neamine by paper chromatography.

The antibiotic is active against several strains of *Mycobacteria* and shows a cross resistance with neomycin. The LD_{50} in mice is 125 mg/kg when given intravenously. Cats exhibit neurotoxicity when given this drug. From the available evidence it appears that catenulin may be used in medicine in the same manner as neomycin (q.v.). It has been shown to be identical with paromomycin (q.v.).

Davisson, *Antibiotics & Chemotherapy*, **2**, 460 (1952)
Szybalski, *Bact. Proc.*, 40 (1952)

CEFAMANDOLE
$C_{18}H_{18}N_6O_5S_2$

A semi-synthetic cephalosporin, cefamandole is used primarily as the sodium salt. It has a broad spectrum activity against gram-positive and gram-negative bacteria, gram-positive cocci except *Streptococcus faecalis*, and also against penicillin-G resistant strains of *Staphylococcus aureus*. Cefamandole is highly active against strains of *Haemophilus influenzae* and although most strains of *Escherichia coli*, *Klebsiella* and *Proteus* are inhibited at low concentrations, an increasing resistance has been observed with larger inocula. It is effective against *Salmonella typhi* but most strains of *Pseudomonas* are resistant to the antibiotic.

Meyers *et al.*, *Antimicrobial Agents & Chemotherapy*, **8**, 737 (1975)
Hirschman, Meyers, Miller, *ibid.*, **11**, 369 (1977)

CEFATRIZINE
$C_{18}H_{18}O_5N_6S_2$

A semi-synthetic cephalosporin antibiotic, cefatrizine is orally active and has a broad spectrum antibiotic activity comparable with cefazolin and cephalexin. It is active against gram-positive and gram-negative bacteria and also a number of enterobacter and enterococcus species. When given to mice either orally or parenterally, it has a higher peak serum level and longer biological half-life than most cephalosporin antibiotics and yields a pronounced *in vivo* protective activity in mice against *Enterobacter cloacae*, *Escherichia coli*, *Hemophilus influenzae*, *Klebsiella pneumoniae*, *Proteus morganii* and *Staphylococcus aureus*.

Actor *et al.*, *J. Antibiotics* (Japan), **28**, 594 (1975)
Stilwell, Adams, Turck, *Antimicrobial Agents & Chemotherapy*, **8**, 751 (1975)

CEFAZAFLUR
$C_{13}H_{12}N_6O_4S_3F_3$

A semi-synthetic cephalosporin, cefazaflur possesses a high activity against most Enterobacteriaceae and also against *Staphylococcus aureus*. It has found little use in medicine at present since it exhibits significant variations in activity depending upon such variables as inocula size, culture media and the method of testing.

Counts *et al.*, *Antimicrobial Agents & Chemotherapy*, **11**, 708 (1977)

CEFAZOLIN (*Cephazolin*)
$C_{14}H_{14}O_4N_8S_3$
M.p. 198–200°C (*dec.*)

A semi-synthetic antibiotic, cefazolin is obtained as colourless needles and is characterized as the sodium salt which exists in two crystal modifications: the α-form with m.p. 185–186°C and the β-form, m.p. 188–189°C. Cefazolin is highly active in the treatment of infections of the urinary tract and finds use in obstetrical and gynaecological fields. A dose of 1 g daily given intramuscularly effectively cures cases of puerperal fever, pyelonephritis and genital infections. In dermatology, it is effective in the treatment of staphylococcal skin infections. Pain is minimal following intramuscular injection and thrombophlebitis has not been observed in those patients given the antibiotic intravenously. Renal clearance has been shown to be essentially the same as the serum clearance and almost 100 per cent of the administered dose is recovered in the urine within 24 hours.

Kariyone *et al.*, *J. Antibiotics* (Japan), **23**, 137 (1970)
Nishida *et al.*, *ibid.*, **23**, 137, 184 (1970)
Mine *et al.*, *ibid.*, **23**, 195 (1970)
Ishiyama *et al.*, *Antimicrobial Agents & Chemotherapy*, 476 (1970)
Nishimura *et al.*, *Nippon Kagaku Ryohogakukai Zasshi*, **18**, 688 (1970)
Nakayama *et al.*, *ibid.*, **18**, 703 (1970)
Shibata *et al.*, *ibid.*, **18**, 714 (1970)
Ohkoshi *et al.*, *ibid.*, **18**, 734 (1970)
Mizuno *et al.*, *ibid.*, **18**, 763 (1970)
Cho *et al.*, *ibid.*, **18**, 770 (1970)
Seiga *et al.*, *ibid.*, **18**, 778 (1970)
Kawamura *et al.*, *ibid.*, **18**, 795 (1970)
Tanioku *et al.*, *ibid.*, **18**, 803 (1970)
Iwazawa, *ibid.*, **18**, 812 (1970)
Kashiwazaki, Hirose, Kikuta, *ibid.*, **18**, 826 (1970)
Sambe *et al.*, *ibid.*, **18**, 831 (1970)
Reller *et al.*, *Antimicrobial Agents & Chemotherapy*, **3**, 488 (1973)
Bergeron *et al.*, *ibid.*, **4**, 396 (1973)
Kirby, Regamey, *J. Inf. Diseases*, **128**, S341 (1973)
Birkhead *et al.*, *ibid.*, **128**, S379 (1973)
Kanazawa, Kuramata, *Chemotherapy* (Tokyo), **21**, 1851 (1973)
Renzini *et al.*, *Antibiotica*, **11**, 5 (1973)
Nicholas *et al.*, *J. Clin. Pharmacol.*, **13**, 325 (1973)
Regamey, Gordon, Kirby, *Arch. Intern. Med.*, **133**, 407 (1974)
Periti *et al.*, *Future Trends Chemother.*, *Proc. Int. Symp.*, 63 (1974)
Welling *et al.*, *Clin. Pharmacol. Ther.*, **15**, 344 (1974)
Actor *et al.*, *J. Antibiotics* (Japan), **28**, 594 (1975)

CEFOXITIN
$C_{16}H_{18}O_7N_3S_2$
M.p. Indefinite

A semi-synthetic antibiotic, this compound is normally isolated and used as the crystalline sodium salt. It is highly effective against gram-positive and gram-negative bacteria, being more active than caphalothin (q.v.) against *Bacteroides fragilis*, *Enterobacter* and *Klebsiella* species and is also active against a large number of indole-producing *Proteus* strains. It also has the advantage that it is completely resistant to hydrolysis by the lactamases elaborated by strains of gram-negative bacteria resistant to cephalosporin antibiotics.

Kosmidis *et al.*, *Brit. Med. J.*, **4** (5893), 653 (1973)
Hamilton-Miller, Kerry, Brumfitt, *J. Antibiotics* (Japan), **27**, 42 (1974)
Miller *et al.*, *Antimicrobial Agents & Chemotherapy*, **5**, 33 (1974)
Onishi *et al.*, *ibid.*, **5**, 38 (1974)
Onishi *et al.*, *Ann. N.Y. Acad. Sci.*, **235**, 406 (1974)

CEFTEZOLE
$C_{13}H_{12}N_8O_4S_3$

A semi-synthetic cephalosporin, ceftezole has the structure shown above. It has broad spectrum antibiotic activity against both gram-positive and gram-negative bacteria and the development of organism resistance has been shown to be significantly less than with most other antibiotics. It has been suggested as a therapeutic agent against *Escherichia coli* and *Klebsiella* species.

Noto *et al.*, *J. Antibiotics* (Japan), **29**, 1058 (1976)
Nehashi *et al.*, *Chemotherapy* (Tokyo), **24**, 635 (1976)

CEFUROXIME-A
$C_{16}H_{16}N_4O_8S$

A broad spectrum semi-synthetic cephalosporin, cefuroxime-A is useful for administration by injection. It is active against gram-positive bacteria including penicillinase-producing staphylococci and against many gram-negative bacteria including most indole-positive *Proteus* species and *Enterobacter*. It is highly effective against *Haemophilus influenzae* and *Neisseria gonorrhoeae* and is stable to most β-lactamases. No evidence has been found of toxicity in human volunteers and the blood level of the antibiotic is both high and prolonged. Some short-lived pain has been experienced following intramuscular injection but cefuroxime-A is well tolerated when administered intravenously.

O'Callaghan *et al.*, *J. Antibiotics* (Japan), **29**, 29 (1976)

CELBENIN
See Methicillin

CELESTICETIN
$C_{24}H_{36}O_9N_2S$
M.p. Indefinite
This antibiotic, obtained from *Streptomyces celestis*, forms a colourless glass which is hygroscopic and cannot be crystallized. It is dextrorotatory with a specific rotation of $[\alpha]_D^{24} + 126 \cdot 6°$ (c 0·5, $CHCl_3$). The oxalate is crystalline with m.p. 147–152°C and $[\alpha]_D^{24} + 106 \cdot 6°$ (c 0·5, H_2O).

de Boer *et al.*, *Antibiotics Annual*, 831 (1954–55)
Hoeksema, Crum, Williams, *ibid.*, 837 (1954–55)
Revised structure
Hoeksema, *J. Amer. Chem. Soc.*, **86**, 4224 (1964)
Hoeksema, *ibid.*, **90**, 755 (1968)

CELESTICETIN I
$C_{24}H_{36-40}O_9N_2S$
A further antibiotic elaborated by *Streptomyces celestis*, this substance is closely allied to the preceding compound although it may be obtained in a crystalline form. With bromine water, mercuric chloride and Millon reagent, it yields white precipitates. It gives positive Ekkert and Molisch tests and forms a crystalline oxalate, m.p. 149–154°C and a salicylate, m.p. 139°C.

Hoeksema, Crum, deVries, *Antibiotics Annual*, **2**, 837 (1954–55)
de Boer, Dietz, Hoeksema, *U.S. Patent*, 2,928,844

CELESTICETIN B
$C_{21}H_{38}O_8N_2S$
Recently, a further series of antibiotics have been obtained from cultures of *Streptomyces celestis*, all having similar structures. Celesticetin B is normally isolated as the crystalline hydrochloride which is dextrorotatory having a specific rotation of $[\alpha]_D^{25} + 146°$ (c 1·0, H_2O).

Argoudelis, Brodasky, *J. Antibiotics* (Japan), **25**, 194 (1972)

CELESTICETIN C
$C_{24}H_{37}O_8N_3S$
Streptomyces celestis produces this antibiotic which differs in structure from the preceding substance only in the nature of the sugar side chain. It has

CELESTICETIN D (Antibiotic SKF 60771)
$C_{19}H_{34}O_8N_2S$

A third antibiotic isolated from cultures of *Streptomyces celestis*, the structure of this substance has been shown to be desalicetin-2′-acetate.

Argoudelis, Brodasky, *J. Antibiotics* (Japan), **25**, 194 (1972)

CELIOMYCIN
See Viomycin

CELLOCIDIN (*Aquamycin*)
$C_4H_4O_2N_2$
M.p. 216–218°C (dec.)

$$H_2NCOC{\equiv}CCONH_2$$

This acetylenic antibiotic is elaborated by *Streptomyces chibaensis* and *S. reticuli* var. *aquamyceticus*. It forms white crystals when purified by recrystallization from CH_3OH. The structure has been established by chemical methods. It is active against a number of gram-positive organisms.

Suzuki *et al.*, *J. Antibiotics* (Japan), **11A**, 81 (1958)
Taniyama *et al.*, *J. Pharm. Soc.*, *Japan*, **79**, 1510 (1959)
Biosynthesis
Sir Ewart R. H. Jones *et al.*, *J. Chem. Soc., Perkin I*, 148 (1973)

CELLVIBRIOCIN
M.p. Indefinite
A bacteriocin, this compound has recently been described. It is produced by at least six strains of *Cellvibrio*, particularly species 9916, and is not easily detectable or inducible in liquid media, nor extractable from agar cultures. It is thermolabile, not affected by DNase, RNase, catalase or lysozyme, but is completely inactivated by proteases and by such solvents as EtOH, $CHCl_3$ and $(CH_3)_2CO$ which are protein denaturants.

Halliwell, Sweet, *J. Gen. Microbiol.*, **77**, 363 (1973)

CEPHACETRILE
$C_{13}H_{13}O_6N_3S$
M.p. Indefinite

A semi-synthetic antibiotic of the cephalosporin type, this compound readily attains therapeutic intrauterine levels in healthy pregnant women during labour, the intravenous injection of 1 g every 2 hours giving peak maternal serum levels of 65–90 μg/ml and cord serum and amniotic fluid levels of 19 and 22–25 μg/ml respectively.

Hirsch *et al.*, *Arch. Gynaekol.*, **216**, 1 (1974)

CEPHALEXIN
$C_{16}H_{17}O_4N_3S$
M.p. Indefinite

A cephalosporanic acid derivative, cephalexin is formed by treatment of 7-aminodeacetoxycephalosporanic acid with D-phenylglycine in an aqueous medium in the presence of an acylating enzyme elaborated by strains of *Achromobacter* B 402-2 (NRRL B-5393), *Alcaligenes faecalis* (ATCC 8750); *Bacillus megaterium* (NRRL B-5385), *Beneckea hyperoptica* (ATCC 15,803) or *Flavobacterium aquatile* (NRRL B-5394). It is normally isolated as the monohydrate. Cephalexin has been examined for its antibacterial activity against a number of organisms. Those which have been found to be sensitive include *Enterobacter aerogenes*, *Ent. cloacae*, *Escherichia coli*, *Klebsiella pneumoniae*, *Proteus morganii*, *P. rettgeri*, *P. vulgaris*, *Salmonella* species, *Staphylococcus* species sensitive to penicillin G, *Streptococcus pneumoniae* and *Strep. pyogenes* A. A few strains of these organisms are resistant as are also *Pseudomonas* species, *Serratia marsecens* and *Streptococcus fecalis*.

Foz, *Prensa Med. Mex.*, **35**, 1 (1970)
Fujii *et al.*, *German Patent*, 2,241,091 (1973)

CEPHALOGLYCIN (*Kefglycin*)

$C_{18}H_{19}O_6N_3S$
M.p. 223–250°C (*dec.*)

A semi-synthetic antibiotic, cephaloglycin is formed from 7-aminocephalosporanic acid and D-phenylglycine in the presence of an acylase produced by strains of *Achromobacter*, *Alcaligenes*, *Bacillus*, *Beneckea*, *Escherichia* or *Flavobacterium*. The antibiotic is obtained by adsorbing the activity on activated carbon, eluting with $(CH_3)_2CO$—AcOH and crystallizing from aqueous acetonitrile. The ultraviolet spectrum in dimethylformamide has a single absorption maximum at 258 nm. It is similar in its activity to the preceding antibiotic.

Kurita *et al.*, *J. Antibiotics* (Japan), **19A**, 243 (1966)
Fujii *et al.*, *Japanese Patent*, 7,447,594 (1974)

CEPHALORIDINE (*Ceporin, Keflordin*[R])

$C_{19}H_{17}O_3N_3S_2$
M.p. Indefinite

The structure of this broad-spectrum antibiotic has been shown to be 7-[(2-thienyl)acetamido]-3-(1-pyridylmethyl)-3-cephem-4-carboxylic acid betaine. The ultraviolet spectrum in H_2O exhibits absorption maxima at 238 and 251 nm. Among the salts formed with inorganic acids are the hydriodide having an ultraviolet spectrum in H_2O with absorption maxima at 237 and 255 nm and the thiocyanate with a similar ultraviolet spectrum showing absorption maxima at 236 and 255 nm. Cephaloridine is active against a number of gram-positive and gram-negative bacteria and has a powerful antibacterial activity when added to chicken embryonic cultures infected with *Staphylococcus aureus*. The LD_{50} for mice is 4·7–5·2 g/kg when given intravenously and for chicken embryonic fibroblasts it varied between 778 and 2216 µg/ml.

Spencer *et al.*, *J. Org. Chem.*, **32**, 500 (1967)
Mandell, *Ann. Intern. Med.*, **79**, 561 (1973)
Zak, Ermolova, Navalotskaya, *Antibiotiki*, **18**, 1037 (1973)

CEPHALOSPORIN C

$C_{16}H_{21}O_8N_3S$
M.p. Indefinite

Cephalosporium species IMI 49137 produces this antibiotic which is also elaborated by *Streptomyces lactamgenes* and *Azotobacter* 5685. The structure has been shown to be 7-(5-amino-5-carboxyvaleramido)-cephalosporanic acid. It gives a purple colour with ninhydrin and on acid hydrolysis furnishes D-α-aminoadipic acid and carbon dioxide. The sodium salt forms colourless crystals of the dihydrate and is dextrorotatory with $[\alpha]_D + 103°$. The antibiotic is active against a range of gram-positive and gram-negative bacteria.

Newton, Abraham, *Biochem. J.*, **62**, 651 (1956)
Abraham, Newton, *ibid.*, **79**, 377 (1961)
Hodgkin, Maslen, *ibid.*, **79**, 393 (1961)
Sciavolino, *German Patent*, 2,157,693 (1972)
Gargiuolo, *German Patent*, 2,239,321 (1973)
Nakao *et al.*, *Japanese Patent*, 7,569,294 (1975)
Kanzaki, Fujisawa, Suide, *German Patent*, 2,445,615 (1975)
Takeda, Maysumoto, Naito, *Japanese Patent*, 7,569,293 (1975)

CEPHALOSPORIN N

See D-4-amino-4-carboxybutylpenicillinic acid

CEPHALOSPORIN P₁

$C_{30}H_{44}O_8$
M.p. 147°C

A number of related antibiotics have been obtained from an unidentified species of *Cephalosporium*. Cephalosporin P₁ forms colourless crystals from aqueous MeOH and has a specific rotation of $[\alpha]_D + 28°$ (CHCl$_3$). It is readily soluble in most organic solvents but only sparingly so in light petroleum. In H$_2$O it is inactivated slowly at pH 8·0 and more rapidly at pH 9·6. It is also inactivated by penicillinase. This antibiotic, and the following cephalosporins, are active against gram-positive and some gram-negative bacteria.

Burton, Abraham, *Biochem. J.*, **50**, 168 (1951)
Burton, Abraham, Caldwell, *ibid.*, **62**, 171 (1956)
Baird *et al.*, *Proc. Chem. Soc.*, 257 (1961)

CEPHALOSPORIN P$_2$
M.p. 151°C
Also elaborated by a species of *Cephalosporium*, this antibiotic forms colourless crystals from aqueous CH$_3$OH. It is freely soluble in (CH$_3$)$_2$CO, EtOH and butyl acetate and sparingly soluble in C$_6$H$_6$ and di*iso*propyl ether. Like the preceding antibiotic it is inactivated by penicillinase.

Burton, Abraham, *Biochem. J.*, **50**, 168 (1952)

CEPHALOSPORIN P$_3$
M. p. Indefinite
An amorphous antibiotic obtained from a species of *Cephalosporium*. this substance is soluble in most organic solvents but insoluble in H$_2$O. It is also deactivated by penicillinase.

Burton, Abraham, *Biochem. J.*, **50**, 168 (1952)

CEPHALOSPORIN P$_4$
M.p. 220–230°C
A further antibiotic isolated from cultures of an unclassified species of *Cephalosporium*, cephalosporin P$_4$ forms light fawn-coloured crystals when recrystallized from aqueous CH$_3$OH. It dissolves readily in (CH$_3$)$_2$CO, but is only slightly soluble in H$_2$O and Et$_2$O. Like the foregoing antibiotics, it is inactivated by penicillinase.

Burton, Abraham, *Biochem. J.*, **50**, 168 (1952)
Burton, Abraham, Caldwell, *ibid.*, **62**, 171 (1956)
Baird *et al.*, *Proc. Chem. Soc.*, 257 (1961)

CEPHALOTHIN
$C_{16}H_{16}O_6N_2S_2$

A semi-synthetic antibiotic, cephalothin is formed enzymatically by acylation of 7-aminocephalosporanic acid, the enzyme being produced by *Bacillus megaterium* B-400 (NRRL B-5385) grown aerobically on a medium containing peptone, corn steep liquor, yeast extract, ammonium salts, molasses, glucose and starch. Cephalothin is usually employed as the sodium salt and is active against gram-positive and gram-negative bacteria, particularly *Salmonella* strains. The LD$_{50}$ in mice is 5670 mg/kg given intraperitoneally and greater than 20,000 mg/kg given orally. Some pathological changes in the liver and pancreas have been observed with doses greater than 500 mg/kg in rats. Combinations of cephalothin and aminoglycosidic antibiotics are ineffective against enterococci since the concentration of cephalothin falls below the minimum inhibitory concentration against enterococci during the *in vivo* metabolism and excretion of the antibiotic when given in the normal doses for endocarditis.

Moreno *et al.*, *Arq. Inst. Biol.*, Sao Paulo, **40**, 39 (1973)
Kuramo *et al.*, *J. Antibiotics* (Japan), **27**, 746 (1974)
Kuramoto *et al.*, *ibid.*, **28**, 195 (1975)
Weinstein, Moellering, *Antimicrobial Agents & Chemotherapy*, **7**, 522 (1975)
Fujii, Shibuya, *German Patent*, 2,353,107 (1975)

CEPHAMYCIN A
$C_{25}H_{31}O_{15}N_3S_2$
A penicillin type antibiotic, cephamycin A has been isolated from cultures of *Streptomyces griseus* and *S. viridochromogenes* SF-1584. This antibiotic

is the sulphate of caphamycin B (q.v.) and is active against gram-positive bacteria.

Albers-Schonberg, Arison, Smith, *Tetrahedron Lett.*, 2911 (1972)
Kondo *et al.*, *Japanese Patent*, 7, 564, 489 (1975)

CEPHAMYCIN B
$C_{25}H_{29}O_{11}N_3S$

Streptomyces griseus and *S. viridochromogenes* SF-1584 also produced this antibiotic when grown aerobically at 28°C for 3 days in a medium containing glycerol, soybean flour and calcium carbonate. The structure has been elucidated by chemical and spectroscopic methods. Cephamycin B is also effective against gram-positive bacteria.

Albers-Schonberg, Arison, Smith, *Tetrahedron Lett.*, 2911 (1972)
Kondo *et al.*, *Japanese Patent*, 7,564,489 (1975)

CEPHAMYCIN C
M.p. Indefinite
A penicillin type antibiotic, cephamycin C is produced by culturing *Streptomyces lactamdurans* in a medium containing added D-lysine or DL-lysine, incubating at 28°C for 4 days. Reduced yields are obtained in the absence of lysine. The antibiotic is effective against a range of gram-positive bacteria.

Inamine, Birnbaum, *U.S. Patent*, 3,886,044 (1975)

CEPHAPIRIN
$C_{17}H_{17}O_6N_3S_2$
M.p. Indefinite

A cephalosporin derivative, this antibiotic has been described by Japanese workers. When tested against gram-positive bacteria *in vitro* it is as active as cefazolin (q.v.) but less so than cephaloridine, whereas against gram-negative organisms the two antibiotics are equal in activity. Clinically-isolated staphylococcal strains are sensitive to cephapirin in the range 0·09–25 µg/ml and the antibiotic is stable against β-lactamase produced by *Escherichia coli*. Cephapirin shows a cross resistance with cephaloridine against most clinically isolated strains. *Pseudomonas* and most *Proteus* isolates are resistant to the antibiotic. Cephapirin is not inactivated by staphylococcal penicillinase but is inactivated by cephalosporinase produced by gram-negative bacteria. The therapeutic effect of the antibiotic for *Escherichia coli* infections is greater than that of cephalothin at doses less than 50 mg/kg but no differences have been observed at higher doses.

The LD_{50} has been given as ~ 6 g/kg after intravenous, subcutaneous, intraperitoneal and oral administration in both mice and rats. Following the administration of toxic doses, symptoms reported include tonic convulsions, paralysis of the hind legs, stimulation of the reflexes and pain response and respiratory paralysis leading to death. In trials with rats and rabbits of both sexes doses up to one half LD_{50} were given intraperitoneally and subcutaneously for periods of between 3 and 6 months. Death was observed only after administration of one half LD_{50}. In doses greater than one eighth LD_{50} degenerative changes were found in the kidneys and liver together with inhibition of body weight increase. With doses below one thirty-second LD_{50} there was no serious change before 3 months, but thereafter the blood serum nitrogen levels rose without any histological change. From these observations, it appears that cephapirin possesses a relatively lower nephrotoxicity level than other cephalosporin derivatives.

Miyamura *et al.*, *J. Antibiotics* (Japan), **27**, 148 (1974)
Mitsuhashi *et al.*, *ibid.*, **27**, 152 (1974)
Nakazawa *et al.*, *ibid.*, **27**, 164 (1974)
Ito, Irie, Sumiyama, *Toho Igakkai Zasshi.*, **21**, 211, 279 (1974)
Tsubura *et al.*, *Oyo Yakuri*, **9**, 11 (1975)
Renzini, Ravagnan, *Chemotherapy*, **21**, 285 (1975)

CEPHAZOLIN
See Cefazolin

CEPHEMIMYCIN
$C_{16}H_{22}N_4O_9S$

A cephalosporin antibiotic, cephemimycin is produced by culturing *Streptomyces jumonjinensis* 3008 (NRRL 5741) in a common nutrient medium at 25–30°C for 40–45 hours. The antibiotic is separated by extraction of the culture medium with organic solvents and purified by column and thin layer chromatography. It possesses bactericidal and fungicidal activity.

Arai *et al.*, *German Patent*, 2,344,020 (1974)

CEPHRADINE
$C_{16}H_{19}O_4N_3S$

A further semi-synthetic cephalosporin derivative, this antibiotic has similar *in vitro* and *in vivo* activities to cephalexin (q.v.). Cephradine has a greater activity against *Escherichia coli*, *Klebsiella* and *Staphylococcus* strains but otherwise its antibacterial activity is equivalent to cephalexin. The LD_{50} in mice is 4571 mg/kg (intravenous) and in rats greater than 2500 mg/kg. No abnormalities have been observed in the post-natal development in mice or rat foetuses to which the antibiotic was given orally. The effect of cephradine on the central nervous system in animals has also been examined and no toxic effects have been found.

Renzini, Filadoro, *Farmaco, Ed. Prat.*, **28**, 659 (1973)
Arnow *et al.*, *Antimicrobial Agents & Chemotherapy*, **5**, 49 (1974)
Renzini *et al.*, *Future Trends Chemother., Proc. Int. Symp.*, 75 (1974)
Otsuki *et al.*, *Chemotherapy*, **23**, 1 (1975)
Aratani *et al.*, *ibid.*, **23**, 19 (1975)
Yamanaka, Kono, Aratani, *ibid.*, **23**, 29 (1975)
Masuda, Suzuki, Okonogi, *ibid.*, **23**, 37 (1975)

CEPORIN
See Cephaloridine

CEREVIOCCIDIN
$C_{22}H_{39}O_4N_5$
M.p. 249°C (dec.)

An antibiotic produced by a species of *Streptomyces*, this compound forms colourless needles from EtOH. The structure is not yet completely known. It is active against bacteria and fungi.

Yamashita *et al.*, *J. Antibiotics* (Japan), **8A**, 42 (1955)

CEREXIN A
Decomp. > 190°C

Cultures of *Bacillus cereus* yield two antibiotics, cerexins A and B which have been separated and purified by chromatographic methods. This antibiotic forms a white amorphous powder which decomposes without melting. It is dextrorotatory having a specific rotation of $[\alpha]_D^{28} + 19.5°$ (c 0.172, dimethylfuran). It is active against gram-positive bacteria.

Shoji *et al.*, *J. Antibiotics* (Japan), **28**, 56 (1975)
Shoji, Hinoh, *ibid.*, **28**, 60 (1975)

CEREXIN B
Decomp. > 190°C

A second antibiotic isolated from cultures of *Bacillus cereus*, this compound is also an amorphous white powder which decomposes above 190°C. It is dextrorotatory having a specific rotation of $[\alpha]_D^{23} + 19.8°$ (c 0.263, dimethylfuran). It possesses an antibiotic activity similar to that of cerexin A.

Shoji, *et al.*, *J. Antibiotics* (Japan), **28**, 56 (1975)
Shoji, Hinoh, *ibid.*, **28**, 60 (1975)

CEREXIN C
The culture broth of *Bacillus cereus* strain 60-6 contains this peptide antibiotic which is effective gram-positive bacteria. It possesses a structure

similar to those of cerexins A and B but contains a lysine residue in place of γ-hydroxylysine.

Shoji et al., *J. Antibiotics* (Japan), **29**, 1288 (1976)

CEREXIN D

This antibiotic has been isolated from cultures of *Bacillus cereus* strain Gp-3. It resembles the preceding antibiotic in having a lysine residue in the molecule in place of the γ-hydroxylysine of cerexins A and B.

Shoji et al., *J. Antibiotics* (Japan), **29**, 1288 (1976)

CERULENIN
$C_{12}H_{17}O_3N$
M.p. Indefinite

A species of *Helicoceras* elaborates this antibiotic which has also been isolated from cultures of *Sartorya fumigata*. In the latter case, the culture filtrate is extracted with AcOEt and the extract chromatographed on an alumina column to yield the pure product. Cerulenin is active against a number of yeasts, particularly *Saccharomyces cerevisiae*.

Yamano et al., *Japanese Patent*, 7,224,156 (1972)
Ohno et al., *Biochem. Biophys. Res. Commun.*, **57**, 1119 (1974)

CERVICARCIN
$C_{19}H_{20}O_9$
M.p. 205°C

Streptomyces ogaensis yields this antitumour antibiotic which has the structure given above. It forms colourless crystals and is laevorotatory with a specific rotation of $[\alpha]_D^{26} - 60\cdot1°$ (c 1·4, EtOH). The ultraviolet spectrum has absorption maxima at 227, 264 and 323 nm. The compound forms a methyl ether as the hemihydrate, m.p. 227°C, characterized as the tri-acetate, m.p. 256°C. Cervicarcin exhibits some activity against experimental tumours.

Ohkuma et al., *J. Antibiotics* (Japan), **15**, 152 (1962)
Ohkuma et al., *ibid.*, **15**, 247 (1962)
Itakura, Sega, Sumiki, *ibid.*, **16**, 231 (1963)
Marumo, Sasaki, Sazuki, *J. Amer. Chem. Soc.*, **86**, 4507 (1964)
Structure
Marumo et al., *Agr. Biol. Chem.*, **32**, 209 (1968)

CHAETOMIDIN
See Oosporein

CHAININ
$C_{33}H_{54}O_{10}$
Dec. 230°C

Produced by a species of *Chainia* (isolate No. 3047), chainin is obtained in the form of colourless, silky needles when recrystallized from CH_3OH—$CHCl_3$. It is laevorotatory having a specific rotation of $[\alpha]_D - 124\cdot4°$ (c 0·2, CH_3OH). The ultraviolet spectrum in EtOH has absorption maxima at 338 and 357 nm. Catalytic hydrogenation furnishes the dihydro derivative as an amorphous solid, m.p. 115°C.

Gopalkrishnan et al., *Nature*, **218**, 597 (1968)
Structure
Pandey et al., *J. Amer. Chem. Soc.*, **94**, 4306 (1972)

CHARTREUSIN
$C_{32}H_{32}O_{14}$
M.p. 184–186°C

Isolated from several species of *Streptomyces*, particularly *S. chartreusis*, chartreusin forms yellow plates from aqueous $(CH_3)_2CO$. It has specific rotations of $[\alpha]_D^{25} - 36\cdot2°$ (c 0·3, AcOH) and $+127\cdot5°$ (c 0·3, pyridine). When hydrolysed with dilute acids it furnishes D-fucose, D-digitalose and an aglycone, $C_{19}H_8O_6$, as yellow crystals with m.p. 310–311°C.

Leach et al., *J. Amer. Chem. Soc.*, **75**, 4011 (1953)
Berger et al., *ibid.*, **80**, 1636, 1639 (1958)
Simonitsch et al., *Helv. Chim. Acta*, **43**, 58 (1960)

CHELOCARDIN
$C_{23}H_{23}O_8N$
Dec. 215–230°C

An antibiotic isolated from *Nocardia sulphurea*, chelocardin crystallizes in the form of yellow needles which decompose over a wide range of temperature without melting. The hydrochloride, $C_{23}H_{22}O_7NCl$, also decomposes without melting at 220–230°C and is dextrorotatory with $[\alpha]_D^{22} + 570°$ (c 1·0, CH_3OH).

Oliver et al., *Antimicrobial Agents & Chemotherapy*, 583 (1962)
Sinclair et al., *ibid.*, 592 (1962)

CHETOMIN (*Chaetomin*)
$C_{16}H_{17}O_4N_3S_2$
M.p. 218–222°C

Chetomin, originally named chaetomin by Waksman and his colleagues, has been derived from *Chaetomium cochliodes* and is also elaborated by *C. elatum*, *C. funiculum*, *C. spirale* and *Verticillium cinnabarinum* (*Acrostalagmus cinnabarinum*). The antibiotic is normally prepared from *C. cochliodes* by surface and submerged culture being incubated for 10 days surface and 10–14 days submerged. The yield has been recorded by Geiger, Conn and Waksman as 200 *Staphylococcus aureus* units/ml in the culture filtrate and 10,000 *Staph. aureus* units/ml from the mycelium. From the filtrate, the crude antibiotic is isolated by extraction with AcOEt, followed by concentration *in vacuo*, washing with sodium bicarbonate solution, sodium carbonate solution and H_2O until neutral in reaction and then evaporation *in vacuo* to yield a brownish gum. Extraction of the mycelium is carried out with $(CH_3)_2CO$, the extract concentrated and then extracted with AcOEt, the procedure then being exactly the same as outlined above for the culture filtrate. Purification may be carried out by dissolving the crude material in C_6H_6, adsorbing the activity on an activated carbon column, washing with C_6H_6 and eluting with 1 per cent anhydrous CH_3OH in C_6H_6. The combined eluates are then evaporated to dryness and the residue is dissolved in $CHCl_3$, the pure antibiotic being precipitated with cold petroleum ether. Chetomin forms colourless crystals and is dextrorotatory with a specific rotation of $[\alpha]_D^{22} + 360°$ (c 1·0, $CHCl_3$). The ultraviolet spectrum shows a single absorption maximum at 287 nm. It is soluble in AcOEt, $(CH_3)_2CO$, C_6H_6, $CHCl_3$, pyridine and dioxan, sparingly so in CH_3OH, EtOH and Et_2O and insoluble in H_2O and petroleum ether. Chetomin is stable in dilute acid but unstable in alkalies. It is also stable in aqueous suspension in the presence of gum acacia and is not precipitated by picric acid or mercuric chloride. It gives a negative Millon and biuret reaction and a positive indole and Hopkins-Cole reaction. It is inactivated by oxidizing agents but not by penicillinase.

Chetomin may be assayed by agar streak using the antibiotic in aqueous suspension at a 5 per cent concentration with gum acacia using *Bacillus mycoides*, *B. subtilis*, *Sarcina lutea* and *Staphylococcus aureus* as test organism or by serial dilution with *Bacillus subtilis* and *Staphylococcus aureus*. Inhibition concentrations of the crude antibiotic have been determined *in vitro* against a variety of organisms by Waksman and Bugie, typical values being: *Bacillus cereus* (1500); *B. megatherium* (60,000); *B. mesentericus* (60,000); *B. mycoides* (40,000); *B. subtilis* (30,000–175,000); *Clostridium butyricum* (6000); *Escherichia coli* (>2000); *Mycobacterium phlei* (20,000); *Myco. tuberculosis avium* (3000–17,000); *Myco. tuberculosis hominis* (3000–17,000); *Pseudomonas fluorescens* (1000); *Sarcina lutea* (200,000); *Staphylococcus aureus* (500,000). Measurements by Geiger, Conn and Waksman using pure chetomin show the following inhibition dilutions: *Bacillus mycoides* (100,000); *B. subtilis* (500,000); *Sarcina lutea* (1,000,000) and *Staphylococcus aureus* (500,000).

Experiments have shown that chetomin is ineffective *in vivo*, no protection being afforded in experimental infections in animals against those organisms which are sensitive to chetomin *in vitro*.

Waksman, Horning, *Mycologia*, **35**, 47 (1943)
Waksman, Bugie, Reilly, *Bull. Torrey Bot. Club.*, **71**, 107 (1944)
Waksman, Bugie, *J. Bact.*, **48**, 527 (1944)
Geiger, Conn, Waksman, *ibid.*, **48**, 531 (1944)
Geiger, *Arch. Biochem.*, **21**, 125 (1949)
Gaumann, Personal Commun. to S. A. Waksman, *Arch. Biochem.*, **21**, (1949)

CHILAPHYLIN

A recently discovered antibiotic, chilaphylin is elaborated by *Streptomyces melanosporofaciens* strain Chilea. It forms a neutral white powder and is aliphatic in nature. The structure of the compound is not yet known. It is active *in vitro* against gram-positive bacteria and mycobacteria. Chemical and biological comparisons indicate that chilaphylin is not identical with melanosporin, an antibiotic produced by *Streptomyces melanosporofaciens* ISP 5318, similar to the organism producing chilaphylin.

Rez, Arrieta, *J. Antibiotics* (Japan), **26**, 126 (1973)

CHINOSPORIN C

Bacillus coagulans elaborates two antibiotics, chinosporins C and S when fermented in a medium consisting of corn steep liquor, sucrose, inorganics salts at 28°C for 48 hours at pH 7·0. Selective extraction and concentration of the successive extracts, followed by treatment with Me_2CO and EtOH yields crude chinosporin C. This antibiotic is soluble in H_2O, moderately soluble in dioxan and sparingly soluble in alcohols and Me_2CO. It possesses an acute toxicity of 5000 mg/kg in mice when given intravenously and is non-toxic *per os*. Chinosporin C has been shown to act as a *p*-aminosalicylic acid and peptone factor competitive antagonist.

Simon, *Hung. Teljes*, 12, 252 (1976)

CHINOSPORIN S

$C_{25}H_{41}N_3O_{10}$
M.p. 138°C (*dec.*)

Formed with chinosporin C by culturing *Bacillus coagulans*, this antibiotic forms colourless crystals when pure and is soluble in the lower alcohols, Et_2O, $CHCl_3$ and silute alkalis but sparingly soluble in H_2O. It exhibits synergism with penicillin G and has LD_{50} in rats of 69 gm/kg when given intravenously.

Simon, *Hung. Teljes*, 12, 252 (1976)

CHLAMYDOCIN

$C_{28}H_{38}O_6N_4$

A macrocyclic polypeptide, chlamydocin is produced by *Diheterospora chlamydosporia*, grown on a common nutrient medium at 28°C for 5 days. The antibiotic is extracted from the culture filtrate with organic solvents and purified by chromatographic techniques. The structure has been determined by NMR studies, Erdman degradation and degradation with carboxypeptidase, L-aminoacid oxidase and leucinaminopeptidase.

Chlamydocin has cytostatic activity and when tested in cultures of mouse mastocytoma cells, this activity is higher than that of actinomycin D (q.v.). The oncostatic activity in mice is comparatively low, possibly due to the inactivation of the drug in blood. The toxicity in mice is 226 mg/kg given intravenously. The antibiotic is considerably more toxic to rats when given as a continuous or interrupted intravenous or intraarterial infusion than when given intraperitoneally. Inhibition of Walker tumour is, however, better by infusion and attained with lower doses.

Close, Huguenin, *Helv. Chim. Acta*, **57**, 533 (1974)
Staehelin, Trippmacher, *Eur. J. Cancer.*, **10**, 801 (1974)

CHLORAMPHENICOL (*Chloromycetin*^{R})

$C_{11}H_{12}O_5N_2Cl_2$
M.p. 149·7–150·7°C

An antibiotic derived from *Streptomyces venezuelae* and also prepared by synthesis, chloramphenicol is obtained by submerged growth in shaker flasks, an average yield being 80 µg/ml after 5 days fermentation. The antibiotic may be isolated by extraction of the culture filtrate with Et_2O and evaporating the ethereal extract to dryness, by adsorbing the activity on activated carbon and eluting with various organic solvents, or by extracting the filtrate with AcOEt, concentrating the extract and adding kerosene, washing with dilute H_2SO_4, dilute sodium bicarbonate and distilled H_2O, drying over anhydrous sodium sulphate, concentrating the solution, chilling and allowing crystallization to take place. Various methods of purification are available. The crude ethereal extract may be chromatographed over alumina, the eluate evaporated to dryness, the residue extracted with H_2O, the aqueous fraction washed with petroleum ether, concentrated and allowed to crystallize, followed by recrystallization from ethylene dichloride. The crude crystals obtained during the isolation process may be dissolved in ethylene dichloride, treated with activated carbon and recrystallized.

Chloramphenicol forms colourless needles or elongated plates. It is laevorotatory with a specific rotation of $[\alpha]_D^{25} - 25\cdot5°$ (AcOEt) or $[\alpha]_D^{25} - 19\cdot0°$ (EtOH). The ultraviolet spectrum in H_2O or 0·1 *N*-HCl has a single absorption maximum at 278 nm. Chloramphenicol is readily soluble in CH_3OH, EtOH, AcOEt, $(CH_3)_2CO$ or BuOH, sparingly so in H_2O and Et_2O and insoluble in C_6H_6 and petroleum ether. It is stable between pH 0·5 and 9.56, gives a negative Molisch, biuret, Benedict, Pauly, Sakaguchi and ferric chloride test and is not hydrolysed by chromotrypsin, pepsin, papain or trypsin, but is hydrolysed by the bacterial enzymes from old cultures of *Bacillus mycoides*, *B. subtilis*, *Escherichia coli* and *Proteus vulgaris*. The antibiotic yields a series of crystalline derivatives including the 3-hydrogen succinoyl, m.p. 127°C; 3-hexanoyl, m.p. 175°C; 3-nonanoyl, m.p. 101°C; 3-hexadecanoyl, m.p. 79–80°C; 3-tetradecanoyl, m.p. 84°C; 3-hexadecanoyl, m.p. 90°C; $[\alpha]_D^{26} + 24\cdot 6°$ (c 5·0, EtOH); 3-octadecanoyl, m.p. 91–92°C; 3-benzoyl, m.p. 175°C and the 1-hexadecanoyl derivative, m.p. 105–106°C. The structure has been shown to be D(−)-*threo*-1-*p*-nitrophenyl-2-dichloroacetamido-1:3-propanediol.

The methods used for assay of chloramphenicol include colorimetric, serial dilution with *Shigella sonnei*, cylinder plate with *Sarcina lutea*, turbidimetric with *Salmonella paradysenteriae* and *Shigella sonnei* and paper disc-plate with *Bacillus subtilis*.

The spectrum *in vitro* has been examined by several workers, the inhibition concentrations (µg/ml) which have been reported including: *Aerobacter aerogenes* (0·5–2·5); *Bacillus anthracis* (0·75–5·0); *B. mycoides* (2·5); *B. subtilis* (10); *Borrelia recurrentis* (2·5); *Brucella abortus* (2·0–10); *Br. brochisepticus* (10); *Br. melitensis* (0·5–5·0); *Clostridium diphtheriae* (0·5); *Cl. diphtheroides* (1·0); *Corynebacterium pyogenes* (2·5); *Diplococcus pneumoniae* (1·0–2·5); *Escherichia coli* (2·5); *Gaffkya tetragena* (2·5); *Hemophilia pertussis* (0·2–0·3); *Klebsiella pneumoniae* (0·5–15·0); *Mycobacterium phlei* (25); *Myco. tuberculosis* (6·25–25); *Neisseria catarrhalis* (0·5–2·5); *N. meningitidis* (2·5); *Pasteurella avicida* (0·25–0·5); *P. oviseptica* (2·5); *P. tularensis* (0·4–10); *Proteus vulgaris* (1·0–5·0); *Pseudomonas aeruginosa* (10); *Salmonella enteriditis* (0·75–2·5); *S. paratyphi* (0·75); *S. schottmuelleri* (0·25–0·5); *S. typhimurium* (2·5–5·0); *S. typhosa* (0·75–5·0); *Sarcina aurantica* (1·0); *Serratia marcescens* (2·5–5·0); *Shigella dysenteriae* (0·75); *Sh. sonnei* (2·5–5·0); *Streptococcus hemolyticus* (0·75–2·5); *Strep. infrequens* (2·5); *Strep. non-hemolyticus* (0·25–0·75) and *Vibrio comma* (1·0).

Chloramphenicol immobilizes *Borrelia novyi* and *B. recurrentis* at concentrations of 1·5–50 µg/ml and possibly inhibits *Endameba histolytica*, but other species are not inhibited by the antibiotic and it has no activity against yeasts, protozoa or fungi.

When tested against experimental infections in animals, favourable results have been obtained against lymphogranuloma, murine typhus, psittacosis, Q fever, rickettsial pox, Rocky Mountain spotted fever, scrub typhus and typhus, all in chick embryos, mice and guinea pigs. In mice, between 35 and 50 mg/kg protected 50 per cent against *Klebsiella pneumoniae* but approximately twice this dose was required to protect against hemolytic streptococcus A. Smadel and Jackson have demonstrated that 1·0 mg in embryonic eggs and 1·5 mg in mice, given orally or intraperitoneally, afford protection against *Dermocentroxenus rickettsi*, *Rickettsia akari*, *R. mooseri*, *R. orientalis*, *R. prowazeki* and psittacosis virus.

Clinical tests against Rocky Mountain spotted fever at a dose of 50–128 mg/kg followed by 0·5 g every 3 hours, given orally, have shown the antibiotic to be effective. Similar favourable results have been obtained against bacterial pneumonias, brucellosis, acute gonorrheal arthritis in males and salmonellosis. No toxic symptoms occur when patients are given a single dose of 2 g or 1 g daily for 10 days.

Chloramphenicol is relatively non-toxic; the LD_{50} in mice being given as 245 mg/kg (intravenous), 2640 mg/kg (oral), 1320 mg/kg (intraperitoneal) while 100 mg/kg given subcutaneously each day is tolerated.

The antibiotic is absorbed rapidly when given orally, diffusing through the placenta and into the spinal fluid. When given rectally to infants it is readily absorbed into the circulation. Pathological studies in animals have been carried out by Gruhzit and his colleagues who have demonstrated that up to 25 mg/kg given intravenously to dogs produces no change in the blood pressure whereas 100 mg/kg causes a fall in the blood pressure, decreased amplitude and an increase in the rate of respiration. Aplastic anaemia has been observed as a side effect of this antibiotic and Grey syndrome has also been observed.

Ehrlich, Bartz, Smith, *Science*, **106**, 417 (1947)
Carter, Gottlieb, Anderson, *ibid.*, **107**, 113 (1948)
Gottlieb *et al.*, *J. Bact.*, **55**, 409 (1948)
Ehrlich *et al.*, *ibid.*, **56**, 467 (1948)
Bartz, *J. Biol. Chem.*, **172**, 445 (1948)
Bartz, *J. Clin. Invest.*, **28**, 1051 (1949)
Rebstock *et al.*, *J. Amer. Chem. Soc.*, **71**, 2458 (1949)
Synthesis
Controulis, Rebstock, Crooks, *J. Amer. Chem. Soc.*, **71**, 2463 (1949)
Long, Troutman, *ibid.*, **71**, 2473 (1949)
Olive, *Chem. Eng.*, **56**, 107 (1949)
Assay
Randall *et al.*, *J. Clin. Invest.*, **28**, 940 (1949)
Joslyn, Ehrlich, Schwab, *ibid.*, **28**, 1051 (1949)

Glazko, Dill, Wolf, *ibid.*, **28**, 1051 (1949)
Joslyn, Galbraith, *J. Bact.*, **54**, 26 (1947)
Bacteriological studies
Smadel, Jackson, *Science*, **106**, 418 (1947)
Woodward *et al.*, *Ann. Int. Med.*, **29**, 131 (1948)
Pincoffs *et al.*, *ibid.*, **29**, 656 (1948)
Youmans, Youmans, Osborne, *Proc. Soc. Exper. Biol. Med.*, **67**, 426 (1948)
Smadel, Jackson, *ibid.*, **67**, 478 (1948)
Ley, Smadel, Crocker, *ibid.*, **68**, 9 (1948)
Smadel *et al.*, *ibid.*, **68**, 12 (1948)
Alexander, Leidy, Redman, *J. Clin. Invest.*, **28**, 867 (1949)
Yow, Spink, *ibid.*, **28**, 871 (1949)
MacLean *et al.*, *ibid.*, **28**, 953 (1949)
Bliss, Todd, *ibid.*, **28**, 1044 (1949)
Gauld, *J. Bact.*, **57**, 349 (1949)
Ross *et al.*, *J. Clin. Invest.*, **28**, 1050 (1949)
Knight, McDermott, Ruiz-Sanchez, *ibid.*, **28**, 1952 (1949)
Chittenden *et al.*, *ibid.*, **28**, 1052 (1949)
Smadel *et al.*, *Science*, **108**, 160 (1949)

CHLORELLIN
This antibiotic was first isolated in 1940 by the action of photosynthesis due to visible light on *Chlorella pyranoidosa* or *Ch. vulgaris* grown on a medium containing carbon dioxide and inorganic salts. The culture liquor is extracted with an organic solvent such as $CHCl_3$, C_6H_6 or dichloroethane, the solvent evaporated and the residue taken up into aqueous solution.

Chlorellin inhibits the growth of *Bacillus subtilis*, *Chlorella vulgaris* itself, *Escherichia coli*, *Pseudomonas aeruginosa*, *Staphylococcus aureus* and *Streptococcus pyogenes*.

Pratt, *Amer. J. Bot.*, **27**, 52 (1940)
Pratt, Fong, *ibid.*, **27**, 431 (1940)
Pratt, *ibid.*, **29**, 142 (1942)
Pratt *et al.*, *Science*, **99**, 351 (1944)

CHLOROBIOCIN
$C_{35}H_{37}O_{11}N_2Cl$

A chlorinated antibiotic, chlorobiocin is produced by a number of *Streptomyces* species including *S. albocinerescens*, *S. hygroscopicus* and *S. roseochromogenes* var. *oscitans*. Structurally the antibiotic resembles novobiocin (q.v.) and the coumermycins, but has a greater antibacterial activity both *in vitro* and *in vivo* than these antibiotics against *Micrococcus* and *Neisseria* with no increase in toxicity. When tested in mice it has a marked therapeutic action against meningococcal and staphylococcal infections.

Ninet *et al.*, *C. R. Acad. Sci.*, **275C**, 455 (1972)

CHLOROCARCIN A
$C_{24}H_{26}N_3O_9Cl$

Streptomyces lavendulae strain No. 314 yields three closely-related chlorine-containing antibiotics which have been separated and purified by column and thin layer chromatography. This compound is a basic powder which is active against gram-positive bacteria and also against Ehrlich carcinoma and L1210 leukemia in mice.

Arai *et al.*, *J. Antibiotics* (Japan), **29**, 398 (1976)

CHLOROCARCIN B
$C_{29}H_{32}N_3O_6Cl$

A second component of the antibiotic complex isolated from cultures of *Streptomyces lavendulae* No. 314, this antibiotic is also a white amorphous powder. It exhibits a similar activity towards gram-positive bacteria, Ehrlich carcinoma and L1210 leukemia as the preceding antibiotic.

Arai *et al.*, *J. Antibiotics* (Japan), **29**, 398 (1976)

CHLOROCARCIN C
$C_{30}H_{34}N_3O_6Cl$

Also present in the mixture of antibiotics obtained by fermentation of *Streptomyces lavendulae* No. 314, this basic antibiotic is an amorphous powder effective against gram-positive bacteria, Ehrlich carcinoma and L1210 leukemia in mice.

Arai *et al.*, *J. Antibiotics* (Japan), **29**, 398 (1976)

7-CHLORO-7-DEOXYLINCOMYCIN
See Clindamycin

CHLORFLAVONIN
$C_{18}H_{15}O_7Cl$
M.p. 212°C

A chlorinated flavone, this antibiotic is produced by certain strains of *Aspergillus candidus*, particularly *A. candidus* ATCC 20022. The spores are incubated in a medium of sucrose, corn steep liquor, corn oil and calcium carbonate with aeration at 26°C for 100 hours. The pH is then adjusted to 4·0, the mycelium separated and extracted with hydrocarbon solvents, concentrated under reduced pressure and the residue crystallized from petroleum ether. The antibiotic yields a dimethyl ether, m.p. 114–115°C and a diacetate which has no definite melting point. Chlorflavonin is highly active against gram-positive and gram-negative bacteria and various species of *Aspergillus* which produce mycotic diseases, including *A. amstelodami*, *A. fumigatus* and *A. ochraceus*, the minimum inhibition concentration against these fungi being 0·08 μg/ml. It is also active against *Aspergillus niger*, *Botrytis cinerea* and *Fusarium oxysporum* but to a much lesser extent.

Richards, Bird, Munden, *J. Antibiotics* (Japan), **22**, 388 (1969)
Richards, Munden, *British Patent*, 1,139,041 (1969)

CHLOROMYCETIN
See Chloramphenicol

CHLOROMYCORRHIZIN A
$C_{14}H_{14}O_4Cl_2$
M.p. 122–123°C

A fungus D37 found on the roots of *Monotropa hypopitys* produces two antibiotics, chloromycorrhizin A and mycorrhizin A (q.v.) when cultivated in a medium containing asparagine, thiamine hydrochloride and inorganic salts at pH 5·8 and 28°C for 11 days. Extraction of the culture filtrate with AcOEt followed by chromatography yields the pure antibiotics. Chloromycorrhizin A forms bright yellow crystals when crystallized from $CHCl_3$-hexane and is laevorotatory with a specific rotation of $[\alpha]_D^{29} - 21·6°$ (c 11·1, EtOH). It gives an ultraviolet and visible spectrum having absorption maxima at 246 and 305 mm. It is stable in acid solution but labile under alkaline conditions. Chloromycorrhizin A is particularly active against the root rot fungus *Fomes annosus*.

Trofast, Wickberg, *Tetrahedron*, **33**, 875 (1977)

CHLORONECTRIN
$C_{23}H_{33}O_6Cl$
M.p. Indefinite

Chloronectrin has been obtained from cultures of *Nectria coccinea*. Even when highly purified it forms a gum that cannot be crystallized. The structure has been established by chemical degradation and spectroscopic investigations. It is active against a number of gram-positive bacteria.

Aldridge *et al.*, *J. Chem. Soc.*, *Perkin I*, 2136 (1972)

6-CHLORO-2-QUINOXALINECARBOXYLIC ACID-1:4-DIOXIDE
$C_9H_5O_4N_2Cl$

A novel antibiotic elaborated by *Streptomyces ambofaciens* NRRL 3455, this antibiotic substance is active against gram-positive bacteria. It yields a number of crystalline salts and derivatives, all of which exhibit a similar antibiotic activity.

Stapley *et al.*, *U.S. Patent*, 3,692,633 (1972)

CHLORORAPHIN

$C_{28}H_{20}O_2N_6$
M.p. 225–230°C (dec.)

This antibiotic has been isolated from cultures of a species of *Chromobacterium* although it had earlier been prepared by synthesis from anthranilic acid and nitrobenzene. The structure is that of a quinhydrone compound of phenazine-*o*-carboxylic acid and its dihydro derivative. The antibiotic forms green crystals and is active *in vitro* at an inhibition concentration greater than 100 µg/ml against *Eberthella typhi*, *Escherichia coli*, *Proteus vulgaris*, *Staphylococcus aureus* and *Streptococcus hemolyticus*.

McIlwain, *Nature*, **148**, 628 (1941)
Synthesis
Richter, *The Chemistry of the Carbon Compounds*, Vol. II, 474 Nordemann, New York (1939)

CHLOROTHRICIN

$C_{50}H_{63}O_{16}Cl$

A complex antibiotic, chlorothricin is elaborated by *Streptomyces antibioticus*. The compound is a carboxylic acid having the structure shown above which is based primarily upon chemical and spectroscopic data. Hydrolysis yields the aglycon chlorothricolide. Chlorothricin is active against a number of gram-positive and gram-negative bacteria and some fungi.

Muntwyler, Keller-Schlierlein, *Helv. Chim. Acta*, **55**, 2071 (1972)
Brufani *et al.*, *ibid.*, **55**, 2094 (1972)

CHLORTETRACYCLINE

See Aureomycin

CHROMIN

An antibiotic produced by an organism related to *Streptomyces antibioticus*, chromin is formed as a yellow-brown precipitate on the addition of Et_2O to a concentrated BuOH extract of the broth. It is readily soluble in $CHCl_3$ and $(CH_3)_2CO$ and is labile in both acidic and alkaline media. The ultraviolet spectrum has absorption maxima at 289, 303 and 317 nm. The antibiotic is active against a large number of yeasts and filamentous fungi but not against bacteria. Although the toxicity is somewhat variable it has shown promise in the treatment of diseases caused by *Candida albicans*.

Wakaki *et al.*, *J. Antibiotics* (Japan), **5**, 677 (1952)

CHROMOCYCLOMYCIN

$C_{48}H_{62}O_{21}$
M.p. Indefinite

This glycosidic antibiotic is related to olivomycin (q.v.) and has been isolated from cultures of *Streptomyces* LA-7017 by cultivating on a common nutrient medium at 27–28°C for 5 days. The structure has been determined from a chemical and spectroscopic study of the hydrolysis and benzoylated products and the result of periodic acid oxidation. The antibiotic is active against a number of tumours but has a somewhat high degree of toxicity.

Berlin, Kolosov, Yartseva, *Khim. Prir. Soedin.*, **9**, 539 (1973)

CHROMOMYCIN A$_2$ (*Aburamycin A*)
$C_{59}H_{86}O_{26}$
M.p. Indefinite

Streptomyces griseus produces a number of cancerostatic antibiotics which consist of chromomycinone linked to a number of sugar moieties. This particular substance is obtained as a yellow powder of the monohydrate which has a specific rotation of $[\alpha]_D^{23} - 61°$ (c 1·0, EtOH) and an ultraviolet spectrum with absorption maxima at 229, 317, 331 and 412 nm. Its identity with aburamycin A has been established by Berlin and his colleagues. It is active in inhibiting the growth of a number of tumours in animals.

Miyamoto et al., *Tetrahedron Lett.*, 545 (1966)
Revised structure
Berlin et al., *Tetrahedron Lett.*, 1643 (1966)
See also
Berlin et al., *Nature*, **218**, 193 (1968)

CHROMOMYCIN A$_3$ (*Aburamycin B, Toyomycin*)
$C_{57}H_{82}O_{26}$
M.p. 187°C (*dec.*)

The major component of the group of cancerostatic antibiotics produced by *Streptomyces griseus*, this compound forms yellow crystals when recrystallized from EtOH. It has a specific rotation of $[\alpha]_D^{20} - 26°$ (c 1·0, EtOH) and on hydrolysis yields chromomycinone, two moles of chromose C and one mole each of chromose A, chromose B and chromose D. It may be characterized as the tri-*p*-toluenesulphonyl derivative, colourless crystals with m.p. 117°C (*dec.*).

Shibata et al., *J. Antibiotics* (Japan), **13B**, 1 (1960)
Mizuni, *ibid.*, **16A**, 22 (1963)
Miyamoto et al., *Tetrahedron Lett.*, 2367 (1964)
Berlin et al., *Nature*, **218**, 193 (1968)
Revised structure
Berlin et al., *Tetrahedron Lett.*, 1643 (1966)

CHROMOMYCIN A$_4$ (*Aburamycin D*)
$C_{48}H_{68}O_{22}$

A third cancerostatic antibiotic from *Streptomyces griseus*, this substance is also produced from chromomycin A$_3$ by partial hydrolysis. It is obtained as an amorphous yellow powder of the monohydrate and has a specific rotation of $[\alpha]_D^{21} - 47°$ (c 1·0, EtOH).

Miyamoto et al., *Tetrahedron Lett.*, 545 (1966)
Berlin et al., *Nature*, **218**, 193 (1968)
Revised structure
Berlin et al., *Tetrahedron Lett.*, 1643 (1966)

CHROTHIOMYCIN
M.p. Indefinite

Streptomyces pluricolorescens yields this antibiotic pigment which forms blackish-purple crystals. It is isolated from the fermentation broth by extraction with organic solvents. Chrothiomycin inhibits the growth of a number of gram-positive bacteria, the following minimum inhibition concentrations (µg/ml) having been determined: *Bacillus anthracis* (100); *Micrococcus flavus* (50); *Sarcina lutea* (25) and strains of *Staphylococcus aureus* (50–100). Even at concentrations of 100 µg/ml, gram-negative bacteria are not inhibited. Chrothiomycin also inhibits the activities of oxygenases which are involved in catechol amine biosynthesis. Chemical evidence indicates that the antibiotic is a quinone containing sulphur.

Ayukawa et al., *J. Antibiotics* (Japan), **22**, 303 (1969)

CHUANGHSINMYCIN
$C_{12}H_{11}NO_2S$

A novel antibiotic isolated from cultures of *Actinoplanes jinanensis*, this compound has been described by Chinese workers. The structure has been established from a study of the infrared, NMR and mass spectra.

Liang et al., *Hua Hsueh Hsueh Pao*, **34**, 129 (1976)

CIBA 36278-Ba
$C_{12}H_{13}O_6N_3S$
M.p. Indefinite

A semi-synthetic cephalosporin derivative, this antibiotic has the structure given above. It is active *in vitro* against gram-positive and gram-negative bacteria, the minimum inhibition concentration for the former being 0·1–0·4 µg/ml and for the latter 3·0–15 µg/ml. It is as active as cephalothin (q.v.) against several strains of *Proteus*, *Staphylococcus aureus* and *Streptococcus fecalis*, but less active against *Escherichia coli*. On proliferating cells of *Escherichia coli* and *Staphylococcus aureus* it exerts a bactericidal action, the former being more readily killed. Ciba 36278-Ba is degraded by cephalosporinases to form a deep red pigment and this may therefore be used as an indicator for the presence of β-lactamase.

Knuesel, Gelzer, Rosselet, *Antimicrobial Agents & Chemotherapy*, 140 (1970)

CICLACILLIN
$C_{15}H_{23}O_4N_3S$
M.p. Indefinite

A semi-synthetic penicillin type antibiotic, this compound is less active than either ampicillin or carbenicillin against 101 strains of *Escherichia coli* and 50 strains each of *Proteus mirabilis* and *Staphylococcus aureus*. It has a toxicity similar to the penicillin antibiotics.

Wewalka et al., *Zentralbl. Bakteriol., Parasitenk., Infektionskr. Hyg., Orog., Reihe A*, **225**, 187 (1973)

CINERUBIN A
$C_{42}H_{52}O_{16}N$
M.p. Indefinite

A glycosidic anthracycline antibiotic elaborated by various *Streptomyces* species, this compound is active against gram-positive bacteria, some fungi and has antitumour properties. Mild hydrolysis furnishes pyrromycin, a basic red pigment. The structure has been determined as that given above.

Keller-Schlierlein, Richle, *Antimicrobial Agents & Chemotherapy*, 68 (1970)

CINNAMYCIN
M.p. Indefinite

A complex basic polypeptide, this antibiotic is produced by *Streptomyces cinnamoneus*. It is soluble in hydrated alcohols and glacial AcOH but insoluble in Et_2O. The ultraviolet spectrum shows an absorption maximum at 230 nm with a shoulder at 250–260 nm. Cinnamycin is stable in solution over the range from pH 2·0 to 9·0. Paper chromatography of the basic and acid hydrolysates indicates the presence of eight aminoacids including lanthionine and the aminoacid $C_7H_{14}O_2N_2S$ obtained from subtilin (q.v.).

Cinnamycin is active against gram-positive rods and mycobacteria at a concentration of 5–55 µg/ml and against *Clostridium botulinum* at a concentration of 0·085 µg/ml. It shows no activity against gram-negative bacteria, gram-positive cocci or yeasts. The toxicity is not yet known and so far it has found no use in medicine.

Benedict *et al.*, *Antibiotics & Chemotherapy*, **2**, 591 (1952)

CIRCULIN
M.p. Indefinite

Derived from *Bacillus circulans*, circulin is a basic polypeptide produced by submerged growth in shaker flasks or deep tanks. A maximum yield of 1260 *Salmonella typhosa* units/ml is obtained when the organism is grown in a 100-gallon tank run at 270 rpm with 0·6 volume air per min/vol medium ratio. The antibiotic is normally isolated by adjusting the pH of the culture filtrate to 6·5 with dilute H_2SO_4, adsorbing on activated carbon, washing the cake with H_2O and then 50 per cent aqueous tertiary butanol, eluting the activity with 25 per cent aqueous tertiary butanol at pH 2·5–4·0, concentrating the eluates *in vacuo*, neutralizing with barium hydroxide, filtering and freeze-drying. Purification is usually done by chromatographing circulin sulphate over activated carbon with 25 per cent aqueous tertiary butanol as the developer. Circulin forms a pale yellow powder which is soluble in H_2O and the lower aliphatic alcohols, insoluble in ether, hydrocarbons and chlorinated hydrocarbons. It readily dialyses through cellophane membranes. On acid hydrolysis it furnishes L-threonine, D-leucine, L-α,γ-diaminobutyric acid and an optically active isomer of pelargonic acid. It gives a positive biuret, formalin and Van Slyke reaction, reacts with 2:4-dinitrofluorobenzene and a negative ninhydrin reaction. In aqueous solution it is unstable above pH 7·0, stable between pH 2·5 to 6·5, thermostable, inactivated by crude trypsin but not by pepsin. It may be characterized as the crystalline hydrochloride, helianthate and reineckate.

Circulin is assayed either by the plate method using filter paper discs with *Escherichia coli* as the test organisms or by serial dilution with *Salmonella typhosa*. Murray and his colleagues have determined the inhibition concentrations (µg/ml) *in vitro* against a number of organisms, e.g. *Aerobacter aerogenes* (3·1); *Bacillus anthracis* (100); *B. subtilis* (>100); *Brucella abortus* (0·3); *Escherichia coli* (0·8); *Klebsiella pneumoniae* (3·1); *Micrococcus pyogenes* var. *aureus* (100); *Mycobacterium avium* (100); *Myco. tuberculosis hominis* (30); *Neisseria catarrhalis* (3·1); *Proteus vulgaris* (67); *Pseudomonas aeruginosa* (3·1); *Salmonella gallinarum* (0·4); *S. paratyphi* (6·2); *S. pullorum* (0·8); *S. schottmuelleri* (6·2); *S. typhimurium* (1·6); *S. typhosa* (3·1); *Serratia marcescens* (30); *Shigella dysenteriae* (>0·4) and *Streptococcus fecalis* (10).

The antibiotic is also active *in vivo* providing complete protection in mice infected with *Salmonella typhosa* at a dosage of 10 mg/kg, against *Klebsiella pneumoniae* at 16 mg/kg and against *Vibrio cholera* with one seventh to one quarter of the LD_{50} dose.

The LD_{50} in mice using a concentration of 2700 µg/ml has been given as 150–180 mg/kg (subcutaneous), 23 mg/kg (intravenous) and 68 mg/kg (intraperitoneal). No evidence has been found of any chronic toxicity in mice or guinea pigs with repeated doses although some skin sloughing is sometimes apparent at the site of the injection. When given to cats and dogs, circulin intravenously lowered the blood pressure but had no effect upon the heart or respiratory rate.

Murray, Tetrault, *Proc. Soc. Amer. Bact.*, **2**, 20 (1948)
Murray *et al.*, *J. Bact.*, **57**, 305 (1949)
Garson *et al.*, *ibid.*, **58**, 115 (1949)
Brook, Richmond, *J. Clin. Invest.*, **28**, 1032 (1949)
Peterson, Reinecke, *ibid.*, **28**, 1053 (1949)
Tetrault *et al.*, *ibid.*, **28**, 1053 (1949)
Peterson, Reinecke, *J. Biol. Chem.*, **181**, 95 (1949)

CITRININ
$C_{13}H_{14}O_5$
M.p. 178–179°C (*dec.*)

This antibiotic was first obtained in a pure form from *Penicillium citrinum* in 1931 by Raistrick and his colleagues. It has also been isolated from *Aspergillus terreus*, *Aspergillus* species of the *Candidus* group, *Penicillium chrzaszszi*, *P. expansum*, *P. citreo-sulphutatum*, *P. implicatum*, *P. lividum* and *P. phoeo-janthinellum*. The antibiotic also occurs in the leaves of *Crotolaria crispata*, a flowering shrub of Northern Australia. It forms colourless crystals when recrystallized from CH_3OH and has a specific rotation of $[\alpha]_{5461} - 42·8°$. Citrinin may be characterized as the methyl ester which gives colourless prisms from either $(CH_3)_2CO$ or C_6H_6, m.p. 138°C (*dec.*); $[\alpha]_D^{20} + 96·9°$ ($CHCl_3$) and the phenylhydrazide, m.p. 207°C (*dec.*).

Raistrick *et al.*, *Trans. Roy. Soc.*, **220B**, 269, 297 (1931)
Hirschy, Ruoff, *J. Amer. Chem. Soc.*, **64**, 1490 (1942)
Oxford, *Ann. Rev. Biochem.*, **14**, 757 (1945)
Gore *et al.*, *Nature*, **157**, 333 (1946)
Sprenger, Ruoff, *J. Org. Chem.*, **11**, 189 (1946)
Wyllie, *Chem. Abstr.*, **40**, 2190 (1946)
Gore *et al.*, *J. Amer. Chem. Soc.*, **70**, 2287 (1948)
Robertson *et al.*, *J. Chem. Soc.*, 859, 867, 1563 (1949)
Fry, Wallis, Dougherty, *J. Org. Chem.*, **14**, 397 (1949)
Cartwright, Robertson, Whalley, *Nature*, **163**, 94 (1949)
Cartwright, Robertson, Whalley, *J. Chem. Soc.*, 1563 (1949)
Warren, Dougherty, Wallis, *J. Amer. Chem. Soc.*, **71**, 3422 (1949)
Robertson *et al.*, *J. Chem. Soc.*, 2971 (1950)
Mehta, Whalley, *ibid.*, 3777 (1963)

CLADOSPORIN
$C_{16}H_{20}O_5$

This antibiotic has been isolated from the mycelium of *Cladosporium cladosporoides* and shown to have the structure given above. It yields a monoacetate which, like the parent antibiotic, completely inhibits the growth of a number of dermatophytes on agar medium at a concentration of 75 µg/ml. The antibiotic also inhibits the germination of the spores of a range of *Aspergillus* and *Penicillium* species at concentrations less than 40 µg/ml in liquid media.

Van Walbeek, *J. Antibiotics* (Japan), **24**, 747 (1971)

CLAVULANIC ACID
$C_8H_9NO_5$

A simple antibiotic isolated from cultures of *Streptomyces clavuligerus*, this compound has the structure shown above based upon chemical and spectroscopic examination. Clavulanic acid is a powerful irreversible β-lactamase inhibitor and is highly active against a number of ampicillin-resistant strains of *Escherichia coli*, *Klebsiella aerogenes*, *Serratia marcescens* and *Staphylococcus aureus* when used in combination with ampicillin.

Brown *et al.*, *Spec. Publ. Chem. Soc.*, **28**, 295 (1977)

CLINDAMYCIN (*7-chloro-7-deoxylincomycin*)
$C_{18}H_{33}O_5N_2SCl$

The structure of this antibiotic has been shown to be 7-chloro-7-deoxylincomycin. It is used in medicine either as the base compound or the 2-palmitate or 2-phosphate. All of these compounds are active against a range of gram-positive and gram-negative bacteria but not against gram-negative rods. They are effective *in vivo* against *Bacteriodes, Clostridium, Hemophilus influenzae, Peptococcus, Peptostreptococcus, Sphaerophorus, Veillonella* and *Toxoplasma*. They also protect mice from infection with *Diplococcus pneumoniae, Staphylococcus aureus* and *Streptococcus pyogenes*. The antibiotic is relatively non-toxic, the LD_{50} being 179 mg/kg given subcutaneously to the neonatal rat and greater than 2000 mg/kg given to the adult rat.

Nakatsuka *et al.*, *Nippon Kagaku Ryohogakukai Zasshi*, **17**, 747 (1969)
Kitamoto, Fukaya, Tomori, *ibid.*, **17**, 822 (1969)
Matsen, *J. Lab. Clin. Med.*, **77**, 378 (1971)
Ito *et al.*, *Toho Igakkai Zasshi.*, **20**, 360 (1973)
Ninomiya *et al.*, *J. Antibiotics* (Japan), **26**, 157 (1973)
Ono *et al.*, *ibid.*, **26**, 321 (1973)
Kono *et al.*, *ibid.*, **26**, 325 (1973)
Liberman, FitzGerald, Robertson, *Antimicrobial Agents & Chemotherapy*, **5**, 458 (1974)
Araujo, Remington, *ibid.*, **5**, 647 (1974)
Barker, *Med. Lab. Technol.*, **31**, 171 (1974)
Gray *et al.*, *Toxicol. Appl. Pharmacol.*, **27**, 308 (1974)
Bollert *et al.*, *ibid.*, **27**, 322 (1974)

CLITOCYBIN
M.p. 77°C

An antibiotic obtained from *Clitocybe gigantea* var. *candida*, clitocybin consists of two components, clitocybins A and B. It is normally produced by fermentation on a yeast extract medium and isolated by extracting the mycelium with organic solvents and H_2O. The Et_2O-soluble portion is then chromatographed on an alumina column and the H_2O-soluble fraction precipitated with ammonium sulphate. When purified by recrystallization from EtOH, clitocybin forms colourless rhombic crystals. It is freely soluble in H_2O, Et_2O, $(CH_3)_2CO$, $CHCl_3$, EtOH and amyl acetate. It diffuses readily and is unstable at temperatures of 70–80°C.

Clitocybin is generally assayed by the cylinder plate method with *Staphylococcus aureus* and typical inhibition dilutions, determined by several workers are: *Bacillus anthracis* (3,000,000); *Brucella abortus* (4,000,000); *Escherichia coli* (3,000,000); *Mycobacterium tuberculosis* (8,000,000); *Salmonella paratyphi* (3,000,000); *Streptococcus lactis* (6,000,000) and *Strep. pyogenes* (6,000,000). At dilutions between 400,000 and 800,000 it is active against a variety of organisms including *Bacillus anthracis, Clostridium perfringens, Erysipelothrix rhusiopathiae, Malleomyces mallei, Mycobacterium tuberculosis bovis, Pasteurella avicida, Pseudomonas aeruginosa, Salmonella schottmuelleri* and *Staphylococcus aureus*.

In vivo, it is of use in the treatment of *Pasteurella*, staphylococcus, streptococcus, tuberculosis and the virus of foot-and-mouth disease.

The toxicity depends upon the activity of the antibiotic preparation. In the guinea pig, 20 mg is tolerated but the use of impure preparations results in haemorrhage, edema and ulceration when administered subcutaneously.

Hollande, *Compt. rend. acad. sci.*, **221**, 361 (1945)
Hollande, *ibid.*, **224**, 1534 (1947)
Riviere, Thely, Gautron, *ibid.*, **225**, 1386 (1947)
Riviere, Thely, Cautron, *Bull. soc. chim. biol.*, **29**, 857 (1947)
Riviere *et al.*, *Ann. Inst. Pasteur*, **74**, 118 (1948)
Hollande, *Compt. rend. acad. sci.*, **228**, 1758 (1949)

CLOMOCYCLINE
$C_{23}H_{25}O_9N_2Cl$
M.p. 145–170°C (*dec.*)

A minor antibiotic isolated from cultures of *Streptomyces aureofaciens* Duggar, clomocycline forms an amorphous yellow solid which melts, with decomposition, over a wide range of temperature. It is active against gram-positive and gram-negative bacteria.

Leo Industrie Chimiche Farmaceutiche, *Belgian Patent*, 628,142 (1964)
Chinoin Gyogysze Vegyeszeti Termekek Gyara, *Hungarian Patent*, 151,295 (1964)

CLOTRIMAZOLE
$C_{22}H_{17}N_2Cl$

A synthetic antibiotic substance, clotrimazole is only weakly active against bacteria but possesses a marked antifungal activity. It is inhibitory against most fungal pathogens, inhibiting *Blastomyces dermatitidis*, *Coccidioides immitis*, *Cryptococcus neoformans*, *Histoplasma capsulatum* and *Sporothrix schenkii* at a concentration of 0 20–3 13 μg/ml. It is less active against *Aspergillus fumigatus* and *Candida albicans* than amphotericin B (q.v.) but inhibited an isolate of *Allescheria boydii* which was resistant to the latter antibiotic.

Shadomy, *Infec. Immunity*, **4**, 143 (1971)

CLOXACILLIN
$C_{19}H_{18}O_5N_3SCl$

A semi-synthetic antibiotic, this compound is effective in the treatment of subclinical mastitis in cattle, decreasing the incidence of the disease by 73·3 per cent. It is also effective against staphylococcal mastitis and is widely used in human medicine against staphylococcal infection, being stable towards staphylococcal β-lactamase.

Walser, Frieding, Scgmid, *Berlin, Muenchen. Tieraerztl. Wochenschr.*, **86**, 101 (1973)

CNICIN
$C_{19}H_{26}O_7$

An antibiotic substance of plant origin, this compound has been isolated from *Cnicus benedictus*. The terpene structure has been established from chemical and spectroscopic data. Cnicin is active against a number of organisms, the minimum bactericidal concentrations which have been determined being: *Bordetella bronchiseptica* (75 μg/ml); *Brucella abortus* (125); *Pseudomonas aeruginosa* (100) and *Staphylococcus aureus* (175). The LD_{50} against KB cell cultures is 3·4 μg/ml.

Vanhaelen-Fastre, *J. Pharm. Belg.*, **27**, 683 (1972)

COCHLIODINOL
$C_{32}H_{32}N_2O_4$

A fungistatic and fungicidal antibiotic, cochliodinol has been isolated from cultures of *Chaetomium cochliodes* and *C. globosum*. The organism is typically cultured on a common nutrient medium at 25°C for 2–8 days and the antibiotic extracted from the culture medium and purified by chromatography.

Brewer, Taylor, Jerram, *Canadian Patent*, 941,323 (1974)

COELICOLORIN
M.p. 142–146°C

Produced by *Streptomyces coelicolor*, this antibiotic is extracted from the solid culture with $(CH_3)_2CO$ in dilute acid followed by precipitation with H_2O and extraction with C_6H_6. The substance may then be further purified by chromatography on an alumina column. It is very soluble in $CHCl_3$, $(CH_3)_2CO$, and AcOEt, less soluble in CH_3OH, EtOH, Et_2O and C_6H_6 and insoluble in petroleum ether. It is primarily active against gram-positive bacteria and has LD_{50} in mice of about 500 mg/kg on intra-peritoneal administration. So far, it has found no use in medicine.

Hatsuta, *J. Antibiotics* (Japan), **2**, 276 (1949)

COFORMYCIN
$C_{11}H_{16}O_5N_4$
M.p. 182–184°C
This antibiotic has been obtained from *Nocardia interforma* ATCC 21072 and is also isolated from *Streptomyces kaniharaensis* and *S. lavendulae*. It is dextrorotatory with a specific rotation of $[\alpha]_D^{24} + 34°$ (c 1·0, H_2O). Coformycin is active against a range of bacteria.

Umezawa et al., *Japanese Patent*, 7,012,278 (1970)

COGOMYCIN
$C_{35}H_{58}O_{12}$
M.p. 190–210°C (*dec.*)

A macrocyclic antibiotic obtained from cultures of *Streptomyces fradiae*, this substance forms colourless crystals and is laevorotatory having a specific rotation of $[\alpha]_D^{25} - 157°$ (c 0·25, MeOH). It gives an ultraviolet spectrum in EtOH with absorption maxima at 295, 309, 322, 329 and 357 nm. The structure has been established from chemical analysis and spectroscopic evidence.

Pozsgay, Tamas, Czira, *Acta Chem. Acad. Sci. Hung.*, **85**, 215 (1975)
Pozsgay et al., *J. Antibiotics* (Japan), **29**, 472 (1976)

COLICINS
Various strains of *Escherichia coli* yield an antibiotic complex, colicin, which has been separated into a number of individual antibiotics. All appear to possess a polypeptide structure and among those that have been isolated and examined are colicins A, B, C, D, E_1, E_2, E_3, F_1, F_2, F_3, F_4, F_5, I, Ia, Ib, K, N, P, Q and CA42-E_2. A colicin V has also been described. The antibiotics are soluble in H_2O and AcOH, sparingly so in pyridine and aqueous phenol, and generally dialyse through a cellophane membrane. They are fairly stable to heat in neutral or acid solution but less stable in alkali and are usually completely destroyed by pepsin, trypsin and streptococcal pus. They may be assayed by the cylinder plate method using a sensitive strain of *Escherichia coli* as the test organism. Most are bactericidal *in vitro* against *Corynebacterium xerosis*, *Mycobacterium phlei*, *Pseudomonas aeruginosa*, *Salmonella newport*, *S. typhimurium*, *S. typhi*, *S. paratyphi*, *Shigella shigae*, *Sh. sonnei* and *Vibrio comma*. In tests with *Escherichia coli*, it has been shown that the action of these antibiotics occurs in two stages, the first being reversible and not leading to the death of the bacterial cell, the second being irreversible and bactericidal. There is evidence that these antibiotics produce lysis of the cell. The toxicity of the antibiotics is variable in mice, 18 mg being tolerated in one experiment while 5 mg proved lethal with a different batch of culture liquor. With most of these compounds there is no hemolysis of human red blood cells, nor are human leucocytes affected at a dilution of 1:1000.

Heatley, Florey, *Brit. J. Exptl. Path.*, **27**, 378 (1946)
Gratia, Fredericq, *Congress. Chin. Biol. Liege, Resumes des Commun.*, **IV**, 2 (1946)
Gratia, Joiris, Weerts, *Rept. Proc. 4th Intern. Congr. Microbiol.*, 141 (1947)
Faguet, *C.R. Acad. Sci.*, **265D**, 822 (1967)
Cavard et al., *ibid.*, **265D**, 1255 (1967)
Faguet, Hamon, *ibid.*, **267D**, 1176 (1968)
Levisohn, Konisky, Nomura, *J. Bact.*, **96**, 811 (1968)
Reynolds, Reeves, *ibid.*, **100**, 301 (1969)

COLIMYCIN M
M.p. Indefinite
A broad-spectrum antibiotic, this substance is highly effective against strains of *Enterobacter* and *Pseudomonas aeruginosa*. When administered to dogs it potentiates the neuromuscular blockade induced by pancuronium bromide.

Lus et al., *Medicamenta*, 61 (509), **197** (1973)
Chinyanga, Stoyka, *Can. Anaesth. Soc. J.*, **21**, 569 (1974)

COLISTATIN

An antibiotic substance obtained by Gause from an unclassified aerobic sporulating bacillus found in a soil sample, colistatin is produced by surface culture. It is isolated by adjusting the pH of the culture filtrate to 3·5, treating with activated carbon, neutralizing, adsorbing the active fraction on activated carbon, eluting with 80 per cent aqueous EtOH, neutralizing, removing the organic solvent *in vacuo* at 50°C and precipitating the crude material from the aqueous fraction with $(CH_3)_2CO$. Colistatin is stable at 100°C for 5 minutes in the culture liquor, is soluble in acidified CH_3OH, less soluble in acid EtOH and insoluble in BuOH. It may be precipitated from the acid CH_3OH solution with Et_2O but here there is partial deactivation.

Colistatin is assayed by serial dilution with *Staphylococcus aureus* and, *in vitro*, inhibits *Bacillus dysenteriae* Shiga, *B. paratyphosus*, *B. proteus*, *B. typhi abdominalis*, various pneumococci and *Staphylococcus aureus*.

In vivo it possesses a chemotherapeutic activity against *Borrellia sogdianum*. When administered to mice infected with this disease, a total dose of 90,000 units/kg resulted in the total absence of spirochetes in the blood on the day following administration. It is not toxic for mice in a concentrated aqueous solution at 100,000 units/kg when given intramuscularly, intravenously or subcutaneously.

Gause, *Science*, **104**, 289 (1946)
Gause, *Byull. eksper. biol. i. med.*, **22**, No. 3, 17 (1946)

COLISTIN
$C_{45}H_{85}O_{10}N_{13}$
M.p. Indefinite

A macrocyclic polypeptide antibiotic, colistin has been reported by Japanese workers. It forms an amorphous powder with no definite melting point. The structure has been established from chemical investigations, particularly from the nature of the hydrolysis products. Colistin is normally employed as the sulphate or the sulphomethate sodium derivative. The antibiotic is active against a wide range of gram-negative bacilli except *Proteus* species, resembling polymyxin B in its antimicrobial activity. It is particularly active against *Escherichia coli* and *Enterobacter* but gives less satisfactory results against *Shigella* and *Salmonella*.

The sulphate is poorly absorbed from the gastro-intestinal tract and as a result toxic effects rarely follow oral administration. It is given orally for the treatment of gastroenteritis due to susceptible organisms. The sulphomethate sodium derivative is the form used for parenteral administration and this salt has also been employed for topical application or as an aerosol for respiratory infections. Nephrotoxicity has been observed in many cases where this derivative has been used.

Kayama et al., *J. Antibiotics* (Japan), **3**, 457 (1950)
Ito et al., *ibid.*, **3**, 147 (1950)
Kayama, *Japanese Patent*, 1546 (1952)
Oda et al., *J. Pharm. Soc., Japan*, **74**, 1234, 1246 (1954)

COLISTIN A (*Polymyxin E₁*)
$C_{53}H_{100}O_{13}N_{16}$

```
    C2H5
    |
    CHCH3                              L-Dbu—D-Leu—L-Leu
    |                                  |
(CH2)4CO—L-Dbu—L-Thr—L-Dbu—L-Dbu
                                       |
                                  L-Thr—L-Dbu—L-Dbu
```

Colistin (q.v.) has recently been separated into three components by countercurrent distribution techniques. The structure of this antibiotic has been elucidated by means of chemical and spectroscopic determinations, particularly from the nature of the hydrolysis products.

Suzuki et al., *J. Biochem.*, **54**, 25 (1963)
Suzuki et al., *ibid.*, **54**, 173 (1963)
Suzuki et al., *ibid.*, **54**, 412 (1963)
Wilkinson, Lowe, *Nature*, **200**, 1008 (1963)
Wilkinson, Lowe, *J. Chem. Soc.*, 4107 (1964)
Wilkinson, Lowe, *Nature*, **204**, 993 (1964)

COLISTIN B
$C_{52}H_{98}O_{13}N_{16}$

```
        CH3
        |
        CHCH3                              L-Dbu—D-Leu—L-Leu
        |                                  |
(CH2)4CO—L-Dbu—L-Thr—L-Dbu—L-Dbu
                                  |
                        L-Thr—L-Dbu—L-Dbu
```

The structure of this polypeptide component of colistin has also been established by investigation of the hydrolysis products. It closely resembles that of colistin A.

Suzuki, Fukjikawa, *J. Biochem.*, **56**, 182 (1964)

COLISTIN C
This antibiotic is a minor component of colistin and is separated by counter-current distribution. So far, little is known concerning its structure.

Wilkinson, Lowe, *Nature*, **204**, 993 (1964)
Suzuki *et al.*, *J. Biochem.*, **56**, 182 (1964)

COLLINOMYCIN
$C_{25}H_{20}O_{11}$?
M.p. 280–282°C

Isolated from cultures of *Streptomyces collinus*, this substance crystallizes from $CHCl_3$—CH_3OH as orange prisms. The acetate forms light yellow needles, m.p. 228–230°C and the benzoate, lemon-yellow needles, m.p. 226°C. With sodium carbonate the antibiotic gives a violet precipitate of the sodium salt. It is active against a number of gram-positive bacteria.

Brockmann, Renneberg, *Naturwiss.*, **40**, 166 (1953)

COMPOUND 593A
See 3,6-Bis-(5-chloro-2-piperidyl)-2,5-piperazinedione

CONOCANDIN
$C_{18}H_{30}O_3$
B.p. Indefinite

Hormococcus conorium elaborates this antibiotic which is a viscous oil and possesses the epoxy structure given above based upon chemical and spectroscopic evidence. Conocandin is highly specific *in vitro* against fungi and has been isolated and purified by counter-current and silica gel chromatography.

Mueller *et al.*, *Helv. Chim. Acta*, **59**, 2506 (1976)

COPIAMYCIN
Dec. 144°C

Streptomyces hygroscopicus var. *chrystallogenes*, or a mutant strain, yields this antibiotic when aerobically cultured in a medium containing soybean flour, starch, yeast and inorganic salts at pH 7·2 and 25°C for 90 hours. The compound is obtained by extraction of the moist mycelium with CH_3OH, concentrating *in vacuo*, dissolving the residue in $CHCl_3$—CH_3OH and chromatographing on a silica gel column. Copiamycin forms colourless small plates, soluble in AcOH, pyridine and dimethylformamide. It has a specific rotation of $[\alpha]_D^{25·5} + 14·4°$ (c 4·15, CH_3OH) and although having no activity against bacteria, is fungicidal to a number of fungi and also yeasts at a concentration of 10 µg/ml. It is relatively non-toxic, mice tolerating a dose of 1 g/kg given intraperitoneally for 14 days.

Arai, *French Patent*, 1,483,731 (1967)

CORALINOMYCIN
M.p. Indefinite

An amorphous antibiotic, coralinomycin is produced by *Streptomyces coralineus*. It forms a number of salts, e.g. the hydrochloride and sulphate, all of which are amorphous. Coralinomycin is a broad-spectrum antibiotic, active against both gram-positive and gram-negative bacteria.

Fernandes de Albuquerque *et al.*, *Rev. Inst. Antibiot., Univ. Fed. Pernambuco, Recife*, **12**, 41 (1972)

CORIOLIN
$C_{14}H_{20}O_5$

A tricyclic antibiotic, coriolin is produced, together with similar antibiotics by the cultivation of *Coriolus consors* under submerged conditions in a common nutrient medium at 25–27°C for 5 days. The structure of the antibiotic has been determined primarily from spectroscopic studies. Coriolin is active in inhibiting the growth of gram-positive bacteria, *Trichomonas* and Yoshida sarcoma cells.

Umezawa, Takeuchi, *Japanese Patent*, 7,316,630 (1973)
Umezawa et al, *Japanese Patent*, 7,401,795 (1974)

CORIOLIN B
$C_{22}H_{34}O_6$

A further antibiotic elaborated by *Coriolus consors*, this substance has structure given above. Oxidation with CrO_3 yields the diketo derivative which is, like the parent antibiotic, active against gram-positive bacteria, leukaemia L1210 and Ehrlich ascites sarcoma.

Umezawa et al., *German Patent*, 2,106,696 (1971)
Umezawa et al., *Japanese Patent*, 7, 410, 795 (1974)

CORIOLIN C
$C_{22}H_{32}O_6$

Also produced by fermentation of a nutrient medium by *Coriolus consors*, this antibiotic shows a similar activity against Ehrlich ascites sarcoma, leukaemia L1210 cells and gram-positive bacteria as the preceding antibiotics.

Umezawa et al., *Japanese Patent*, 7,401,795 (1974)

CORTICIN
An antibiotic substance of this name has been described by Robbins and his coworkers. It is obtained from an unclassified species of *Basidiomycetes*.

Robbins, Kavanagh, Hervey, *J. N.Y. Bot. Gardens*, **46**, 130 (1945)

CORYLOPHILIN
See Penatin

CORYNECINS
An antibiotic complex consisting of three kinds of antibiotic, tentatively named corynecins, is produced by cultivation of *Corynebacterium* KY 4339 on a medium containing C_{12-14} paraffins as the sole carbon source. The compounds are isolated from the culture broth by extraction with AcOEt followed by chromatography on a silica gel column. The antibacterial activities of these substances are very similar to that of chloramphenicol but not so marked.

Suzuki, Honda, Katsumata, *Agr. Biol. Chem.*, **36**, 2223 (1972)

COUMERMYCIN A_1
$C_{55}H_{57}O_{20}N_5$

A complex antibiotic, this compound is formed, together with the following substance by *Streptomyces rishiriensis*, *S. spinichromogenes* and *S. spinicoumarensis*. The organisms are typically fermented aerobically on a common nutrient medium for 6 days at 27–28°C and the antibiotic extracted from the culture broth. The antibiotic decomposes at 240–245°C. It is active *in vitro* against several strains of *Mycobacterium tuberculosis* at inhibition concentrations of 0·3–2·5 µg/ml. It is also highly effective against *Neisseria meningitidis* when given subcutaneously and orally but active against meningopneumonitis agent only when administered subcutaneously. Numerous semi-synthetic coumermycins have been prepared, some of which are active against *Diplococcus pneumoniae*, *Klebsiella pneumoniae*, *Pseudomonas aeruginosa*, *Staphylococcus aureus* and *Streptococcus pyogenes*.

Grunberg, Cleeland, Titsworth, *Antimicrobial Agents & Chemotherapy*, 397 (1966)
Schmitz et al., *J. Antibiotics* (Japan), **21**, 603 (1968)
Keil, Hooper, *U.S. Patent*, 3,454,548 (1969)
Duma, Warner, *Appl. Microbiol.*, **18**, 404 (1969)
Keil et al., *Antimicrobial Agents & Chemotherapy*, 200 (1969)
Michaeli et al., *ibid.*, 95 (1970)
Umezawa et al., *Japanese Patent*, 7,115,675 (1971)
Batcho et al., *U.S. Patent*, 3,706,729 (1972)

COUMERMYCIN A$_2$
$C_{53}H_{53}O_{20}N_5$

A further antibiotic isolated from cultures of *Streptomyces rishiriensis*, *S. spinichromogenes* and *S. spinicoumarensis*, this compound is the dimethyl derivative of the preceding antibiotic. It possesses an antibacterial activity almost identical with that of coumermycin A$_1$.

Keil, Hooper, *U.S. Patent*, 3,454,548 (1969)

CREMEOMYCIN
M.p. Indefinite

Actinomyces cremeus NRRL 3241 elaborates this antibiotic when grown on a medium containing black strap molasses, cottonseed flour, lard oil and calcium carbonate in tap water at pH 8·0 and 25°C for 110 hours. The antibiotic is obtained by adjusting the pH of the broth to 4·0, filtering, washing the cake with H$_2$O, combining the filtrates, adjusting to pH 4·0 and extracting with Skellysolve B, discarding the extracts. The filtrate is then extracted with CHCl$_3$, the extract concentrated *in vacuo* below 30°C. Purification is carried out by silica gel chromatography and concentration *in vacuo*, followed by crystallization from cyclohexane. Cremeomycin is active against a number of gram-positive bacteria and some gram-negative organisms, particularly *Proteus vulgaris* which is used as the test organism in the assay of the antibiotic.

Bergy, Pyke, *U.S. Patent*, 3,350,269 (1967)

CREPIN
$C_{15}H_{18}O_4$
Dec. 300°C

A plant antibiotic, crepin is found in the buds, flowers, roots and inflorescence stems of *Crepis taraxacifolia* and *C. virens*. In the plant it is present as an antibiotically inactive precursor. The active form is obtained by incubating an aqueous extract with a concomitant enzyme which is found in the yellow petals and, to a lesser extent, in the root. Crepin is isolated by macerating the dried flowers and buds, extracting with H$_2$O, acidifying to pH 2·5–3·0 with HCl and stirring the precipitated material with 0·01 N-HCl and centrifuging. The activity is found in the supernatant liquid and is adsorbed on activated carbon and eluted with 80 per cent aqueous (CH$_3$)$_2$CO. After concentrating *in vacuo*, it is extracted with Et$_2$O, the ethereal extract passed through an alumina column and chilled when crepin is precipitated. When purified by re-crystallization from absolute EtOH it forms colourless monoclinic or orthorhombic crystals which darken, without melting, at 300°C. The antibiotic is soluble in EtOH, Et$_2$O, pyridine and glycerol, slightly soluble in H$_2$O. It is stable under acid conditions, unstable in alkaline solution and gives no typical ultraviolet spectrum. The unsaturated nature is shown by decolourizing bromine water, potassium permanganate and its ease of hydrogenation.

It is active against a number of bacteria *in vitro*, typical inhibition dilutions obtained by Heatley, being: *Bacillus subtilis* (16,000); *Pseudomonas pyocyanea* (>4000); *Salmonella typhi* (4000); *Staphylococcus aureus* (32,000) and *Streptococcus pyogenes* (8000).

Crepin is fairly toxic. At a dilution of 1:4500 it is rapidly lethal while it inhibits human leucocytes at 1:4,500,000.

Osborn, *Brit. J. Exptl. Path.*, **24**, 227 (1943)
Heatley, *ibid.*, **25**, 208 (1944)
Rogers, *ibid.*, **25**, 212 (1944)

CROTOCIN (*Antibiotic-T*)

$C_{19}H_{24}O_5$
M.p. 126°C

This antifungal antibiotic has been isolated from cultures of *Cephalosporium crotocinigenum*. It forms colourless prisms from CH_3OH and has a specific rotation of $[\alpha]_D^{20} + 13.5°$ (c 1.0, $CHCl_3$). When hydrolysed with dilute acids it yields crotocol and *iso*crotonic acid. It is active against gram-positive bacteria.

Glaz et al., *Nature*, **184**, 908 (1959)
Glaz et al., *ibid.*, **212**, 1665 (1967)
Structure
Gyimesi, Melera, *Tetrahedron Lett.*, 1665 (1967)

2-CROTONYLOXYMETHYL-(4R,5R,6R)-4,-5,6-TRIHYDROXYCYCLOHEX-2-ENONE

$C_{11}H_{14}O_6$

Streptomyces griseosporeus strain MD287-CF-49 elaborates this simple antibiotic which has been shown to possess anticancer activity. The LD_{50} in mice is 90 mg/kg when administered intravenously.

Matsuda et al., *Japanese Patent*, 77 113,946 (1977)

CRYOMYCIN

M.p. 214–217°C (*dec.*)
This antibiotic is produced by *Streptomyces griseus* subsp. *psychrophilus*, type strain AKU 2881. The antibiotic is formed by cultivation on a medium, preferably containing hexamethylenediamine dihydrochloride at 28°C for 4 days followed by 7 days at 12°C. Cryomycin is a polypeptide antibiotic and contains a large proportion of glycine. It is highly effective against gram-positive bacteria *in vitro*. The LD_{50} in mice is 150 mg/kg when given intravenously.

Yoshida et al., *J. Antibiotics* (Japan), **25**, 546, 653 (1972)
Yoshida, Ogata, *ibid.*, **27**, 138 (1974)

CRYPTOMYCIN

M.p. Indefinite
A heptaene antibiotic, this compound is elaborated by *Actinomyces bulgaricus* LIA-0179 grown under submerged conditions in a medium containing glucose, soybean flour and inorganic salts at 27°C for 4 days. The mycelium is filtered, extracted with BuOH, concentrated, and the crystalline compound washed with $(CH_3)_2CO$. Cryptomycin contains 6 or 7 heptaene units and on hydrolysis yields mycosamine, *p*-aminoacetophenone and N-methyl-*p*-aminoacetophenone. It has little activity against bacteria but is highly effective in inhibiting both fungi and yeasts.

Tsyganov et al., *Antibiotiki*, **17**, 1067 (1972)

CRYPTOSPORIOPSIN

$C_{10}H_{10}O_4Cl_2$
M.p. 133–137°C

A species of *Cryptosporiopsis* isolated from the yellow birch yields this simple antibiotic which is extracted from the mycelium with $CHCl_3$, the extract being evaporated to dryness and purified by column chromatography on alumina. Cryptosporiopsin forms a dihydro derivative, m.p. 75–91°C and has a specific rotation of $[\alpha]_D^{25} + 129°$ (c 1.35, $CHCl_3$). The ultraviolet spectrum consists of a single absorption maximum at 292 nm. It inhibits a large variety of organisms *in vitro* including Ascomycetes, Basidiomycetes, imperfect fungi, Phycomycetes and bacteria, particularly *Phytophthora infestans* and *Staphylococcus aureus*.

Stilwell, *Can. J. Bot.*, **44**, 259 (1966)
Stilwell, Wood, Strunz, *Can. J. Microbiol.*, **15**, 501 (1969)

CYATHIN A_3
$C_{20}H_{30}O_3$
M.p. 148–150°C

Cyathus helenae Brodie yields a number of related terpenoid antibiotics when grown at room temperature for 25 days on a chemically defined medium in static culture. The complex and individual antibiotics are active against gram-positive and gram-negative bacteria, actinomycetes and some fungi including dermatophytes. This compound forms colourless crystals from CH_3OH and is laevorotatory with a specific rotation of $[\alpha]_D - 160°$ (CH_3OH).

Allbutt *et al.*, *J. Microbiol.*, (Canada), **17**, 1401 (1971)
Ayer, Taube, *Tetrahedron Lett.*, 1917 (1972)
Ayer, Taube, *Can. J. Chem.*, **51**, 3842 (1973)

allo-CYATHIN A_4
$C_{20}H_{30}O_4$

Also present in the cyathin complex produced by *Caythus helenae*, this antibiotic has also been described. It has a similar antibiotic activity as the other antibiotics of this group.

Allbutt *et al.*, *Can. J. Microbiol.*, **17**, 1401 (1971)

CYATHIN A_4
$C_{20}H_{30}O_4$

A further antibiotic obtained from the complex elaborated by *Cyathus helenae*, this compound is very similar to the preceding antibiotic.

Allbutt *et al.*, *Can. J. Microbiol.*, **17**, 1401 (1971)

CYATHIN B_3
$C_{20}H_{28}O_3$
M.p. 131–133°C

Also produced by *Cyathus helenae*, this antibiotic forms a mixture with cyathin C_3 having the above melting point. So far, it has proved extremely difficult to separate these two compounds.

·Allbutt *et al.*, *Can. J. Microbiol.*, **17**, 1401 (1971)
Ayer, Carstens, *Can J. Chem.*, **51**, 3157 (1973)

CYATHIN B_4
$C_{20}H_{28}O_4$

A further terpenoid antibiotic isolated from the cyathin complex formed by *Cyathus helenae*, this substance has an antibiotic activity similar to those of the accompanying antibiotics.

Allbutt *et al.*, *Can. J. Microbiol.*, **17**, 1401 (1971)

CYATHIN C_3
$C_{20}H_{26}O_8$
M.p. 131–133°C

This substance occurs as an intimate mixture with cyathin B_3 from which it is virtually impossible to separate it.

Allbutt *et al.*, *Can. J. Microbiol.*, **17**, 1401 (1971)
Ayer, Carstens, *Can. J. Chem.*, **51**, 3157 (1973)

CYATHIN C_5
$C_{20}H_{26}O_5$

Also present in the antibiotic complex elaborated by *Cyathus helenae*, this compound almost certainly possesses a terpenoid structure similar to that of the associated compounds of this group.

Allbutt *et al.*, *Can. J. Microbiol.*, **17**, 1401 (1971)

CYCLAMIDOMYCIN
See Pyracrimycin A

CYCLOHEPTAMYCIN
$C_{48}H_{68}O_{12}N_8$
M.p. 256–258°C

A polypeptide antibiotic produced by an unclassified *Streptomyces* species, this substance crystallizes from EtOH and has a specific rotation of

$[\alpha]_D^{20} + 37°$ (c 1·0, CHCl$_3$). The ultraviolet spectrum in EtOH has absorption maxima at 276·5, 282, 296·5 and 308 nm. Cycloheptamycin is active against some gram-positive bacteria.

Godtfredson, Vangedal, Thomas, *Tetrahedron*, **26**, 4931 (1970)

CYCLOHEXIMIDE
See Actidione

CYCLOSERINE
See Oxamycin

CYLINDROCHLORIN
C$_{23}$H$_{27}$O$_4$Cl
M.p. 150–150·5°C

An unclassified species of *Cylindrocladium* elaborates this chlorine-containing antibiotic which forms yellow crystals from EtOH. It gives an ultraviolet spectrum exhibiting absorption maxima at 240, 290 and 346 nm. The full structure is not yet known.

Kato *et al.*, *J. Antibiotics* (Japan), **23**, 168 (1970)

CYLINDROCLADIN A
C$_{22}$H$_{28}$O$_6$
M.p. 173–175°C
One of three closely related antibiotics produced by *Cylindrocladium ilicicola*. This substance forms colourless crystals from EtOH and has a specific rotation of $[\alpha]_D^{20} - 52·3°$ (dioxan). The ultraviolet spectrum in EtOH consists of two absorption maxima at 236 and 353 nm.

Matsushima *et al.*, *Japanese Patent*, 7,018,278 (1970)

CYLINDROCLADIN B
C$_{22}$H$_{30}$O$_6$
M.p. 132–134°C
A second antitumour antibiotic produced by *Cylindrocladium ilicicola*, this compound also forms colourless crystals from EtOH and is slightly dextrorotatory having $[\alpha]_D^{20} + 0·9°$ (dioxan). In ethanol solution, it gives an ultraviolet spectrum having absorption maxima at 229·5, 295·5 and 347 nm.

Matsushima, *Japanese Patent*, 7,018,278 (1970)

CYLINDROCLADIN C
C$_{22}$H$_{26}$O$_6$
M.p. 161–162°C
Also elaborated by *Cylindrocladium ilicicola*, this antitumour antibiotic forms colourless crystals when recrystallized from EtOH and is laevorotatory having a specific rotation of $[\alpha]_D^{20} - 130·4°$ (dioxan). The ultraviolet spectrum in EtOH has three absorption maxima at 237, 295 and 348 nm.

Matsishima, *Japanese Patent*, 7,018,278 (1970)

CYNEMATIN
An antibiotic produced by a strain of *Tilachlidium*, very little is known of its chemical, physical and biological properties.

Gottshall, Roberts, Portwood, *Soc. Amer. Bact.*, **15**, No. 5, 11 (1949)

CYTICILLIN
See Procaine Penicillin G

CYTOCHALASIN A
C$_{29}$H$_{35}$O$_5$N
M.p. 193–195°C

The cytochalasins have been isolated from cultures of various fungi and are important in that they affect animal cells in certain ways thereby allowing examination of cell structures and kinetics. Cytochalasin A is elaborated by *Helminthosporium dematioideum* and has the structure given above. The antibiotic is comparatively stable but is affected by light which isomerizes the conjugated double bond from *trans* to *cis*. It causes a reversible inhibition of cell locomotion, chemotaxis, cell aggregation and a variety of morphogenetic movements. Characteristically, it blocks the process of cytokinesis in animal cells without interfering with nuclear division.

Imperial Chemical Industries, *French Patent*, 1,511,746 (1968)

CYTOCHALASIN B
$C_{29}H_{37}O_5N$
M.p. 221–223°C

A further compound isolated from cultures of *Helminthosporium dematioideum*, this substance has a similar structure to that of the preceding antibiotic. Its action upon animal cells also parallels that of cytochalasin A. It is, however, completely stable both as the solid and in solution.

Imperial Chemical Industries, *French Patent*, 1,511,746 (1968)

CYTOCHALASIN C
$C_{30}H_{37}O_6N$
M.p. 260°C (*dec.*)

This member of the group is elaborated by *Metarrhizium anisopliae* when grown on a medium containing Dextrolact, yeast extract, tartaric acid, ammonium tartrate and inorganic salts at 24°C for 13–15 days. The culture filtrate is extracted with $CHCl_3$, the solvent evaporated, the residue dissolved in $(CH_3)_2CO$ and chromatographed on a silica gel column, being finally purified by crystallizing from $(CH_3)_2CO$. It has a similar effect upon animal cells as the preceding compounds.

Imperial Chemical Industries, *French Patent*, 1,511,746 (1968)

CYTOCHALASIN D
$C_{30}H_{37}O_6N$
M.p. 255°C (*dec.*)

A stereoisomer of cytochalasin C, this compound also occurs in the culture filtrate of *Metarrhizium anisopliae*. It forms colourless crystals and gives similar effects with animal cells.

Imperial Chemical Industries, *French Patent*, 1,511,746 (1968)

CYTOCHALASIN E
$C_{26}H_{30}O_7N$
M.p. 206°C (dec.)

Rosellinia mecatrix yields this compound when grown in a common nutrient medium at 26°C for 10 days. It forms colourless crystals from $(CH_3)_2CO$ and is stable in the solid form and reasonably stable in solution. Cytochalasin E produces effects on cells similar to cytochalasins A and B but these are morphologically distinct. Multinuclear cells are produced due to failure of cytokinesis but these tend to have characteristically scalloped margins. Nuclear extrusion is not a feature of the activity of this compound.

Broadbent *et al.*, *German Patent*, 2,121,168 (1971)

CYTOTETRINS
The culture broth of *Streptomyces griseoflavus* yields an antibiotic complex named cytotetrin which forms a basic red powder, separable by chromatography and countercurrent distribution into five active components, cytotetrins A, B, C, D and E. The complex and individual constituents are active against gram-positive bacteria and some tumours.

Berdy *et al.*, *J. Antibiotics* (Japan), **24**, 209 (1971)

CYTRIMYCIN
$C_{60}H_{88}O_{26}$
M.p. 178–181°C

A complex antibiotic, cytrimycin has been isolated from the culture filtrate of *Streptomyces katsunumaensis* (FERM-P 2071) when cultured at pH 6·4 and 28°C for 3 days on a medium comprising starch, yeast and inorganic salts. The filtrate is extracted with AcOEt, concentrated to a yellow-brown powder and separated from the accompanying antibiotics by silica gel thin layer chromatography. It is soluble in the lower alcohols, Me_2CO, MeCOEt, AcOEt, $CHCl_3$ and dioxan. The antibiotic is active against gram-positive bacteria, particularly *Xanthomonas*. It is toxic to mice, the LD_{50} being 1·0–1·5 mg/kg given intraperitoneally.

Oki *et al.*, *Japanese Patent*, 75 13,593 (1975)

D

DACTINOMYCIN
See Actinomycin D

DACTYLARIN
$C_{16}H_{16}O_6$

This recently isolated antibiotic is obtained from the culture filtrate of *Dactylaria lutea* Routien. It is extracted from the filtrate with organic solvents and purified by chromatography on an alumina column. Dactylarin exhibits a slight activity against gram-positive bacteria but is primarily active against protozoa including *Entamoeba invadens* and *Leishmania brasiliensis*.

Kettner *et al.*, *J. Antibiotics* (Japan), **26**, 692 (1973)

DAUNOMYCIN (*Daunorubicin*)
$C_{27}H_{29}O_{10}N$
M.p. Indefinite

This antibiotic has been isolated from *Streptomyces peucetius*. On hydrolysis it furnishes daunosamine and daunomycinone. The former is characterized as the hydrochloride, m.p. 168°C; $[\alpha]_D - 54.5°$ (H_2O) and the latter forms colourless crystals, m.p. 213–214°C; $[\alpha]_D + 193°$ (dioxan). Daunomycin hydrochloride forms thin red needles, m.p. 188–190°C and is dextrorotatory with a specific rotation of $[\alpha]_D + 253°$ (c 0.15, CH_3OH). It gives an ultraviolet spectrum in CH_3OH with absorption maxima at 234, 252, 290, 480 and 532 nm.

Bossa and his colleagues have demonstrated that the antibiotic inhibits the respiration of Ehrlich ascites tumour cells *in vitro* at a concentration of 0.5 µg/ml and that the inhibition is greater at a temperature of 42°C than at 37°C. In addition, both the cell permeability and the binding of the antibiotic to the nuclei and mitachondria are greater at the higher temperature.

A number of *in vivo* experiments have been carried out with daunomycin. Biswas and his coworkers have found that when injected intraperitoneally into sarcoma-bearing mice, the antibiotic increases the alkaline RNase activity in the kidney, liver and spleen whereas in normal mice the enzyme activity is inhibited. When administered to pigs by extracorporeal liver perfusion with a shunt between the external jugular vein and the portal vein, a dose of 3 mg/kg caused no damage to normal liver cells, the antibiotic being rapidly eliminated, none being present in the perfusate after 10 minutes. Daunomycin does, however, significantly prolong the initial *in vitro* blood clotting rate of canine blood plasma without affecting either the reaction time or the maximum amplitude. At an increased concentration (25 µg/200 µg plasma) there was a significantly increased initial clotting rate and a reduction in the maximum amplitude. It would appear that these latter effects are related to changes in the platelet function.

Compounds in which daunomycin hydrochloride is modified in structure have led to substantial modifications in antiviral, antitumour and cytotoxic activity. Of those prepared, only 13-dihydrodaunomycin hydrochloride exhibits significant antitumour activity *in vivo*.

Di Marco *et al.*, *Nature*, **201**, 706 (1964)
Arcamone *et al.*, *J. Amer. Chem. Soc.*, **86**, 5334 (1964) Structure
Arcamone *et al.*, *Tetrahedron Lett.*, 3349 (1968)
Iwamoto *et al.*, *ibid.*, 3891 (1968)

Absolute configuration
  Arcamone et al., *Tetrahedron Lett.*, 3353 (1968)
Synthesis
  Acton, Fujiwara, Henry, *J. Med. Chem.*, **17**, 659 (1974)
Studies *in vitro*
  Bossa et al., *G. Ital. Chemioter.*, **20**, 52 (1973)
  Bossa, Galatulas, Montanari, *IRCS Med. Sci. Libr. Compend.*, 3, (1975)
Studies *in vivo*
  Di Marco et al., *Cancer Chemother. Rep., Part 1*, **57**, 269 (1973)
  Rimal et al., *Indian J. Cancer*, **11**, 301 (1974)
  Toennesen et al., *Acta Chir. Scand.*, **140**, 631 (1974)

DAUNORUBICIN
See Daunomycin

11-DEACETOXYWORTMANNIN
$C_{21}H_{22}O_6$

A highly fungistatic and antiinflammatory antibiotic, this compound is produced by culturing *Aspergillus janus* NRRL 3807 or *Penicillium funiculosum* NRRL 3363 on a medium containing cerulose, malt extract, yeast extract and inorganic salts at 27°C for 112 hours, or by the base-catalysed isomerization of $\Delta^{9(11)}$-8:9-dihydro-11-deacetoxywortmannin. The structure of the antibiotic has been shown to be that given above based upon chemical and spectroscopic evidence. It possesses a marked edema-inhibiting activity.

  Hauser, *German Patent*, 2,022,452 (1970)

DEACETYLCEPHALOSPORIN C
$C_{14}H_{19}O_6N_3S$
A cephalosporin antibiotic, this compound is obtained from the cultures of a number of species, e.g. *Cephalosporium* C-28 ATCC 20,370, *C. acremonium* 132 ATCC 20,371, *C. chrysogenum* ATCC 14,615, *Diheterospora chlamydosporia* NRRL 5728, *Emericellopsis* species NRRL 5446, NRRL 5447 and NRRL 5714, *Paecilomyces carneus* NRRL 5711 and *Scopulariopsis* NRRL 5715. The antibiotic is normally purified by penicillinase treatment followed by chromatography on an alumina column. It is active against a range of gram-positive and gram-negative bacteria.

  Kanzaki et al., *German Patent*, 2,318,650 (1973)
  Hamill, Higgens, *German Patent*, 2,320,696 (1973)

4″-O-DEACETYLDELTAMYCIN
$C_{37}H_{59}NO_{15}$

A macrocyclic antibiotic isolated from cultures of *Streptomyces deltae* when grown on a medium of corn steep liquor, dried yeast and glucose at 20°C for 2 days, this antibiotic has the structure given above based upon chemical correlations and spectroscopic data. It is primarily active against gram-positive bacteria.

  Okamura et al., *J. Ferment. Technol.*, **55**, 347 (1977)

9-DEHYDRODEMYCAROSYL PLATENOMYCIN
$C_{31}H_{49}NO_{11}$
A platenomycin derivative, this antibiotic has been isolated from the culture broth of *Streptomyces platensis* subsp. *malvinus* MCRL 0388 by extraction with polar solvents followed by column chromatography. It is effective against gram-positive bacteria.

Furumai, Suzuki, *J. Antibiotics* (Japan), **28**, 775 (1975)

DEISOVALERYLBLASTMYCIN
$C_{21}H_{28}N_2O_8$
M.p. 186–188°C

The fermentation broth of *Streptomyces* species 5140-A yields this blastmycin derivative which exhibits a high activity against *Piricularia oryzae*. It has a lower toxicity against killifish than the antimycin-A-blastmycin range of antibiotics.

Ishiyama *et al.*, *J. Antibiotics* (Japan), **29**, 804 (1976)

DEKAMYCIN
A basic H_2O-soluble antibiotic isolated from the culture broth of *Streptomyces fradiae*, this antibiotic is active against both gram-positive and gram-negative bacteria. It has no activity against fungi or protozoa. It has been suggested that dekamycin belongs to the aminoglycoside group of antibiotics.

Truong Cong Quyen *et al.*, *Biologic* (Bratislava), **32**, 217 (1977)

DELTAMYCIN A$_1$
$C_{39}H_{61}NO_{16}$

Streptomyces deltae yields a number of macrocyclic antibiotics when cultured on a medium consisting of corn steep liquor, dried yeast, glucose and $CaCO_3$ at 20°C for 2 days. The components have been separated and purified chromatographically and their structures determined from chemical and spectroscopic data. This component has the structure given above and is effective against gram-positive bacteria.

Okamura *et al.*, *J. Ferment. Technol.*, **55**, 347 (1977)

DELTAMYCIN A$_2$
$C_{40}H_{63}NO_{16}$

A further component of the deltamycin complex obtained from cultures of *Streptomyces deltae*, this antibiotic has a structure similar to that of the preceding substance. It is also active against gram-positive bacteria.

Okamura *et al.*, *J. Ferment. Technol.* **55**, 347 (1977)

DELTAMYCIN A₃
$C_{41}H_{65}NO_{16}$

This antibiotic also occurs in the culture broth of *Streptomyces deltae* when grown on a medium of corn steep liquor, yeast, glucose and $CaCO_3$. It has the structure shown above and is effective against gram-positive bacteria.

Okamura et al., *J. Ferment. Technol.*, **55**, 347 (1977)

7-O-DEMETHYLCELESTICETIN
$C_{23}H_{34}O_9N_2S$
M.p. Indefinite

This antibiotic from a mutant strain of *Streptomyces celestis* has been obtained as the crystalline hydrochloride which is dextrorotatory with a specific rotation of $[\alpha]_D^{25} + 115°$ (c 0·84, H_2O). The structure has been determined by chemical and spectroscopic studies and by comparison with that of celesticetin (q.v.). The antibacterial activity of the hydrochloride is equivalent *in vitro* to that of celesticetin.

Argoudelis et al., *J. Antibiotics* (Japan), **25**, 445 (1972)

Argoudelis et al., *German Patent*, 2,262,626 (1973)
Argoudelis, Coats, Sebek, *U.S. Patent*, 3,812,096 (1974)

N-DEMETHYLLINCOMYCIN
See Antibiotic V-II, 973

11-DEMETHYLTOMAYMYCIN
$C_{15}H_{18}O_4N_2$
M.p. Indefinite

An antibiotic produced by cultivation of *Streptomyces achromogenes* var. *tomaymyceticus* on a common nutrient medium. The compound possesses marked antiviral activity.

Kariyone et al., *Chem. Pharm. Bull.*, **19**, 2289 (1971)
Arima et al., *J. Antibiotics* (Japan), **25**, 437 (1972)
Biosynthesis
Hurley, Gaivola, Zmijewski, *Chem. Commun.*, 120 (1975)

DEMETRIC ACID
M.p. Indefinite

Streptomyces umbrosus var. *suragaoensis* yields this antibiotic when cultivated under aerobic conditions in a medium containing cerelose, Pharmamedia, corn steep liquor and inorganic salts. Demetric acid forms colourless crystals and is assayed by ultraviolet examination and HeLa cell plate methods. It is active in inhibiting HeLa cells.

Schmitz, DeVault, *U.S. Patent*, 3,629,407 (1961)

DEMYCAROSYL PLATENOMYCIN
$C_{31}H_{51}NO_{11}$

A macrocyclic antibiotic isolated from the fermentation broth of blocked mutants of *Streptomyces platensis* subsp. *malvinus* MCRL 0388, this antibiotic has been isolated by solvent extraction of the filtered broth followed by column chromatography. It has been shown to be active against gram-positive organisms.

DENAMYCIN
M.p. 226–228°C

An antibiotic elaborated by several species of *Streptomyces*, denamycin forms yellow needles when purified by recrystallization from CH_3OH. It has a specific rotation of $[\alpha]_D^{20} + 41°$ (CH_3OH) and gives an ultraviolet spectrum in EtOH consisting of a single absorption maximum at 311 nm.

Miyazaki et al., *J. Antibiotics* (Japan), **22A**, 393 (1969)

DEOXYBOUVARDIN
$C_{40}H_{48}N_6O_9$

Furumai, Suzuki, *J. Antibiotics* (Japan), **28**, 775 (1975)

The plant antibiotic has been isolated, together with bouvardin (q.v.) from the flowers, leaves and stems of *Bouvardia ternifolia*, from which it is extracted with MeOH. Like bouvardin it shows an inhibitory activity against P388 lymphocytic leukemia and B16 melanotic melanoma.

Jolad et al., *J. Amer. Chem. Soc.*, **99**, 8040 (1977)

5-DEOXYBUTIROSAMINE
$C_{12}H_{26}N_4O_5$

A mutasynthetic antibiotic, this compound is elaborated by the D⁻ strain of *Bacillus circulans* when cultured in the presence of 2,5-dideoxystreptamine as the mutasython. It has the structure shown above and is active against gram-positive organisms.

Claridge et al., *Dev. Ind. Microbiol.*, **15**, 101 (1974)
Taylor, Schmitz, *J. Antibiotics* (Japan), **29**, 532 (1976)

6β-DEOXY-5-HYDROXYTETRACYCLINE
$C_{22}H_{24}O_8N_2$

This epimer of the preceding antibiotic is also obtained as the crystalline hydrochloride which has m.p. 250–251°C (*dec.*) and is laevorotatory with a specific rotation of $[\alpha]_D^{25} - 251°$ (c 0·9, 0·1 N-H_2SO_4). The salt gives an ultraviolet spectrum in CH_3OH—HCl with absorption maxima at 244 and 267 nm.

Stephens *et al.*, *J. Amer. Chem. Soc.*, **80**, 5324 (1958)
McCormick *et al.*, *ibid.*, **82**, 3381 (1960)
McCormick, Jensen, *U.S. Patent*, 3,019,260 (1961)
Wittenau *et al.*, *J. Amer. Chem. Soc.*, **84**, 2645 (1962)
Beereboom, Butler, *U.S. Patent*, 3,069,467 (1963)
Stephens *et al.*, *J. Amer. Chem. Soc.*, **85**, 2643 (1963)

10-DEOXYMETHYLMYCIN
See Antibiotic YC-17

DEOXYNYBOMYCIN
$C_{16}H_{14}O_3N_2$
Dec. >335°C

Streptomyces hyalinum produces this antibiotic which forms crystals that decompose above 335°C without melting. The structure given above has been determined from chemical and spectroscopic evidence.

Rinehart, Renfroe, *J. Amer. Chem. Soc.*, **83**, 3729 (1961)
Naganawa *et al.*, *J. Antibiotics* (Japan), **23**, 365 (1970)
Rinehart *et al.*, *J. Amer. Chem. Soc.*, **92**, 6994 (1970)
Forbis, Rinehart, *ibid.*, **92**, 6995 (1970)

6-DEOXYPAROMOMYCIN I
$C_{23}H_{44}N_4O_{13}$

Streptomyces rimosus forma *paromomycinus* normally produces the paromomycins but a mutant strain has been developed which, on culturing in the presence of 2,6-dideoxystreptamine yields two stereoisomeric mutasynthetic antibiotics, 6-deoxyparomomycins I and II. These have been separated and purified chromatographically. The structure of this antibiotic has been shown to be that given above. It has a similar antibiotic activity to that of the paromomycins.

Cleophax *et al.*, *J. Amer. Chem. Soc.*, **98**. 7110 (1976)

6-DEOXYPAROMOMYCIN II
$C_{23}H_{44}N_4O_{13}$

A second antibiotic obtained by culturing a mutant strain of *Streptomyces rimous* forma *paromomycinus* on a medium containing added 2,6-dideoxy-streptamine, this compound has the structure given above. It has an antibiotic activity similar to that of the paromomycins.

Cleophax *et al.*, *J. Amer. Chem. Soc.*, **98**, 7110 (1976)

DEOXY-(O-8)-SALINOMYCIN
$C_{42}H_{70}O_{10}$

This antibiotic, and its 17-epimer (q.v.) are formed by *Streptomyces albus* ATCC 21838 when grown in a common nutrient medium. The components have been separated and purified by column and thin layer chromatography. It is active gram-positive bacteria but is principally effective against coccidia in poultry, particularly *Eimeria tenella* infections.

Westley *et al.*, *J. Antibiotics* (Japan), **30**, 610 (1977)

DEOXY-(O-8)-17-*epi*-SALINOMYCIN
$C_{42}H_{70}O_{10}$

The 17-epimer of the preceding salinomycin derivative, this antibiotic has also been isolated from cultures of *Streptomyces albus* ATCC 21838. It has a similar antibiotic spectrum against gram-positive bacteria and *Eimeria tenella* in poultry.

Westley *et al.*, *J. Antibiotics* (Japan), **30**, 610 (1977)

1-DEOXY-D-THREO-PENTULOSE
$C_5H_{10}O_4$

Streptomyces hygroscopicus strain UC-5601 elaborates this simple antibiotic, the structure of which has been established by chemical and spectroscopic methods. It possesses only weak antibiotic properties but exhibits a specific inhibition of the growth of the UC-159 strain of *Mycobacterium avium*.

Slechta, Johnson, *J. Antibiotics* (Japan), **29**, 658 (1976)
Structure
Hoeksema, Baczynskyj, *J. Antibiotics* (Japan), **29**, 688 (1976)

DERINAMYCIN
$C_{51}H_{93}NO_{23}$

A complex antibiotic, derinamycin has been obtained from the wet mycelia of *Streptomyces venezuelae* by solvent extraction and column chromatography. It is effective in inhibiting the growth of gram-positive, some gram-negative bacteria and fungi but is less active against yeasts. The action of the antibiotic on macromolecular synthesis of intact *Bacillus subtilis* has been examined and it has been demonstrated that derinamycin supresses both RNA and DNA syntheses but protein synthesis is less affected. No selective inhibition between RNA and DNA syntheses in a double-isotope experiment to assess the comparative effects of the antibiotic has been discovered.

Uchida, Zahner, *J. Antibiotics* (Japan), **28**, 266 (1975)

DERMADIN
M.p. Indefinite

An antibiotic substance produced by *Trichoderma viride* NRRL 3153 when cultivated under aerobic conditions. Dermadin forms an amorphous powder which inhibits the growth of gram-positive bacteria, particularly *Bacillus subtilis* and also that of *Aerobacter aerogenes*.

Coats, Meyer, Pyke, *U.S. Patent*, 3,627,882 (1971)

DERMOSTATIN A
$C_{40}H_{64}O_{11}$

A polyene antibiotic produced by a species of *Streptomyces*, this antibiotic occurs with dermostatin B in the culture filtrate. It is active against gram-positive bacteria.

Narasimhachari, Swami, *J. Antibiotics* (Japan), **22**, 566 (1970)
Pandey *et al.*, *ibid.*, **26**, 475 (1973)

DERMOSTATIN B
$C_{41}H_{66}O_{11}$

A further component isolated from the dermostatin complex, this compound is the homologue of the preceding antibiotic and possesses a similar antibiotic spectrum.

Narasimhachari, Swami, *J. Antibiotics* (Japan), **22**, 566 (1970)
Pandey *et al.*, *ibid.*, **26**, 475 (1973)

DESALICITIN
$C_{17}H_{32}O_7N_2S$
M.p. Indefinite

Produced by *Streptomyces celestis*, this antibiotic is isolated as the hydrochloride which forms colourless crystals having a specific rotation of $[\alpha]_D^{25} + 150°$ (c 1·0, H_2O). The 2″-acetate of this antibiotic is celesticetin (q.v.). It is active against gram-positive bacteria.

Argoudelis, Brodasky, *J. Antibiotics* (Japan), **25**, 194 (1972)

DESDANINE
See Pyracrimycin A

DESFERRITRIACETYLFUSIGENIN
$C_{38}H_{60}N_6O_{14}$

A macrocyclic antibiotic produced by *Aspergillus deflectus* CBS 109-55 when cultivated on an iron-free nutrient medium, this substance inhibits the growth of gram-positive and some gram-negative bacteria. Fungi and yeasts are only weakly affected by the antibiotic. The structure has been established from chemical and spectroscopic evidence.

Anke, *J. Antibiotics* (Japan), **30**, 125 (1977)

DESTOMYCIN A
$C_{20}H_{37}O_{13}N_3$
M.p. 180–190°C (*dec.*)

An antibiotic produced, together with the two following compounds, from *Streptomyces rimofaciens*. It forms a white, amorphous powder having a specific rotation of $[\alpha]_D^{22} + 7°$ (c 2·0, H_2O). Destomycin A has been used as an anthelmintic added to the feed stock of various domestic animals. It has been shown to inhibit phosphofructokinase obtained from the homogenate of *Ascaris* muscle, but it does not inhibit the fumarate reductase or malic enzyme obtained from *A. lumbricoides*.

Kondo et al., *J. Antibiotics* (Japan), **18A**, 38 (1965)
Kondo et al., ibid., **19A**, 139 (1966)
Murakoshi et al., *Nihon Daigaku Yakugaku Kenkyu Hokoku*, **12**, 1 (1972)

DESTOMYCIN B

$C_{21}H_{39}O_{13}N_3$
M.p. 140–200°C (*dec.*)

A further antibiotic obtained from cultures of *Streptomyces rimofaciens*, this compound is also a white amorphous powder decomposing over a wide range of temperature. The structure is not yet known with certainty. It has a specific rotation of $[\alpha]_D^{21} + 6°$ (c 1·0, H_2O) and forms an N-acetate with m.p. 220–240°C (*dec.*). It has a similar activity to that of the preceding substance.

Kondo et al., *J. Antibiotics* (Japan), **18A**, 38 (1965)

DESTOMYCIN C

$C_{21}H_{39}O_{13}N_3$

This antibiotic has been isolated from cultures of *Streptomyces rimofaciens*. The structure given above has been established by C-13 ultraviolet absorption, infrared and NMR studies. It has antimicrobial properties similar to those of destomycin A and also shows anthelmintic activity against round worm in domestic fowls. The LD_{50} in mice is 6·5–12·5 mg/kg when administered intravenously.

Shimura et al., *J. Antibiotics* (Japan), **28**, 83 (1975)

DETOXINS

Streptomyces caespitosus var. *detoxicus* yields an antibiotic complex, detoxin, which has been separated by chromatography into at least 8 components, all of which appear to be mixtures. The most active of these are detoxins C and D and these have been further purified to yield a number of components of which those described below have been isolated in a state of reasonable purity. The compounds have inhibitory activity against a number of gram-positive organisms.

Otake, Kakinuma, Yonehara, *J. Antibiotics* (Japan), **21**, 371 (1968)

DETOXIN C_1

$C_{29-30}H_{44-46}O_9N_4$
M.p. 142–144°C

This compound is amphoteric with pK_a 8·0 and 3·9. It is laevorotatory with a specific rotation of $[\alpha]_D - 23°$ (c 1·0, CH_3OH) and had an activity of 2200 units/ml.

Otake, Kakinuma, Yonehara, *J. Antibiotics* (Japan), **21**, 371 (1968)

DETOXIN D_1
$C_{30}H_{46}O_9N_4$
M.p. 168°C

Also amphoteric, this antibiotic has pK_a 8·0 and 4·0 and a specific rotation of $[\alpha]_D - 16°$ (c 1·0, CH_3OH). The activity of the compound was 5500 units/ml.

Otake, Kakinuma, Yonehara, *J. Antibiotics* (Japan), **21**, 371 (1968)

DEXTROMYCIN

An antibiotic resembling streptomycin and streptothricin, this substance is produced by an unclassified species of *Streptomyces*. It is a stable, basic substance, soluble in H_2O and insoluble in organic solvents. It has a specific rotation of $[\alpha]_D^{25} + 61·0°$ (c 1·0, H_2O) and is slowly diffusible. It gives a negative Maltol reaction.

The biological activity is the same as that of streptomycin (q.v.) and the LD_{50} in mice is 50 mg/kg (intravenous) and 750–100 mg/kg when given subcutaneously. There is no evidence of any delayed toxicity in mice.

Ogata, *J. Antibiotics* (Japan), **3**, 440 (1950)

4,5-DIACETYLVERRUCAROL
See Antibiotic A-2

DIATETRYNE II (*Nudic acid B*)
$C_8H_3O_2N$
M.p. 179°C (*dec.*)

HOOC—CH=CH—C≡C—C≡C—CN

This highly unsaturated acetylenic acid has been isolated from cultures of *Clitocybe diatreta* and shown to possess the structure given above. It forms colourless crystals which decompose explosively at the melting point. The ultraviolet spectrum in 95 per cent EtOH has absorption maxima at 228, 238, 268, 283, 299 and 322 nm.

Anchel, *J. Amer. Chem. Soc.*, **75**, 1588 (1952)
Anchel, *ibid.*, **76**, 4621 (1953)
Anchel, *Science*, **121**, 607 (1955)
Ashworth *et al.*, *J. Chem. Soc.*, 950 (1958)

2:6-DIBROMO-4-CARBAMOYLMETHYL-4-HYDROXYCYCLOHEXA-2:5-DIEN-1-ONE
$C_8H_7O_3NBr_2$
M.p. 193–195°C

The marine sponge *Verongia cauliformis* yields this antibiotic which forms yellowish crystals and gives an ultraviolet spectrum consisting of a single absorption maximum at 257 nm. The substance furnishes a monoacetate, m.p. 185°C, with an ultraviolet spectrum having an absorption maximum at 266 nm.

Sharma, Burkholder, *J. Antibiotics* (Japan), **20A**, 200 (1967)
Synthesis
Sharma, Burkholder, *Tetrahedron Lett.*, 4147 (1967)

S-2,3-DICARBOXYAZIRIDINE
$C_4H_5NO_4$
Decomp. 178°C

An unclassified species of *Streptomyces* yields this simple aziridine antibiotic, the structure of which has been elucidated from chemical and spectroscopic evidence. It forms colourless plates and is dextrorotatory with a specific rotation of $[\alpha]_D^{24} + 54°$. It is active against gram-positive and gram-negative bacteria and fungi and is particularly effective against *Aeromonas salmonecida*.

Naganawa *et al.*, *J. Antibiotics* (Japan), **28**, 828 (1975)

DICLOXACILLIN
$C_{19}H_{17}O_5N_3SCl_2$

A semi-synthetic penicillin, this antibiotic has been shown to be the most effective of the *isoxazolyl* penicillins in treating *Staphylococcus* infections in humans. It has a marked synergistic action with ampicillin (a.v.) against *Aerobacter*, *Proteus*, *Klebsiella*, and *Shigella* species and *Pseudomonas pyocyanea*, *Escherichia coli*, *Staphylococcus aureus* and *Streptococcus fecalis*. Dicloxacillin is not, however, used clinically with ampicillin against *Pseudomonas aeruginosa*. It also inhibits the degradation of ampicillin by penicillinase isolated from ampicillin-resistant *Escherichia coli* or *Staphylococci*.

Yoshioka *et al.*, *J. Antibiotics* (Japan), **20B**, 34 (1967)
Fomina *et al.*, *Antibiotiki*, **16**, 153 (1971)
De Azevedo e Silva *et al.*, *Univ. Fed. Pernambuco, Inst. Biocienc., Publ. Avulsa*, 9 (1973)
Suda *et al.*, *J. Antibiotics* (Japan), **26**, 504 (1973)
Ambrosoli, Menozzi, Mandras, *Ig. Mod.*, **66**, 339 (1973)
Ito *et al.*, *J. Antibiotics* (Japan), **27**, 490 (1974)

DI-2,4-DIACETYLFLUOROGLUCYLMETHANE
$C_{21}H_{20}O_{10}$

A dimeric antibiotic, this compound has been isolated from the culture broth of *Pseudomonas aurantica*. It has the symmetrical structure shown above which is based upon chemical analysis and a study of the infrared, NMR and mass spectra. The antibiotic is effective against gram-positive bacteria in concentrations of 0·1–1·0 µg/ml. It also exhibits some fungistatic and antiviral activity.

Esipov *et al.*, *Antibiotiki*, **20**, 1077 (1975)

3′:4′-DIDEOXYBUTIROSIN B
$C_{21}H_{41}O_{10}N_5$
M.p. Indefinite

A semi-synthetic antibiotic produced from butirosin B by classical chemical methods, this compound has an antibacterial activity similar to that of butirosin B but is also effective against *Escherichia coli* strain K-12 JR 66/W 677 and *Klebsiella pneumoniae* type 22 3038 which are resistant to the parent antibiotic.

Ikeda *et al.*, *J. Antibiotics* (Japan), **26**, 307 (1973)

3′:4′-DIDEOXYKANAMYCIN B
$C_{18}H_{37}O_8N_5$
M.p. Indefinite

A semi-synthetic antibiotic, this compound is bactericidal for a range of organisms but has no inhibitory effect upon fungi. The inhibiting action is greater under alkaline conditions and although the activity against *Staphylococcus aureus* is not affected by bovine, horse or rabbit serum it is decreased by high concentrations of rabbit serum against *Pseudomonas aeruginosa*. This antibiotic has proved to be more effective than gentamycin in protecting mice against infections from *Escherichia coli*, *Klebsiella pneumoniae* and *Pseudomonas aeruginosa*. The LD_{50} in mice has been given as 180 mg/kg given intravenously. Some chronic toxicity has been observed in rats and female dogs given doses of 5–200 mg/kg over a period.

Umezawa et al., *German Patent*, 2,135,191 (1972)
Koeda et al., *J. Antibiotics* (Japan), **26**, 28, 40, 228, 247 (1973)
Komiya et al., *ibid.*, **26**, 49 (1973)
Fujita et al., *ibid.*, **26**, 55 (1973)
Mitsuhashi et al., *ibid.*, **26**, 89 (1973)
Ichikawa et al., *ibid.*, **26**, 262 (1973)
Nakazawa et al., *ibid.*, **26**, 454 (1973)
Shimizu, *ibid.*, **26**, 522 (1973)
Akiyoshi et al., *ibid.*, **27**, 15, 735 (1974)
Mizuno et al., *Japanese Patent*, 9,529,530 (1975)

3′,4′-DIDEOXYRIBOSTAMYCIN
$C_{17}H_{34}N_4O_8$

A mutasynthetic antibiotic produced by a deoxystreptamine lacking mutant of *Streptomyces ribosidificus* cultured in the presence of added neamine, this compound has the structure given above. It is active against gram-positive bacteria and also against kanamycin and ribostamycin-resistant strains of *Escherichia coli* and *Pseudomonas aeruginosa*.

Umezawa et al., *J. Antibiotics* (Japan), **24**, 711 (1971)
Kojima, Satoh, *ibid.*, **26**, 784 (1973)

DIENOMYCIN A
$C_{20}H_{27}O_2N$

One of three antibiotics produced by a strain MC67-C1, this substance may be crystallized from CH_3OH—AcOEt. It is characterized as the hydrochloride, colourless crystals from CH_3OH—AcOEt—H_2O with m.p. 212–214°C and a specific rotation of $[\alpha]_D^{20} + 84°$ (c 1·0, CH_3OH). The ultraviolet spectrum of this salt in CH_3OH has absorption maxima at 211, 220, 227, 234, 287 and 307 nm with shoulders at 280 and 297 nm.

Umezawa et al., *J. Antibiotics* (Japan), **23A**, 20 (1970)

DIENOMYCIN B
$C_{18}H_{23}O_2N$

A further antibiotic isolated from cultures of strain MC67-C1, this substance also crystallizes from CH_3OH—AcOEt. The hydrochloride forms colourless crystals from CH_3OH—AcOEt—H_2O with m.p. 280–281°C (sealed tube). It is dextrorotatory with a specific rotation of $[\alpha]_D^{20} + 80°$ (c 1·0, CH_3OH).

Umezawa et al., *J. Antibiotics* (Japan), **23A**, 20 (1970)

DIENOMYCIN C
$C_{16}H_{21}ON$
M.p. 130–131°C

A third antibiotic elaborated by strain MC67-C1, this compound forms colourless crystals from CH_3OH—$(CH_3)_2CO$. It has $[\alpha]_{589}^{20} + 85°$ (c 1·0, CH_3OH). The hydrochloride may also be crystallized from CH_3OH—AcOEt—H_2O with m.p. 252–253°C and $[\alpha]_D^{20} + 65°$ (c 1·0, CH_3OH).

Umezawa et al., *J. Antibiotics* (Japan), **23A**, 20 (1970)

7β,8β-2′,3′-DIEPOXYRORIDIN H
$C_{29}H_{34}O_{10}$

One of a group of roridin type antibiotics produced by the aerobic culture of *Cylindrocarpon* strain PF-60 on a medium of boiled potato extract and sucrose, this antibiotic has been separated and purified by extraction of the

Dihydroabikoviromycin

fermentation broth with AcOEt followed by silica gel column and preparative thin layer chromatography. It is active against a number of gram-positive and gram-negative bacteria.

Matsumoto et al., *J. Antibiotics* (Japan), **30**, 681 (1977)

DIHYDROABIKOVIROMYCIN
$C_{10}H_{13}ON$
M.p. Indefinite

An antiviral antibiotic, dihydroabikoviromycin is obtained by the aerobic culture of *Streptomyces olivaceus*, *S. reticuli* or *S. viridochromogenes* on a medium containing glucose, vegetable protein, wheat embryo and sodium chloride at 28°C and pH 7·0 for 2 days. It is isolated by the repeated extraction of the filtrate with an organic solvent at an acidic pH. The probable structure is that given above.

Shomura et al., *Japanese Patent*, 7,311,040 (1973)

5,6-DIHYDRO-5(S)-ACETOXY-6(S)-(1',2'-*trans*-EPOXYPROPYL)-2H-PYRAN-2-ONE
$C_{10}H_{12}O_5$

Aspergillus strain NRRL 5769 yields three closely related pyran antibiotics when cultivated on a medium comprising corn steep liquor, cottonseed meal, glucose, hydrochloric acid and sitosterol. The culture filtrate is extracted with CH_2Cl_2 and the individual compounds separated and purified by silica gel chromatography. This substance has the structure shown above based upon chemical and spectroscopic data. It is effective against *Candida albicans*.

Jiu, Kraychy, Mizuba, *U.S. Patent*, 3,909,362 (1975)

5,6-DIHYDRO-5(R)-ACETOXY-6(S)-(1',2'-*trans*-EPOXYPROPYL)-2H-PYRAN-2-ONE
$C_{10}H_{12}O_5$

A stereoisomer of the preceding antibiotic, this compound is a further constituent of the antibiotic complex produced by *Aspergillus* strain NRRL 5769. The structure has been determined from chemical and spectroscopic evidence. It is active against *Candida albicans*.

Jiu, Kraychy, Mizuba, *U.S. Patent*, 3,909,362 (1975)

5,6-DIHYDRO-5(S)-ACETOXY-6(S)-(1',2'-*trans*-PROPYL)-2H-PYRAN-2-ONE
$C_{10}H_{12}O_4$

5-DIHYDROCORIOLIN C
$C_{22}H_{36}O_7$
M.p. Indefinite

A further antibiotic isolated from cultures of *Aspergillus* strain NRRL 5769, this substance has the structure given above which has been elucidated from chemical examination and the infrared, NMR and mass spectra.

Jiu, Kraychy, Mizuba, *U.S. Patent*, 3,909,362 (1975)

This derivative of coriolin C is formed by the aerobic fermentation of *Coriolus consors* ATCC 20,305 in a common nutrient medium at pH 7·0 and 27°C for 3 days. It has, bactericidal and neoplasmic activity comparable with coriolin C.

Umezawa *et al.*, *German Patent*, 2,261,832 (1973)

DIHYDROMOCIMYCIN
$C_{43}H_{62}N_2O_{10}$
M.p. 123°C

Streptomyces namocissimus yields this antibiotic which is crystalline and is laevorotatory with a specific rotation of $[\alpha]_D - 85°$. It is produced by culturing the organism on a nutrient medium containing a source of assimilable carbohydrate at a pH of 4·0–7·0, with aeration and stirring. The structure has been established from chemical and spectroscopic examination.

Jongsma *et al*, *German Patent*, 2,621,615 (1976)

9-DIHYDRONIDDAMYCIN
$C_{40}H_{67}O_{13}N$
M.p. 120–122°C

This antibiotic compound is formed by conversion of a medium containing niddamycin sulphate by *Streptomyces albireticulia* NRRLB 1670 or *S. eurocidicus* NRRLB 1676. The structure has been elucidated by means of NMR and mass spectrometry. The antibiotic is active against a range of gram-positive bacteria.

Theriault, Hager, *U.S. Patent*, 3,817,836 (1974)

10,11-DIHYDROPICROMYCIN
$C_{28}H_{49}NO_7$

A derivative of picromycin, this antibiotic has been isolated from cultures of *Streptomyces venezuelae*. It exhibits activity against gram-positive bacteria.

Majer *et al.*, *J. Antibiotics* (Japan), **29**, 769 (1976)

DIHYDROSTREPTOMYCIN
$C_{21}H_{41}O_{12}N_7$
M.p. 215–225°C

This synthetic antibiotic is produced by hydrogenation of streptomycin in H_2O with a platinum catalyst at atmospheric pressure. Chemical investigation shows that the aldehyde group in the streptose moiety in the molecule is reduced. The antibiotic forms a white granular powder and has a specific rotation of $[\alpha]_D^{25} - 88.7°$ (c 1·0, H_2O). It is not inactivated by either cysteine or hydroxylamine. The biological activity is virtually identical to that of streptomycin. The toxicity is similar to that of streptomycin although auditory impairment is more common and vestibular disturbance less. It finds very little use in medicine as streptomycin.

Peck *et al.*, *J. Amer. Chem. Soc.*, **68**, 1390 (1946)

Heck *et al.*, *Minutes 12th V. A. Conf. Chemotherapy of Tuberculosis*, Atlanta, **125**, 294 (1953)

11:11′-DIHYDROXYCHAETOCIN
$C_{30}H_{28}O_8N_6S_4$
M.p. 233–234°C (*dec.*)

This antimicrobial metabolite is produced by *Verticillium tenerum*. It is strongly dextrorotatory having a specific rotation of $[\alpha]_D^{20} + 758°$ (c 1·02, $(CH_3)_2SO$). The dimeric structure given above is based upon chemical degradative studies and spectroscopic data.

Hauser, Loosli, Niklaus, *Helv. Chim. Acta*, **55**, 2182 (1972)

3′,8-DIHYDROXY-4′,6,7-TRIMETHOXYISOFLAVONE
$C_{18}H_{16}O_7$

An isoflavone isolated from cultures of a *Streptomyces* species, this antibiotic is a specific inhibitor of catechol-O-methyl transferase. It exhibits no hypotensive action. The structure has been deduced from chemical analysis and a study of the infrared, NMR and mass spectra.

Chimura *et al.*, *J. Antibiotics* (Japan), **28**, 619 (1975)

DIMOCILLIN
See Methicillin

DIPLOCOCCIN
$C_{16}H_{10}O_5Cl_4$
M.p. 232°C

The antibacterial properties of a substance produced by an unclassified lactic-acid producing streptococcus was first observed by Whitehead, but the compound itself was not isolated until 1944 by Oxford. Diplococcin is produced by surface growth on a culture medium containing inorganic salts, sucrose and heart broth. It may be isolated by decanting the supernatant liquor, centrifuging the cells and drying them *in vacuo*. The dried bacteria are then milled, washed with H_2O containing a small amount of AcOH and extracted by refluxing with 0·4 per cent aqueous AcOH. The picrate is then obtained and the antibiotic purified by decomposing this salt with AcOH in EtOH. Diplococcin appears to be a polypeptide. It gives positive tests for proteins except Millon and Hellers. It is soluble in H_2O, insoluble in absolute EtOH and is precipitated by protein reagents such as ammonium sulphate and tannic acid. It gives a negative Molisch test, but positive tests for arginine, tryptophane and tyrosine. The antibiotic is stable in acid solutions but unstable under alkaline conditions.

Diplococcin is assayed by serial dilution using a streptococcus normally employed as a 'cheese-starterd' as test organism. The activity *in vitro* has been examined by Oxford, typical inhibition dilutions being: *Staphylococcus aureus* (10,000); *Streptococcus cremoris* (200,000); *Strep. hemolyticus* (20,000) and *Strep. lactis* (10,000). It has no activity against *Escherichia coli*. Diplococcin is unusual in that the organism which is most sensitive to the antibiotic is a streptococcus almost indistinguishable from that which produces the antibiotic.

Whitehead, *Biochem. J.*, **27**, 1793 (1933)
Oxford, *ibid.*, **38**, 178 (1944)

DIPLOICIN
$C_{16}H_{22}O_5Cl_4$

Diploicin is elaborated by the lichen *Buellia canescens* and has the probable structure given above. Inhibition dilutions *in vitro* determined by Barry are *Corynebacterium diphtheriae mitis* (100,000); *Mycobacterium smegmatis* (70,000) and *Myco. tuberculosis* (100,000).

Barry, *Nature*, **158**, 131 (1946)

DISTAMYCIN A
$C_{22}H_{27}O_4N_5$
M.p. Indefinite

A trimeric peptide antibiotic produced by a *Streptomyces* species, this substance yields a crystalline hydrochloride from dilute HCl with m.p. 184–187°C. The ultraviolet spectrum of this salt has two absorption maxima at 237 and 303 nm. The structure has been established by chemical and spectroscopic analysis. Distamycin has antiviral properties, inhibiting the plaque formation and replication of Aujeszky's virus at 0·05–0·20 mM. Addition of the antibiotic to a DNA-dependent RNA polymerase system instantly halted the initiation of new RNA chains although it was found that growing chains were resistant to the drug.

Puschendorf *et al.*, *Biochem. Biophys. Res. Commun.*, **43**, 617 (1971)
Chandra *et al.*, *Collect. Pap. Annu. Symp. Fundam. Cancer Res.*, **25**, 290 (1974)
Pancheva, *Acta Microbiol. Virol. Immunol.*, **2**, 69 (1975)

DIUMYCIN A'
M.p. 165–170°C (*dec.*)

Streptomyces umbrinus ATCC 15,972 yields two phosphorus containing antibiotics which may be separated by silica gel chromatography or countercurrent distribution. This antibiotic is a colourless compound having a specific rotation of $[\alpha]_D$ + 13° (c 1·0, H_2O). It is active against a wide range of gram-positive bacteria.

Slusarchyk *et al.*, *J. Antibiotics* (Japan), **26**, 391 (1973)
Slusarchyk, Weisenborn, *German Patent*, 2,255,563 (1973)

DIUMYCIN B'

M.p. 170°C (dec.)

A second phosphorus-containing antibiotic elaborated by *Streptomyces umbrinus* ATCC 15,972, this compound has a specific rotation of $[\alpha]_D + 13°$ (c 1·0, H_2O) and has the same antibiotic properties as the preceding substance.

Slusarchyk et al., *J. Antibiotics* (Japan), **26**, 391 (1973)
Slusarchyk, Weisenborn, *German Patent*, 2,255,563 (1973)

DORICIN

$C_{43}H_{52}O_{11}N_8$
M.p. 170–190°C

Produced by *Streptomyces loidensis*, this antibiotic belongs to the macrocyclic polypeptide class. It is laevorotatory with a specific rotation of $[\alpha]_D^{20} - 92°$ (c 1·0, CH_3OH) and is active against a range of gram-positive and gram-negative bacteria.

Bodansky, Sheehan, *Antimicrobial Agents & Chemotherapy*, 38 (1963)
Charles-Sigler, Gil-Av, *Tetrahedron Lett.*, 4231 (1966)

DOXORUBICIN

See Adriamycin

DOXYCYCLINE

$C_{22}H_{24}O_8N_2$

A semi-synthetic tetracycline antibiotic, this substance differs from most of the other antibiotics of this class in being quantitatively absorbed in man when given orally. It is active against both gram-positive and gram-negative bacteria, inhibiting the growth of *Bacillus*, *Shigella*, *Staphylococcus* and *Streptococcus* strains and *Escherichia coli*. It also has a high curative rate against gonorrhoea. The antibacterial activity is greater and has a longer duration than that of tetracycline hydrochloride. Experiments with mice show that it also reduces the acute toxicity associated with daunomycin (q.v.). Doxycycline is a very useful tetracycline antibiotic as it can be used in cases of renal failure and is lipid soluble.

Stephens et al., *J. Amer. Chem. Soc.*, **80**, 5324 (1958)
McCormick et al., *ibid.*, **82**, 3381 (1960)
McCormick, Jensen, *U.S. Patent*, 3,019,260 (1961)
von Wittenau et al., *J. Amer. Chem. Soc.*, **84**, 2645 (1962)
Beereboom, Butler, *U.S. Patent*, 3,069,467 (1963)
Stephens et al., *J. Amer. Chem. Soc.*, **85**, 2643 (1963)
Monnier, Bourse, Onfray, *Int. Congr. Chemother., Proc. 5th*, **1**, 785 (1967)
Magliardi, Schach Von Wittenau, *ibid.*, **4**, 165 (1967)
Annunziata, Aulisio, Romito, *Arch. Ital. Laringol.*, **76**, 295 (1968)
Ciceri et al., *Bull. Chim. Farm.*, **109**, 605 (1970)
Fabre et al., *Advan. Antimicrob. Antineoplas. Chemother., Proc. Int. Congr. Chemother., 7th*, **1**, 29 (1971)
Tarvainen et al., *ibid.*, **1**, 1429 (1971)
Mannhart, Dettli, Spring, *Schweiz. Med. Wochenschr.*, **101**, 123 (1971)
Leibowitz et al., *Curr. Ther. Res., Clin. Exp.*, **14**, 820 (1972)
Yakovlev, *Antibiotiki*, **18**, 1041 (1973)
Arena et al., *J. Antibiotics* (Japan), **26**, 339 (1973)
Guiti, Abtahi, *Chemotherapy*, **19**, 65 (1973)

DROSOPHILIN B

See Pleuromutilin

E

E129 COMPLEX
See Ostreogrycin

ECHINOCANDIN
See Antibiotic SL 7810

ECHINOMYCIN (*Quinomycin A*)
$C_{50}H_{60}O_{12}N_{12}S_2$
M.p. 217–218°C

A macrocyclic peptide antibiotic, echinomycin is elaborated by *Streptomyces echinatus* and *Streptomyces* strains X-53 and X-63. From the latter it may be formed from cell-free extracts of the fungus grown in the presence of mercaptoethanol, ATP and magnesium salts which act as precursors. The structure has been established by chemical degradation and spectroscopic examination. Echinomycin forms somewhat hygroscopic crystals and is laevorotatory with $[\alpha]_D^{20} - 310°$ (c 0·86, $CHCL_3$). It possesses a neutral reaction and is active against a wide range of gram-positive organisms. The LD_{50} in mice is 0·4 mg/kg given intraperitoneally.

Corbaz *et al.*, *Helv. Chim. Acta*, **40**, 199 (1957)
Dhar *et al.*, *Pure Appl. Chem.*, **28**, 469 (1971)
Structure
  Keller-Schlierlein, Mihailovic, Prelog, *Helv. Chim. Acta*, **42**, 305 (1959)

EDEINE A₁
$C_{32}H_{58}O_{10}N_{10}$

Bacillus brevis Vm4, mutant strain 587, yields two polyamine antibiotics when grown on a medium containing glycerol, yeast extract, L-asparagine and inorganic salts at 34°C and pH 7·2–7·4 for 30 hours. The antibiotic induces the formation of mutants which are resistant to streptomyces when added to cultures of *Bacillus subtilis* and *Escherichia coli* and exerts a powerful bactericidal action. Edeine A₁ has been shown to bind reversibly to polynucleotides *in vitro* and inhibits DNA and protein synthesis *in vivo*. The antibiotic activity appears to be related to the ability to combine with nucleic acids.

Borowski, Chmara, *Acta Microbiol. Pol.*, **16**, 159 (1967)
Hettinger *et al.*, *Ann. N.Y. Acad. Sci.*, **171**, 1002 (1970)
Sander-Tabaczynska, Tabaczynski, *Acta Microbiol. Pol.*, **3A**, 29 (1971)

EDEINE B₁
$C_{33}H_{60}O_{10}N_{12}$

Also present in the culture of *Bacillus brevis* Vm4, mutant strain 587, this antibiotic has a structure very similar to that of edeine A₁. This has been determined by complete partial acid hydrolysis and by digestion of the compound with carboxypeptidase B. It has a similar binding effect to polynucleotides and also inhibits DNA and protein synthesis.

Borowski, Chmara, *Acta Microbiol. Pol.*, **16**, 159 (1967)
Hettinger *et al.*, *Ann. N.Y. Acad. Sci.*, **171**, 1002 (1970)
Sander-Tabaczynska, Tabaczynski, *Acta Microbiol. Pol.*, **3A**, 29 (1971)

EFROTOMYCIN
$C_{59}H_{88}N_2O_{20}$

This antibiotic has been obtained by culturing *Streptomyces lactamdurans* under submerged conditions for 4 days at 28°C in a medium of glucose, yeast, distillers solubles, corn starch and L-phenylalanine. The fermentation broth is extracted with $CHCl_3$ followed by petroleum ether. Efrotomycin is effective against gram-positive and gram-negative bacteria and also coccidiosis in mice and chickens.

Wax *et al.*, *J. Antibiotics* (Japan), **29**, 670 (1976)
Maiese *et al.*, *U.S. Patent*, 4,024,251 (1977)

EFSIOMYCIN
See Fluvomycin

EHRLICHIN
An antibiotic produced by *Streptomyces lavendulae*, this compound is obtained by adjusting the culture filtrate to pH 2·0 with concentrated HCl and collecting the filtrate by centrifuging. The antibiotic is a dark brown amorphous powder which is non-dialysable. It is stable in neutral and alkaline solutions and although inactivated by horse serum *in vitro* it is not affected by tryptic digestion.

Ehrlichin is active against influenza B *in vivo* and inhibits both influenza A and B *in vitro*. It is, however, inactive against bacteria, fungi, bacterial and pox viruses and *Chlamydozoaceae*. The antibiotic is only moderately toxic with LD_{50} in mice of 300 mg/kg administered subcutaneously and 100 mg/kg when given intraperitoneally. So far, it has found no use in medicine.

Groupe *et al.*, *J. Immunol.*, **67**, 471 (1951)

ELAIOMYCIN
$C_{13}H_{26}O_3N_2$
B.p. Indefinite

Streptomyces hepaticus yields this antibiotic which forms a pale yellow oil having no definite boiling point. The compound is dextrorotatory with a specific rotation of $[\alpha]_D^{26} + 38\cdot4°$ (c. 2·8, EtOH) and gives an ultraviolet spectrum with a single absorption maximum at 237·5 nm.

It is stable in air and light, sparingly soluble in H_2O but soluble in all common organic solvents. The monoacetate is an oil, b.p. 84–90°C/0·5 mm with a specific rotation of $[\alpha]_D^{27} + 25·3°$ (c 3·0, EtOH). Elaiomycin inhibits the growth of a number of bacteria, particularly *Mycobacterium tuberculosis* var. *hominis in vitro*.

Haskell et al., *Antibiotics & Chemotherapy*, **4**, 141 (1954)
Ehrlich et al., ibid., **4**, 338 (1954)
Anderson et al., ibid., **6**, 100 (1956)
Structure
Stevens et al., *J. Amer. Chem. Soc.*, **78**, 3229 (1956)
Configuration
Stevens et al., *J. Amer. Chem. Soc.*, **81**, 1435 (1959)

EMERICID
$C_{44}H_{76}O_{14}$

A member of the family of polyether monocarboxylic acid antibiotics, emericid has recently been isolated from cultures of *Streptomyces hygroscopicus* DS 24 367. It forms a sodium and silver salt which are virtually isomorphous, the structure of the antibiotic having been determined from X-ray crystallographic examination of these salts. Emericid is active against gram-positive bacteria and has shown promise in the treatment of coccidial infections in poultry.

Benazet et al., *Int. Congr. Chemother., 9th*, M432 (1975)
Riche, Pascard-Billy, *Chem. Commun.*, 951 (1975)

EMERIMICINS
A recently discovered group of antibiotics, the emericidins are produced by *Emericellopsis microspora* when 4-*trans*-n-propyl-L-proline is added to the fermentation medium. Little is known at present of their chemical constitution although it appears that this particular aminoacid is not incorporated into the molecular structures of the antibiotics but merely serves to induce their formation in the medium.

Argoudelis, Johnson, *J. Antibiotics* (Japan), **27**, 274 (1974)

ENDOMYCIN
The mycelium of a *Streptomyces* species allied to *S. albus* elaborates this antibiotic. It is normally extracted with BuOH, concentrated to a gum, re-extracted with Et_2O followed by evaporation to dryness and the residue suspended in H_2O. Further extraction with Et_2O removes any impurities and the active precipitate is formed by adjusting the pH of the aqueous solution to 4·5. Endomycin is soluble in the lower alcohols and methyl cellosolve but insoluble in Et_2O, C_6H_6, $CHCl_3$, AcOEt, H_2O and solvents for fats. It is thermostable at 100°C for at least 30 minutes. The antibiotic is active against bacteria, being more active against gram-positive than gram-negative organisms and also active against yeast-like fungi, more so than against the filamentous type. It is relatively non-toxic, mice surviving a dose of 0·5 g/kg but being killed by 1·0 g/kg.

Gottlieb et al., *Phytopathology*, **41**, 393 (1951)

ENDOSUBTILYSIN
An antibiotic substance isolated from *Bacillus subtilis*, endosubtilysin is obtained by extracting the culture liquor pellicle with EtOH at a pH of 3·0. $CHCl_3$ and half-saturated saline are then added to the extract, the $CHCl_3$ layer extracted with dilute alkali at pH 8·0–9·0, the aqueous fraction concentrated, adjusted to pH 3·0 once more and extracted with $CHCl_3$. Petroleum ether is then added to the $CHCl_3$ fraction, the aqueous phase separated and neutralized.

Endosubtilysin is normally assayed by the serial dilution technique using *Staphylococcus aureus* as test organism. The antibiotic is highly active *in vitro* against *Eberthella typhi*, *Escherichia coli*, *Mycobacterium tuberculosis* and *Staphylococcus aureus*. It possesses a very low toxicity towards both rabbit and man.

Saint-Rat, Olivier, *C.R. Acad. d. sc.*, **222**, 296 (1946)

ENDURACIDINS
Streptomyces fungicidicus yields a complex of polypeptide antibiotics when grown under submerged aerobic conditions. The complex has been separated into enduracidins A and B and, when *S. fungicidicus* strain B-5477 is grown on a medium under somewhat different conditions, two further members, enduracidins S_A and S_B are produced. The latter two antibiotics apparently have the same structures as enduracidins A and B but with α-amino-3:5-dichloro-4-hydroxyphenylacetic acid replaced by α-amino-3-chloro-4-hydroxyphenylacetic acid. The antibiotics are active against both gram-positive and acid-resistant bacteria, especially *Bacillus subtilis*

and *Staphylococcus aureus*. Typical LD_{50} values for mice are 60 mg/kg given intravenously and 880 mg/kg when administered intraperitoneally.

Tanayama *et al.*, *J. Antibiotics* (Japan), **21**, 313 (1968)
Takeda Chem. Indust., *Fr. Patent*, 1,514,139 (1968)
Mizuno *et al.*, *Antimicrobial Agents & Chemotherapy*, 6 (1970)
Sugita *et al.*, *Takeda Kenkyusho Ho*, **31**, 313 (1972)

ENHYGROFUNGIN
M.p. Indefinite

An antibiotic isolated from cultures of *Streptomyces hygroscopicus*, this compound has not yet been obtained in a state of purity. It is active against *Bacillus subtilis*, *Cryptococcus neoformans* and *Saccharomyces cerevisiae*.

Bergy, Hoeksema, Johnson, *German Patent*, 2,028,934 (1970)

ENNIATIN A (*Lateritiin I*)
$C_{36}H_{63}O_9N_3$
M.p. 122–122·5°C

Fusarium orthoceras var. *enniatinum* elaborates two, possibly three, closely related antibiotics, enniatins A, B and C. This particular substance is also produced by *F. sciroi*. From both organisms, the antibiotic is obtained by surface culture on a medium containing glucose and inorganic salts. From *Fusarium orthoceras* var. *anniatinum* a product containing 1000 *Mycobacterium tuberculosis* units/ml is obtainable from the mycelium, very little activity being found in the culture filtrate. The mycelium is pressed dry, milled with anhydrous sodium sulphate and extracted with Et_2O, the ethereal extract being dried and evaporated to yield a reddish-brown oil. This may be purified by adsorbing on a neutral alumina column, eluting with Et_2O, $Et_2O-C_6H_6$ and $Et_2O-AcOH$, combining the eluates, diluting with CH_3OH and cooling to $-15°C$. On addition of distilled H_2O, enniatin A is precipitated. Pure enniatin A forms colourless needles when recrystallized from aqueous EtOH. It is soluble in most common organic solvents but insoluble in H_2O. It is optically active with the following specific rotations: $[\alpha]_D^{18} - 90°$ (c 1·0, $CHCl_3$) and $-91·9°$ (c 0·926, $CHCl_3$). It may be sublimed *in vacuo* without any significant loss of activity and gives no typical absorptions in the ultraviolet spectrum. Enniatin A is a thermostable substance but rapidly becomes deactivated by alkalies although only slowly by acids.

The antibiotic is assayed by serial dilution using *Mycobacterium paratuberculosis* as the test organism. Typical inhibition dilutions ($\times 1000$) determined by Gaueumann and his colleagues are: *Bacillus subtilis* (320); *Escherichia coli* ($>1·0$); *Mycobacterium paratuberculosis* (1200); *Myco. phlei* (310); *Myco. tuberculosis hominis* (100–500) and *Staphylococcus aureus* (160).

Gauemann *et al.*, *Experientia*, **9**, 202 (1947)
Plattner, Nager, *ibid.*, **9**, 326 (1947)
Cook *et al.*, *Nature*, **160**, 31 (1947)
Plattner, Nager, Boller, *Helv. Chim. Acta*, **31**, 594 (1948)
Plattner, Nager, *ibid.*, **31**, 2192 (1948)

ENNIATIN B
$C_{33}H_{57}O_9N_3$
M.p. 174·5–175·5 and 173–173·5°C

This antibiotic is isolated from *Fusarium orthoceras* var. *enniatinum* and is obtained from the pressed and dried mycelium in the same manner as the preceding antibiotic. It is purified by chromatography on alumina when crystalline fractions are obtained. The proposed structure is very similar to that of enniatin A. From the chromatographic purification, two crystalline forms have been obtained having the above melting points. The higher melting modification has a specific rotation of $[\alpha]_D - 106·3°$ (CH_3OH-H_2O) and the lower $[\alpha]_D - 107·5°$ (petroleum ether). Enniatin B is slightly soluble in H_2O and on acid hydrolysis yields 2 moles each of N-methyl-(+)-

valine and D-α-hydroxyvaleric acid. Alkaline hydrolysis furnishes D-α-hydroxy*iso*valeryl-N-methyl-(+)-valine, the corresponding lactone and 4-methyl-3:6-di*iso*propyl-2:5-dioxo-morpholine.

The antibiotic is assayed by serial dilution with *Mycobacterium paratuberculosis* and has an antibiotic spectrum *in vitro* very similar to that of the preceding antibiotic.

Plattner, Nager, Boller, *Helv. Chim. Acta*, **31**, 594 (1948)
Plattner, Nager, *ibid.*, **31**, 665 (1948)

ENNIATIN C

This substance, isolated from *Fusarium orthoceras* var. *enniatinum*, was originally believed to be a mixture of enniatins A and B although somewhat later work indicates that it may be an isomer of anniatin A.

Plattner, Nager, Boller, *Helv. Chim. Acta*, **31**, 594 (1948)
Plattner, Nager, *ibid.*, **31**, 2203 (1948)

ENOCIN

An antibiotic produced by the fermentation of *Streptomyces salivarius* ATCC 31,067 on a common nutrient medium for 7–8 hours at 37°C, enocin is particularly active against group A streptococci and most other pantothenate-requiring organisms.

Sanders, Sanders, *U.S. Patent*, 3,925,160 (1975)

ENSHUMYCIN
$C_{39}H_{49}N_8O_{11}S$
M.p. 215–219°C

Enshumycin has been obtained by culturing *Streptomyces enshuensis* FERM-P 2444 aerobically on a medium of dried yeast, glucose, cottonseed powder and inorganic salts at 27–28°C and pH 7·0 for about 40 hours. It is separated by extraction of the culture filtrate with an organic solvent and purified by silica gel and alumina column chromatography. The antibiotic is an amorphous white powder and is laevorotatory with a specific rotation of $[\alpha]_D^{20} - 217·4°$. It is freely soluble in MeOH, EtOH, AcOEt, AcOBu, Me_2CO, $CHCl_3$ and C_6H_6, but insoluble in H_2O and hexane. Enshumycin has been shown to be effective against *Bacillus*, *Staphylococcus*, *Streptococcus*, *Sarcina* and *Xanthomonas*. It has LD_{50} in mice of > 650 mg/kg when given orally.

Minowa et al., *Japanese Patent*, 75 111,289 (1975)

ENTEROCIN
$C_{22}H_{22}O_{10}$

This antibiotic has been isolated from cultures of *Streptomyces candidus* var. *enterostaticus* WS-8096 and also from variant M-127 of *Streptomyces viridochromogenes*. It possesses a bacteriostatic action against gram-positive and gram-negative bacteria but is without activity against fungi or yeasts. The structure has been elucidated from chemical and spectroscopic data.

Miyairi et al., *J. Antibiotics* (Japan), **29**, 227 (1976)
Structure
Tokuma, Miyairi, Morimoto, *J. Antibiotics* (Japan), **29**, 1114 (1976)

ENTEROMYCIN
$C_6H_8O_5N_2$
M.p. Indefinite

A simple antibiotic, enteromycin is produced by *Streptomyces albireticuli*. It has the structure N-(O-methyl-*aci*-nitroacetyl)-3-aminoacrylic acid. Enteromycin crystallizes from CH_3OH in two interchangable crystal forms and in thermolabile and also unstable in acids or alkalies. It is only sparingly soluble in H_2O and other common solvents. The ultraviolet spectrum in CH_3OH has absorption maxima at 230, 275 and 298 nm. The methyl ester forms colourless crystals from CH_3OH with m.p. 141°C. Enteromycin is active against a range of gram-positive bacteria and has LD_{50} in mice of 1·35 mg/10 g.

Nakazawa, *Chem. Abstr.*, **51**, 10647 (1957)
Structure
Mizuno, *Bull. Chem. Soc., Japan*, **34**, 1419, 1425, 1631, 1633 (1961)

EPIDERMIDINS

A number of closely related antibiotics have been isolated from *Staphylococcus epidermidis* strains 29297 and 36534. Purification of the antibiotics has been carried out by treatment with dilute acid and barium hydroxide followed by precipitation with zinc chloride. Epidermidins A_1 and A_2 are the Zn-precipitable and Zn-soluble components derived from strain 29297 and epidermidins B_1 and B_2 are the corresponding fractions isolated from strain 36534. All components are active against gram-positive bacteria.

Hsu, Wiseman, *Can. J. Microbiol.*, **17**, 1223 (1971)

EPOFORMIN
$C_7H_8O_3$
M.p. 75°C

A simple epoxy-5:6-unsaturated ketone, epoformin has been isolated from the culture filtrate of *Penicillium claviforme*. It forms colourless crystals and is dextrorotatory with a specific rotation of $[\alpha]_D^{23}$ + 114·3° (c 1·0, EtOH). The structure has been deduced from its physicochemical properties and its conversion into known benzoquinone derivatives.

Epoformin has little activity against bacteria but possesses a strong cytotoxic activity against PS cells and a somewhat lower activity against L-1210 sarcoma.

Yamamoto et al., *Takeda Kenkyusho Ho*, **32**, 532 (1973)

7β,8β-EPOXYISORORIDIN E
$C_{29}H_{36}O_9$

A derivative of isororidin E (q.v.), this antibiotic has been obtained from the culture broth of *Cylindrocarpon* strain PF-60 by extraction with AcOEt followed by separation and purification by silica gel column and preparative thin layer chromatography. The antibiotic is active against gram-positive and some gram-negative bacteria.

Matsumoto et al., *J. Antibiotics* (Japan), **30**, 681 (1977)

1:2-EPOXYPROPYLPHOSPHONIC ACID (*Phosphonomycin*)
$C_3H_7O_4P$
M.p. 94°C

The antibiotic produced by *Streptomyces fradiae*, *S. viridochromogenes* and *S. wedmorensis*, grown in the presence of phosphates, has been shown to be the (−)-*cis* form of the above acid. The structure has been determined by chemical methods and confirmed by synthesis.

Hendlin et al., *French Patent*, 1,574,556 (1969)
Hendlin et al., *Science*, **166**, 122 (1969)
Christensen et al., *ibid.*, **166**, 123 (1969)
Synthesis
Glamkowski et al., *J. Org. Chem.*, **35**, 3510 (1970)

7β,8β-EPOXYRORIDIN H
$C_{29}H_{34}O_9$

An antibiotic obtained from aerobic cultures of *Cylindrocarpon* strain PF-60, this compound has the structure shown above which is based upon chemical correlations and spectroscopic data. It is active against a number of gram-positive and gram-negative bacteria.

Matsumoto et al., *J. Antibiotics* (Japan), **30**, 681 (1977)

EQUISETIN
$C_{22}H_{31}NO_4$
M.p. 65–66°C

A white amorphous powder, equisetin has been obtained from cultures of *Fusarium equiseti* NRRL 5537. It has the structure shown above and gives an ultraviolet spectrum in ethanolic solution having absorption maxima at 235, 250 and 292 nm. Equisetin is active against a range of gram-positive bacteria.

Burmeister, *U.S. Patent, Appl.*, 457,548 (1974)

ERICAMYCIN
$C_{31}H_{23}O_8N$
M.p. 260–265°C

An antibiotic pigment, this substance is produced by deep aerated submerged culture of *Streptomyces varius* ATCC 19562 at pH 7·0–8·0 and 27–28°C for 3–4 days. Ericamycin is a thermostable compound and there is no significant change in its antibacterial activity when a solution in dimethylformamide is heated at 100°C for 1 hour. It is active mainly against gram-positive bacteria, in particular it inhibits the growth of *Staphylococcus aureus*. It shows synergistic activity in combination with a number of antibiotics including chloramphenicol, erythromycin, kanamycin, the penicillins and streptomycin. It is comparatively non-toxic, no abnormal symptoms being observed in mice following an oral administration of 100 mg/kg. The LD_{50} in mice is 0·5–1·0 mg/kg given intraperitoneally.

Hara *et al.*, *U.S Patent*, 3,769,403 (1973)

ERIZOMYCIN
M.p. Indefinite

Isolated from a culture of *Streptomyces griseus* var. *erizensis* NRRL 3242, erizomycin has been obtained in a crystalline form. The formula and structure are not yet known with certainty. The antibiotic is active against *Escherichia coli*, *Klebsiella pneumoniae*, *Proteus vulgaris* and a number of *Salmonella* and *Streptococcus* species at 125–250 μg/ml. It has also been shown to inhibit the growth of KB cell cultures.

Herr, Reusser, *U.S. Patent*, 3,367,833 (1968)
Herr, Reusser, *French Patent*, 1,545,790 (1968)

ERYTHRIN
M.p. Indefinite

An antibiotic substance isolated from animal tissues, presumably from erythrocytes, erythrin must not be confused with the erythritol ester of lecanoric acid, derived from the lichen *Rocella tinctoria* and given the same name. The antibiotic may be obtained from the blood of a variety of animals or human blood by extracting with a phosphate buffer at pH 7·6, precipitating with HCl and extracting the precipitate with $(CH_3)_2CO$. When the extract is concentrated by evaporation *in vacuo* and then poured into saline solution, the antibiotic is obtained as a dark brown amorphous powder with no definite melting point. It is soluble in organic solvents, sodium carbonate solution, but insoluble in H_2O. It is stated to be thermostable.

Erythrin is effective against a number of organisms, typical inhibition concentrations (μg/ml) being *Bacillus brevis* (15–31); *Corynebacterium diphtheriae* (15–31); Staphylococcus (31–62); Streptococcus (31–62) and intestinal bacteria (>250).

When applied to the conjunctiva of monkeys which had been traumatized and then infected with diphtheria, erythrin brought about a disappearance of the infection and similar results have been obtained in trials on the oral-nasal cavity with the same disease. Experiments with guinea pigs have also demonstrated that they are protected against experimental diphtheria infections when 0·25 per cent solution is simultaneously given at a dose of 0·1 ml. If the therapeutic dose is delayed, however, there is no protection, apparently due to the non-diffusibility of the antibiotic.

Zil'ber, Yakobson, *Zhur. Mikrobiol. Epidemiol. Immunobiol.*, **12**, 3 (1946)

ERYTHROCIN
See Erythromycin

ERYTHROMYCIN (*Erythrocin, Ilotycin*)
$C_{37}H_{67}O_{13}N$
M.p. 136–140°C (190–193°C)

A number of closely related macrocyclic antibiotics have been isolated from *Streptomyces erythreus*. This particular compound forms colourless crystals from either $CHCl_3$ or aqueous $(CH_3)_2CO$ which melt at 136–140°C, resolidify and then remelt at the higher figure given above. The antibiotic is laevorotatory having specific rotations of $[\alpha]_D^{25} - 73.5°$ (CH_3OH) and $[\alpha]_D^{25} - 78°$ (c 1·99, EtOH). It yields a series of crystalline derivatives including the benzoate, m.p. 184–188°C; *p*-chlorobenzoate, m.p. 190–193°C; $[\alpha]_D^{24} - 84°$ (c 1·0, $CHCl_3$); succinate, m.p. 153–157°C; hexadecanoate, m.p. 73–76°C; allyl carbonate, m.p. 115–118°C; ethyl carbonate, $[\alpha]_D^{24} - 75°$ (c 1·0, $CHCl_3$); benzyl carbonate, m.p. 117–128°C; $[\alpha]_D^{24} - 82.6°$ (c 1·0, $CHCl_3$) and the N-oxide, m.p. 220–223°C. The nitrogen is present in the form of a dimethylamino group.

Erythromycin is an antibiotic which, like the propionate, does not cause hepatic damage in patients on administration. Two of the derivatives of this antibiotic, the estolate and the lactobionate do, however, cause liver damage. In the case of the former it has been shown that this toxic property is due to the propionyl ester linkage at the 2'-position in the molecule. The effect of these derivatives is both dose- and time-dependent. When added to an incubation medium containing human liver cells, a concentration of the estolate of 5×10^{-6} molar induced leakage of malate dehydrogenase and aspartate aminotransferase from the cells. Such a leakage of enzyme did not occur with erythromycin or the propionate until the concentration reached a level of 5×10^{-4} molar.

McGuire *et al.*, *Antibiotics & Chemotherapy*, **2**, 281 (1952)
Murphy, *Antibiotics Annual* (1953–54)
Murphy, *Proc. Symp. Antibiotics*, 500, 514 (1953), Washington, D.C.
Bunch, McGuire, *U.S. Patent*, 2,653,899 (1954)
Flynn *et al.*, *J. Amer. Chem. Soc.*, **76**, 3121 (1954)
Flynn, Murphy, McMahon, *ibid.*, **77**, 3104 (1955)
Clark, Taterka, *Antibiotics & Chemotherapy*, **5**, 206 (1955)
Wiley, Weaver, *J. Amer. Chem. Soc.*, **77**, 3422 (1955)
Wiley *et al.*, *ibid.*, **77**, 3676 (1955)
Sigal *et al.*, *ibid.*, **78**, 388 (1956)
Gerzon *et al.*, *ibid.*, **78**, 6396 (1956)
Wiley *et al.*, *ibid.*, **79**, 6062 (1957)
Configuration
  Hofheinz, Grisebach, *Chem. Ber.*, **96**, 2867 (1963)
  Celmer, *J. Amer. Chem. Soc.*, **87**, 1799, 1801 (1965)
Crystal structure
  Harris, McGeachin, Mills, *Tetrahedron Lett.*, 679 (1965)
Cytotoxicity
  Zimmerman, Kendler, Libber, *Proc. Soc. Exptl. Biol. Med.*, **144**, 759 (1973)
  Tolman, Sannella, Freston, *Ann. Intern. Med.*, **81**, 58 (1974)
  Carevic, Prpic, Sverko, *Biochim. Biophys. Acta*, **381**, 269 (1975)

ERYTHROMYCIN B
$C_{37}H_{67}O_{12}N$
M.p. 191–195°C (202–203°C)

Also isolated from *Streptomyces erythreus*, this macrocyclic antibiotic crystallizes as colourless plates from $(CH_3)_2CO$. It is laevorotatory with a specific rotation of $[\alpha]_D^{25} - 78°$ (c 2·0, EtOH). It forms several crystalline salts and derivatives, e.g. the hydrochloride, m.p. 149–150°C; sulphate, m.p. 154–156°C; benzoate, m.p. 102–104°C, octadecanoate, m.p. 54–57°C; the *p*-(*p*-hydroxyphenylazo)-benzene sulphonate, m.p. 165–167°C and the ethyl carbonate, m.p. 117–118°C. It is a broad-spectrum antibiotic, particularly active against *Staphylococcus aureus* and *Streptococcus fecalis*.

Pettinga, Stark, van Abeele, *J. Amer. Chem. Soc.*, **76**, 569 (1954)
Clark, Teterka, *Antibiotics & Chemotherapy*, **5**, 206 (1955)
Gerzon *et al.*, *J. Amer. Chem. Soc.*, **78**, 6412 (1956)
Wiley *et al.*, *ibid.*, **79**, 6070 (1957)
Predicted absolute configuration
Celmer, *J. Amer. Chem. Soc.*, **87**, 1799, 1801 (1965)

ERYTHROMYCIN B 9-(O-METHYLOXIME)
$C_{38}H_{70}O_{12}N_2$

This semi-synthetic antibiotic has been prepared from erythromycin B by reaction with methylhydroxylamine hydrochloride in aqueous CH_3OH. It forms colourless crystals and is active against *Staphylococcus aureus* and *Streptococcus fecalis*.

Von Esch, *German Patent*, 2,200,940 (1972)

ERYTHROMYCIN C
$C_{36}H_{63}O_{13}N$
M.p. 121–125°C

A third macrocyclic antibiotic obtained from cultures of *Streptomyces erythreus*, this compound forms colourless needles when recrystallized from $CHCl_3$. The most probable structure is that given above which is based upon chemical evidence and comparison with the two preceding antibiotics. It is active against gram-positive bacteria.

Wiley *et al.*, *J. Amer. Chem. Soc.*, **79**, 6074 (1957)

ERYTHROMYCIN D
$C_{36}H_{65}NO_{12}$

This erythromycin has been isolated from the mother liquors from the culture of *Streptomyces erythreus* after the crystallization of erythromycin A and has been separated from the other erythromycins by preparative thin layer chromatography. The structure has been determined by chemical and spectroscopic examination. It is a broad spectrum antibiotic and does not cause hepatic damage to patients on administration.

Majer *et al.*, *J. Amer. Chem. Soc.*, **99**, 1620 (1977)

ERYTHROMYCIN E

This macrocyclic antibiotic has recently been isolated from a culture of *Streptomyces erythreus* NRRL 3887 grown on a medium containing monosaccharides, a source of nitrogen and a buffer. The biological activity is similar to that of erythromycin A.

Martin, Goldstein, *U.S. Patent*, 3,801,465 (1974)

ERYTHRONOLIDE B
M.p. 223–225°C

Streptomyces erythreus elaborates this antibiotic which forms colourless crystals from $CHCl_3$. It is active against gram-positive bacteria.

Petzoldt, Kieslich, *German Patent*, 1,900,647 (1970)

ESKACILLIN V
See Penicillin V

ESPERINE
$C_{39}H_{67}O_{11}N_3$
M.p. 238°C (*dec.*)

Bacillus mesentericus elaborates this peptide antibiotic which forms colourless needles which decompose on melting. It has a specific rotation of $[\alpha]_D^{15} - 24°$ (c 0·66, CH_3OH) and forms a sodium salt as colourless needles from aqueous EtOH with m.p. 268–269°C. Treatment with sodium hydroxide hydrolyses the substance with the formation of esperidine, m.p. 195°C; *trans*-2-tridecenoic acid, DL-leucine, L-aspartic acid and L-valine. It is inhibitory against a range of gram-positive organisms.

Ogawa, Ito, *J. Agr. Chem. Soc., Japan*, **24**, 191 (1950)
Kochi *et al.*, *Japanese Patent*, 2497 (1951)
Ogawa, Ito, *J. Agr. Chem. Soc., Japan*, **26**, 432 (1952)
Ogawa, Ito, *Bull. Agr. Chem. Soc., Japan*, **23**, 536 (1959)

ETAMYCIN (*Viridogrisein*)
$C_{44}H_{62}O_{11}N_8$

A cyclic polypeptide antibiotic, this compound has been isolated from various species of *Streptomyces*. It forms colourless crystals and has the following specific rotations: $[\alpha]_D^{25} + 59°$ ($CHCl_3$), $+28°$ (EtOH) and $-10°$ (EtOH, H_2O 1:1). The hydrochloride forms colourless crystals with m.p. 163–170°C (*dec.*). Acid hydrolysis yields 3-hydroxypyridine-2-carboxylic acid, D-leucine, L-valine and D-*allo*hydroxyproline. With $FeCl_3$ the antibiotic gives a red-brown colour.

Heinemann *et al.*, *Antibiotics Annual*, 728 (1954–55)
Bartz *et al.*, *ibid.*, 777 (1954–55)
Sheehan, Zachau, Lawson, *J. Amer. Chem. Soc.*, **79**, 3973 (1954)

ETRUSCOMYCIN
See Lucensomycin

EULICIN
$C_{24}H_{52}O_8N_2$
M.p. Indefinite

This antifungal antibiotic is derived from a species of *Streptomyces* allied to

Eumycin

H$_2$NCNH(CH$_2$)$_8$CHCH(CH$_2$)$_3$NH$_2$ (with NH, OH, and NHCO(CH$_2$)$_8$NHCNH$_2$, NH substituents)

S. parvus. It is characterized as the trihydrochloride, a hygroscopic white powder which is H$_2$O-soluble and the helianthate, colourless crystals from CH$_3$OH, decomposing at 154–156°C after sintering at 142°C. The compound is active against a number of gram-positive bacteria and a range of pathogenic fungi.

Charney *et al.*, *Antibiotics Annual*, 228 (1955–56)
Charney *et al.*, *U.S. Patent*, 2,998,438 (1961)
Structure
Harman *et al.*, *J. Amer. Chem. Soc.*, **80**, 5173 (1958)

EUMYCIN
M.p. Indefinite

Eumycin has been obtained from a strain of *Bacillus subtilis* by surface growth on a buffered peptose-proteose-yeast extract broth, incubated for 5 days at 30°C. The culture filtrate is acidified to form a precipitate which is filtered, extracted with EtOH, the alcoholic extract evaporated and the residue dissolved in NaOH at pH 7·0. Eumycin is thermostable, unstable above pH 8·0, soluble in EtOH, (CH$_3$)$_2$CO and BuOH but insoluble in Et$_2$O or amyl acetate.

The antibiotic inhibits the growth of *Actinomyces*, *Epidermophyton floccosum* and related fungal species, *Microsporum gypseum*, *Mycobacterium tuberculis* (avian and human), *Trichophyton mentagrophytes*; less active against *Hormodendrum* species and *Sporotrichum*. It has only a slight activity against Staphylococcus aureus and none against *Cryptococcus*, *Monilia* and the colon-typhoid bacilli. It is most active against *Corynebacterium diphtheriae*, concentrations as low as 0·005 mg/ml being bacteriostatic. When tested *in vivo* in mice it exhibits a very low toxicity.

Johnson, Burdon, *J. Bact.*, **51**, 590 (1946)

EVERNINOMICIN B
C$_{66}$H$_{99}$NO$_{36}$Cl$_2$
M.p. 184–185°C

A complex antibiotic isolated from cultures of *Micromonospora carbonaceae*, this substance is laevorotatory with a specific rotation of $[\alpha]_D - 33 \cdot 1°$ (CHCl$_3$). The structure has been determined from chemical and spectroscopic examination. It is active against gram-positive bacteria.

Ganguly, Saksena, *J. Antibiotics* (Japan), **28**, 707 (1975)

EVERNINOMICIN C
C$_{63}$H$_{93}$NO$_{34}$Cl$_2$
M.p. 181–184°C

A further antibiotic obtained from the culture medium of *Micromonospora carbonaceae*, this compound has a specific rotation of $[\alpha]_D - 33 \cdot 7°$. The structure is very similar to that of everninomicin B.

Ganguly, Szmulewicz, *J. Antibiotics* (Japan), **28**, 710 (1975)

EVERNINOMICIN D
$C_{66}H_{99}NO_{35}Cl_2$
M.p. Indefinite
An amorphous white powder having no definite melting point, this antibiotic is produced by *Micromonospora carbonaceae*. It is laevorotatory having a specific rotation of $[\alpha]_D - 32.4°$. The structure has been established from chemical and spectroscopic data and comparison with those of the other everninomicins.

Ganguly *et al.*, *J. Amer. Chem. Soc.*, **97**, 1984 (1975)

EXFOLIATIN
$C_{27}H_{40}O_{16}Cl$
M.p. 172°C
An antibiotic isolated from *Streptomyces exfoliatum*, exfoliatin is obtained by extraction of the broth with AcOEt followed by concentration *in vacuo* to a syrup which is washed with petroleum ether. The crude antibiotic thus obtained is purified by recrystallization from EtOH. It forms colourless needles when pure, is soluble in CH_3OH, EtOH, $(CH_3)_2CO$, Et_2O and AcOEt and insoluble in petroleum and H_2O.

The antibiotic is active against gram-positive bacteria but shows little, if any, activity against gram-negative organisms with the exception of *Hemophilus*. The LD_{50} in mice is approximately 500 mg/kg when given subcutaneously.

Umezawa *et al.*, *J. Antibiotics* (Japan), **5**, 466 (1952)

Umezawa *et al.*, *Japan. J. Med. Sci. Biol.*, **5**, 311 (1952)

EZOMYCIN A₁
$C_{26}H_{38}O_{15}N_8S$
M.p. Indefinite
An unclassified *Streptomyces* species produces two aminoglycosidic antibiotics, ezomycins A_1 and A_2. This compound forms a white amorphous powder with no definite melting point. It is inactive against bacteria but is effective against phytopathogenic fungi such as *Botrytis* and *Sclerotinia*.

Ezomycin A₂

Sakata, Sakurai, Tamura, *Agr. Biol. Chem.*, **37**, 697 (1973)
Sakata, Sakurai, Tamura, *Tetrahedron Lett.*, 4327 (1974)

EZOMYCIN A$_2$
C$_{19}$H$_{26}$O$_{12}$N$_6$
M.p. Indefinite

A second antifungal antibiotic isolated from cultures of an unclassified *Streptomyces* species. This substance also forms an amorphous powder and has an antibiotic activity limited to phytopathogenic fungi such as *Botrytis* and *Sclerotinia*.

Sakata, Sakurai, Tamura, *Agr. Biol. Chem.*, **37**, 697 (1973)
Sakata, Sakurai, Tamura, *Tetrahedron Lett.*, 4327 (1974)
Sakata, Sakurai, Tamura, *Agr. Biol. Chem.*, **39**, 885 (1975)

EZOMYCIN B$_1$
C$_{26}$H$_{37}$N$_7$O$_{16}$S
M.p. >200°C (*dec.*)

A further component of the ezomycin complex elaborated by a strain of *streptomyces*, this substance has the structure given above which has been elucidated from chemical and spectroscopic evidence. It melts, with decomposition, above 200°C and is laevorotatory with a specific rotation of $[\alpha]_D^{22} - 5.5°$ (c 0.83, H$_2$O). It possesses antifungal properties.

Sakata *et al.*, *Agr. Biol. Chem.*, **38**, 1883 (1974)
Sakata *et al.*, *Tetrahedron Lett.*, 3191 (1975)

EZOMYCIN B$_2$
C$_{19}$H$_{25}$N$_5$O$_{13}$
M.p. >205°C (*dec.*)

Also isolated from the ezomycin complex by chromatographic methods, this antifungal antibiotic forms colourless prisms of the monohydrate and is dextrorotatory having a specific rotation of $[\alpha]_D^{16} + 10.8°$ (c 1.02, MeOH). The structure has been established from chemical analysis and a study of the infrared, NMR and mass spectra.

Sakata *et al.*, *Agr. Biol. Chem.*, **38**, 1883 (1974)
Sakata *et al.*, *Tetrahedron Lett.*, 3191 (1975)

EZOMYCIN C$_1$
C$_{26}$H$_{37}$N$_7$O$_{16}$S
M.p. >200°C (*dec.*)

An amorphous white powder, this ezomycin antibiotic has been obtained as the monohydrate by chromatography of the antibiotic complex produced

Ezomycin C₂

by an unclassified species of *Streptomyces*. It melts above 200°C with decomposition and has a specific rotation of $[\alpha]_D^{22} - 76.4°$ (c 0.9, H$_2$O). The structure has been elucidated from chemical and spectroscopic data. Ezomycin C$_1$ possesses an antifungal activity but is only weakly active against bacteria.

Sakata *et al.*, *Tetrahedron Lett.*, 3191 (1975)

EZOMYCIN C$_2$
$C_{19}H_{25}N_5O_{13}$
M.p. >200°C (*dec.*)

This antibiotic has been obtained from the ezomycin complex by column and thin layer chromatography. It forms colourless needles and is laevorotatory with a specific rotation of $[\alpha]_D^{18} - 100°$ (c 0.52, NH$_4$OH). It has been assigned the above structure on the basis of chemical and spectroscopic evidence. It is active against a range of fungi.

Sakata *et al.*, *Tetrahedron Lett.*, 3191 (1975)

EZOMYCIN D$_1$
$C_{26}H_{39}N_7O_{17}S$
M.p. >200°C (*dec.*)

A further component isolated by column and thin layer chromatography

Ezomycin D₂

of the ezomycin complex, this antibiotic is an amorphous white powder and has a specific rotation of $[\alpha]_D^{22} - 62.1°$ (c 0.84, H$_2$O). It has the structure shown above based upon chemical analysis and a study of the infrared, NMR and mass spectra.

Sakata *et al.*, *Tetrahedron, Lett.*, 3191 (1975)

EZOMYCIN D$_2$
$C_{19}H_{27}N_5O_{14}$
M.p. >200°C (*dec.*)

The ezomycin complex obtained from cultures of an unclassified species of *Streptomyces* also yields this antibiotic when subjected to column and thin layer chromatography. It has been obtained as colourless needles and is dextrorotatory with a specific rotation $[\alpha]_D^{18} + 58.8°$ (c 0.87, NH$_4$OH). The structure has been determined from chemical correlations and spectroscopic examination. It is active against a number of fungi.

Sakata *et al.*, *Tetrahedron Lett.*, 3191 (1975)

F

FARCINICIN
See Thiolutin

FELDAMYCIN
$C_{17}H_{25}N_7O_5$

Streptomyces ficellus yields this antibiotic which has been obtained as an amphoteric white powder. The structure has been established from a study of the infrared, NMR and mass spectra. Feldamycin has been shown to inhibit a wide range of bacteria *in vitro* but it has no effect in the treatment of experimental bacterial infections in mice.

   Argoudelis *et al.*, *J. Antibiotics* (Japan), **29**, 1007 (1976)
Structure
   Argoudelis *et al.*, *J. Antibiotics* (Japan), **29**, 1117 (1976)

FENACILIN
See Penicillin V

FERRIMYCIN A
$C_{41}H_{65}O_{14}N_{10}Fe$
M.p. Indefinite

This complex iron-containing antibiotic is produced by *Streptomyces griseoflavus* (Stamm ETH 9578). It is normally isolated as the hydrochloride which is an amorphous hygroscopic solid giving an ultraviolet spectrum with absorption maxima at 229, 319 and 430 nm. It is active against a number of gram-positive organisms.

   Bickel *et al.*, *Helv. Chim. Acta*, **43**, 2105 (1960)
Structure
   Bickel *et al.*, *Tetrahedron*, 8th Suppl., 171 (1966)

FERVENULIN (*Planomycin*)
$C_7H_7O_2N_5$
M.p. 178–179°C

The culture filtrates of *Streptomyces fervens* yield this simple antibiotic which has the structure 6:8-dimethyl-5:7-dioxo-5:6:7:8-tetrahydropyrimido[5,4-e-]-*as*-triazine. Fervenulin forms yellow orthorhombic crystals and gives an ultraviolet spectrum in EtOH with absorption maxima at 238, 275 and 340 nm. It is slightly soluble in cold H_2O, more soluble in hot, readily soluble in most common organic solvents but insoluble in hydrocarbons. Fervenulin is active against a range of gram-positive bacteria.

Eble *et al.*, *Antibiotics Annual*, 227 (1959–60)
Structure
Daves *et al.*, *J. Org. Chem.*, **26**, 5256 (1961)
Synthesis
Pfleiderer, Schündhütte, *Annalen*, **615**, 42 (1958)
Tanabe *et al.*, *Chem. Abstr.*, **60**, 13242 (1964)

FICELLOMYCIN
$C_{13}H_{24}N_6O_3$

An antibiotic isolated from cultures of *Streptomyces ficellus*, this substance has been shown to inhibit the growth of gram-positive bacteria *in vitro*. Tests have demonstrated that it is also effective in the treatment of experimental infections due to *Staphylococcus aureus* in mice.

Argoudelis *et al.*, *J. Antibiotics* (Japan), **29**, 1001 (1976)

FIGAROIC ACID

An antibiotic complex elaborated by *Streptosporangium* strain C-31751 when cultured in a common nutrient medium with stirring at 27°C for 210 hours and the pH adjusted to 3·35, this substance has been purified by fractional precipitation using organic solvents. The structure is not yet known.

Bradner, Buph, Nettleton, *German Patent*, 2,628,487 (1977)

FILIMARISIN (*Filipin*)
$C_{35}H_{58}O_{11}$
M.p. 195–205°C (147°C)

A macrocyclic antibiotic, filimarisin has been isolated from cultures of *Streptomyces filipinensis* obtained from Philippine soil samples. It forms feathery yellow needles when crystallized from $CHCl_3$ and is sensitive to air. A rare, and less stable modification, having the lower melting point given above is sometimes encountered. The antibiotic is laevorotatory with a specific rotation of $[\alpha]_D^{22} - 148\cdot3°$ (c 0·89, CH_3OH) and gives an ultraviolet spectrum with absorption maxima at 322, 338 and 355 nm. Filimarisin is freely soluble in pyridine, dimethylformamide, AcOEt and amyl acetate and insoluble in H_2O, $CHCl_3$ and CH_2Cl_2. It possesses marked antifungal properties and also produces arthritis rapidly when given to rabbits. The LD_{50} in mice is 17 mg/kg when administered intraperitoneally.

Whitfield *et al.*, *J. Amer. Chem. Soc.*, **77**, 4799 (1955)
Structure
Dhar *et al.*, *Proc. Chem. Soc.*, 310 (1960)
Djerassi *et al.*, *Tetrahedron Lett.*, 383 (1961)
Dhar *et al.*, *J. Chem. Soc.*, 842 (1964)
Golding, Richards, *Tetrahedron Lett.*, 2615 (1964)
Pras, Weissman, *Drug Trade News*, **40**, July 4, 1966

FILIPIN
See Filimarisin

FLAMBAMYCIN
$C_{61}H_{90}O_{34}Cl_2$
M.p. 226–228°C

A highly complex antibiotic, flambamycin has been isolated from cultures of *Streptomyces hygroscopicus*. It forms colourless crystals from CH_3OH, EtOH or $(CH_3)_2CO$ and is laevorotatory with a specific rotation of $[\alpha]_D^{20} - 11\cdot4°$ (c 1·0, $CHCl_3$). The structure is not yet known. Flambamycin is active against a number of gram-positive bacteria and some tumours.

Ninet *et al.*, *Experientia*, **30**, 1270 (1974)

FLAVEOLIN
M.p. Indefinite

A *Streptomyces* species resembling *S. flaveolus* yields this antibiotic which is obtained by adsorption from the culture filtrate on charcoal, followed by elution with acidified $(CH_3)_2CO$, concentration *in vacuo*, extraction with BuOH at pH 8·0 and back extraction of the solution with dilute HCl. Further purification may be carried out, but countercurrent distribution between BuOH and phosphate buffer at pH 5·5. Flaveolin is an amorphous yellow, basic substance normally obtained as the hydrochloride which is freely soluble in H_2O, CH_3OH or EtOH, slightly soluble in BuOH, $CHCl_3$, C_6H_6 and $(CH_3)_2CO$ but insoluble in AcOEt, Et_2O and petroleum ether. It has a maximum stability at pH 2·0 and gives negative biuret, Millon and Sakaguchi reactions.

Flaveolin is a broad-spectrum antibiotic, active against gram-positive and gram-negative bacteria, fungi and mycobacteria. It shows a higher degree of activity in acid than in alkaline media. An activity of 25–30 times greater than streptomycin has been claimed. The LD_{50} in mice is approximately 30 mg/kg given intravenously; 10 mg/kg administered in the same manner caused no deaths.

Takahashi, *J. Antibiotics* (Japan), **6A**, 11 (1953)

(-)-FLAVIPUCINE
$C_{12}H_{15}NO_4$
M.p. 130–131°C

A strain of *Aspergillus flavipes* yields this antibiotic which forms white needles when purified by recrystallization from C_6H_6. It is laevorotatory with a specific rotation of $[\alpha]_D^{21} - 71·8°$ (c 1·0, 95% EtOH) and gives an ultraviolet spectrum in ethanolic solution having a single absorption maximum at 330 nm. The structure has been established from chemical and spectroscopic evidence.

Casinovi *et al.*, *Tetrahedron Lett.*, 3175 (1968)
Casinovi *et al.*, *Ann. Ist. Super. Sanita.*, **5**, 523 (1969)
Revised structure
Findlay, Radics, *J. Chem. Soc., Perkin I*, 2071 (1972)
Findlay, Kavan, *ibid.*, 2962 (1972)

FLAVOFUNGIN
$C_{36}H_{58}O_{10}$
M.p. 210°C

Streptomyces flavofungini produces this antibiotic substance which has been shown to be a mixture of the *iso*propyl and the 1-methylpropyl derivatives which are present in a ratio of approximately 10:1. At present, these two components have not been resolved. The ultraviolet spectrum in EtOH has two absorption maxima at 261 and 374 nm.

Bognar *et al.*, *Tetrahedron Lett.*, 471 (1970)

FLAVOMYCIN
See Neomycin

FLAVOMYCOINE
$C_{41}H_{68}O_{10}$
M.p. 161–163°C

Flavomycoine is a polyene antibiotic with marked antifungal properties which has been isolated from cultures of *Streptomyces roseoflavus* var. *jenensis*, being extracted primarily from the mycelium. When crystallized from EtOH it forms yellow-green needles and is laevorotatory with a specific rotation of $[\alpha]_D^{23} - 45°$ (c 1·0, dioxan) and $[\alpha]_D^{23} - 4°$ (c 4·0, pyridine). The ultraviolet spectrum has two absorption maxima at 262 and 363 nm. On catalytic hydrogenation the antibiotic furnishes a decahydro derivative, oxidative degradation of this compound resulting in the formation of 2-methyltridecane-1:13-dioic acid, identified by gas chromatography and mass spectrometry. Chemical and spectroscopic studies indicate that the antibiotic contains a pentaene chromophore which is conjugated with a lactone carbonyl group.

Flavomycoine exhibits inhibitory activity against fungi, protozoa and yeasts.

Schlegel, Thrum, *Experientia*, **24**, 11 (1968)
Schlegel, Thrum, *J. Antibiotics* (Japan), **24**, 360, 368 (1971)

FLAVOVIRIDOMYCIN
M.p. Indefinite

A tetraene antibiotic, flavoviridomycin has been isolated by Russian workers from *Streptomyces flavoviridis fungicidicus* var. nov. Ultraviolet and infrared spectroscopy have demonstrated that this substance is a new antibiotic. The structure is still unknown.

Mitskavich *et al.*, *Antibiotiki*, **18**, 867 (1973)

FLORIMYCIN
See Viomycin

FLUCLOXACILLIN
$C_{19}H_{17}O_5N_3SClF$

This halogen-substituted *iso*xazolyl penicillin antibiotic has recently been prepared and found to be as effective as cloxacillin, dicloxacillin and oxacillin against a wide range of gram-positive cocci *in vitro*. The total and free serum levels following oral administration in humans are generally greater than with these other antibiotics and the extent of binding to human serum protein is very similar. Flucloxacillin has the important property of being stable towards staphylococcal β-lactamase.

Sutherland, Croydon, Rolinson, *Brit. Med. J.*, **4** (5733), 455 (1970)
Renzini *et al.*, *Farmaco, Ed. Sci.*, **28**, 733 (1973)

FLUOPSIN B (*Fluopsin F*)
$C_6H_{12}O_3N_3S_3Fe$
M.p. Indefinite

Japanese workers have recently isolated three unique metal-containing antibiotics by cultivating *Pseudomonas fluorescens* KY 4032 on a paraffin-containing medium at 25–37°C in the presence of inorganic salts. Similar results have been obtained utilizing other carbon sources such as alcohols, glucose, organic acids and sorbitol. The pH is maintained at 4·0–10·0 during the fermentation by the addition of ammonium hydroxide, ammonium carbonate or a solution of urea. This antibiotic is isolated from the culture broth by extraction with $CHCl_3$ or AcOEt and separated from the accompanying components by chromatography on a silica gel column. The antibiotic has a powerful inhibitory effect against most gram-positive and gram-negative bacteria and also exhibits antineoplastic activity.

Ito *et al.*, *J. Antibiotics* (Japan), **23**, 542 (1970)

Shirahata *et al.*, *ibid.*, **23**, 546 (1970)
Tanaka *et al.*, *Japanese Patent*, 7,310,554 (1973)

FLUOPSIN C
$C_4H_8O_2N_2S_2Cu$
M.p. Indefinite

A copper-containing antibiotic also isolated from cultures of *Pseudomonas fluorescens* KY 4032 grown on a paraffin-containing medium. The formation of this antibiotic is dependent upon the amount of cupric ion present in the medium since, if too little is present, fluopsin C is replaced by fluopsin B. The antibiotic also possesses a marked activity against both gram-positive and gram-negative bacteria.

Ito *et al.*, *J. Antibiotics* (Japan), **23**, 542 (1970)
Shirahata *et al.*, *ibid.*, **23**, 546 (1970)

FLUOPSIN F
See Fluopsin B

FLUOPSIN N
$C_4H_8O_2N_2S_2Ni$
M.p. Indefinite

A third antibiotic isolated from *Streptomyces fluorescens* grown on a paraffin-containing medium, fluopsin N contains nickel in the molecule. It is also active in inhibiting the growth of gram-positive and gram-negative bacteria and has a marked antineoplastic activity.

Tanaka *et al.*, *Japanese Patent*, 7,310,554 (1973)

FLUOROPOLYOXIN L
$C_{16}H_{22}O_{12}N_5F$
M.p. Indefinite

Streptomyces cacoi yields two closely related fluorinated antibiotics when grown on a medium to which 5-fluorouracil is added. Alkaline hydrolysis furnishes 5-fluorouracil, 5-fluorouracil polyoxin C, 2-amino-2-deoxy-L-xylonic acid, ammonia and carbon dioxide. The compound inhibits the growth of *Escherichia coli* and *Streptococcus fecalis*.

Isono et al., *J. Amer. Chem. Soc.*, **95**, 5788 (1973)

FLUOROPOLYOXIN M
$C_{16}H_{22}O_{11}N_5F$
M.p. Indefinite

A further antibiotic obtained from cultures of *Streptomyces cacaoi* when grown in a medium containing 5-fluorouracil, this compound yields 5-fluorouracil, 5-fluorouracil polyoxin C, 2-amino-2:3-dideoxy-L-xylonic acid, carbon dioxide and ammonia. It has a lower activity against bacteria than the preceding compound.

Isono et al., *J. Amer. Chem. Soc.*, **95**, 5788 (1973)

FLUVOMYCIN (*Efsiomycin, Riomycin, Vivicil*)
M.p. Indefinite
This antibiotic has been obtained from cultures of *Bacillus subtilis* isolated from fresh river mud at Lawrenceberg, Indiana, U.S.A. It forms a white amorphous powder with no definite melting point and is soluble in H_2O and dilute aqueous CH_3OH and EtOH, but insoluble in Et_2O, $(CH_3)_2CO$, $CHCl_3$ and amyl acetate. It diffuses through agar and dialyzes through a cellophane membrane. The antibiotic is more stable in acid solution than in alkalies.

Although devoid of activity *in vivo*, fluvomycin is active against a large number of pathogenic fungi, gram-positive and gram-negative bacteria *in vitro*. It is normally assayed against *Staphylococcus aureus* strain FDA 209. The LD_{50} in mice is 1·3 g/kg when administered intravenously.

Carvajal, *Antibiotics & Chemotherapy*, **3**, 765 (1953)
Carvajal, *British Patent*, 722,433 (1955)

FOMECIN A
$C_8H_8O_5$
Dec. 160°C

A simple aromatic antibiotic, this substance has been isolated from several strains of *Fomes juniperinus* Schrenk (*Basidiomycete*) cultured on a medium containing corn steep liquor. It forms a cream-coloured to orange crystalline mass from several solvents including aqueous EtOH, AcOEt and $(CH_3)_2CO—C_6H_6$ which decomposes without melting. The ultraviolet spectrum in EtOH exhibits two absorption maxima at 241 and 304 nm. Fomecin A is optically inactive in EtOH, is stable in aqueous solutions at neutral or acid pH but rapidly loses its activity at pH 8·0.

The antibiotic is active *in vitro* against *Bacillus mycoides*, *B. subtilis*, *Escherichia coli*, *Klebsiella pneumoniae*, *Mycobacterium smegmatis*, *Pseudomonas aeruginosa* and *Staphylococcus aureus*.

Fomecin A is comparatively non-toxic, mice tolerating doses up to 50 mg/kg given intravenously. The activity of the antibiotic is considerably reduced in the presence of human blood.

Anchel et al., *Proc. Nat. Acad. Sci. U.S.*, **38**, 655 (1952)
Structure
McMorris, Anchel, *Can. J. Chem.*, **42**, 1595 (1964)

FORMYCIN
$C_{10}H_{12}O_4N_5$
Dec. 144°C
An antibiotic produced by *Streptomyces lavendulae* 6600 GC-1, this com-

pound is prepared by culturing the organism with shaking on a medium containing glycerol, soybean flour and inorganic salts at 27°C for 3 days. The antibiotic is adsorbed from the culture filtrate on activated carbon, eluted with ammoniacal 60 per cent CH_3OH and purified with Dowex 50w-XI and chromatography on a cellulose column. It is primarily active against *Xanthomonas oryzae*, the inhibition concentration being 6μg/ml.

Ishizuka *et al.*, *J. Antibiotics* (Japan), **21**, 1 (1968)
Sumiki, *Japanese Patent*, 6,806,996 (1968)

FORMYCIN B
$C_{10}H_{11}O_5N_4$
M.p. 247°C (*dec.*)

Formycin B may be prepared by enzymic deamination of the preceding antibiotic and is also produced, with formycin, by *Nocardia interforma*. It is more active against *Xanthomonas oryzae* than formycin, the inhibition concentration being 2 μg/ml. Formycin B is laevorotatory with a specific rotation of $[\alpha]_D^{20} - 51\cdot5°C$ (c 1·0, H_2O) and is more soluble in H_2O.

Umezawa, *Japanese Patent*, 21,755 (1967)
Ishizuka *et al.*, *J. Antibiotics* (Japan), **21**, 1 (1968)
Umezawa, *Japanese Patent*, 759 (1968)

FOROMACIDIN A (*Spiromycin A, Spiromycin I*)
$C_{43}H_{74}O_{14}N_2$

One of three macrocyclic antibiotics, the structure of this compound has been revised twice. That given above is the one now generally accepted.

Kuehne, Benson, *J. Amer. Chem. Soc.*, **87**, 4660 (1965)
Paul, Tchelitcheff, *Bull. Soc. Chim. Fr.*, 650 (1965)
Revised structure
Omura *et al.*, *J. Amer. Chem. Soc.*, **91**, 3401 (1969)

FOROMACIDIN B (*Spiromycin B, Spiromycin II*)
$C_{45}H_{76}O_{15}N_2$

This macrocyclic antibiotic has been shown to be the 3-acetyl derivative of foromacidin A.

Kuehne, Benson, *J. Amer. Chem. Soc.*, **87**, 4660 (1965)
Paul, Tchelitcheff, *Bull. Soc. Chim. Fr.*, 650 (1965)
Revised structure
Omura *et al.*, *J. Amer. Chem. Soc.*, **91**, 3401 (1969)

FOROMACIDIN C (*Spiromycin C, Spiromycin III*)
$C_{46}H_{78}O_{15}N_2$

Chemical analysis has shown this antibiotic to be the 3-propionyl derivative of foromacidin A.

Kuehne, Benson, *J. Amer. Chem. Soc.*, **87**, 4660 (1965)
Paul, Tchelitcheff, *Bull. Soc. Chim. Fr.*, 650 (1965)
Revised structure
Omura *et al.*, *J. Amer. Chem. Soc.*, **91**, 3401 (1969)

FORTIMICIN A
$C_{17}H_{35}N_5O_6$

An aminoglycoside antibiotic isolated from *Micromonospora olivoasterospora*, this compound, together with fortimicin B has also been obtained from the fermentation broth of *Micromonospora* species MK-70 and separated and purified by a combination of paper, silica gel column and thin layer chromatography. It forms a white, basic amorphous powder which is soluble in H_2O. Acid hydrolysis yields one mole of glycine. The structure has been established from a study of the proton and ^{13}C NMR and mass spectra. It is active against a range of gram-positive bacteria.

Nara *et al.*, *Japanese Patent*, 75 29,789 (1975)
Okachi *et al.*, *J. Antibiotics* (Japan), **30**, 541 (1977)
Structure
Egan *et al.*, *J. Antibiotics* (Japan), **30**, 552 (1977)

FORTIMICIN B
$C_{15}H_{32}N_4O_5$

This antibiotic also occurs in the culture broth of *Micromonospora* species MK-70 and has been separated from the preceding antibiotic by chromatography. It is also a basic, white amorphous powder soluble in H_2O. It may be differentiated from fortimicin A in not yielding glycine on acid hydrolysis. It is active against gram positive bacteria.

Okachi *et al.*, *J. Antibiotics* (Japan), **30**, 541 (1977)
Structure
Egan *et al.*, *J. Antibiotics* (Japan), **30**, 552 (1977)

FRADICIN
$C_{30}H_{34}O_4N_4$

One of a number of antibiotics which have been isolated from *Streptomyces fradiae*, this compound is obtained by extraction of the broth with BuOH, concentration *in vacuo*, further extraction with EtOH, concentration *in vacuo* and precipitation of the oily substance with a mixture of $(CH_3)_2CO$ and petroleum ether. The oil may then be dissolved in *tert*-BuOH and lyophilized. Fradicin is weakly basic and has the above tentative empirical formula. It is soluble in alcohols, propylene glycol and $CHCl_3$ and insoluble in $(CH_3)_2CO$, CCl_4, C_6H_6, Et_2O and H_2O. It is active against most common fungi, particularly under alkaline conditions but has no activity against bacteria. It is comparatively toxic, the LD_{50} in mice being 4 mg/kg when given both orally and intraperitoneally. The antibiotic has a very irritating action upon rabbit skin.

Swart et al., Proc. Soc. Exptl. Biol. Med., **73**, 376 (1950)
Hickey, Hidy., Science, **113**, 361 (1951)

FRAMYCETIN
See Neomycin B

FRENOLICIN
$C_{18}H_{18}O_7$
M.p. 161–162°C

One of several antibiotics isolated from *Streptomyces fradiae*, this substance forms pale yellow crystals from EtOH. It is laevorotatory having a specific rotation of $[\alpha]_D^{25} - 37·7°$ (c 1·5, CH_3OH). The ultraviolet spectrum in CH_3OH consists of absorption maxima at 234 and 362 nm with a shoulder at 284 nm. In 0·01 N-CH_3OH—NaOH solution there are two absorption maxima at 280 and 425 nm. The antibiotic forms a crystalline acetyl derivative, m.p. 161–163°C and the methyl ester, m.p. 82–83°C, the latter giving a methyl ether, m.p. 109–110°C. The structure has been elucidated primarily from the NMR spectrum.

Van Meter, Dann, Bohonos, *Antibacterial Agents Annual*, 77, Plenum Press, New York (1961)
NMR spectrum
Ellestad, Whaley, Patterson, *J. Amer. Chem. Soc.*, **88**, 4109 (1966)
Ellestad et al., ibid., **90**, 1325 (1968)

FUCOTHRICIN
Streptomyces MYC-19-A elaborates this streptothricin antibiotic which is isolated from the culture broth. In general, the characteristics of this substance resemble those of known streptothricins but it contains a new aminosugar designated fucosamine. Fucothricin is a broad-spectrum antibiotic.

Thirumalachar et al., *Hindustan Antibiotics Bull.*, **14**, 4 (1971)

FULVOPLUMIERIN
$C_{14}H_{12}O_4$
M.p. 151–152°C (dec.)

This simple antibiotic has been obtained from the rind of *Plumeria acutifolia* and forms orange needles when crystallized from a mixture of EtOH and $CHCl_3$. The structure has been established as methyl 7-crotonylidenecyclopenta[c]-pyran-1(7H)-one-4-carboxylate. The solution in EtOH gives a deep red colour on the addition of alkalies. The structure of the antibiotic has been confirmed by synthesis.

Schmid, Bencze, *Helv. Chim. Acta*, **36**, 205, 1468 (1953)
Albers-Schönberg et al., ibid., **45**, 1406 (1962)
Synthesis
Buchi, Carlson, *J. Amer. Chem. Soc.*, **90**, 5336 (1968)

FUMAGILLIN (*Amebacilin, Fumidil, Phagopedin sigma*)
$C_{26}H_{34}O_7$
M.p. 189–194°C

The culture of *Aspergillus fumigatus* H3 yields this antibiotic which crystallizes as colourless prisms from aqueous CH_3OH. It is laevorotatory with a specific rotation of $[\alpha]_D^{25} - 26·6°$ (c 0·25, CH_3OH) and is soluble in most organic solvents but insoluble in H_2O, dilute acids and saturated hydrocarbons. On hydrolysis it furnishes 2:4:6:8:decatetraenedioic acid and fumagillol. The latter has the structure oxiranspiro-2-(3-isopent-2′-enyl-1′-methoxyoxiranyl)-3-methoxycyclohexan-4-ol, m.p. 55–56°C and $[\alpha]_D$ − 68°. Several crystalline amine salts and other derivatives have been prepared; e.g. diamylamine salt, m.p. 143–144°C; decylamine salt, m.p.

163–165°C; dodecylamine salt, m.p. 147–149°C; dicyclohexylamine salt, m.p. 147–148°C (dec.); the methyl ester, m.p. 151–152°C; the octabromo derivative, m.p. 118–122°C and the di-2:4-dinitrophenylhydrazone, m.p. 123–126°C. The antibiotic has both amoebicidal and antiphage properties.

Eble, Hanson, *Antibiotics & Chemotherapy*, **1**, 54 (1951)
Schenck et al., *J. Amer. Chem. Soc.*, **75**, 2274 (1953)

FUMARAMIDMYCIN
$C_{12}H_{12}N_2O_3$

A colourless, crystalline antibiotic, fumaramidmycin has been obtained from cultures of *Streptomycin kurssanovii* NR-7GG1. The structure given above has been confirmed by synthesis from fumaramic acid. The antibiotic is effective against gram-positive and some gram-negative bacteria.

Suhara et al., *J. Antibiotics* (Japan), **28**, 648 (1975)

FUMARYLCARBOXYAMIDO-L-2:3-DIAMINOPROPIONYL-L-ALANINE

A dipeptide antibiotic, this compound has been prepared by culturing *Streptomyces collinus* NRRL 5332 aerobically and under submerged conditions and isolated from the culture filtrate by chromatography on an alumina column. The structure has been determined from an investigation of the hydrolysis products.

The antibiotic is active against *Salmonella gallinarum* and *Trichomonas vaginalis*. The activity against gram-negative organisms is inhibited by D-glucosamine and, to a somewhat lesser extent, by N-acetylglucosamine.

Molloy et al., *J. Antibiotics* (Japan), **25**, 137 (1972)
Gale, Lively, *U.S. Patent*, 3,780,016 (1973)

FUMIDIL
See Fumagillin

FUMIGACHLORIN
$C_{16}H_{25}O_4NCl_2$
M.p. 112–113°C

Sartorya fumigata var. *spinosa* elaborates this antibiotic which forms colourless needles when recrystallized from CCl_4-hexane. It is laevorotatory with a specific rotation of $[\alpha]_D^{26} - 77\cdot5°$ (c 1·0, $CHCl_3$) and gives an ultraviolet spectrum in CH_3OH with absorption maxima at 238, 273 and 325 nm. Fumigachlorin is active primarily against fungi and has only a weak activity against bacteria.

Atsumi et al., *J. Antibiotics* (Japan), **23**, 223 (1970)

FUMIGACIN (*Helvolic acid*)
$C_{32}H_{44}O_8$
M.p. 212°C (215–220°C dec.)

This antibiotic isolated from *Aspergillus fumigatus* was described and named helvolic acid by Chain and his colleagues who isolated it from *Aspergillus fumigatus, mut helvola* Yuill. The identity of the two substances was demonstrated by Menzel and his coworkers in 1944. Fumigacin may be obtained either by surface growth on various media or by submerged growth in shaker flasks and aerated tanks. In both methods, fumigatin (q.v.) and gliotoxin (q.v.) are also produced. Various means of isolation are available including acidifying the culture filtrate with HCl to pH 4·0, adsorbing the activity on activated carbon, eluting with 80 per cent $(CH_3)_2CO$, removing the solvent *in vacuo* and dissolving the residue in $CHCl_3$ or by precipitating the crude fumigacin by acidification of the culture filtrate. The antibiotic may be purified by crystallizing from C_6H_6 and recrystallization from CH_3OH. Fumigacin forms four- and six-sided monoclinic crystals or long colourless needles and is laevorotatory with specific rotations of $[\alpha]_D^{20} - 49\cdot4°$ (c 3·5, $CHCl_3$) and $[\alpha]_D^{25} - 132°$ (c 0·4, $CHCl_3$). The antibiotic is soluble in warm EtOH, $CHCl_3$, $(CH_3)_2CO$, AcOEt, C_6H_6, Et_2O, dioxan, pyridine and glacial AcOH, sparingly so in cold EtOH, CH_3OH, H_2O and petroleum ether. Fumigacin is thermostable, stable in acid solution but less so in alkaline media. It gives negative Molisch, Tollens, Rosenheim, Fehling, Jaffe-Tortelli and digitonin reactions, positive bile acid and Liebermann-Burchard reactions. Catalytic hydrogenation over PtO_2 in EtOH gives the hexahydro derivative, in glacial AcOH, the octahydroderivative is formed.

Fumigacin may be assayed by serial dilution with *Staphylococcus* aureus and by cylinder plate with *Staphylococcus*. Inhibition concentrations (μg/ml) *in vitro* have been measured by Menzel and his colleagues, e.g. *Bacillus anthracis* (6·0); *B. subtilis* (156); *Micrococcus tetragenus* (60); *Staphylococcus albus* (4·0); *Staph. aureus* (14–15); *Staph. citreus* (4·0); *Streptococcus hemolyticus* (5–25) and *Strep. viridans* (312).

Inhibition dilutions ($\times 1000$) have been measured by several groups of investigators against a larger number of organisms, typical figures being: *Bacillus anthracis* (160); *B. cereus* (500); *B. megatherium* (1250); *B. mycoides* (1250); *Corynebacterium diphtheriae* (640); *Clostridium septique* (80); *Cl. welchii* (320); *Diplococcus pneumoniae* III (10); *Escherichia coli* (0·5–1200); *Mycobacterium smegmatis* ($>0·5$); *Myco. tuberculosis* (10–100); *Neisseria intracellularis* (40); *Pseudomonas aeruginosa* (0·5); *Salmonella cholerae-suis* (>40); *S. schottmuelleri* (>40); *S. typhi* (0·5); *Shigella dysenteriae* ($>2·5$); *Sh. paradysenteriae* ($>2·5$); *Sh. sonnei* ($>2·5$); *Staphylococcus aureus* (80–2000); *Streptococcus pyogenes* (40); *Strep. viridans* (>160).

A slight decrease in activity has been noted due to the action of various agents including bacterial extract, liver extract, pus, serum and yeast extract. Both staphylococcus and streptococcus show a resistance to the antibiotic with successive transfers in a medium containing fumigacin. The antibiotic possesses a moderate activity *in vivo*. When administered to mice experimentally infected with staphylococcus and streptococcus it prolonged the survival period while 2–4 mg given subcutaneously afforded a 50 per cent protection against *Streptococcus hemolyticus*.

Fumigacin has a moderately low toxicity. Waksman and Geiger have shown that 16 mg given intraperitoneally to mice is tolerated. An experiment in which 1·0 mg proved lethal has been attributed to the presence of gliotoxin in the fumigacin given. The LD_{50} in mice is 400 mg/kg given intraperitoneally. A dose of 4 mg given intraperitoneally caused necrosis of the liver whereas 20 mg given orally was tolerated. Repeated oral doses, however, caused severe liver damage. Fumigacin is absorbed from the gastrointestinal tract and after intravenous administration it is found in both the blood and urine although none has been detected in the spinal fluid.

Waksman, Horning, Spencer, *Science*, **96**, 202 (1942)
Wilkins, Harris, *Brit. J. Exptl. Path.*, **23**, 166 (1942)
Chain *et al.*, *ibid.*, **24**, 108 (1943)
Crowfoot, Low, *ibid.*, **24**, 120 (1943)
Waksman, Norning, Spencer, *J. Bact.*, **45**, 233 (1943)
Waksman, Geiger, *ibid.*, **47**, 391 (1944)
Menzel, Wintersteiner, Hoogerhide, *J. Biol. Chem.*, **152**, 419 (1944)
Birkinshaw, Bracken, Raistrick, *Biochem. J.*, **39**, 70 (1945)
Jennings, *Nature*, **156**, 633 (1945)
Elliott *et al.*, *Fed. Proc.*, **6**, 250 (1947)

FUMIGATIN
$C_8H_8O_4$
M.p. 116°C

Aspergillus fumigatus elaborates this simple antibiotic which may also be conveniently produced by synthesis from 3:4:5-trimethoxybenzene. It is obtained naturally by surface growth on a medium containing tartaric acid and inorganic salts and incubated at 24°C for between 31 and 37 days. Fumigatin is isolated by aerating the culture filtrate to produce the quinone form, acidifying with dilute HCl, extracting with $CHCl_3$, evaporating the extract to dryness *in vacuo* and extracting the residue with petroleum ether in a Soxhlet. Purification is best carried out by recrystallization from petroleum ether. The antibiotic forms maroon-coloured crystals which can be sublimed unchanged in a high vacuum. It is soluble in Et_2O, $(CH_3)_2CO$, C_6H_6, $CHCl_3$, AcOEt and EtOH, moderately soluble in H_2O, only slightly so in petroleum ether. It is unstable in aqueous solution and readily reduced to the corresponding quinol. The structure, as 3-hydroxy-4-methoxy-2:5-toluquinone, has been confirmed by synthesis.

Like the preceding antibiotic, fumigatin is assayed by serial dilution using *Staphylococcus aureus* as the test organism. Typical inhibition dilutions ($\times 1000$) are: *Bacillus anthracis* (33–50); *B. subtilis* (40); *Escherichia coli* (1·2–12); *Sarcina lutea* (100); *Salmonella typhimurium* ($>2·0$); *Staphylococcus aureus* ($>1·2$–200); *Streptococcus viridans* (1·2–20) and *Vibrio comma* (100).

Anslow, Raistrick, *Biochem. J.*, **32**, 687 (1938)
Raistrick, *Chem. Ind.*, **57**, 293 (1938)
Anslow, Raistrick, *Biochem. J.*, **32**, 2288 (1938)
Baker, Raistrick, *J. Chem. Soc.*, 670 (1941)
Oxford, Raistrick, *Chem. Ind.*, **61**, 128 (1942)
Waksman, Geiger, *J. Bact.*, **47**, 391 (1944)
Menzel, Wintersteiner, Hoogerheide, *J. Biol. Chem.*, **152**, 419 (1944)

FUNGICHROMIN
$C_{35}H_{58}O_{12}$
M.p. 205–210°C

A macrocyclic antibiotic, fungichromin has been isolated from cultures of *Streptomyces cellulosae* found in Texan soil. It forms a very stable monohydrate as colourless crystals with the above melting point. The antibiotic is laevorotatory with a specific rotation of $[\alpha]_D - 172°$ (c 0·25, CH_3OH) and gives an ultraviolet spectrum in CH_3OH with absorption maxima at 322·5, 338·5 and 356·5 nm. It is soluble in CH_3OH, EtOH, BuOH, $(CH_3)_2CO$, dimethylformamide and pyridine, insoluble in H_2O and aliphatic hydrocarbons.

Fungichromin is active against a large number of pathogenic fungi. It has no oral toxicity in mice at 1 g/kg but is toxic at a dose of 16·4 mg/kg when administered intraperitoneally.

Tytell et al., Antibiotics Annual, 716 (1954–55)
Structure
Cope, Johnson, J. Amer. Chem. Soc., **80**, 1504 (1958)
Cope et al., ibid., **84**, 2170 (1962)

FUNGICIDIN
See Nystatin

FUNGICIDIN RAW
See Antimycoin

FUNGIMYCIN NC-1968
See Perimycin A

FUNGISPORIN
$C_{56}H_{72}O_8N_8$
M.p. 355–360°C (dec.)
Several *Penicillium* and *Aspergillus* species elaborate this macrocyclic polypeptide antibiotic which forms colourless crystals that sublime from 250°C and possess the rather indefinite melting point given above. The structure has been established primarily from an investigation of the hydrolysis products.

Sumiki, Miyao, J. Agr. Chem. Soc., Japan, **26**, 27 (1952)

Sumiki, Miyao, Bull. Agr. Chem. Soc., Japan, **19**, 86 (1955)
Miyao et al., ibid., **24**, 23 (1960)

FUNGOSIN
See Bacillomycin A

FUNICULOSIN
$C_{27}H_{41}O_7N$
M.p. Indefinite
An antifungal and antiviral antibiotic, funiculosin is derived from *Penicillium funiculosum*, the fungus being cultivated on a common nutrient medium at 26·5°C for 4 days. It is obtained by extraction of the mycelium with $(CH_3)_2CO$ followed by chromatography on a silica gel column. The antibiotic is insoluble in H_2O and forms colourless crystals from $(CH_3)_2CO$. It has no activity against bacteria but is effective against *Candida albicans* and *Piricularia oryzae* and also inhibits the growth of a number of viruses. The LD_{50} in mice is given as 2 mg/kg when administered intraperitoneally.

Tamura et al., Japanese Patent, 7,128,829 (1971)

FURANOMYCIN
$C_7H_{11}O_3N$
M.p. Indefinite

A neutral aminoacid, furanomycin is elaborated from the culture filtrate of *Streptomyces* L-803 (ATCC 15,795). It is active against *Escherichia coli*, the inhibitory activity being completely reversed by *iso*leucine. It also inhibits the growth of T-even coliphage.

Katagiri et al., J. Med. Chem., **10**, 1149 (1967)

FUSAFINGINE (*Locabiotal*)

$C_{29}H_{51}O_8N_2$
M.p. 125–129°C

This antibiotic has been isolated from cultures of *Fusarium lateritium*. It forms colourless crystals when purified by recrystallization from EtOH or CH_3OH.

Couchoud, *French Patent*, 1,164,181 (1960)
Servier, *Belgian Patent*, 612,474 (1962)

FUSCIN

$C_{15}H_{16}O_4$
M.p. 230°C

A quinonoid metabolite obtained from *Oidiodendron fuscum* Robak, this compound is formed by surface growth on a Czapek-Dox medium incubated for 24–30 days at 24°C. In the culture filtrate it is present as the colourless reduced form and is converted into the active quinonoid form by aeration in the presence of ferrous sulphate at pH 9·0. The crude material is extracted with boiling EtOH, the extract being cooled and the pure fuscin allowed to crystallize. Fuscin forms bright orange diamond-shaped plates which can be sublimed in a high vacuum between 160 and 180°C. It is soluble in $(CH_3)_2CO$, $CHCl_3$, AcOEt, AcOH and hot EtOH; moderately so in C_6H_6 and Et_2O, slightly soluble in cold EtOH and insoluble in H_2O and petroleum ether. It forms a sodium salt as deep purple cubic crystals and a stable crystalline salt with thioglycollic acid, colourless needles, m.p. 193°C which is also antibiotically active.

Assayed by serial dilution with *Staphylococcus aureus*, it has the following inhibition dilutions ($\times 1000$) *in vitro*: *Bacillus anthracis* (320–1280); *B. subtilis* (80); *Corynebacterium diphtheriae gravis* (160); *C. diphtheriae intermedium* (320); *C. diphtheriae mitis* (320); *Escherichia coli* (5·0); *Mycobacterium phlei* (10); *Myco. smegmatis* (20); *Proteus vulgaris* (5·0); *Salmonella enteriditis* (>5·0); *S. paratyphi* (>5·0); *S. typhi* (10); *Shigella flexneri* (>5·0); *Sh. shigae* (10); *Staphylococcus albus* (80); *Staph. aureus* (80–1280); *Staph. citreus* (1280); *Streptococcus pyogenes* (640); *Strep. viridans* (640) and *Vibrio comma* (80).

Marcus has determined similar inhibition dilutions for the derivative with thioglycollic acid: *Bacillus subtilis* (40); *Escherichia coli* (>5·0); *Corynebacterium diphtheriae mitis* (640); *Proteus vulgaris* (5·0); *Staphylococcus aureus* (40–160) and *Vibrio comma* (20). From these observations, fuscin has found some use as an antibacterial.

Michael, *Biochem. J.*, **42**, xl (1948)
Michael, *ibid.*, **43**, 528 (1948)
Marcus, *ibid.*, **43**, 532 (1948)
Birkinshaw *et al.*, *ibid.*, **48**, 67 (1951)
Barton, Hendrickson, *J. Chem. Soc.*, 1028 (1956)

FUSIDIC ACID (*Fusidin*)

$C_{31}H_{48}O_6$
M.p. 192–193°C

Isolated from a strain of *Fusidium*, this antibiotic belongs to the steroidal class and crystallizes from C_6H_6 as colourless needles of the solvate which have the melting point given above. The specific rotation is $[\alpha]_D^{20} - 9°$ (c 1·0, $CHCl_3$) and the ultraviolet spectrum consists of an absorption maximum at 204 nm with a shoulder at 210 nm. The compound may be characterized as the crystalline 3-acetate, m.p. 121°C; $[\alpha]_D^{20} - 23°$ ($CHCl_3$), forming an acetate as colourless needles, m.p. 119–120°C; $[\alpha]_D^{20} - 26°$ ($CHCl_3$).

Fusidic acid is active mainly against gram-positive bacteria, e.g. *Bacillus subtilis*, *Staphylococcus aureus* and against certain gram-negative organisms such as *Escherichia coli*. In the case of *B. subtilis*, Guha and Szulmajster have demonstrated that the antibiotic inhibits both spore formation and protein synthesis when added to either the log phase or to sporulating cells. With *Escherichia coli* or *Staphylococcus aureus*, or chick embryonic fibroblasts, it has been shown by Gerastimova and Gershanovich that maximum absorption of the antibiotic into the cells occurs during the first few minutes after the introduction of fusidic acid into the incubation medium. Accumulation of the antibiotic is inhibited by low temperature.

Fusidin

    Godtfredson et al., *Nature*, **193**, 987 (1962)
    Godtfredson, Vangedal, *Tetrahedron*, **18**, 1029 (1962)
    Arigoni et al., *Experientia*, **19**, 521 (1963)
    Melera, *ibid.*, **19**, 565 (1963)
    Bucourt et al., *Compt. Rend.*, **257**, 2679 (1963)
Stereochemistry
    Arigoni et al., *Experientia*, **20**, 344 (1964)
    Godtfredson et al., *Tetrahedron*, **21**, 3505 (1965)
Mass spectrum
    Lynch et al., *Experientia*, **19**, 211 (1963)
Crystal structure
    Cooper, *Tetrahedron*, **22**, 1379 (1966)
    Cooper, Hodgkin, *ibid.*, **24**, 909 (1968)
Biological activity
    Kiryushchenkov et al., *Antibiotiki*, **18**, 723 (1973)
    Gerastimova, Gershanovich, *ibid.*, **18**, 918 (1973)
    Guha, Szulmajster, *Fed. Eur. Biochem. Soc., Lett.*, **38**, 315 (1974)

FUSIDIN
    See Fusidic acid

G

GARLANDOSUS

This antibiotic is produced by *Streptomyces althioticus* var. *garlandosus* NRRL 3109 and is obtained by first using a soil stock of the fungus to inoculate a sterile medium containing glucose and cottonseed meal for 3 days at 28°C. This culture is then used to inoculate a sterile medium containing liquid corn sugar, cottonseed meal and lard oil which is incubated with aeration at 28°C for 2 days. A second inoculum of this material is then used to inoculate a medium consisting of dextrin, blackstrap molasses, fish meal, lard oil, wheat grits and H_2O and the culture grown at 28°C, with aeration, for 63 hours. At the end of this procedure the broth assay against *Sarcina lutea* was found to be 386 µg of garlandosus/ml. The antibiotic is extracted by filtering the broth through diatomaceous earth and extracting with CH_2Cl_2, the extract being concentrated when crystallization occurs. The crystalline material has a potency of 1200 µg/mg. Garlandosus is active against gram-negative bacteria and inhibits the growth of gram-positive organisms.

Bergy, De Boer, *U.S. Patent*, 3,642,984 (1972)

GATAVALIN

M.p. 245–248°C

A bacis polypeptide antibiotic, gatavlin is elaborated by *Bacillus polymyxa* subsp. *colistinus* ATCC 21,830. The antibiotic is obtained by aerobic fermentation of the organism on common media at pH 7·0 and 28°C for 3–5 days. Gatavalin is isolated from both the culture filtrate and bacterial cells by heating at pH 2·0–5·0 and 70°C for 10–15 minutes and extracting with BuOH, the extract being concentrated under reduced pressure and crude gatavalin being precipitated with Et_2O. Purification is carried out by dissolving the crude antibiotic in an aqueous mixture of BuOH and CH_3OH and chromate graphing on an alumina column. The crystalline compound has a molecular weight of about 2000 and is dextrorotatory with a specific rotation of $[\alpha]_D^{23} + 22\cdot4°$ (c 0·65, 50 per cent CH_3OH). Hydrolysis shows the presence of aspartic acid, alanine, glutamic acid, threonine and valine.

Gatavalin is active against gram-positive bacteria, mycobacteria, moulds and yeasts. The LD_{50} in mice and rats when given intraperitoneally are 22·5 mg/kg and >50 mg/kg respectively.

Bergy, De Boer, *U.S. Patent*, 3,642,984 (1972)
Nakatsugawa *et al.*, *German Patent*, 2,251,916 (1974)
Nakajima, Chihara, Koyama, *J. Antibiotics* (Japan), **25**, 243 (1972)
Nakajima *et al.*, *Japanese Patent*, 7,329,150 (1973)
Nakajima *et al.*, *Japanese Patent*, 7,332,353 (1973)
Nakajima *et al.*, *British Patent*, 1,346,972 (1974)
Nakajima *et al.*, *French Patent*, 2,203,620 (1974)

GELBECIDIN

M.p. 169–170°C

Certain *Streptomyces* species have been found to elaborate this antibiotic which forms colourless crystals from EtOH. The substance is dextrorotatory with a specific rotation of $[\alpha]_D^{26} + 140°$ (c 1·0, $CHCl_3$).

Robinson *et al.*, *German Patent*, 1,942,694 (1970)

GELDANAMYCIN

$C_{29}H_{40}O_9N_2$
M.p. 252–255°C

A macrocyclic antibiotic produced by *Streptomyces hygroscopicus*, this compound forms yellow needles when recrystallized from $CHCl_3$. It has a specific rotation of $[\alpha]_D^{25} + 55°$ (c 0·6, $CHCl_3$). The structure has been established from chemical and spectroscopic evidence.

Genipic acid

De Boer et al., *J. Antibiotics* (Japan), **23**, 442 (1970)
Structure
Sasaki et al., *J. Amer. Chem. Soc.*, **92**, 7591 (1970)

GENIPIC ACID
$C_9H_{12}O_4$
M.p. Indefinite

A plant antibiotic, isolated from *Genipa americana* L., this antibiotic forms an amorphous white powder with no definite melting point. It is laevorotatory having a specific rotation of $[\alpha]_D^{27} - 105°$ (c 1·0, EtOH) and gives an ultraviolet spectrum in EtOH consisting of a single absorption maximum at 203 nm. It has been characterized as the crystalline ammonium salt, m.p. 125–130°C (dec.) and the methyl ester which is a colourless oil that cannot be crystallized.

Tallent, *Tetrahedron*, **20**, 1781 (1964)

GENTAMICIN

A bactericidal antibiotic complex isolated from a number of *Micromonospora* species, this compound has been separated into a number of aminoglycosidic components which are described below. The gentamicins show, in general, a higher antibacterial action than streptomycin, kanamycin or neomycin.

They are effective against several gram-negative bacteria including *Enterobacter*, *Escherichia*, *Klebsiella*, *Salmonella*, *Serratia*, some *Proteus* species and *Pseudomonas aeruginosa* with minimum inhibitory concentrations of between 0·06 and 8·0 micrograms/millilitre. Among the gram-positive bacteria only *Straphylococcus aureus* is highly sensitive to these antibiotics, the minimum inhibitory concentration against this organism being between 0·125 and 1·0 micrograms/millilitre. Other gram-positive organisms are less sensitive although *Bacillus*, *Clostridium* and *Corynebacterium* species are susceptible and *Listeria monocytogenes* may be inhibited at normal concentrations.

The sulphate is the salt normally used clinically to treat septicaemia and other systemic infections due to susceptible organisms and this may be given intramuscularly or intravenously. The gentamicins are also used topically and sometimes systemically in the treatment of staphylococcal infections but the topical use has been shown to lead to the emergence of resistance strains.

Boyce, *Brit. J. Clin. Pract.*, **22**, 197 (1968)
Washington et al., *Mayo Clin. Proc.*, **45**, 146 (1970)
Klatersky et al., *Amer. J. Med. Sci.*, **262**, 283 (1971)
Klatersky, *Antimicrobial Agents & Chemotherapy*, **1**, 441 (1972)
Washington, *Ann. Intern. Med.*, **76**, 611 (1972)
Davis, Iannetta, *Appl. Microbiol.*, **23**, 775 (1972)

GENTAMICIN A₁ (*Gentamicin A*)
$C_{18}H_{36}O_{10}N_4$
Dec. 200°C

This aminoglycosidic antibiotic is elaborated by *Micromonospora species*, particularly *M. echinospora* and *M. purpurea*. The culture filtrate at pH 2·0 is treated with oxalic acid to precipitate calcium ions and the supernatant liquor passed through an Amberlite IRC-50 column and eluted with 2N-ammonium hydroxide followed by gel chromatography which separates the components of the antibiotic complex. The original gentamicin A has now been separated by countercurrent distribution into four constituents. Gentamicin A_1 is obtained as colourless prismatic needles of the sesquihydrate which sinter at 150°C and slowly decompose above 200°C. The antibiotic is dextrorotatory with a specific rotation of $[\alpha]_D^{23} + 136°$ (c 1·0, H_2O). It is soluble in H_2O, slightly so in CH_3OH and insoluble in EtOH. On hydrolysis it furnishes glucosamine and 2-deoxystreptomine. Gentamicin A_1 is a broad-spectrum antibiotic, active against bacteria and protozoa and possesses anthelmintic properties.

Maehr, Schaffner, *J. Chromatog.*, **30**, 572 (1967)
Cooper, Waitz, *German Patent*, 2,130,113 (1972)
Structure
Maehr, Schaffner, *J. Amer. Chem. Soc.*, **89**, 6787 (1967)
Maehr, Schaffner, *ibid.*, **92**, 1697 (1970)
Nagabhushan et al., *J. Org. Chem.*, **40**, 2830 (1975)

GENTAMICIN A₂
$C_{17}H_{33}O_9N_3$
M.p. Indefinite

The structure of this component of the gentamicin A complex has been determined by mass spectrometry and chemical examination of the hydrolysis products. It has a similar antibiotic activity to that of the preceding compound.

Nagabhushan et al., *J. Org. Chem.*, **40**, 2835 (1975)

GENTAMICIN A₃
$C_{18}H_{36}O_{10}N_4$
M.p. Indefinite

An isomer of gentamicin A₁, this antibiotic also occurs in the complex forms by *Micromonospora echinospora* and *M. purpurea*. It is a broad-spectrum antibiotic, active against gram-positive and gram-negative bacteria, protozoa, some fungi and also possessing anthelmintic properties.

Nagabhushan et al., *J. Org. Chem.*, **40**, 2830 (1975)

GENTAMICIN A₄
$C_{19}H_{36}O_{11}N_4$
M.p. Indefinite

A fourth component of the gentamicin A complex produced by *Micromonospora echinospora* and *M. purpurea*, the structure of this antibiotic is that given above based upon mass spectrometry and chemical degradation studies.

Nagabhushan et al., *J. Org. Chem.*, **40**, 2830 (1975)

GENTAMICIN B
$C_{19}H_{38}O_{10}N_4$

A further aminoglycosidic antibiotic separated from the complex isolated from cultures of *Micromonospora echinospora* and *M. purpurea*, this component also possesses antibacterial, antiprotozoal and anthelmintic activity. The structure has been determined primarily from a study of the hydrolysis products.

Cooper, Waitz, *German Patent*, 2,130,113 (1972)

GENTAMICIN B₁
$C_{20}H_{40}O_{10}N_4$

Also isolated from the antibiotic complex produced by culturing *Micromonospora echinospora* or *M. purpurea* on common media followed by isolation and purification by chromatography on silica gel, this compound is the methyl derivative of the preceding antibiotic. Its biological activity is similar to that of all the gentamicins.

Cooper, Waitz, *German Patent*, 2,130,113 (1972)

GENTAMICIN C *Garamycin*ᴿ)

Gentamicin C is a broad-spectrum antibiotic complex isolated from *Micromonospora purpurea* NRRL 2953. Column chromatography separates the complex into three active components which are described below. All possess antibacterial, antiprotozoal and anthelmintic properties characteristic of this group of antibiotics.

GENTAMICIN C$_1$
C$_{21}$H$_{43}$O$_7$N$_5$
M.p. 94–100°C

This component of the gentamicin C complex forms colourless crystals and is dextrorotatory with a specific rotation of $[\alpha]_D^{25}$ + 158° (H$_2$O). It is characterized as the triacetate, m.p. 206–225°C which is also dextrorotatory with $[\alpha]_D^{25}$ + 143° (CH$_3$OH). The structure given has been determined by mass spectrometry.

Weinstein et al., *Antimicrobial Agents & Chemotherapy*, 1 (1963)
Weinstein et al., *J. Med. Chem.*, **6**, 463 (1963)
Cooper et al., *J. Chem. Soc.*, C, 2876, 3126 (1971)
Marquez, Wagman, Cooper, *U.S. Patent*, 3,651,042 (1972)

GENTAMICIN C$_{1a}$
C$_{19}$H$_{39}$O$_7$N$_5$

A minor component of the gentamicin C complex, the structure given above has been established by mass spectrometry.

Cooper et al., *J. Chem. Soc.*, C, 2876, 3126 (1971)
Marquez, Wagman, Cooper, *U.S. Patent*, 3,651,042 (1972)

GENTAMICIN C$_2$
C$_{20}$H$_{41}$O$_7$N$_5$
M.p. 107–123°C

A third constituent of gentamicin C, obtained from *Micromonospora purpurea* NRRL 2953, this antibiotic forms colourless crystals and is dextrorotatory with $[\alpha]_D^{25}$ + 160° (H$_2$O). It yields a crystalline triacetate with m.p. 206–222°C and a specific rotation of $[\alpha]_D^{26}$ + 151° (CH$_3$OH).

Weinstein et al., *Antimicrobial Agents & Chemotherapy*, 1 (1963)
Weinstein et al., *J. Med. Chem.*, **6**, 463 (1963)
Cooper et al., *J. Chem. Soc.*, C, 2876, 3126 (1971)
Marquez, Wagman, Cooper, *U.S. Patent*, 3,651,042 (1972)

GENTAMICIN X
C$_{19}$H$_{38}$O$_{10}$N$_4$

Elaborated by both *Micromonospora echinospora* and *M. purpurea*, the structure of this antibiotic has been determined by hydrolysis experiments and mass spectrometry. It has anthelmintic activity and is active against gram-positive and gram-negative bacteria and protozoa.

Cooper, Waitz, *German Patent*, 2,130,113 (1972)

GENTISYL ALCOHOL
C$_7$H$_8$O$_3$
M.p. 100–101°C

A simple compound, this antibiotic substance is produced by *Penicillium patulum* Bainier, *P. divergens* Bainier and from an unclassified *Penicillium* species. When obtained from *P. urticae* it is found in the quinhydrone form. Gentisyl alcohol is obtained naturally by surface culture on Raulin-Thom solution and isolated by concentrating the culture filtrate *in vacuo* to a syrup, distributing this between H$_2$O and Et$_2$O, separating the ethereal fraction, evaporating and dissolving the crude residue in CH$_3$OH when the pure product is precipitated in a crystalline form on the addition of CH$_3$OH. It may be further purified by recrystallization from hot CHCl$_3$.

Gentisyl alcohol forms colourless needles which sublime at 70–80°C in a high vacuum. It is soluble in EtOH, Et_2O and H_2O, slightly so in $CHCl_3$ and C_6H_6 and insoluble in light petroleum. The aqueous solution is neutral to litmus and a molecular compound, formed from three moles of hentisyl alcohol and one mole of hydroxymethyl-*p*-benzoquinone as a quinhydrone has also been isolated from a culture filtrate of *Penicillium urticae*.

Gentisyl alcohol itself almost completely inhibits the growth of *Staphylococcus aureus* at a concentration of 1:500 whereas the quinhydrone complex has the same effect at a concentration of 1:5000.

Birkinshaw, Bracken, Raistrick, *Biochem. J.*, **37**, 726 (1943)
Braek, *Helv. Chim. Acta*, **30**, 1 (1947)
Renz, *ibid.*, **30**, 124 (1947)
Engel, Brzeski, *ibid.*, **30**, 1472 (1947)
Barta, Mecir, *Experientia*, **4**, 277 (1948)

GEODIN
$C_7H_{12}O_7Cl_2$
M.p. 235°C (*dec.*)

This antibiotic was first described by Raistrick and Smith in 1935. It is derived from *Aspergillus terreus* and obtained by surface growth in a medium containing glucose and inorganic salts, being incubated at 24°C for 26 days. Isolation consists of acidifying the culture filtrate, washing the flocculent brown precipitate with H_2O and drying *in vacuo*. The residue is then extracted with boiling $CHCl_3$, filtered hot, diluted with Et_2O and cooled when crystalline geodin is precipitated. The crude product is then purified by recrystallization from a variety of solvents including AcOEt, CH_3OH, $CHCl_3$—Et_2O and aqueous $(CH_3)_2CO$.

Geodin formed pale yellow needles when recrystallized from a solvent and yellow microcrystals when sublimed. It is soluble in EtOH, AcOEt, $(CH_3)_2CO$, $CHCl_3$, dioxan and sodium bicarbonate solution, slightly soluble in Et_2O and C_6H_6, insoluble in H_2O and petroleum ether. It is dextrorotatory with $[\alpha]_{5461}^{20} + 179°$ and $[\alpha]_{5790}^{20} + 149°$ (c 0·8, $CHCl_3$).

Marcus has determined inhibition dilutions ($\times 1000$) *in vitro* for the antibiotic: *Bacillus anthracis* (32–128); *B. subtilis* (32–1000); *Corynebacterium diphtheriae* (23–128); *Escherichia coli* (40); *Mycobacterium smegmatis* (4·0–20); *Pseudomonas viridans* (20); *Shigella dysenteriae* (1·0); *Staphylococcus albus* (8·0); *Staph. aureus* (8·0–200); *Staph. citreus* (128); *Streptococcus pyogenes* (128); *Strep. viridans* (8·0) and *Vibrio comma* (2·0). The activity of geodin is decreased by cysteine and by serum.

Raistrick, Smith, *Biochem. J.*, **29**, 606 (1935)
Raistrick, Smith, *ibid.*, **30**, 1315 (1936)
Clutterbuck, Koerber, Raistrick, *ibid.*, **31**, 1089 (1937)
Calam *et al.*, *ibid.*, **33**, 579 (1938)
Calam *et al.*, *ibid.*, **41**, 458 (1947)
Marcus, *ibid.*, **41**, 462 (1947)
Rinderknecht *et al.*, *ibid.*, **41**, 463 (1947)

GEOMYCIN
$C_6H_{12}O_2N_2$
M.p. Indefinite

This antibiotic isolated from cultures of *Streptomyces xanthophaeus* has been described by a number of workers. It is usually isolated as the crystalline helianthate and also forms a hydrochloride as colourless crystals. It has only a weak activity against bacteria but is effective against *Entameba histolytica* in rats. When tested *in vivo* it produces a nephrotoxicity of a similar order to that found with neomycin and streptothricin.

Brockmann, Musso, *Naturwiss.*, **41**, 451 (1954)
Brockmann *et al.*, *German Patent*, 913,687 (1954)
Brockmann, Musso., *Ber.*, **88**, 648 (1955)
Brockmann, Cölln., *ibid.*, **92**, 114 (1959)

GLADIOLIC ACID
$C_{11}H_{10}O_5$
M.p. 160°C

An antibiotic substance isolated from *Penicillium gladioli*, gladiolic acid is obtained by surface culture on Raulin-Thom medium yielding 32 *Botrytis allii* units/ml. Isolation of the antibiotic is carried out by acidifying the culture filtrate to pH 4·0, adsorbing on activated carbon, drying the cake at room temperature and extracting with Et_2O. The ethereal extract is then evaporated to yield a yellow-brown paste. Purification of gladiolic acid is best done by recrystallization from H_2O and drying *in vacuo*.

Gladiolic acid forms colourless silky needles and is a monobasic acid which is stable for 10 days at 25°C at pH 3·0–8·0 as an aqueous solution in McIlvaine's buffer.

The antibiotic is assayed by inhibition of the germination of *Botrytis allii* conidia. It inhibits *Staphylococcus aureus in vitro* at a concentration of 250 g/ml but is ineffective against either *Escherichia coli* or *Salmonella typhi* even at twice this concentration. It possesses quite marked fungistatic properties.

Wilkins, Harris, *Brit. J. Exptl. Path.*, **24**, 141 (1943)
Wilkins, Harris, *ibid.*, **25**, 135 (1944)
Brian et al., *Nature*, **157**, 698 (1946)

GLIOTOXIN
$C_{13}H_{14}O_4N_2S_2$
M.p. 192–193°C (215–220°C dec.)

This antibiotic was first described as long ago as 1932 by Weindling and named after *Gliocladium fimbricatum*, the name erroneously assigned to the antibiotic-producing organism, now known to be *Trichoderma viride*. It has also been isolated from *Aspergillus fumigatus*, *Penicillium jenseni*, *P. obscurum* and other species of *Penicillium*. It may be produced by both surface growth and submerged culture and isolated by various methods including extraction of the culture filtrate with $CHCl_3$, evaporating, dissolving the residue in CH_3OH, treating the solution with activated carbon and allowing to crystallize and extracting the culture filtrate with C_6H_6 at pH 2·0, concentrating the extract and adding petroleum ether to precipitate the crude gliotoxin. Purification is by recrystallization from a number of solvents, e.g. CH_3OH, EtOH, C_6H_6 and AcOEt.

Gliotoxin forms colourless needles or elongated plates. It is soluble in $CHCl_3$, AcOH, acetonitrile, dioxan, dimethylformamide and pyridine, moderately so in AcOEt, EtOH, $(CH_3)_2CO$, C_6H_6 and *tert*-BuOH. Gliotoxin is laevorotatory with the following specific rotations: $[\alpha]_D^{25} - 290°$ $\pm 10°$ (c 0·078, EtOH); $[\alpha]_D^{19} - 239°$, $[\alpha]_D^{20} - 256°$ and $[\alpha]_D^{22} - 245°$ (all in $CHCl_3$). The ultraviolet spectrum has absorption maxima at 270 and 450 nm. In acid solution, the antibiotic is stable, but unstable in alkalies.

Gliotoxin is assayed by serial dilution with *Rhizoctonia solani* which is inhibited at a concentration of 1 : 300,000 using crystalline gliotoxin. Inhibition concentrations *in vitro* against a number of organisms vary according to the medium used. Brian et al. and Johnson and his colleagues have determined inhibition concentration (μg/ml) in broth: *Aerobacter aerogenes* (4·8); *Boletus bovinus* (5·0); *Bol. elegans* (19–20); *Epidermophyton* sp. (15·6); *Escherichia coli* (12·7); *Micrococcus lysodeikticus* (0·15); *Mycorrhizum radicis atrovirens* (5·0–10); *Phoma radicis callunae* (20–40); *Pneumococcus* I (0·312); *Pneumococcus* III (0·234); *Rhizoctonia* sp. (5·0–10); *Salmonella enteriditis* (3·9); *Staphylococcus aureus* (0·234) and *Streptococcus pyogenes* (0·936). Determinations carried out by Johnson and his coworkers in agar media are: *Eberella typhi* (2·5); *Epidermophyton* sp. (0·8); *Escherichia coli* (5·0–10); *Hemophilus pertussis* (1·0–2·5); *Neisseria catarrhalis* (0·2); *Salmonella paratyphi* (2·5–5·0); *S. schottmuelleri* (10); *Staphylococcus albus* (1·0–2·5); *Staph. aureus* (0·5) and *Streptococcus viridans* (0·5).

In addition to the above, gliotoxin is active *in vitro* against *Blastomycoides dermatiditis*, *Fomes annosus*, *Penicillium italicum* and *Rhizopus* species but not against *Aspergillus niger*, *Penicillium digitatum* or *Trichoderma* species. There is a small decrease in activity by rabbit serum and the antibiotic is antagonized by both cysteine and oxyhemoglobin. *Clostridium welchii*, *Salmonella typhi* and *Staphylococcus aureus* all show a marked resistance to the antibiotic when transferred on gliotoxin-containing media.

The action of gliotoxin *in vivo* is disappointing. When given 0·5 mg subcutaneously, mice gain no protection against streptococcus. It does, however, find some use in the treatment of cereals, barley being protected against *Ustilego hordei*, oats against *Helmintosporium avenae* and wheat against *Tilletia caries*. In all cases, no phytocidal effect has been recorded.

In both mice and rats, the lethal dose is stated to be 50–65 mg/kg when given intraperitoneally or orally, the corresponding intravenous dose in rabbits being 45 mg/kg.

Weindling, *Phytopath.*, **22**, 839 (1932)
Weindling, *ibid.*, **24**, 1153 (1934)
Weindling, *ibid.*, **27**, 1175 (1937)
Weindling, *ibid.*, **31**, 991 (1941)
Dutcher, *J. Bact.*, **42**, 815 (1941)
Johnson, Bruce, Dutcher, *J. Amer. Chem. Soc.*, **65**, 2005 (1943)
Brian, *Nature*, **154**, 667 (1944)
Menzel, Wintersteiner, Hoogerheide, *J. Biol. Chem.*, **152**, 419 (1944)
Waksman, Geiger, *J. Bact.*, **47**, 391 (1944)
Johnson, McCrone, Bruce, *J. Amer. Chem. Soc.*, **66**, 501 (1944)
Bruce et al, *ibid.*, **66**, 614 (1944)
Dutcher, Johnson, Bruce, *ibid.*, **66**, 617, 619 (1944)
Brian, Hemming, *Ann. Appl. Biol.*, **32**, 214 (1945)
Mull, Towmley, Scholz, *J. Amer. Chem. Soc.*, **67**, 1626 (1945)
Dutcher, Johnson, Bruce, *ibid.*, **67**, 1736 (1945)
Brian, Hemming, McGowan, *Nature*, **155**, 637 (1945)
Kidd, *Science*, **105**, 411 (1947)

GLUTAMYCIN
$C_{12}H_{15}O_4N$
M.p. 130–131°C

Aspergillus flavipes elaborates this simple diketonic antibiotic which crystallizes from EtOH. The structure has been determined as 4-acetyl-1:2:3:6-tetrahydro-3-*iso*valerylpyridine-2:6-dione.

Casinovi *et al.*, *Ann. Int. Super. Sanita.*, **5**, 523 (1969)

GLUTINOSIN
$C_{48}H_{60}O_{16}$
Dec. 300°C

Glutinosin is obtained from *Metarrhizium glutinosum* and produced by surface growth on Raulin-Thom medium, yielding 265 *Botrytis allii* units/ml. The activity of the culture filtrate may be adsorbed on activated carbon and eluted with boiling C_6H_6. The antibiotic is readily purified by recrystallization from hot EtOH. The compound forms colourless plates which darken at 300°C without melting. It is dextrorotatory with a specific rotation of $[\alpha]_D^{20}$ + 54° (c 0·2, C_6H_6).

Glutinosin is normally assayed by the inhibition of spore germination of *Botrytis allii*, 0·2 µg/ml of the antibiotic being equivalent to 1 unit. Even at high concentrations has no effect on bacteria but is effective against a large number of fungi and yeasts. Brian and his colleagues have distinguished between the concentration necessary for inhibition of growth and inhibition of spore germination. Typical growth inhibition concentrations given are: *Aspergillus oryzae* (200); *Botrytis allii* (5·0–25); *Byssochlamys fulva* (1·0); *Chaetomium elatum* (5·0–25); *Endomycopsis albicans* (25–100); *Fusarium coerulum* (>100); *Gibberella saubinetti* (>100); *Hydnum coralloides* (>1·0); *Melanospora pampeana* (>100); *Monilia sitophila* (100); *Mucor mucedo* (1·0–5·0); *Neurospora crassa* (1·0); *Penicillium digitatum* (1·0–5·0); *P. gladioli* (25–100); *Phoma betae* (1·0); *Phytophthora palmivora* (5·0–25); *Saccharomyces cerevisiae* (5·0–25); *Stachybotrys atra* (>100); *Stereum purpureum* (1·0); *Thamnidium elegans* (5·0–25); *Torulopsis utilis* (100); *Trichoderma viride* (>100); *Trichothecium roseum* (>100); *Verticillium dahliae* (100).

Similar concentrations required for inhibition of spore germination given by the same workers are: *Aspergillus niger* (20–25); *Fusarium graminearum* (3·1); *Mucor mucedo* (1·6); *Penicillium digitatum* (1·0–3·1); *P. gladioli* (3·1); *Stachybotrys atra* (1·6); *Stemphylium* spp. (50); *Syncephalastrum racemosum* (12·5); *Thamnidium elegans* (0·4); *Trichoderma viride* (>50); *Trichothecium roseum* (0·8) and *Verticillium cinnabarinum* (25).

Brian, McGowan, *Nature*, **157**, 334 (1946)
Brian, Curtis, Hemming, *Proc. Roy. Soc.*, **135B**, 106 (1947)

GLYCINOTHRICIN
$C_{18}H_{31}N_7O_8$

Streptomyces griseus elaborates this antibiotic, the structure of which has been elucidated from chemical and spectroscopic evidence. It is active against gram-positive and gram-negative bacteria but has a lower activity than antibiotic LL-AB644 of which it is the deformino derivative.

Sawada *et al.*, *J. Antibiotics* (Japan), **30**, 460 (1977)

GLYCOLIPID A
$C_{26}H_{48}O_9$

Japanese workers have recently isolated two compounds from *Pseudomonas* species which possess antiviral properties. This particular substance is obtained by cultivating *Ps. aeruginosa* or *Ps. fluorescens* in a nutrient medium containing polypeptone and sorbital and inorganic salts at pH 7·3 and 28°C for 24 hours. The solution formed was then used as an inoculum in a medium consisting of biotin, corn steep liquor, meat extract and n-C_{12-15} paraffins together with inorganic salts and fermented at 30°C and pH 6·0–7·5 for 3 days. Glycolipid A is active against a number of viruses.

Suzuki, Itoh, *German Patent*, 2,150,375 (1972)

GLYCOLIPID B
$C_{32}H_{58}O_{13}$
M.p. Indefinite

A second antiviral compound isolated from cultures of *Pseudomonas aeruginosa* and *Ps. fluorescens* and prepared by the method given for the preceding compound. The structure has been determined by chemical and spectroscopic methods.

Suzuki, Itoh, *German Patent*, 2,150,375 (1972)

GOLDINOX
See Antibiotic X-5108

GOUGEROTIN
$C_{16}H_{24}O_8N_7$
M.p. 211–217°C (dec.)

An aminoglycosidic antibiotic derived from *Streptomyces gougerotii*, this compound is dextrorotatory with specific rotations of $[\alpha]_D^{27} + 53°$ (c 0·8, H_2O) and $[\alpha]_D^{21} + 45°$ (c 0·8, H_2O). It forms colourless needles when crystallized from H_2 which decompose, with effervescence, at the melting point. The ultraviolet spectrum in H_2O has absorption maxima at 235 and 267 nm. In 0·1 N-HCl, there is a single absorption maximum at 275 nm which is shifted to 267 nm in 0·1 N-NaOH solution.

Gougerotin inhibits *Escherichia coli*, there being 50 per cent inhibition at a dilution of $4·0 \times 10^{-5}$ molar. It has been shown to inhibit protein synthesis by preventing transfer of aminoacids from aminoacyl tRNA to polypeptide and is also an inhibitor of the multiplication of certain viruses.

Kanzaki *et al.*, *J. Antibiotics* (Japan), **15A**, 93 (1962)
Clark, Gunther, *Biochem. Biophys. Acta*, **76**, 636 (1963)
Clark, Chang, *J. Biol. Chem.*, **240**, 4374 (1965)
Sinohara *et al.*, *Biochem. Biophys. Res. Commun.*, **18**, 98 (1965)
Fox, Block, Watanabe, *Progr. Nucl. Acid Res. Mol. Biol.*, **5**, 251 (1966)
Thiry, *J. Gen. Virol.*, **2**, 143 (1968)
Kyoichi, Watanabe, Falco, *J. Amer. Chem. Soc.*, **94**, 3272 (1972)

GRAMICIDIN (*Tyrothricin*)
Certain strains of *Bacillus brevis* elaborate a mixture of antibiotics which are all polypeptides, originally named tyrothricin. This was later separated into two main classes of antibiotics, the tyrocidins (q.v.) forming approximately 80 per cent of the mixture and the gramicidins which make up the remaining 20 per cent. The gramicidins described below are all broad-spectrum antibiotics and have been obtained in a state of reasonable purity.

Hotchkiss *et al.*, *J. Biol. Chem.*, **132**, 791 (1940)
Hotchkiss *et al.*, *ibid.*, **141**, 155 (1941)
Hotchkiss *et al.*, *Advances in Enzymol.*, **4**, 153 (1944)
Tishler *et al.*, *J. Biol. Chem.*, **141**, 197 (1944)
Gregory, Craig, *ibid.*, **172**, 839 (1948)
Synge, *Biochem. J.*, **44**, 542 (1949)
Craig, Gregory, Barry, *Cold Springs Harbour Symposium on quantitative biology*, **14**, 24 (1950)
James, Synge, *Biochem. J.*, **50**, 109 (1951) (*Bibl.*)

GRAMICIDIN C
See Gramicidin S

GRAMICIDIN D (*Gramicidin Dubos*)
M.p. 229°C (*dec.*)
A crystalline antibiotic obtained from the original tyrothricin (see above), this macrocyclic peptide is made up of the following aminoacids, L-tryptophane (4 mols), D-leucine (4 mols), D-valine (2 mols), L-valine (2 mols), L-alanine (2 mols) and 1 mole each of glycine and ethanolamine. The manner in which these aminoacids are linked in the molecule is not yet fully established.

Dubos, Hotchkiss, *J. Exptl. Med.*, **73**, 629 (1941)
Gordon, Martin, Synge, *Biochem. J.*, **37**, 86 (1943)
Hotchkiss, *Advances in Enzymol.*, **4**, 153 (1944)
Synge, *Biochem. J.*, **39**, 355 (1945)

GRAMICIDIN DUBOS
See Gramicidin D

GRAMICIDIN J_1
$C_{44}H_{65}O_7N_9$

D-Orn → L-Val → L-Orn
↑   ↓
L-Pro
↑   ↓
L-Phe ← D-Leu ← D-Phe

This antibiotic has been isolated and described by Japanese workers who have proposed that the constituent aminoacids are linked in the manner shown above.

Otani, Saito, *Proc. Japan. Acad.*, **30**, 991 (1954)
Otani, Saito, *Congr. intern. biochim., Resumes communs.*, 3ᵉ *Congr. Brussels*, 88 (1955)

GRAMICIDIN J_2
$C_{35}H_{56}O_6N_8$

D-Orn → L-Val → L-Orn
↑   ↓
L-Pro ← D-Phe ← D-Leu

This somewhat simpler antibiotic contains the six aminoacids linked in the form given above.

Otani, Nagano, Saito, *Osaka Shiritsu Daigaku Igaku Zasshi*, **7**, 640 (1958)

GRAMICIDIN S (*Gramicidin C, Soviet gramicidin*)
$C_{60}H_{92}O_{10}N_{12}$
M.p. 77°C (*dec.*)

L-Val → L-Orn → L-Val → D-Phe
↑   ↓
L-Pro   L-Pro
↑   ↓
D-Phe ← L-Val ← L-Orn ← L-Val

This macrocyclic polypeptide antibiotic has been obtained from the strain *Bacillus brevis* var. Gause-Brazhnikova and may be purified by crystallization from aqueous $(CH_3)_2CO$ when it forms colourless needles. It has more recently been isolated from cultures of *B. brevis* mutants 204, 777 and U-32. Advantages of using these mutant strains are lower fermentation temperatures of 26–27°C and a higher yield. The U-32 mutants, for example, yield 33 times as much antibiotic as the parent strain. Gramicidin S is laevorotatory with a specific rotation of $[\alpha]_D^{18} - 289°$ (c 0.43, 70 per cent EtOH) and is freely soluble in EtOH, Et_2O and $(CH_3)_2CO$ but insoluble in H_2O, acids and alkalies. The compound is thermostable, gives a bright blue colour with ninhydrin and also gives positive biuret and xanthoproteic reactions.

Gause, Brazhnikov, *Chem. Abstr.*, **39**, 1893, 1894 (1945)
Synge, *Biochem. J.*, **39**, 363 (1945)
Hausze et al., *Chem. Abstr.*, **40**, 918 (1946)
Sanger, *Biochem. J.*, **40**, 261 (1946)
Consden et al., *ibid.*, **40**, xlii (1946)
Consden et al., *ibid.*, **41**, 596 (1947)
Schwyzer, Sieber, *Helv. Chim. Acta*, **40**, 624 (1957)
Myaskovskaya et al., *Antibiotiki*, **17**, 38 (1972)
Synthesis
Losse, Neubert, *Tetrahedron Lett.*, 1267 (1970)
Crystal structure
Camilletti, De Santis, Rizzo, *Chem. Commun.*, 1073 (1970)

GRAMICIDIN S-A
$C_{60}H_{92}O_{10}N_{12}$

L-Pro → L-Val → L-Orn → D-Leu
↑   ↓
D-Phe   D-Phe
↑   ↓
D-Leu ← L-Orn ← L-Val ← L-Pro

This antibiotic has a polypeptide structure similar to that of gramicidin S but with 2 moles of valine replaced by 2 moles of leucine.

Stern, Gobbinos, Craig, *Proc. U.S. Nat. Acad. Sci.*, **61**, 734 (1968)
Gibbons et al., *Nature*, **227**, 840 (1970)

GRANATACIN
$C_{22}H_{20}O_{10}$
M.p. 204–206°C (*dec.*)

Corbaz and his colleagues have isolated this antibiotic from *Streptomyces olivaceus* (Waksman) Waksman & Henrici as pomegranate-red crystals from

EtOH. The ultraviolet spectrum in EtOH has absorption maxima at 223 and 286 nm and there are absorptions in the visible at 532 and 576 nm. With acids, the antibiotic gives a red colour whereas the solutions in alkalies are blue. The compound may be characterized as the tetraacetate which forms pale yellow crystals from EtOH with m.p. 242–243°C and $[\alpha]_D^{20} - 100°$ (c 0·818, CHCl$_3$). It is active against gram-positive and gram-negative bacteria.

Corbaz et al., Helv. Chim. Acta, **40**, 1262 (1957)

GRANATICIN B
$C_{28}H_{30}O_{12}$
M.p. Indefinite

An antibiotic produced by a strain of *Streptomyces violaceoruber*, this compound is obtained in the form of a red, amorphous powder with no definite melting point. The ultraviolet and visible spectra contain absorption maxima at 223, 285, 527 and 566 nm with a shoulder at 498 nm. The tetraacetate is crystalline with m.p. 257–259°C and gives an ultraviolet spectrum in EtOH with absorption maxima at 242 and 356 nm.

Barcza et al., Helv. Chim. Acta, **49**, 1736 (1966)

GRANEGILLIN
$C_{12}H_{20}O_2N_2$
M.p. 99–100°C

Both *Aspergillus effussu* and *A. plavus* elaborate this antibiotic which is obtained as light yellow needles from EtOH. It has been suggested that it is identical with aspergillic acid.

Csillag, Acta Microbiol. Acad. Sci. Hung., **1**, 321 (1954)

GRASSERIOMYCIN
M.p. Indefinite

An unidentified species of *Streptomyces* produces this antibiotic which has been characterized as the hydrochloride, a pale yellow precipitate soluble in H_2O and CH_3OH, the helianthate, yellow crystals, decomposing at 215–255°C and the reineckate, also crystalline, decomposing at 187–190°C. It has found some use in the control of virus jaundice in silkworms.

Ueda et al., J. Antibiotics (Japan), **8A**, 91 (1955)
Sumiki et al., Japanese Patent, 6266 (1957)

GRATIZIN
M.p. 274–276°C (dec.)

A mutant of *Bacillus brevis*, strain Y-33, elaborates this antibiotic. The organism is cultivated on a yeast substrate with shaking at 40°C for 2 days. The cells are then dried and extracted with EtOH followed by chromatography on an alumina column. Gratizin forms colourless crystals and gives a characteristic ultraviolet spectrum in 0·1 N-HCl having a single absorption maximum at 270 nm. Chromatography of the acid hydrolysis products of the antibiotic show that it contains leucine, ornithine, phenylalanine, proline, tyrosine and valine in the molecule. Biologically it is more active than gramicidin C.

Zharikova, Myaskovskaya, Silaev, Vestn. Mosk. Univ., Biol., Pochvoved., **27**, 110 (1972)

GRISAMINE
$C_{28}H_{38}O_{10}N_6$ ($C_{20}H_{30}O_7N_4$)
M.p. 167–170°C

Isolated from an unidentified species of *Streptomyces*, this antibiotic substance crystallizes as colourless needles from EtOH. The chemical analysis does not allow a distinction between the two empirical formulae given above.

Sawazaki et al., J. Antibiotics (Japan), **8A**, 39 (1955)

GRISEIN
$C_{40}H_{61}O_{20}N_{10}SFe$
M.p. Indefinite

A highly complex antibiotic containing both sulphur and iron in the molecule, grisein is elaborated by *Streptomyces griseus* and forms an amorphous red powder with no definite melting point. The antibiotic is usually isolated from the culture filtrate by adsorption on activated carbon and elution with 95 per cent EtOH followed by precipitation with CH_3OH and $(CH_3)_2CO$. Grisein is soluble in H_2O, slightly so in 95 per cent EtOH and virtually insoluble in $(CH_3)_2CO$, Et_2O and absolute EtOH. It is quite a stable substance withstanding 10 minutes at 100°C. It is inactivated by iron but not by cysteine.

Grisein is assayed by both plate and serial dilution methods using a streptomycin-resistant strain of *Escherichia coli* as the test organism. The inhibition (units/mg) has been measured by Reynolds and Waksman using a potent preparation of the antibiotic: *Bacillus cereus* (1000); *B. subtilis* (300); *B. megatherium* (1000); *Escherichia coli* (1800); *Micrococcus lysodeikticus* (30,000); *Pseudomonas aeruginosa* (>100); *Salmonella alkalescens* (1800); *S. dysenteriae* (18,000); *S. paradysenteriae* (18,000); *S. pullorum* (30,000) and *Staphylococcus aureus* (3000). The development of resistance to the antibiotic is quite rapid.

When tested *in vivo* in the mouse, protection was given against *Salmonella schottmuelleri* and *Staphylococcus aureus* at a dosage of 800–1600 units. Grisein appears to be comparatively non-toxic. In several tests, experimental animals tolerated up to 500,000 units/kg of the antibiotic.

Reynolds, Schatz, Waksman, *Proc. Soc., Exptl. Biol. Med.*, **55**, 66 (1944)
Reynolds, Schatz, Waksman, *ibid.*, **64**, 50 (1947)
Raynolds, Waksman, *J. Bact.*, **55**, 739 (1948)
Garson, Waksman, *Proc. U.S. Nat. Acad. Sci.*, **34**, 232 (1948)
Kuehl et al., *J. Amer. Chem. Soc.*, **73**, 1770 (1951)

GRISEOFLAVIN

M.p. 210–215°C (*dec.*)

Streptomyces griseoflavus produces this antibiotic which, when first obtained, is a brownish powder that is purified by chromatography over alumina followed by recrystallization from EtOH when it forms colourless crystals. It is readily soluble in CH_3OH, EtOH, PrOH, phenol, AcOH and dilute alkalies, slightly soluble in AcOEt and H_2O and insoluble in Et_2O, C_6H_6, $CHCl_3$ and petroleum ether. The biuret, ninhydrin, $FeCl_3$, Molisch and Sakaguchi tests are all negative. It is mainly active against gram-positive organisms and shows only a limited activity against gram-negative bacteria. It is highly active against *Vibrio comma* and strains of *Staphylococci* at concentrations of 1–2 µg/ml. The LD_{50} in mice is in excess of 250 mg/kg when given intraperitoneally.

Waga, *J. Antibiotics* (Japan), **6A**, 55 (1953)

GRISEOFULVIN (*Curling factor*)

$C_{17}H_{17}O_6Cl$
M.p. 218–219°C

The (+)-form of this compound is elaborated by *Penicillium griseofulvum* and also occurs in cultures of *P. janczewski* and *P. patulum*. It is produced by surface growth on a medium containing glucose and inorganic salts or on Raulin-Thom or Weindling media. It may be isolated from the culture filtrate by extraction with $CHCl_3$ or adsorbing the activity on activated carbon and eluting with $CHCl_3$ or Et_2O and evaporating the eluate to dryness. On the other hand, it has been isolated from the mycelium by extracting with petroleum ether in a Soxhlet, discarding the extract and re-extracting the mycelium with Et_2O and evaporating the ethereal extract to dryness. Purification is carried out by recrystalling from EtOH when griseofulvin forms colourless crystals. It has the following specific rotations: $[\alpha]_D^{19} + 337°$; $[\alpha]_{5461}^{19} + 417°$; $[\alpha]_{5790}^{19} + 354°$ all in $(CH_3)_2CO$. The compound is only sparingly soluble in $CHCl_3$, C_6H_6, $(CH_3)_2CO$ or AcOEt and insoluble in H_2O. When hydrolysed with dilute acids it yields griseofulvic acid, $C_{16}H_{15}O_6Cl$, which decomposes at 255–258°C and has a specific rotation of $[\alpha]_D^{22} + 399°$. From this observation the structure of the antibiotic has been established as 7-chloro-2′:4:6-trimethoxy-6′-methylgris-2′-en-3:4′-dione. Both the monoxime, m.p. 120°C with the evolution of gas, followed by resolidification and remelting at 224°C and the mono-dinitrophenylhydrazone, bright red needles, m.p. 155–160°C (*dec.*) have been prepared. The (−)-form of this compound has m.p. 216–217°C; $[\alpha]_D - 341°$ (c 1·03, $CHCl_3$) and the (±)-form has m.p. 217–222°C.

Griseofulvin is assayed by serial dilution with *Botrytis allii* spores. The alternative name 'curling factor' was given to this antibiotic since as little as 0·2 µg/ml causes curling of the growing hyphae and stunting of the germ tubes. Griseofulvin is mainly active against fungi and yeasts exhibiting inhibition of growth *in vitro* in all species of *Ascomycetes* (except *Saccharomyces cerevisae*), *Basidiomycetes* (except *Coniophora cerebella*), *Fungi imperfecti* (except *Torulopsis utilis*) and *Zygomycetes* which have been tested, at a concentration of 20 µg/ml. It exhibits no activity against bacteria, *Actinomycetes* or *Oomycetes*. Griseofulvin is toxic to angiosperm seeds at a concentration of 25 µg/ml.

Oxford, Raistrick, Simonart, *Biochem. J.*, **33**, 240 (1939)
Brian, Curtis, Hemming, *Brit. Mycol. Soc. Trans.*, **29**, 173 (1946)

McGowan, *ibid.*, **29**, 188 (1946)
Grove, McGowan, *Nature*, **160**, 574 (1947)
Brian, Curtis, Hemming, *Brit. Mycol. Soc. Trans.*, **32**, 30 (1949)
Brian, *Ann. Bot.*, **13**, 59 (1949)
Grove et al., *Chem. & Ind.*, 219 (1951)
McMillan, *ibid.*, 719 (1951)
Grove et al., *J. Chem. Soc.*, 3949 (1952)
Brassi et al., *Helv. Chim. Acta*, **43**, 1444 (1960)
Day, Nabney, Scott, *J. Chem. Soc.*, 4067 (1961)
Brassi et al., *Helv. Chim. Acta*, **45**, 1292 (1962)
Stork, Tomasz, *J. Amer. Chem. Soc.*, **84**, 310 (1962)
Taub, Kuo, Wendler, *Chem. & Ind.*, 1617 (1962)
Arkley et al., *J. Chem. Soc.*, 1260 (1962)
Taub, Kuo, Wendler, *Tetrahedron*, **19**, 1 (1963)
Arison et al., *J. Amer. Chem. Soc.*, **85**, 627 (1963)
See also
Grove, *Quart. Rev.*, **17**, 1 (1963) (Review)
Rhodes, *Progr. in Industrial Microbiol.*, 165, Heywood & Co. Ltd., London (1963)

GRISEOLUTEIN A
$C_{17}H_{14}O_6N_2$
M.p. 193°C (dec.)

An antibiotic produced by *Streptomyces griseoluteus*, this substance is obtained by extraction of the mycelium with AcOEt followed by chromatography on an alumina column and cooling to 0°C. Griseolutein A forms red-yellow needles, soluble but unstable at alkaline pH, slightly soluble in AcOEt and EtOH and insoluble in Et_2O and H_2O. It has a maximum stability under acid conditions. The antibiotic is active against both gram-positive and gram-negative bacteria and shows no toxicity to mice even when injected subcutaneously at 1000 mg/ml.

Umezawa et al., *J. Antibiotics* (Japan), **4**, 34 (1951)
Nakamura, *Chem. Pharm. Bull.*, **6**, 547 (1958)

GRISEOLUTEIN B
$C_{17}H_{16}O_6N_2$
M.p. >220°C (dec.)

A further antibiotic obtained from *Streptomyces griseoluteus*, this substance is the secondary alcohol corresponding to griseolutein A. It crystallizes from AcOEt in the form of yellow needles.

Umezawa et al., *J. Antibiotics* (Japan), **4**, 34 (1951)
Umezawa, *Japanese Patent*, 2249 (1952)
Osato et al., *J. Antibiotics* (Japan), **7A**, 15 (1954)
Nakamura et al., *ibid.*, **10A**, 265 (1957)
Nakamura, *Chem. Pharm. Bull.*, **6**, 547 (1958)

GRISEOMYCIN (*Lomycin*)
M.p. 76–80°C

This antibiotic, isolated from cultures of *Streptomyces griseolus*, forms white crystals and is dextrorotatory with a specific rotation of $[\alpha]_D^{25} + 32°$ (c 1.0, $CHCl_3$). It has been characterized as the hydrochloride, m.p. 120°C. This salt is freely soluble in H_2O but only slightly so in organic solvents. Griseomycin is active against gram-positive bacteria although a small number of gram-negative organisms, particularly *Neisseria* species, are also susceptible. The LD_{50} in mice is 0.21 g/kg (intraperitoneal), 2.1 g/kg (oral) and 1.33 g/kg (subcutaneous).

Van Dijck, van de Voorde, de Somer, *Antibiotics & Chemotherapy*, **3**, 1243 (1953)
See also
Belgian Patent, 522,647 (1953)

GRISEORHODINE
M.p. Indefinite

An antibiotic pigment, griseorhodine is produced chiefly by *Streptomyces californicus* strain JA 2640 and also, in smaller amounts, by strain ATCC 3312. It shows some inhibitory activity against gram-positive bacteria, but little against gram-negative organisms.

Thrum et al., *Z. Allg. Mikrobiol.*, **7**, 121 (1967)

GRISEOVIRIDIN
$C_{22}H_{27}O_7N_3S$
M.p. 158–166°C; 194–200°C or 230–240°C (dec.)

A tricyclic sulphur-containing antibiotic elaborated by *Streptomyces griseus*, griseoviridin may be recrystallized from CH_3OH and, depending upon the particular crystal modification obtained, has one of the three melting points given above. When crystallized from pyridine it forms colourless plates, m.p. 228–230°C and yields a crystalline diacetate, m.p. 137–140°C (dec.); $[\alpha]_D^{27} - 230°$ (c 0.44, CH_3OH), forming a perchlorate, m.p. >170°C; $[\alpha]_D - 185°$ (c 0.19, dimethylformamide). The antibiotic is active *in vitro* against several strains of *Actinomyces*, *Clostridium*, *Corynebacterium*, *Diplococcus*, *Escherichia*, *Hemophilus*, *Moraxella*, *Neisseria*, *Shigella* and *Streptococcus*. It has a low toxicity in experimental animals and is effective against pertussis infection in mice when given intraperitoneally and when injected locally against clinical bovine coli mastitis.

Bartz *et al.*, *Antibiotics Annual*, **2**, 777 (1954–55)
Ehrlich *et al.*, *ibid.*, **2**, 790 (1954–55)
Ames *et al.*, *J. Chem. Soc.*, 4260 (1955)
Ames, Bowman, *ibid.*, 4264 (1955)
Ames, Bowman, *ibid.*, 2925 (1956)
Fallona *et al.*, *J. Amer. Chem. Soc.*, **84**, 4162 (1962)
Fallona *et al.*, *Can. J. Chem.*, **42**, 371, 394 (1964)

GRISEORIXIN
$C_{40}H_{68}O_{10}$
M.p. 75–80°C

One of a number of antibiotics elaborated by *Streptomyces griseus*, this compound is isolated from the mycelium after fermenting the organism in a medium containing sucrose, soybean flour and potato extract at 27°C for 7 days with shaking. The mycelium is extracted with EtOH, the extract concentrated and purified by chromatography on a silica gel column. It is an amorphous powder which is dextrorotatory with a specific rotation of $[\alpha]_{578}^{20} + 16°$ (c 4.0, $(CH_3)_2CO$). It forms a methyl ester which is also somewhat difficult to crystallize with m.p. 55–63°C. The structure has been elucidated chemically and spectroscopically.

Griseorixin is active against a number of bacteria, filamentous fungi and yeasts in concentrations of 0.1–200 µg/ml. It is phytotoxic at 0.02 per cent, preventing infection of beans by *Colletotrichum lindemuthianum* at a concentration of 0.01 per cent and is also cytotoxic to HeLa cells at 10 µg/ml, inhibiting growth at 1.0 µg/ml.

Gachon *et al.*, *Chem. Commun.*, 1421 (1970)
Crystal structure
    Alleaume, Hickel, *Chem. Commun.*, 1422 (1970)
Biological activity
    Staron *et al.*, *French Patent*, 2,091,913 (1972)

GRISEUSIN A
$C_{22}H_{20}O_{10}$

A strain of *Streptomyces griseus* elaborates two structurally similar antibiotics which have been separated and purified by extraction of the culture broth followed by column and thin layer chromatography. This antibiotic is effective against a range of gram-positive bacteria.

Tsuji *et al.*, *J. Antibiotics* (Japan), **29**, 7 (1976)

GRISEUSIN B
$C_{22}H_{22}O_{10}$

Also present in the culture broth of a strain of *Streptomyces griseus*, the structure of griseus in B is very similar to that of the preceding antibiotic. It possesses a similar activity against gram-positive organisms.

Tsuji *et al.*, *J. Antibiotics* (Japan), **29**, 7 (1976)

GRISIC ACID

An antibiotic derived from a species of *Streptomyces*, the chemical and physical properties of this compound are still in doubt.

Robbins, Kavanagh, Hervey, *J. N.Y. Bot. Gardens*, **45**, 130 (1945)

GUAMYCIN

M.p. Indefinite

Streptomyces strain 6617-IAUFPe elaborates this antibiotic. It gives an ultraviolet spectrum with absorption maxima at 289, 305 and 320 nm and is freely soluble in H_2O, CH_3OH, pyridine and dilute alkalies, slightly so in glacial AcOH and BuOH, insoluble in EtOH, $(CH_3)_2CO$, C_6H_6, $CHCl_3$, hexane and petroleum ether. Guamycin exhibits a marked inhibitory effect against several *Candida* species, *Micrococcus lutea*, *Saccharomyces cerevisiae* and *Sarcina lutea*.

de Alburquerque *et al.*, *Rev. Inst. Antibiot., Univ. Fed. Pernambuco, Recife*, **9**, 39 (1969)

GUANAMYCIN

M.p. Indefinite

A quinoxaline antibiotic, similar to the actinomycins, this compound is produced by *Streptomyces* species 6617-IAUFPe and gives an ultraviolet spectrum having absorption maxima at 243 and 315–318 nm. The infrared spectrum is also characteristic of quinoxaline derivatives. When hydrolysed with HCl at 100°C for 4 hours it gives a positive ninhydrin reaction and paper chromatography shows the presence of L-alanine, N-methylvaline and L-serine. It is active against a wide range of organisms and also shows some antitumour activity. The LD_{50} in mice is about 300 mg/kg when given subctuaneously and 100–200 mg/kg administered intraperitoneally.

de Alburquerque *et al.*, *Rev. Inst. Antibiot., Univ. Recife*, **8**, 3 (1968)

H

HACHIMYCIN (*Trichomycin*)
Dec. 155°C

Streptomyces hachijoensis elaborates this antibiotic which is obtained in the form of pale yellow crystals which decompose without melting. It has been shown to be identical with trichomycin. The antibiotic is active against a range of gram-positive organisms.

Hosoya *et al.*, *Japan. J. Med.*, **22**, 505 (1952)
Hosoya, *Chemotherapy*, **2**, 1 (1954)

HADICIDIN
$C_3H_5O_4N$
M.p. 119–120°C

OHC—N(OH)CH$_2$COOH

An unstable antibiotic, hadicidin has been obtained from cultures of *Penicillium frequentans* Westling and the structure, N-formyl-N-hydroxyglycine, confirmed by synthesis. The antibiotic forms unstable crystals which rapidly turn brown and liquefy on standing in air. It is soluble in H_2O, CH_3OH, EtOH, Et_2O and $(CH_3)_2CO$. The monosodium salt forms colourless crystals, readily soluble in H_2O, from which it yields a hydrate. It has been used experimentally as an antineoplastic agent.

Kaczka *et al.*, *Biochemistry*, **1**, 340 (1962)
Kinnel, Schoenewaldt, *U.S. Patent*, 3,154,578 (1964)
Biosynthesis
Stevens, Emery, *Biochemistry*, **5**, 74 (1966)

HALOMICIN A
$C_{43}H_{58}N_2O_{12}$

A macrocyclic antibiotic isolated from cultures of *Micromonospora halophytica*, this compound has been separated and purified by extraction of the culture broth and column and thin layer chromatography. It forms yellow crystals and has the structure shown above based upon chemical and spectroscopic examination. It is active against gram-positive bacteria and certain fungi.

Weinstein *et al.*, *Antimicrobial Agents & Chemotherapy*, 1435 (1967)
Structure
Ganguly *et al.*, *J. Antibiotics* (Japan), **30**, 625 (1977)

HALOMICIN B
$C_{43}H_{58}O_{12}N_2$
M.p. 178–182°C

A macrocyclic antibiotic, halomicin B is produced by *Micromonospora halophytica*. It may be purified by recrystallization from C_6H_6 when it forms yellow needles. It is dextrorotatory with a specific rotation of $[\alpha]_D$ + 73.1° and gives an ultraviolet spectrum in EtOH with absorption maxima at 238, 298 and 415 nm. The structure has been determined by chemical and spectroscopic methods. Halomycin B is active against gram-positive bacteria and some fungi.

Weinstein et al., *Antimicrobial Agents & Chemotherapy*, 1435 (1967)

HALOMICIN C
$C_{43}H_{58}N_2O_{12}$

A positional isomer of halomicins A and B, this macrocyclic antibiotic has also been isolated from the fermentation broth of *Micromonospora halophytica*. It has the structure given above which has been established from chemical analysis and spectroscopic data. It possesses an antibiotic spectrum similar to those of the preceding antibiotics.

Weinstein et al., *Antimicrobial Agents & Chemotherapy*, 1435 (1967)
Structure
Ganguly et al., *J. Antibiotics* (Japan), **30**, 625 (1977)

HAMYCIN
Dec. 160°C
A heptaene antibiotic produced by *Streptomyces pimprina*, hamycin forms a yellow amorphous powder. It has a specific rotation of $[\alpha]_D^{25}$ + 216° and gives an ultraviolet spectrum in 80 per cent CH_3OH with a single absorption maximum at 383 nm. Hamycin is soluble in basic solvents such as pyridine and in aqueous lower alcohols but virtually insoluble in H_2O, C_6H_6, $CHCl_3$ and Et_2O. The acute toxicity in mice is 6.16 mg/kg of a 0.21–0.52 mg/ml dispersion in sodium carboxymethylcellulose when given intravenously. Given orally to rats in food it produces a dose-dependent hypocholesterolemic effect.

Thirumalachar et al., *Hindustan Antibiot. Bull.*, **3**, 136 (1961)
Thirumalachar, *U.S. Patent*, 3,261,751 (1966)
Toxicity
Williams et al., *Antimicrobial Agents & Chemotherapy*, 737 (1964)
Dave et al., *Proc. Soc. Exp. Biol. Med.*, **149**, 299 (1975)

HELENINE
M.p. Indefinite
A complex antibiotic produced by *Penicillium funiculosum* NRRL 2075, this compound is probably a ribonucleoprotein. It is precipitated by protein reagents such as $(CH_3)_2CO$ and freeze-drying of the broth does not reduce the antibiotic activity. It has been found to contain nitrogen, phosphorus and polysaccharides and is active in mice against both SK and Semliki Forest viruses.

Shope, *J. Exptl. Med.*, **97**, 601, 627, 639 (1953)
Lewis et al., *J. Amer. Chem. Soc.*, **81**, 4115 (1959)
Lewis et al., *ibid.*, **82**, 5178 (1960)

HELIOCERIN
$C_{12}H_{17}O_3N$
M.p. 90–91°C
From its ultraviolet and infrared spectra, this antibiotic from cultures of *Helioceras oryzae* appears to be identical with cerulenin (q.v.).

Kouhei et al., *Ann. Sankyo Res. Lab.*, **19**, 86 (1967)

HELIOMYCIN
An antibiotic possessing bactericidal and vasoconstrictive activity, heliomycin is produced by *Streptomyces variabilis* var. *roseolus* strain 6383 and is isolated by extraction of the mycelium with $(CH_3)_2CO$. The antibiotic has proved useful in medicine in the treatment of burns or pyoderma and also for incorporation into cosmetics. By the use of labelled precursors it has been demonstrated that at 0.05–1.0 μg/ml, heliomycin inhibits RNA formation after 5 minutes incubation and protein formation after 3 minutes, but it does not have any effect upon DNA formation in cells of *Staphylococcus*

aureus. At the same concentration it has bacteriostatic activity against staphylococci and it appears that its antibacterial activity is due to inhibition of RNA formation.

Gauze *et al.*, *German Patent*, 2,212,854 (1972)
Korolev *et al.*, *Antibiotiki*, **20**, 503 (1975)

HELIXIN

An antibiotic produced by a *Streptomyces* species, this substance is closely related to endomycin (q.v.). It is obtained from the culture broth by precipitation at pH 3·0 followed by extraction of the precipitate with EtOH. Helixin is soluble in EtOH, CH_3OH, pyridine and glacial AcOH, slightly soluble in $(CH_3)_2CO$, $CHCl_3$ and BuOH and insoluble in Et_2O, C_6H_6, AcOEt, CCl_4 and petroleum ether. It is somewhat less stable than endomycin and is most active at an alkaline pH. Almost all filamentous and non-filamentous fungi are susceptible at concentrations of less than 15 µg/ml. It is also active against bacteria in concentrations of 30 µg/ml or more. Helixin causes the inhibition of seed germination and is toxic to tomato cuttings at low concentrations of 7–15 µg/ml.

Leben, Stessel, Keitt, *Mycologia*, **44**, 159 (1952)
Leben, Keitt, *Phytopath.*, **42**, 168 (1952)

HELVOLIC ACID

See Fumigacin

HEPCIN

M.p. Indefinite

A new species of fungus, *Actinosporangium griseoroseum* yields this antibiotic when cultivated on a medium consisting of glucose, soybean flour and inorganic salts at 28°C for 4 days. The moist mycelium is extracted with BuOH, the solvent evaporated, the crude antibiotic washed with petroleum ether and purified by countercurrent distribution. Hepcin is dextrorotatory with $[\alpha]_D^{20} + 90°$ (c 0·2, dimethylformamide) and the ultraviolet spectrum in 80 per cent CH_3OH has absorption maxima at 359, 379 and 401 nm. It is primarily active against fungi and has LD_{50} in mice of 0·5 mg/kg when given intravenously.

Tsyganov *et al.*, *Antibiotiki*, **15**, 963 (1970)

HEPTAFUNGIN A

Dec. > 170°C

Streptomyces longisoporolavendulae strain S401 yields an antibiotic complex which, on separation and purification by countercurrent distribution yields 80 per cent of this antibiotic and smaller amounts of heptafungins B and C as minor components. Heptafungin A is a pale yellow amorphous powder decomposing above 170°C. The ultraviolet spectrum in CH_3OH has absorption maxima at 360, 380 and 402 nm. Alkaline hydrolysis gives *p*-aminoacetophenone and acid hydrolysis furnishes mycosamine. It closely resembles candicidin (q.v.) in its chemical and biological properties.

Kalasz *et al.*, *Acta Microbiol.*, **19**, 111 (1972)

2-n-HEPTYL-4-QUINOLINOL

$C_{16}H_{21}NO$

A simple quinolinol derivative, this antibiotic has been obtained from cultures of a marine *Pseudonomad* together with the n-pentyl derivative (q.v.). It exhibits inhibitory activity against *Candida albicans*, *Staphylococcus aureus*, *Vibrio anquillarum* and *V. harveyi*.

Wratten *et al.*, *Antimicrobial Agents & Chemotherapy*, **11**, 411 (1977)

HERBICIDIN A

$C_{23}H_{29}N_5O_{11}$

Streptomyces saganonensis elaborates two similar antibiotics when grown by submerged culture and these have been isolated by adsorption on a resinous adsorbent and eluted with Me_2CO. Purification has been carried out by either silica gel chromatography or counter-current distribution on a Ronor column. This antibiotic is active against a range of gram-positive bacteria.

Haneishi *et al.*, *J. Antibiotics* (Japan), **29**, 870 (1976)

HERBICIDIN B

$C_{18}H_{23}N_5O_9$

A second component of the antibiotic mixture produced by the submerged culture of *Streptomyces saganonensis*, this substance is also active against gram-positive bacteria.

Haneishi *et al.*, *J. Antibiotics* (Japan), **29**, 870 (1976)

HERQUEIN
$C_{19}H_{20}O_8$
M.p. 120–129°C (dec.)

Herquein was first described by Burton in 1949 who obtained it from cultures of *Penicillium herquei*. It is formed by surface growth on a medium containing glucose and inorganic salts and isolated by acidifying the culture filtrate to pH 2·0, suspending the precipitate in H_2O and extracting with $CHCl_3$. The extract is then shaken with H_2O at pH 7·5, the aqueous phase separated and acidified with dilute HCl thereby precipitating the antibiotic as a yellow microcrystalline powder. It may be purified further by recrystallizing from C_6H_6 or aqueous EtOH. Herquein forms brownish-yellow crystals which are soluble in EtOH and $CHCl_3$, sparingly so in EtO_2, CCl_4, C_6H_6 and H_2O and insoluble in petroleum ether. The antibiotic is active against *Mycobacterium phlei*, *Pseudomonas aeruginosa*, *Shigella dysenteriae*, *Staphylococcus albus* and *Streptococcus pyogenes* and inhibits both *Staphylococcus aureus* and *Vibrio comma* at a dilution of 1:2500.

Burton, *Brit. J. Exptl. Path.*, **30**, 151 (1949)

HETACILLIN
$C_{19}H_{23}O_4N_3S$
M.p. Indefinite

A semi-synthetic antibiotic of the penicillin type, this substance is used as the crystalline potassium salt for the treatment of bovine mastitis in lactating cows. In this respect it complies with the requirements of the American Federal Food, Drug and Cosmetic Act with the proviso that the milk from such cows must not be used for at least 3 days. Hetacillin has also found use in clinical medicine. The parent antibiotic decomposes at 182–184°C and has a specific rotation of $[\alpha]_D^{25} + 366°$ (c 1·0 pyridine). The methyl ester has m.p. 101·5–102°C and is soluble in most organic solvents. Minimum inhibitory concentrations (μg/ml) determined by Morita *et al.* are: *Bacillus anthracis* (6·2); *B. Subtilis* (6·2); *Escherichia coli* (3·1–6·3); *Klebsella* spp. (6·2); *Proteus vulgaris* (6·2); *Salmonella* spp. (3·1–6·2); *Shigella* spp. (1·6–6·2); *Staphylococcus aureus* (0·4–1·6) and *Streptococcus fecalis* (6·2). The antibiotic is inactive against *Aerobacter*, *Cloaca*, *Hafnia* and *Pseudomonas*.

Johnson, Panetta, *U.S. Patent*, 3,198,804 (1965)
Hardcastle *et al.*, *J. Org. Chem.*, **31**, 897 (1966)
Shioda *et al.*, *J. Antibiotics* (Japan), **20B**, 94 (1967)
Morita *et al.*, *ibid.*, **20B**, 100 (1967)
Ueda *et al.*, *ibid.*, **20B**, 206 (1967)
Fed. Regist., **38** (217), 31172 (12 November 1973)
Suda *et al.*, *J. Antibiotics* (Japan), **26**, 512 (1973)

HETEROSTROPHIN
$C_{36}H_{62}O_{10}$
M.p. 172–173°C

A complex antibiotic, heterostrophin has been isolated from *Ophiobolus heterostrophus*. When recrystallized from EtOH it forms colourless needles. It is slightly dextrorotatory with a specific rotation of $[\alpha]_D + 15°$ and forms a crystalline sodium salt, m.p. 249–250°C.

Tsuda, Nozoe, Shirasaka, *Japanese Patent*, 7,020,557 (1970)

HEXA-N-BENZYLNEOMYCIN
$C_{65}H_{82}O_{13}N_6$

This antibiotic substance has been prepared chemically from neomycin (q.v.) by reductive alkylation with benzaldehyde. It is active *in vitro* against a number of bacteria including *Staphylococcus aureus* when it has a minimum inhibitory concentration of 3·9 mg/ml. It has no activity, however, *in vivo* when administered to mice infected with *Staph. aureus* at a dose of 40 mg/kg given subcutaneously.

Shier, Rinehart, *J. Antibiotics* (Japan), **26**, 547 (1973)

HIKIZIMYCIN
$C_{13}H_{29}O_{10}N_3$

Streptomyces hikiziensis yields this antibiotic which is normally isolated as the crystalline hydrobromide which forms colourless crystals that become brown at 214–215°C, darken at 230°C and do not melt up to 300°C. An earlier specific rotation for this salt of $[\alpha]_D^{23.5} + 30.9°$ (c 1·0, H_2O) was later revised to $[\alpha]_D^{23.5} - 40.6°$ (c 1·0, H_2O) and it is possible that two stereoisomers are involved here, since in the latter case *Streptomyces* strain A-5 was used in the production of the antibiotic. The base antibiotic has been prepared by culturing the organism at 27–29°C and pH 6·0–8·0 for 10 days. Almost all carbon sources examined were utilized by the organism with the exception of cellulose, dulcitol, raffinose, rhamnose and sorbitol. The base antibiotic is soluble in H_2O but insoluble in organic solvents, the hydrobromide is soluble in H_2O, slightly soluble in CH_3OH but insoluble in EtOH, ACOEt, $CHCl_3$, C_6H_6, AcOH and pyridine. The NMR spectrum and degradative studies indicate the presence of cytosine and 3-amino-3-deoxy-D-glucose (kanosamine) in the molecule.

Hikizimycin is active against *Helminthosporium* and numerous other species of plant-pathogenic fungi. The LD_{50} in mice is 15 mg/kg when administered intravenously.

Uchida et al., *Japanese Patent*, 7,039,038 (1970)
Uchida et al., *J. Antibiotics* (Japan), **24**, 259 (1971)

HIRSUTIC ACID A
$C_{15}H_{20}O_4$
M.p. Indefinite

The fungus *Stereum hirsutum* elaborates a substance, hirsutic acid C, during the early stages of its life cycle which is antibiotically inactive and is the precursor for a series of antibiotics. Hirsutic acid A, however, is formed from the precursor by treatment with dilute alkali at 20–24°C for 30 minutes, acidifying the mixture to pH 2·0, cooling and filtering off any unchanged starting material. It may be purified further by chromatographine on an alumina column after Et_2O extraction and evaporating the ethereal fraction. The antibiotic forms a colourless, brittle glass having no definite melting point. It is soluble in most organic solvents with the exceptions of CCl_4 and n-hexane, decolourizes potassium permanganate solution and gives negative reactions with Fehling's solution, 2:4-dinitrophenylhydrazine and acidified potassium iodide solution.

The antibiotic is assayed by cylinder plate using *Staphylococcus aureus* as the test organism. It shows no activity towards *Escherichia coli* or *Salmonella enteriditis*, has a slight activity against *Streptococcus pyogenes* but is active against *Staphylococcus aureus* at an inhibition dilution of 1:8000. There is, however, no evidence for any lysis of the latter organism. The activity is not affected by either peptone or ox serum.

The intravenous LD_{50} for mice has been given as 15–20 mg/kg while at a dilution of 1:4000 it kills human leucocytes.

Heatley, Jennings, Florey, *Brit. J. Exptl. Path.*, **28**, 35 (1947)

HIRSUTIC ACID N
$C_{15}H_{20}O_4$
M.p. Indefinite

Also obtained from hirsutic acid C, isolated from *Stereum hirsutus*, this antibiotically active substance may be obtained either by incubating hirsutic acid C with washed mycelium or mycelial extract or by continuing the growth and metabolism of the organism when the fungus converts the initially formed hirsutic acid C into this compound. Hirsutic acid N is purified by passing the Et_2O extract through a silica-phosphate buffer column at pH 7·0, washing with more Et_2O, concentrating the percolates by distillation, extracting with H_2O at pH 6·5–7·0, treating the aqueous extracts with activated carbon, acidifying and extracting again into Et_2O. The ethereal extract is then passed through an alumina column, the zone containing the antibiotic showing up with a purple fluorescence under ultraviolet light. It is eluted with a phosphate buffer, acidified, extracted with Et_2O and the solvent evaporated to leave hirsutic acid N as a colourless, transparent glass which cannot be crystallized. The antibiotic is soluble in alkali and most organic solvents with the exception of CCl_4 and n-hexane, slightly soluble in hot H_2O and insoluble in cold H_2O. It is stable indefinitely as the glassy solid or in solution in Et_2O, but has a lower stability in aqueous solution, particularly at an alkaline pH.

Like the preceding antibiotic, it is assayed by the cylinder plate method with *Staphylococcus aureus* as the test organism. It is inhibitory *in vitro* against *Corynebacterium diphtheriae* and *Neisseria meningitidis* at a dilution of 1:40,000 and against *Staphylococcus aureus* and *Streptococcus pyogenes* at a dilution of 1:10,000. It is also active against the following organisms which are arranged in order of increasing sensitivity: *Bacillus subtilis*, *Vibrio comma*, *Sarcina lutea*, *Bacillus anthracis* and *Mycobacterium lysodeikticus*. It has no activity against *Aerobacter aerogenes*, *Escherichia coli*, *Klebsiella pneumoniae*, *Proteus vulgaris*, *Pseudomonas aeruginosa* and *Salmonella typhi*.

The LD_{50} in mice is 1–2 mg when given intravenously although 20 mg is tolerated when administered orally. In cats it causes an irreversible slowing of the isolated heart and an increased blood pressure but has no effect on the respiration. When administered to guinea pigs it caused a cessation of the uterine contractions.

Heatley, Jennings, Florey, *Brit. J. Exptl. Path.*, **28**, 35 (1947)

HISTIDOMYCIN A

An antibiotic derived from *Nocardia histedans* ATCC 21021, this substance is produced by culturing the organism by submerged fermentation in an aqueous-nutrient medium at 28°C for 7–8 days. Purification by chromatography separates the initial mixture into two components, histidomycins A and B. This antibiotic has been proposed for the control of plant diseases, particularly leaf rust of wheat and also for the sterilization of pharmaceutical equipment.

Demny, *U.S. Patent*, 3,657,418 (1972)

HISTIDOMYCIN B

A further antibiotic produced by *Nocardia histedans* ATCC 21021, this substance is separated from the preceding antibiotic by chromatography on an alumina column. It has similar biological properties to histidomycin A.

Demny, *U.S. Patent*, 3,657,418 (1972)

HISTOCILLIN
See Amoxycillin

HODYDAMYCIN
M.p. Indefinite

A peptide antibiotic, hodydamycin has been described by Egyptian workers. It is stated to be active against gram-positive bacteria but has little activity against gram-negative organisms. Its mode of action is to cause DNA scission with subsequent inhibition of protein synthesis. When tested against *Staphylococcus aureus* it brought about the release of nucleic acids and inhibited the formation of protein and DNA but has no effect on RNA synthesis, the cell membrane or the synthesis of the cell wall.

Shimi, Shoukry, *J. Antibiotics* (Japan), **27**, 133 (1974)

HOLOMYCIN
$C_7H_6O_2N_2S_2$
Dec. 268–270°C

Produced by a strain of *Streptomyces griseus* (Krainski) Waksman et Henrici, the structure of this antibiotic is N-demethylthiolutin. When crystallized from CH_3OH—AcOEt it forms orange-yellow flakes which decompose without melting. The ultraviolet spectrum in EtOH has absorption maxima at 245, 302 nm with a shoulder at 290 nm. It is active against a number of gram-positive and gram-negative organisms.

Ettlinger *et al.*, *Helv. Chim. Acta*, **42**, 563 (1959)
Gaumann *et al.*, *U.S. Patent*, 3,014,922 (1961)
Synthesis
Schmidt, Geiger, *Annalen.*, **664**, 168 (1963)
Büchi, Lukas, *J. Amer. Chem. Soc.*, **86**, 5654 (1964)
Okamura *et al.*, *J. Antibiotics* (Japan), **30**, 334 (1977)

HONDAMYCIN (*Albimycin*)
$C_{47}H_{78}O_{13}$
M.p. 149–150°C (*dec.*)

Streptomyces griseochromogenes var. *albicus* elaborates this antibiotic which forms colourless crystals when purified by recrystallization from EtOH. It has a specific rotation of $[\alpha]_D^{13.5} - 48.1°$ (c 1·93 CH_3OH) and gives an ultraviolet spectrum in CH_3OH having absorption maxima at 225 and 232·5 nm with shoulders at 219, 240 and 270-279 nm. The compound forms a crystalline acetate, m.p. 120°C (*dec.*). Hondamycin inhibits the growth of gram-positive bacteria.

Sakagami *et al.*, *J. Antibiotics* (Japan), **22**, 521 (1969)
Sakagami, Yamabayashı, Ueda, *ibid.*, **22**, 528 (1969)
Ueda, Sakagami, *ibid.*, **22**, 536 (1969)

HUMULON
$C_{21}H_{30}O_5$
M.p. 65–66·5°C

A plant antibiotic isolated from the dried cones of *Humulus lupulus* (hop vine), this substance accompanies lupulon (q.v.). It may be obtained by precipitation from a crude petroleum ether extract of hops or from the mother liquor of lupulon crystals with *o*-phenylenediamine, followed by acidification and extraction with Et_2O. The pure material forms yellow crystals and is laevorotatory with a specific rotation of $[\alpha]_D^{20} - 232°$ (c 1·0, C_6H_6). It is moderately soluble in CH_3OH, EtOH, *n*-hexane, *iso*-octane and petroleum ether, and slightly soluble in neutral or acid aqueous solution. The antibiotic is comparatively stable in acid solution but unstable under alkaline conditions and readily oxidized on exposure to air. It decolourises potassium permanganate solution and bromine water, gives a violet-red colour with $FeCl_3$ solution and forms the dihydro derivative on catalytic hydrogenation.

Humulon is assayed by serial dilution with *Sclerotina fructicola* spore germination and by cylinder plate and turbidimetric methods. It is somewhat more active than lupulon (q.v.), the following inhibition dilutions ($\times$ 1000) having been determined by Lewis *et al.*: *Bacillus anthracis* (100); *B. cereus* var. *mycoides* (100); *B. subtilis* (50); *Corynebacterium diphtheriae gravis* (10); *Diplococcus pneumoniae* I (20); *Micrococcus lysodeikticus* (60); *M. pyogenes* var. *aureus* (30); *Mycobacterium phlei* (30); *Myco. tuberculosis hominis* (10); *Sarcina lutea* (30); *Streptococcus fecalis* (30) and *Streptomyces coelicolor* (3·0). There is no synergism with other antitubercular antibiotics.

Walker, Parker, *J. Inst. Brewing*, **43**, 17 (1937)
Shimwell, *ibid.*, **43**, 111 (1937)
Lewis *et al.*, *J. Clin. Invest.*, **28**, 916 (1949)
Michener, Andersen, *Science*, **110**, 68 (1949)

HYALODENDRIN
$C_{14}H_{16}N_2O_3S_2$

A species of *Hyalodendron* yields this antibiotic, the structure of which has been established from chemical and spectroscopic examination. It has been shown to inhibit a broad range of fungi which cause damage and decay of trees. The LD_{50} in mice has been found to be 75 mg/kg when administered intraperitoneally.

Stillwell, Magasi, Strunz, *Can. J. Microbiol.*, **20**, 759 (1974)

HYBRIMYCIN A_1
$C_{23}H_{46}O_{14}N_6$

A number of aminoglycosidic antibiotics are produced by mutant microorganisms which are incapable of synthesizing an aminocyclitol molecule when these organisms are grown in a medium which contains an added aminocyclitol unit. This particular antibiotic is formed by *Streptomyces fradiae* ATCC 21401 mutant when it is cultured in the presence of added streptamine. The structure has been determined by chemical degradation and spectroscopic techniques. Like all of the known hybrimycins, it possesses activity against gram-positive and gram-negative organisms.

Shier, Rinehart, Gottlieb, *U.S. Patent*, 3,669,838 (1972)

HYBRIMYCIN A_2
$C_{23}H_{46}O_{14}N_6$

An isomer of the preceding semi-synthetic antibiotic, this compound is also produced by *Streptomyces fradiae* ATCC 21401 mutant growth in the

HYBRIMYCIN B₁
$C_{23}H_{46}O_{14}N_6$

This antibiotic is an epimer of hybrimycin A₁ and is formed when *Streptomyces fradiae* mutant ATCC 21401 is cultured in the presence of added 2-*epi*streptamine. The structure given has been established by degradative and spectroscopic determination. The antibiotic activity is similar to that of hybrimycin A₁.

Shier, Rinehart, Gottlieb, *U.S. Patent*, 3,669,838 (1972)

HYBRIMYCIN B₂
$C_{23}H_{46}O_{14}N_6$

presence of added streptamine. It is an antibacterial agent and has the structure given above.

Shier, Rinehart, Gottlieb, *U.S. Patent*, 3,669,838 (1972)

A fourth semi-synthetic antibiotic produced by *Streptomyces fradiae* ATCC 21401 mutant grown on a medium containing added 2-*epi*streptamine, the structure of this compound has been shown to be the epimer of hybrimycin A₂.

Shier, Rinehart, Gottlieb, *U.S. Patent*, 3,669,838 (1972)

HYBRIMYCIN C₁
$C_{23}H_{45}O_{15}N_5$

This semi-synthetic antibiotic is produced by *Streptomyces rimosus* forma *paromomycinus* ATCC 21485 mutant grown on a medium to which streptamine has been added. The structure is similar to that of hybrimycin A₁ but with one amino substituent replaced by a hydroxyl group.

Shier, Rinehart, Gottlieb, *U.S. Patent*, 3,669,838 (1972)

HYBRIMYCIN C₂
$C_{23}H_{45}O_{15}N_5$

Hydracillin

A further antibiotic formed by culturing *Streptomyces rimosus* forma *paromomycinus* ATCC 21485 mutant in the presence of added streptamine, this compound has a structure similar to that of hybrimycin A_2 with one amino group replaced by a hydroxyl group in the molecule.

Shier, Rinehart, Gottlieb, *U.S. Patent*, 3,668,838 (1972)

HYDRACILLIN
See Procaine Penicillin G

1-N-(DL-HYDROXY-4-AMINOBUTYRL)RIBOSTAMYCIN
A semi-synthetic antibiotic, this compound has been prepared from ribostamycin by a series of standard chemical reactions. It has been shown to be highly active against *Pseudomonas aeruginosa*.

Akita, Horiuchi, Ito, *Japanese Patent*, 7,378,141 (1973)

N^5-HYDROXY-L-ARGININE
This antibiotic aminoacid is derived from an unclassified species of *Bacillus*. It is active against a number of gram-positive and gram-negative organisms including *Escherichia coli*. The antibiotic activity is reversed by L-arginine and similar compounds.

Maehr et al., *J. Antibiotics* (Japan), **26**, 284 (1973)

2-HYDROXYBUTIROSIN
$C_{17}H_{34}N_4O_{11}$

6′-Hydroxy-6′-deamino-1-N-methylkanamycin A

A mutasynthetic antibiotic produced by a deoxystreptamine-lacking mutant of *Bacillus circulans*, this compound is formed when cultured in the presence of added streptamine. The structure has been shown to be that given above. It has an antibiotic activity similar to that of butirosin.

Claridge et al., *Dev. Ind. Microbiol.*, **15**, 101 (1974)
Taylor, Schmitz, *J. Antibiotics* (Japan), **29**, 532 (1976)

6′-HYDROXY-6′-DEAMINO-2-*epi*-HYDROXYKANAMYCIN A
$C_{17}H_{33}N_3O_{13}$

A mutasynthetic antibiotic having properties similar to those of kanamycin A, this substance is produced by a D^- strain of *Streptomyces kanamyceticus*. The structure has been established as that given above by chemical and spectroscopic examination.

Kojima, Satoh, *J. Antibiotics* (Japan), **26**, 784 (1973)
Shier et al., *Biochemistry*, **13**, 5073 (1974)

6′-HYDROXY-6′-DEAMINO-1-N-METHYLKANAMYCIN A
$C_{18}H_{35}N_3O_{12}$

The D^- mutant of *Streptomyces kanamyceticus* which is unable to synthesize deoxystreptamine, also yields this kanamycin antibiotic, the structure of which has been established as that given above. It possesses an antibiotic activity similar to that of kanamycin.

14-HYDROXYDAUNOMYCIN

See Adriamycin

8-HYDROXYERYTHROMYCIN A

$C_{37}H_{67}O_{14}N$

A synthetic derivative of erythromycin A, this antibiotic has been prepared from the N-oxide of erythromycin A 8:9-anhydro-6-hemiacetal. It is active *in vitro* against *Bacillus pumilus* although it has only about half the activity of the parent antibiotic, the cylinder plate method assaying at 500 μg/mg in erythromycin A units. It has the advantage, however, that its stability under acid conditions is some 500–600 times greater.

Krowicki, Zamojski, *J. Antibiotics* (Japan), **26**, 575 (1973)

(+)-5'-HYDROXYGRISEOFULVIN

$C_{17}H_{17}O_7Cl$

A semi-synthetic antibiotic, (+)-5'-hydroxygriseofulvin is produced from either (+)-griseofulvin or dehydrogriseofulvin by fermentation with *Streptomyces cinereocrocatus*. The compound possesses antifungal properties *in vitro* and also *in vivo*.

Andres, Kunstmann, *U.S. Patent*, 3,557,151 (1971)

1-(L-2-HYDROXY-3-MERCAPTOPROPANOIC ACID)OXYTOCIN

$C_{43}H_{65}O_{13}N_{11}S_2$

This analogue of oxytocin, containing a hydroxyl group in place of the amino group has been prepared by coupling *p*-(nitrophenyl)-L-2-acetoxy-

Kojima, Satoh, *J. Antibiotics* (Japan), **26**, 784 (1973)

3-(benzylthiopropanoyl)-L-tyrosinate with a heptapeptide. Tests have demonstrated that it has three times the oxytocic activity of oxytocin itself.

Waelti, Hope, *J. Chem. Soc., Perkin I*, 1946 (1972)

5-HYDROXYMETHYLTUBERCIDIN
$C_{12}H_{16}O_5N_4$

A semi-synthetic antibiotic, this substance has been prepared from tubercidin-5-carboxylic acid via the methyl ester and the $2':3'$-O-*iso*propylidene derivative followed by reduction with $LiAlH_4$. It resembles toyocamycin (q.v.) in its action but is more selective, giving 50 per cent inhibition of growth of leukemia L-1210 cells at a concentration of 4×10^{-7} M. It does not inhibit the growth of either *Escherichia coli* or *Mycobacterium phlei* cells.

Uematsu, Suhadolnik, *J. Med. Chem.*, **16**, 1405 (1973)

HYDROXYMYCIN
See Paromomycin

HYDROXYNYBOMYCIN
$C_{16}H_{14}N_2O_5$

Streptomyces strain D-57 elaborates this derivative of nybomycin which has been isolated and purified as the dibutyrate. The free antibiotic has been obtained by hydrolysis of this ester with concentrated hydrochloric acid at 25°C. Hydroxynybomycin is active against a number of bacteria, particularly *Bacillus subtilis*, *Klebsiells pneumoniae* and *Mycobacterium avium*. The activity of this antibiotic is lower than that of nybomycin or deoxynybomycin.

Nadzan, Rinehart, Sokolski, *J. Antibiotics* (Japan), **30**, 523 (1977)

1-(*p*-HYDROXYPHENYL)-2:3-DIISOCYANO-4-(*p*-METHOXYPHENYL)-1:3-BUTADIENE
$C_{19}H_{14}O_4N_2$

By means of the paper disc-agar diffusion plaque-inhibition method, this antibiotic is isolated from the mycelium of *Dichotomomyces albus* in a crystalline form. Its structure is the methyl ether of xanthocillin X. The crystals decompose about 116°C. It is active against some gram-positive and gram-negative bacteria, particularly *Proteus vulgaris* and *Shigella flexneri* and also inhibits plaque formation of Newcastle disease virus infected upon primary chick embryo fibroblast cell monolayer. The acute intraperitoneal LD_{50} for mice is 40 mg/kg and the LD_{50} for HeLa cells 0·3 µg/ml.

Ando *et al.*, *J. Antibiotics* (Japan), **21**, 582 (1968)

3-HYDROXYPIROMIDIC ACID
$C_{14}H_{16}O_4N_4$

A new antibiotic, 3-hydroxypiromidic acid is elaborated by *Streptomyces endus* strain 228. It has the structure given above and is active against gram-positive and gram-negative bacteria.

Hironaka, Nishikawa, *Hakko Kogaku Zasshi*, **53**, 372 (1975)

1-(S)-HYDROXY-2-(S,S)-VALYLAMIDO-CYCLOBUTANE-1-ACETIC ACID
$C_{11}H_{20}N_2O_4$

A simple antibiotic obtained from cultures of a strain of *Streptomyces* designated X-1092, this substance inhibits the growth of a range of gram-positive bacteria in a chemically-defined medium. Experiments have shown, however, that the growth inhibition is partially reversed in the presence of L-cysteine.

Pruess *et al.*, *J. Antibiotics* (Japan), **27**, 754 (1974)

HYGROMYCIN A
$C_{23}H_{29}O_{12}N$
M.p. Indefinite

A glycosidic antibiotic, this compound has been obtained from *Streptomyces hygroscopicum* (Jensen) Waksman. It is an amorphous white powder which is laevorotatory with a specific rotation of $[\alpha]_D^{25} - 126°$ (c 1·0, H_2O). It may be characterized as the crystalline 2:4-dinitrophenylhydrazone which crystallizes from H_2O with m.p. 154–156°C.

Mann, Gale, van Abcole, *Antibiotics & Chemotherapy*, **3**, 1279 (1953)
Mann, Wolf, *J. Amer. Chem. Soc.*, **79**, 120 (1957)

HYGROMYCIN B
$C_{20}H_{37}O_{13}N_3$
M.p. Indefinite

A further antibiotic elaborated by *Streptomyces hygroscopicus* (Jensen) Waksman, hygromycin B is also an amorphous white powder with no definite melting point. It has a specific rotation of $[\alpha]_D^{26} + 20·2°$ (c 1·0, H_2O).

Mann, Bromer, *J. Amer. Chem. Soc.*, **80**, 2714 (1958)
Wiley, Sigal, Weaver, *J. Org. Chem.*, **27**, 2793 (1962)
Structure
Neuss *et al.*, *Helv. Chim. Acta*, **53**, 2314 (1970)

HYPERFORIN
$C_{35}H_{52}O_4$
M.p. 79–80°C

This antibiotic has been obtained from cultures of *Hypericum perforatum*. It is dextrorotatory having a specific rotation of $[\alpha]_D^{18} + 41°$ (c 1·0, EtOH). The structure is not yet known with certainty.

Gurevich *et al.*, *Antibiotiki* (Moscow), **16**, 510 (1971)

I

IKARUGAMYCIN
$C_{29}H_{38}O_4N_2$
M.p. Indefinite

A *Streptomyces* antibiotic, this compound has been isolated from *S. phaeochromogenes* var. *ikaruganensis* freshly obtained from soil. The organism is cultivated on a common nutrient medium for 2 days at 30°C, the culture filtrate being stirred with activated carbon at pH 7·6 and the mycelium extracted with CH_3OH—$CHCl_3$, the combined extracts being evaporated to give the crystalline antibiotic. Ikarugamycin is only active against *Trichomonas vaginalis*. It is a fairly non-toxic with mice tolerating a dose of 62·5 mg/kg given intraperitoneally.

Ajisaka *et al., Japanese Patent*, 7,128,833 (1971)

IKUTAMYCIN
$C_{68}H_{114}O_{13}N_2$
M.p. 169–171·5°C

An extremely complex antibiotic, ikutamycin has been obtained from cultures of *Streptomyces diastatochromogenes*. It forms colourless crystals when recrystallized from CH_3OH and is laevorotatory with a specific rotation of $[\alpha]_D^{13 \cdot 5} - 27 \cdot 8°$ (c 1·33, CH_3OH). It is active against gram-positive bacteria and, to a lesser extent, against gram-negative organisms.

Sakagami, *Japanese Patent*, 7,016,793 (1970)

ILCOCILLIN P
See Procaine penicillin G

ILICICOLINS
Cylindrocladium ilicicola elaborates an antibiotic complex which has been separated by chromatography into a number of components, e.g. ilicicolins A, B, C, D, E, F, G and H. All of these antibiotics have only a limited antibacterial activity and only *Bacillus anthracis* is inhibited at a concentration of 6 µg/ml. Possible antiviral activity could not be detected by means of the agar diffusion plaque-inhibition test because of the cytotoxicity of the substances. One characteristic feature of the cytotoxicity of these compounds is the chromosome aggregation in mitotic HeLa cells. Ilicicolin A is tolerated by mice at a dose of 100 mg/kg and the acute LD_{50} of ilicicolin E is given as 37·9 mg/kg when administered intraperitoneally.

Hayakawa *et al., J. Antibiotics* (Japan), **24**, 653 (1971)

ILLICICOLIN
See Ascochlorin

ILICICOLIN H
$C_{27}H_{31}NO_4$
M.p. 144–150°C

This component of the antibiotic complex produced by *Cylindrocladium ilicicola* forms colourless crystals and is laevorotatory having a specific rotation of $[\alpha]_D^{23} - 17 \cdot 4°$. It gives an ultraviolet spectrum in ethanol consisting of two absorption maxima at 248 and 349 nm. The structure given above has been elucidated from chemical analysis and a study of the infrared, NMR and mass spectra.

Hayakawa, Minato, Katagiri, *J. Antibiotics* (Japan), **24**, 653 (1971)
Structure
Matsumoto, Minato, *Tetrahedron Lett.*, 3827 (1976)

ILLUDIN M
$C_{15}H_{20}O_3$
M.p. 216°C

The basidiomycete *Clitocybe illudens* yields two closely related antibiotics, illudins M and S. This compound forms flat, prismatic rods when crystallized from 95 per cent EtOH. The ultraviolet spectrum in EtOH has absorption maxima at 228 and 318 nm. The antibiotic is characterized as the monoacetate, m.p. 75–76°C. Biologically, it is active against *Mycobacterium smegmatis* and *Myco. tuberculosis* H 37R.

Anchel *et al.*, *Proc. Nat. Acad. Sci.*, **36**, 300 (1950)
Structure
McMorris, Anchel, *J. Amer. Chem. Soc.*, **87**, 1594 (1965)
Tada *et al.*, *Chem. Pharm. Bull.*, **12**, 853 (1964)
Matsumoto *et al.*, *Tetrahedron*, **21**, 2671 (1965)
Stereochemistry
Nakanishi *et al.*, *Chem. Pharm. Bull.*, **12**, 856 (1964)
Matsumoto *et al.*, *Bull. Chem. Soc., Japan*, **37**, 1716 (1964)
Nakanishi *et al.*, *Tetrahedron*, **21**, 1231 (1965)

ILLUDIN S (*Lampterol*)
$C_{15}H_{20}O_4$
M.p. 124–126°C

A second antibiotic produced by *Clitocybe illudnes*, this substance forms colourless crystals from EtOH and has an ultraviolet spectrum in EtOH with absorption maxima at 223 and 319 nm. It yields a diacetate, m.p. 99–100°C. It possesses a similar antimicrobial activity to that of the preceding antibiotic.

Anchel *et al.*, *Proc. Nat. Acad. Sci.*, **36**, 300 (1950)
Structure
McMorris, Anchel, *J. Amer. Chem. Soc.*, **87**, 1594 (1965)
Tada *et al.*, *Chem. Pharm. Bull.*, **12**, 853 (1964)
Matsumoto *et al.*, *Tetrahedron*, **21**, 2671 (1965)
Stereochemistry
Nakanishi *et al.*, *Chem. Pharm. Bull.*, **12**, 856 (1964)
Matsumoto *et al.*, *Bull. Chem. Soc., Japan*, **37**, 1716 (1964)
Nakanishi *et al.*, *Tetrahedron*, **21**, 1231 (1965)

ILOTYCIN
See Erythromycin

INDANYLCARBENICILLIN
$C_{26}H_{26}O_6N_2S$

This semi-synthetic penicillin-type antibiotic is normally used in the form of the sodium salt. It has an antibiotic spectrum *in vitro* similar to that of carbenicillin (q.v.) and is active against indole-positive strains of *Proteus* and *Pseudomonas*. Tests carried out *in vivo* show that it has the same therapeutic effect in experimental infections in mice and rats as parenterally administered carbenicillin disodium salt. A single dose of 1·0 g given orally to humans produces serum and urine levels comparable with those found following a similar dose of carbenicillin given intramuscularly. This antibiotic, however, possesses the advantage over both benzylpenicillin and carbenicillin in that it is stable when incubated with gastric juice at 37°C for 1 hour, both of the former antibiotics being totally destroyed by this treatment.

Butler *et al.*, *Infect. Dis. Rev.*, **1**, 157 (1970)

INDOLMYCIN
$C_{14}H_{15}O_2N_3$
M.p. 209–210°C

An indole-type antibiotic derived from *Streptomyces albus*, this compound forms long rectangular prisms when crystallized from CH_3OH or AcOEt. It has a specific rotation of $[\alpha]_D^{25} - 214°$ (c 2·0, CH_3OH) and gives an ultraviolet spectrum with a single absorption maximum at 218 nm. It is a weakly basic substance, thermostable, moderately soluble in $(CH_3)_2CO$ and the lower alcohols, but only slightly soluble in H_2O, C_6H_6 and Et_2O. The picrate forms yellow-red plates from EtOH—Et_2O, m.p. 148–149°C. Indolmycin is active against a range of gram-positive and some gram-negative bacteria.

Rao, *Antibiotics & Chemotherapy*, **10**, 312 (1960)
Marsh *et al.*, *ibid.*, **10**, 316 (1960)
Structure and synthesis
Schach, von Wittenau, Els, *J. Amer. Chem. Soc.*, **83**, 4678 (1961)
Absolute configuration
Chan, Hill, *J. Org. Chem.*, **35**, 3519 (1970)
Biosynthesis
Hornemann *et al.*, *J. Amer. Chem. Soc.*, **93**, 3028 (1971)
See also
Watanabe *et al.*, *Japanese Patent*, 7,412,097 (1974)

INGRAMYCIN

$C_{18}H_{28}O_4$
M.p. 79–81°C

A recently discovered antibiotic, ingramycin is produced by *Streptomyces maizeus* NRRL 3508 cultured under aerobic submerged conditions on an aqueous nutrient medium. When purified by chromatography, the antibiotic forms colourless crystals, soluble in EtOH, CH_3OH, PrOH, BuOH, $(CH_3)_2CO$ and common chlorinated solvents but insoluble in H_2O. It is active against both gram-positive and gram-negative bacteria such as *Proteus vulgaris* and *Staphylococcus aureus* and also inhibits the growth of a number of pathogenic fungi, e.g. *Blastomyces dermatitidis* and *Histoplasma capsulatum*. Among the uses proposed for ingramycin are as a feed supplement for growth in animals, a disinfectant for dental and medical eqiupment and fungal growth in plate assays.

Bergy, Hoeksema, Johnson, *U.S. Patent*, 3,651,219 (1972)

INOLOMIN

M.p. Indefinite

Isolated from the fungus *Inoloma traganum*, this antibiotic substance forms a yellow varnish which is highly hygroscopic and difficult to purify. It is stable at room temperature and is freely soluble in H_2O and neutral phosphate buffer. When autoclaved it turns brown and rapidly loses its activity. It is isolated by crushing the fungi with H_2O, centrifuging and extruding the liquid through filter paper when a pale violet colloid is obtained. This is concentrated by heating to 100°C at pH 5·0–7·0. Purification is carried out by saturating the filtrate with ammonium sulphate, mixing the clear yellow filtrate with animal charcoal, filtering, mixing the filtrate with 'carborafine', refiltering, extracting the moist 'carborafine' with EtOH, filtering the extract and evaporating *in vacuo*.

Impure inolomin has been shown to inhibit the growth of an unclassified species of *Micrococcus*. It is non-toxic to mice at a dose of 1·0 ml of a 10 per cent solution administered intravenously.

Pragner, *Experientia*, **5**, 167 (1949)

INOMYCIN

An antibiotic of the actidione type, inomycin is elaborated by *Streptomyces griseus* var. *inomycini* which is cultured in a deep fermentation medium of glucose, oat flakes and inorganic salts at 27–29°C and pH 6·7–6·9 for 60–80 hours. Inomycin is isolated by adjusting the pH of the spent medium to 3·0, adsorbing the activity on activated carbon, eluting with 90 per cent $(CH_3)_2CO$, removing the solvent under reduced pressure, extracting with $CHCl_3$, chromatographing on an alumina column, eluting with 10:1-$CHCl_3$—$(CH_3)_2CO$, evaporating the solvent and crystallizing the residue from EtOH—C_6H_6-naphtha ether. Inomycin has been shown to inhibit transplantable tumours.

Tyc, *Polish Patent*, 66,256 (1972)

IODININ

$C_{12}H_8O_4N_2$

The antibiotic activity of iodinin was first discovered in 1941 by McIlwain although the compound has been isolated from *Chromobacterium iodinum* three years earlier by Clemo and McIlwain. It is produced by surface growth on media containing meat extract or peptone together with soluble citrates and beerwort. In the presence of sugars and most aminoacids, no antibiotic is formed. The culture is incubated for several days at 28°C followed by further incubation at 15°C. The substance is a dihydroxyphenazine N:N′-dioxide with the probable structure given above. It is readily soluble in $CHCl_3$, CS_2, AcOEt, C_6H_6, toluene and xylene, slightly soluble in hot EtOH, insoluble in cold EtOH, H_2O, Et_2O, amyl alcohol, aqueous and cold EtOH. In C_6H_6 solution it has a general absorption in the visible and near ultraviolet spectrum between 470 and 570 nm. It is stable in strong acid solution but unstable in alkalies. With alkali it forms a water-soluble, blue-green salt.

Inhibition concentrations (μf/ml) *in vitro* have been determined by McIlwain: *Eberalla typhi* (>43–85); *Escherichia coli* (>85); *Proteus vulgaris* (>85–170); *Staphylococcus aureus* (8–43) and *Streptococcus hemolyticus* (0·4–1·7). The activity of iodinin is reduced by both anthraquinone and maphthaquinone derivatives.

Clemo, McIlwain, *J. Chem. Soc.*, 479 (1938)
Davis, *Zbtl. Bakt. Parasitenk, II Abtl.*, **100**, 273 (1939)
McIlwain, *Nature*, **148**, 628 (1941)
McIlwain, *Biochem. J.*, **37**, 265 (1943)

IRPEXIN

This antibiotic is produced, together with corticin, from a species of *Basidiomycetes*. It has not been extensively examined since its discovery.

Robbins, Kavanagh, Hervey, *J. N.Y. Bot. Gardens*, **46**, 130 (1945)

ISEMYCIN
$C_{28}H_{30}O_7N_2$
M.p. 220°C (*dec.*)

Japanese workers have obtained this antibiotic from *Streptomyces flavochromogenes* var. *isensis* by fermentation, with aeration and shaking, in an aqueous medium containing soybean flour, yeast, starch and inorganic salts at 30°C for 3–4 days. Isemycin forms yellow crystals with a neutral reaction, which are thermostable and stable in acids and alkalies. The antibiotic inhibits the growth of *Bacillus megatherium*, *B. subtilis*, *Sarcina lutea* and *Staphylococcus aureus* 209P strain.

Miyoshi *et al.*, *Japanese Patent*, 7,200,038 (1972)

ISOCILLIN
See Penicillin V potassium salt

ISORORIDIN E
$C_{29}H_{38}O_8$

A macrocyclic antibiotic produced by *Cylindrocarpon* strain PF-60, this substance has the above structure based upon chemical and spectroscopic evidence. The organism is fermented for 91 hours at 28°C with aeration and agitation in a medium comprising sucrose and boiled potato extract. Extraction of the culture broth yields an oily residue which possesses antifungal activity. Silica gel column chromatography followed by preparative thin layer chromatography on silica gel gives this compound together with 7β,8β-epoxyisororidin E, 7β,8β-epoxyroridin H and 7β,8β-2′,3′-diepoxyroridin H (q.v.). The antibiotic is active against gram-positive and some gram-negative bacteria.

Matsumoto *et al.*, *J. Antibiotics* (Japan), **30**, 681 (1977)

ISOTENTOXINE
$C_{20}H_{28}N_4O_4$

Alternaria mali Roberts AKI-3 produces this antibiotic which has the structure shown above based upon chemical and spectroscopic studies. The organism is cultured at pH 4·5 and 30°C for 16–28 days and the filtrate extracted with $CHCl_3$ to give an oil which, on column chromatography with silica gel yields this antibiotic and tentoxine (q.v.), separated by high-speed liquid chromatography. Isotentoxine is active against *Piricularia oryzae* and bacterial infections of plants.

Okeino, *Japanese Patent*, 77 118,487 (1977)

ITABASHILLIN
$C_{32}H_{30}O_{14}$
M.p. 264·5–266·5°C
This antibiotic is derived from *Penicillium oxalicum* var. *itabashikum* NRRL 5672 and is obtained by fermentation of the organism in a common medium with aeration at 28°C and pH 5·0 for 6 days. Itabashillin is active against *Bacillus subtilis* and against infections with *Trichophyton* in humans and mice.

Ishida *et al.*, *German Patent*, 2,262,722 (1973)

ITAMYCIN
M.p. 300°C
Itamycin is obtained by growing *Streptomyces* species 5695-IAUFPe in submerged culture in a medium consisting of glucose, soybean flour, dried yeast and inorganic salts at pH 6·6–6·8 and 27°C for 4 days. The antibiotic is isolated by extraction of the culture filtrate and mycelium with BuOH at pH 2·0, 7·0 or 9·0, or with $CHCl_3$ or C_6H_6—AcOEt at pH 7·0 or 9·0. It forms yellow crystals and gives positive Benedict and Tollens reactions, negative tests with Fehlings and Molisch reagents. The acetyl derivative has m.p. 226·5°C. Itamycin is active against gram-positive bacteria and *Brucella* species. The LD_{50} in mice is about 75 mg/kg given intravenously.

Lyra *et al.*, *Rev. Inst. Antibiot., Univ. Recife*, **8**, 49 (1968)

J

JANEIMYCIN
M.p. Indefinite

Cultivation of *Streptomyces macrosporus* ATCC 21,388 under submerged aerobic conditions in a medium containing common assimilable carbon and nitrogen sources for 6 days yields this antibiotic which has a polypeptide structure. Electrophoresis at pH 3·3 in the presence of 30 per cent formamide separates the compound into three active components. The complex is a light tan amorphous powder with no definite melting point, the ultraviolet spectrum in EtOH having absorption maxima at 239 and 272 nm, that in alkaline solution having a single absorption maximum at 253 nm. Janeimycin is active against a number of bacteria including *Bacillus subtilis*, *Staphylococcus aureus* and *Streptococcus pyogenes*, the antibiotic acting by inhibiting cell wall synthesis, more specifically the synthesis of peptidoglycan. A dose of approximately 0·5 mg/kg is sufficient to protect mice given an intraperitoneal dose of 1000 LD_{50} of *Streptococcus pyogenes* C203, 50 per cent of the control animals surviving when the dose was given subcutaneously 1 and 5 hours following infection.

Meyers *et al.*, *German Patent*, 2,035,655 (1971)
Meyers *et al.*, *U.S. Patent*, 3,577,530 (1971)
Brown *et al.*, *Ann. N.Y. Acad. Sci.*, **235**, 399 (1974)

JAVANICIN
$C_{15}H_{14}O_6$
M.p. 207·5–208°C (*dec.*)

A red antibiotic pigment elaborated by *Fusarium javanicum*, javanicin is obtained by surface growth on a medium containing glucose and inorganic salts incubated at pH 6·8–7·0 for 8–12 days at 25°C when the final pH is 3·0. The yield is then 100 *Staphylococcus aureus* units. Various methods have been employed to extract the antibiotic. The mycelium may be separated from the culture medium, dried and powdered and extracted with petroleum ether, the extract being concentrated when crude javanicin is formed. Grinding the dry mycelium and extracting with $(CH_3)_2CO$ also yields the crude product. In most of the methods used, a second antibiotic, oxyjavanicin, is also produced. When purified by extraction of the crude material with hot EtOH—$(CH_3)_2CO$, followed by recrystallization from EtOH, javanicin forms red crystals with a coppery lustre. It is a weakly acidic substance, stable to heat, acids and alkalies, stable in solvents, yielding a deep violet colour with 10 per cent aqueous NaOH and a purple solution with ammonium hydroxide and sodium carbonate.

Javanicin is assayed by serial dilution with *Staphylococcus aureus* as the test organism. Arnstein and his colleagues have determined the inhibition dilutions ($\times 1000$) *in vitro* against a number of organisms, these being as follows: *Bacillus fasciens* (100–200); *B. subtilis* (200); *B. tumefaciens* (10); *Clostridium welchii* (100); *Escherichia coli* (20); *Mycobacterium phlei* (100–400); *Myco. tuberculosis hominis* (50–100); *Pseudomonas aeruginosa* (10); *Ps. fluorescens* (10); *Staphylococcus aureus* (200–400); *Streptococcus hemolyticus* (100) and *Strep. pyogenes* (40). The antibiotic exhibits only a slight activity against fungi. The activity of javanicin *in vitro* is not affected by serum but the compound is decomposed in the presence of blood yielding methemoglobin.

When given to guinea pigs experimentally infected with *Mycobacterium tuberculosis*, the antibiotic has no obvious effect. At low concentrations, e.g. 1:20,000 it inhibits the seed germination and root growth of lettuce, tomato and turnip. It possesses a relatively low toxicity, mice tolerating a dose of 10 mg when given intraperitoneally.

Wilkins, Harris, *Brit. J. Exptl. Path.*, **23**, 166 (1942)
Cook, Lacey, *ibid.*, **26**, 404 (1945)
Arnstein, Cook, Lacey, *Nature*, **157**, 333 (1946)
Arnstein, Cook, Lacey, *Brit. J. Exptl. Path.*, **27**, 439 (1946)
Arnstein, Cook, *J. Chem. Soc.*, **189**, 1021 (1947)

JOLIPEPTIN
M.p. >300°C (*dec.*)

A polypeptide antibiotic, jolipeptin is obtained by aerobic fermentation of *Bacillus polymyxa* subsp. *colistinus* ATCC 21,830 on a medium containing starch, biotin and inorganic salts at pH 7·0 and 30°C for 24 hours. The antibiotic is isolated by addition of benzaldehyde to the culture medium at pH 8·0–8·6 when a precipitate is formed. The precipitate is isolated by centrifuging and extracted with acidified BuOH, the extract is treated with H_2O to remove the accompanying colistin (q.v.), Et_2O added to the mother liquor and the precipitate which is formed is dissolved in CH_3OH, insoluble impurities being removed by filtration. Addition of Et_2O to the filtrate precipitates the antibiotic which is dried to form a white powder that decomposes above 300°C. Further purification may be carried out by chromatography on Sephadex LH-20 with CH_3OH as the developer. Jolipeptin has been shown to contain the aminoacids alanine, α,γ-diaminobutyric acid, glutamic acid, glycine, serine and valine. It is a wide-spectrum antibiotic, active against a range of gram-positive and gram-negative organisms.

Ito, Koyama, *J. Antibiotics* (Japan), **25**, 304 (1972)
Ito, Koyama, *Japanese Patent*, 7,243,291 (1972)
Ito, Koyama, *German Patent*, 2,254,899 (1974)
Ito, Koyama, *British Patent*, 1,346,973 (1974)
Ito, Koyama, *U.S. Patent*, 3,883,649 (1975)

JOSAMYCIN S

$C_{40}H_{67}O_{15}N$
M.p. 208–210°C (*dec.*)

This antibiotic has been isolated by Japanese workers from *Streptomyces narbonensis* var. *josamyceticus*. When crystallized from CH_3OH it forms small, colourless needles. It is laevorotatory with a specific rotation of $[\alpha]_D^{25} - 58\cdot5°$ (c 1·0, CH_3OH) and gives an ultraviolet spectrum in CH_3OH consisting of a single absorption maximum at 234 nm. Josamycin S is a wide-spectrum antibiotic and is employed either as the base compound or the propionate, active both *in vitro* and *in vivo*. The levels of the latter are lower in the blood, kidney and spleen of rats but last longer than with josamycin S. Similar blood levels have been found in the case of dogs and adult humans. In dogs, the antibiotic is metabolized to de*iso*valeryljosamycin S, hydroxyljosamycin S and an unidentified metabolite. Human urine contains only josamycin S and the hydroxylated form. The antibiotic and the propionate are both comparatively non-toxic. In rats, the latter brought about no evidence of hematological or histological abnormalities when administered for 194 days at a daily dosage of 2000 mg/kg given orally.

Umezawa et al., *Japanese Patent*, 7,005,032 (1970)
Mashimo et al., *Nippon Kagaku Ryohogakukai Zasshi*, **17**, 604 (1969)
Ueda et al., *ibid.*, **17**, 610 (1969)
Hazato et al., *J. Antibiotics* (Japan), **26**, 1 (1973)
Tachibana et al., *ibid.*, **26**, 122 (1973)

Takagi, *ibid.*, **26**, 130 (1973)
Oshima, Iwadare, *ibid.*, **26**, 148 (1973)

JUGLOMYCIN A

$C_{14}H_{10}O_6$
Dec. 172°C

When grown aerobically on a medium containing starch, peptone, yeast extract and inorganic salts, *Streptomyces diastatochromogenes*, freshly isolated from soil, yields two closely related antibiotics, juglomycins A and B. The former yields colourless crystals which decompose without melting. It is laevorotatory with a specific rotation of $[\alpha]_D^{25} - 51\cdot9°$ (c 0·42, $(CH_3)_2SO$). The minimum inhibition concentrations (μg/ml) which have been determined are: *Bacillus subtilis* (6·25–12·5); *Diplococcus pneumoniae* (25–50) and *Proteus vulgaris* (25–50).

Irikura et al., *Japanese Patent*, 7,316,197 (1973)

JUGLOMYCIN B

$C_{14}H_{10}O_6$
Dec. 202°C

An isomer of the preceding antibiotic, juglomycin B is separated from it by chromatography on silica gel. It also forms colourless crystals but is dextrorotatory with a specific rotation of $[\alpha]_D^{25} + 227\cdot5°$ (c 0·75, $(CH_3)_2SO$). The minimum inhibition concentrations against the same bacteria are identical to those for juglomycin A.

Irikura et al., *Japanese Patent*, 7,316,197 (1973)

JULIMYCIN B-II

$C_{38}H_{34}O_{14}$
M.p. 215–220°C (*dec.*)

A dimeric anthraquinone type antibiotic isolated from *Streptomyces shiodaensis*, julimycin B-II crystallizes from CH_3OH-H_2O or AcOEt-hexane in the form of orange-red plates. It is laevorotatory with a specific rotation of $[\alpha]_D^{24.5} - 82.9°$ (c 0·06, CH_3OH) and gives an ultraviolet spectrum with absorption maxima at 234 and 456 nm. The diacetate forms crystals from CH_3OH with m.p. 272–274°C.

Shoji, Kimura, Katagiri, *J. Antibiotics* (Japan), **17A**, 156 (1964)
Katagiri, *Chem. Abstr.*, **63**, 2358 (1965)
Structure
 Tsuji, *Tetrahedron*, **24**, 1765 (1968)
Configuration
 Nakai, Shiro, Koyama, *J. Chem. Soc.*, B, 498 (1969)

JULIMYCIN C
$C_{38}H_{38}O_{15}$
M.p. 170°C

A further antibiotic isolated from *Streptomyces shiodaensis*, this compound is produced during the latter stages of culture in a medium containing dextrin, peptone, meat extract and inorganic salts at 27°C for 2 days with shaking. Julimycin C is purified by chromatography and crystallization from CH_3OH when it forms orange needles. It is prophylactic against poliovirus infections in mice at a single dose of 100 mg/kg and cytotoxic to HeLa cells giving 50 per cent inhibition at 15·2 µg/ml.

Katagiri, Tsuji, *Japanese Patent*, 6,805,720 (1968)

JUVENIMICINS
A fat-soluble basic antibiotic complex isolated from *Micromonosporia chalcea* var. *izumensis* grown in a common nutrient medium, the complex is obtained by extraction of the culture filtrate with organic solvents and separated into its components by thin-layer chromatography. Eight components have been isolated so far, juvenimicins A_1 (antibiotic T-1124-a), A_2, A_3, A_4 (antibiotic T-1124-D), B_1, B_2, B_3, B_4. The structures of five of these antibiotics have been firmly established and these are described below.

Shibata *et al.*, *German Patent*, 2,034,245 (1971)

JUVENIMICIN A_2
$C_{30}H_{51}NO_8$

This antibiotic has the structure shown above which is based upon chemical analysis and a study of the infrared, NMR and mass spectra. It is effective against gram-positive and some gram-negative bacteria, particularly *Escherichia coli*.

Kishi *et al.*, *J. Antibiotics* (Japan), **29**, 1171 (1976)

JUVENIMICIN A_3
This component of the juvenimicin complex has been shown to be identical with rosamicin (q.v.).

Kishi *et al.*, *J. Antibiotics* (Japan), **29**, 1171 (1976)

JUVENIMICIN A_4
$C_{31}H_{53}NO_9$

Juvenimicin B₁

A macrocyclic antibiotic, this substance has been assigned the structure shown above which has been established from chemical and spectroscopic evidence. It is especially active against *Escherichia coli*.

Kishi *et al.*, *J. Antibiotics* (Japan), **29**, 1171 (1976)

JUVENIMICIN B₁
$C_{31}H_{53}NO_8$

The structure of juvenimicin B₁ is similar to that of the other members of this complex but it does not possess the epoxy ring.

Kishi *et al.*, *J. Antibiotics* (Japan), **29**, 1171 (1976)

JUVENIMICIN B₃
$C_{31}H_{53}NO_9$

The structure of this component of the juvenimicin complex differs from that of the preceding antibiotic only in having two primary alcoholic groups in the molecule.

Kishi *et al.*, *J. Antibiotics* (Japan), **29**, 1171 (1976)

K

KALAFUNGIN
$C_{16}H_{12}O_6$
M.p. Indefinite

This antibiotic has been obtained from cultures of *Streptomyces tanashiensis* strain Kala UC-5063. The structure is not yet known although it has been shown not to be a polyene compound. Kalafungin has a high degree of inhibitory activity *in vitro* against gram-positive bacteria, fungi, protozoa and yeasts. It is less active towards gram-negative bacteria.

Johnson, Dietz, *Appl. Microbiol.*, **16**, 1815 (1968)
Hoeksema, Krueger, *J. Antibiotics* (Japan), **29**, 704 (1976)

KANAMYCIN (*Resistomycin*)

Streptomyces kanamyceticus elaborates an antibiotic complex when grown aerobically on common media incubated at 37°C for 4–5 days at pH 7·0. The final pH of the medium is then greater than 8·0. The complex has been separated into three components, described below. Both the complex and the individual antibiotics have inhibitory activity against a wide range of gram-positive and gram-negative bacteria.

Umezawa *et al.*, *J. Antibiotics* (Japan), **10A**, 181 (1957)
Umezawa *et al.*, *U.S. Patent*, 2,931,798 (1960)

KANAMYCIN A
$C_{18}H_{36}O_{11}N_4$
M.p. Indefinite

This constituent of the kanamycin complex forms colourless crystals from CH_3OH—EtOH and has $[\alpha]_D^{24}$ + 146° (c 1·0, 0·1N-H_2SO_4). It has LD_{50} in mice of 583 mg/kg given intravenously. The sulphate forms prisms which decompose over a wide range above 250°C. It has negligible gastro-intestinal absorption and is normally given intramuscularly in a dose of 15 mg/kg with a maximum of 1·5 g daily. Side effects which have been observed include neutropenia, skin eruptions, renal and eighth cranial nerve impairment.

Johnson *et al.*, *U.S. Patent*, 2,936,307 (1960)
Rothrock, Putter, *U.S. Patent*, 3,032,547 (1962)
Structure
Ogawa *et al.*, *J. Antibiotics* (Japan), **11A**, 169 (1958)
Cron *et al.*, *J. Amer. Chem. Soc.*, **80**, 4741 (1958)
Absolute configuration
Hichens, Rinehart, *J. Amer. Chem. Soc.*, **85**, 1547 (1963)

KANAMYCIN B
$C_{18}H_{37}O_{10}N_5$
Dec. >170°C

Kanamycin B forms colourless crystals that decompose over a wide range above 170°C. It is dextrorotatory with a specific rotation of $[\alpha]_D^{21} + 114°$ (c 0·98, H_2O). It is soluble in H_2O and formamide, but insoluble in non-polar solvents. The LD_{50} in mice has been given as 136 mg/kg when administered intravenously.

Wakazawa et al., J. Antibiotics (Japan), **14A**, 180, 187 (1961)

KANAMYCIN C
$C_{18}H_{36}O_{11}N_4$
Dec. >270°C

A third component of the kanamycin complex, this antibiotic is a positional isomer of kanamycin A. It yields colourless crystals from CH_3OH—EtOH which have a specific rotation of $[\alpha]_D^{20} + 126°$ (c 1·0, H_2O).

Murase et al., J. Antibiotics (Japan), **14A**, 156 (1961)
Murase, ibid., **14A**, 367 (1961)
Biosynthesis
Umezawa, Asian Med. J., **11**, 69 (1968)

KANCHANOMYCIN (*Antibiotic BA-180265-A*)
M.p. Indefinite
An antibacterial antibiotic, kanchanomycin has been isolated from cultures of *Actinomyces tumemacerans* strain INMI P-42. The organism is cultured on a medium containing wheat flour and the antibiotic extracted from the culture filtrate. Kanchanomycin is active against a number of gram-positive and gram-negative organisms but has only a limited antitumour activity.

Kuimova et al., J. Antibiotics (Japan), **24**, 69 (1971)

KASUGAMYCIN
$C_{14}H_{25}O_9N_3$
M.p. Indefinite

Isolated from cultures of *Streptomyces kasugaensis*, kasugamycin forms a white amorphous powder with no definite melting point. It has shown some use in medicine as a therapeutic in the treatment of *Pseudomonas* infections in humans and is also useful for the prevention of rice blast disease being an ideal agricultural chemical with a very low toxicity to humans, animals and plants.

Umezawa et al., J. Antibiotics (Japan), **18A**, 101 (1965)
Takeuchi et al., ibid., **18A**, 115 (1965)
Umezawa et al., Japanese Patent, 6,808,003 (1968)
Yagai et al., Hakko Kogaku Zasshi, **49**, 117 (1971)
Tahara et al., Japanese Patent, 7,127,351 (1971)
Takaoka et al., Japanese Patent, 7,323,990 (1973)
Structure
Ikekawa, Umezawa, Iitaka, J. Antibiotics (Japan), **19A**, 49 (1966)

KEFGLYCIN
See Cephaloridine

KEFLORDIN
See Cephaloridine

5-KETOCORIOLIN B
$C_{23}H_{34}O_6$

An antibiotic isolated from an unclassified *Basidiomycete* grown aerobically in a medium containing glucose, peptone, silicone oil and inorganic salts at 27°C for 6 days. The compound may be extracted from the culture medium with an organic solvent followed by concentration under reduced pressure. The concentrate is then re-extracted with AcOEt, concentrated, and chromatographed on silica gel when it is separated from the accompanying coriolin (q.v.). 5-Ketocoriolin B inhibits the growth of gram-positive bacteria, Yoshida tumour and mouse ascites tumour.

Umezawa *et al., Japanese Patent*, 7,239,698 (1972)

KIDAMYCIN
$C_{39}H_{48}O_9N_2$
M.p. Indefinite

An antitumour antibiotic, kidamycin is obtained from cultures of *Streptomyces phaeoverticillatus* var. *takatsukiensis*. The organism is incubated in a medium consisting of the usual nutrients together with an anthraquinone sulphonate. The antibiotic forms orange-red crystals and shows some promise in the treatment of various forms of cancer. It demonstrates antitumour activity when given intraperitoneally in mice against Ehrlich ascites carcinoma, leukemia SN-36, sarcoma-180, NF-sarcoma and Yoshida sarcoma. It shows little effect, however, against leukemia L1210.

Kanda, *J. Antibiotics* (Japan), **24**, 599 (1971)
Kanda, Kono, Asano, *ibid.*, **25**, 553 (1972)
Structure
Furukawa, Iitaka, *Tetrahedron Lett.*, 3287 (1974)

KINAMYCIN A
$C_{23}H_{19}O_{11}N_2$

Streptomyces murayamaensis ATCC 21,414 produces an antibiotic complex when cultivated on a medium containing glucose, soybean flour and aspartic acid. Extraction of the culture filtrate with C_6H_6 yields the crude mixture of antibiotics which may be separated and purified by chromatography on silica gel. This compound is active against gram-positive bacteria and is moderately toxic with LD_{50} in mice of 20–50 mg/kg when administered intraperitoneally. Chemical evidence shows that the antibiotic possesses a quinoid structure.

Hata *et al., J. Antibiotics* (Japan), **24**, 353 (1971)
Hata *et al., Japanese Patent*, 7,202,556 (1972)

KINAMYCIN B
A further quinoid antibiotic obtained from cultires of *Streptomyces murayamaensis*, this compound is separated from the preceding antibiotic by silica gel chromatography. It has a similar bacteriostatic spectrum *in vitro* to kinamycin A and a comparable toxicity.

Hata *et al., J. Antibiotics* (Japan), **24**, 353 (1971)
Hata *et al., Japanese Patent*, 7,202,556 (1972)

KINAMYCIN C
Also isolated from the culture filtrate of *Streptomyces murayamaensis*, this antibiotic is a minor component of the complex and is isolated by chromatography on a silica gel column. The LD_{50} in mice when given intraperitoneally is 20–55 mg/kg.

Hata *et al., J. Antibiotics* (Japan), **24**, 353 (1971)
Hata *et al., Japanese Patent*, 7,202,556 (1972)

KINAMYCIN D
A fourth constituent of the antibiotic complex produced by *Streptomyces murayamaensis*, this antibiotic has a similar antibacterial activity and toxicity in mice to the preceding antibiotics.

Hata *et al., J. Antibiotics* (Japan), **24**, 353 (1971)
Hata *et al., Japanese Patent*, 7,202,556 (1972)

KOBENOMYCIN
M.p. Indefinite
A crystalline polypeptide antibiotic, kobenomycin is produced by *Strepto-*

myces kobenensis. It forms colourless crystals and has a specific rotation of $[\alpha]_D^{21 \cdot 5} - 87 \cdot 5°$ (CH$_3$OH). The antibiotic is inhibitory against aerobic sporulating bacilli, slightly less so against acid-fast bacteria and protozoa but inactive against other bacteria. Minimum inhibition concentrations that have been determined are: *Bacillus* spp. 0·5–5·0 µg/ml and for *Mycobacterium* and *Trichomonas* spp. 12·5–200 µg/ml. Kobenomycin is toxic to mice with LD$_{50}$ of 25 mg/kg (intraperitoneal), 15 mg/kg (intravenous) and greater than 100 mg/kg given subcutaneously. The last value is somewhat misleading since the antibiotic does not appear to be well absorbed when given by this means. A dose of 30 µg/ml completely lyses rabbit red blood cells.

Okamoto et al., *J. Antibiotics* (Japan), **21**, 320 (1968)

KOJIC ACID
$C_6H_{10}O_4$
M.p. 152°C

Kojic acid was first isolated by Saito from *Aspergillus oryzae* in 1907 and its antibiotic activity noted by Yabuta in 1912. It is produced by a large number of fungi, e.g. *Aspergillus albus, A. awamori, A. candidus, A. clavatus, A. flavus, A. fumigatus, A. giganteus, A. glaucus, A. gymnosardae, A. nidulans, A. parasiticus, A. tamarii* and *Penicillium dahlae*, and also by *Acetobacter effusus, Acetobacter. luteo-virescens* and *Acetobact. lutescens*. When *Aspergillus flavus* is used, it is obtained by surface growth on a medium containing glucose or xylose, dextrins, starches, di- and mono-saccharides, pentoses, dulcitol, sorbitol, inositol, glycerol, gluconic acid, tartaric acid or dihydroxyacetone as the carbon source, ammonium nitrate as the nitrogenous constituent and various inorganic salts. The medium is incubated for 9–20 days at 29–35°C. Using *Acetobacter luteo-virescens*, a Raulin-Thom medium is employed containing glucose and with *Acetobacter effusus*, a medium containing maltose, peptone and malt extract. Kojic acid is purified by recrystallizing from hot H$_2$O or (CH$_3$)$_2$CO, or by sublimation *in vacuo*. The antibiotic forms large, colourless crystals, reduces Fehling's solution and gives a deep red colour with FeCl$_3$. The structure is 5-hydroxy-2-hydroxymethyl-γ-pyrone.

Kojic acid is assayed by cylinder plate with *Staphylococcus aureus*, isolation of the copper salt or by a colourimetric determination with FeCl$_3$. When tested *in vitro* it has only a slight activity against bacteria, fungi and yeasts, being somewhat more active against gram-negative organisms. However, *Leptospira icterohemorrhagiae* is inhibited at a dilution of 1:100,000 and *L. canicola* at 1:1,000,000. The antibiotic has proved disappointing *in vivo*, giving no protection to mice against poliomyelitis or St. Louis encephalitis.

The antibiotic has a relatively high toxicity. An intravenous dose of 150 mg/kg administered to dogs, rabbits and rats was toxic and lethal at a dose of 1 g/kg. When given orally to mice, 80 mg/kg was lethal. Human leucocytes are killed at a dilution of 1:100.

Saito, *Japan. J. Bot.*, **21**, 7 (1907)
Yabuta, *8th Int. Congr. Pure Appl. Chem.*, **25**, 455 (1912)
Yabuta, *J. Chem. Soc., Japan*, **37**, 1185, 1234 (1916)
Friedmann, *Science*, **80**, 34 (1934)
May et al., *U.S. Patent*, 2,006,086 (1935)
Prescott, Dunn, *Industrial Microbiology*, McGraw-Hill Co. (1940)
Oxford, *J. Chem. Ind.*, **61**, 48 (1942)
Wilkins, Harris, *Brit. J. Exptl. Path.*, **23**, 166 (1942)
Kramer, Greer, Szobel, *J. Immunol.*, **49**, 273 (1944)
Cook, Lacey, *Nature*, **155**, 790 (1945)
Foster, Karow, *J. Bact.*, **49**, 19 (1945)
Morton, Kocholaty, *ibid.*, **50**, 579 (1945)
Marston, *Nature*, **164**, 961 (1949)

KOMAMYCIN A
M.p. 150–156°C (*dec.*)
One of two closely related polypeptide antibiotics isolated from cultures of *Streptomyces* sp. nova, this compound has been separated from the following antibiotic by column and thin layer chromatography. It is dextrorotatory having a specific rotation of $[\alpha]_D^{22} + 64°$ (MeOH) and is active against gram-positive bacteria.

Oda, Mori, Kamemoto, *Japanese Patent*, 70 08,636 (1970)

KOMAMYCIN B
M.p. 149–158°C (*dec.*)
A second antibiotic of the polypetide group isolated from the culture filtrate of an unclassified species of *Streptomyces*, this compound is also dextrorotatory with a specific rotation of $[\alpha]_D^{25} + 56°$ (MeOH). It is active in inhibiting the growth of gram-positive bacteria.

Oda, Mori, Kamemoto, *Japanese Patent*, 70 08,636 (1970)

KOTOMYCIN
$C_{29}H_{28}O_4N_4$

A *Streptomyces* antibiotic isolated from *S. candidus* var. *kotohiranensis* freshly obtained from a soil sample, this organism is cultured on a common medium and isolated by extraction of the mycelium with $(CH_3)_2CO$. The extract is then chromatographed over silica gel to give the pure antibiotic. Kotomycin is insoluble in H_2O but soluble in organic solvents. It has been shown to be active against *Tetrahymena pyriformis* and *Trichomonas vaginalis*.

Kuroda *et al.*, *Japanese Patent*, 7,202,558 (1972)

KUNDRYMYCIN

A crystalline antibiotic, kundrymycin has been isolated from *Streptomyces metachromogenes* ATCC 21,440 grown in a medium containing glucose, soybean flour, cottonseed embryo meal, H_2O and calcium carbonate at 27°C for 3 days. The antibiotic bears a close resemblance to aquayamycin (q.v.) but differs from this substance in molecular weight.

Kundrymycin is assayed by cylinder type agar diffusion with *Bacillus subtilis* as the test organism. It possesses antitumour activity against transplanted mouse tumours and Walker 256 carcinoma.

Bush *et al.*, *J. Antibiotics* (Japan), **24**, 143 (1971)
Nettleton, Bush, Bradner, *U.S. Patent*, 3,663,691 (1972)

KUWAITIMYCIN
M.p. 158–159°C

A polypeptide antibiotic, kuwaitimycin is produced by *Streptomyces kuwaitinensis* nov. species isolated from Kuwait soil. When pure it forms yellowish needles and is dextrorotatory with a specific rotation of $[\alpha]_D^{28}$ + 60° (c 2·0, EtOH). Hydrolysis yields arginine, alanine, glutamic acid, lysine, serine and an unsaturated aliphatic acid which has an *iso*hexadeca-3:6-dienoic structure. It possesses an *in vitro* activity against gram-positive bacteria but little activity against gram-negative organisms.

Shimi, Dewedar, Shoukry, *J. Antibiotics* (Japan), **26**, 593 (1973)

L

LACTAROVIOLIN
$C_{15}H_{14}O$
M.p. Indefinite

Lactarius deliciosus elaborates this pigment which has been shown to be active against *Mycobacterium tuberculosis* at a concentration of 0·31 nM/l.

Willstaedt, Zetterberg, *Svensk. Kemisk. Tidskr.*, **58**, 306 (1946)

LACTEROSPORAMINE
$C_{17}H_{35}O_4N_7$

This antibiotic has been described by Japanese workers who have isolated it from cultures of *Bacillus lacterosporus*. It forms a water-soluble basic white powder and has a non-peptide structure and the probable empirical formula given above. It is active against gram-positive and gram-negative bacteria both *in vitro* and *in vivo*.

Shoji et al., *J. Antibiotics* (Japan), **29**, 390 (1976)

LACTOSIN 27
M.p. Indefinite

Lactobacillus helveticus strain LP27 produces this potent bacteriocin which has been obtained from the culture supernatant fluid and shown to be a protein-lipopolysaccharide complex. The activity, however, is present in a small glycoprotein. When purified, the aminoacid composition of lactosin 27 has been demonstrated to be very similar to that of bacteriocin isolated from *Lactobacillus fermentii*.

Upreti, Hinsdill, *Antimicrobial Agents & Chemotherapy*, **4**, 487 (1973)

LADAKAMYCIN
$C_8H_{12}O_5N_4$

This recently discovered antibiotic is elaborated by *Streptoverticillium ladakanus* var. *ladakanus*. It forms colourless crystals and is soluble in H_2O and only slightly soluble in CH_3OH, $CHCl_3$, $(CH_3)_2CO$, hexane and $(CH_3)_2SO$. It inhibits the growth of a number of gram-negative bacteria.

Bergy et al., *U.S. Patent*, 3,816,619 (1974)

LADERCILLIN
See Procaine Penicillin G

LAGOSIN (*Antibiotic A 246, Pentamycin*)
$C_{35}H_{58}O_{12}$
Dec. 230–240°C

An antifungal antibiotic, lagosin, has been isolated from cultures of *Streptomyces roseo-luteus* and is possibly identical with pentamycin, obtained from *Streptomyces penticus* by Umezawa and Tanaka. The antibiotic forms pale yellow needles when crystallized from CH_3OH and is laevorotatory with a specific rotation of $[\alpha]_D^{20} - 160°$ (c 0·2, CH_3OH). The ultraviolet spectrum has absorption maxima at 323, 339 and 357 nm. The structure of lagosin is the same as that of fungichromin with which it may also be identical. It is active against a number of pathogenic fungi and has LD_{50} in mice of 2100 mg/kg when given orally, the corresponding value for rats being 1750 mg/kg.

Umezawa, Tanaka, *J. Antibiotics* (Japan), **11A**, 26 (1958)
Bessel et al., *U.S. Patent*, 3,013,947 (1961)
Dhar et al., *Proc. Chem. Soc.*, 310 (1960)
Cope et al., *J. Amer. Chem. Soc.*, **84**, 2170 (1962)
Dhar et al., *J. Chem. Soc.*, 842 (1964)
Berry, Whiting, *ibid.*, 862 (1964)

LAIDLOMYCIN
$C_{37}H_{62}O_{12}$

A polycyclic polyether monocarboxylic acid, laidlomycin has been isolated from cultures of *Streptomyces* species S-822 cultured on a common nutrient medium. It is a broad spectrum antibiotic, active against gram-positive bacteria, some gram-negative bacteria, and fungi. It also possesses cytotoxic and antimycoplasmal activity.

Kitame *et al.*, *J. Antibiotics* (Japan), **27**, 884 (1974)

LAMBDAMYCIN

A yellow-green pigment isolated from cultures of *Streptomyces glaucoachromogenes* strain IMET 31118, this antibiotic is obtained from the mycelium and culture filtrate by extraction with one of the lower alcohols followed by gel filtration. It has been shown to contain digitalose and fucose. Lambdamycin is active against gram-positive bacteria and also has antiviral and cancerostatic properties. It finds some use as a growth stimulant and is relatively non-toxic with LD_{50} in mice > 125 mg/kg given intraperitoneally.

Fleck *et al.*, *Z. Allg. Mikrobiol.*, **16**, 521 (1976)

LAMPTEROL
See Illudin S

LANKACIDINOL A
See Antibiotic T-2636D

LANKACIDINOL F
See Antibiotic T-2636F

LANKAMYCIN
$C_{42}H_{72}O_{16}$
M.p. 147–150°C and 181–182°C

A macrocyclic glycosidic antibiotic, lankamycin has been isolated from cultures of *Streptomyces violaceoniger* obtained from a sample of soil from Ceylon. Acid hydrolysis yields lankavose and acetylarcanose and the aglycon monoacetyllankolid. The antibiotic crystallizes from Et_2O-petroleum ether as colourless needles having the double melting point given above. It is laevorotatory with a specific rotation of $[\alpha]_D^{29} - 94°$ (c 1·23, EtOH) and gives an ultraviolet spectrum consisting of a single absorption maximum at 289 nm. The antibiotic has been shown to be active in inhibiting the growth of a number of gram-positive and gram-negative bacteria.

Gaumann *et al.*, *Helv. Chim. Acta*, **43**, 601 (1960)
Keller-Schlierlein, Roncari, *obod.*, **45**, 148 (1962)
Keller-Schlierlein, Roncari, *ibid.*, **47**, 78 (1964)
Configuration
Muntwyler, Keller-Schlierlein, *ibid.*, **55**, 460 (1972)

LASALOCID
See Antibiotic X-537A.

LASALOCID B
$C_{35}H_{56}O_8$

Streptomyces lasaliensis elaborates a series of four isomeric homologues of lasalocid A (Antibiotic X-537A). These have been extracted from the fermentation broth and separated and purified by column and thin layer chromatography. This component has the structure given above which is based upon chemical and spectroscopic evidence. It is active against gram-positive bacteria.

Westley *et al.*, *J. Antibiotics* (Japan), **27**, 744 (1974)

LASALOCID C
$C_{35}H_{56}O_8$

A second component of the antibiotic complex isolated from cultures of *Streptomyces lasaliensis*, this compound has the structure shown above which has been established from chemical analysis, the infrared, NMR and mass spectra and comparison with the other lasalocids. It is effective against gram-positive bacteria.

Westley et al., *J. Antibiotics* (Japan), **27**, 744 (1974)

LASALOCID D
$C_{35}H_{56}O_8$

A positional isomer of the preceding two antibiotics, lasalocid D has been isolated from the culture broth of *Streptomyces lasaliensis* and shown to have the above structure. It possesses a similar antibiotic activity to the other lasalocids.

Westley et al., *J. Antibiotics* (Japan), **27**, 744 (1974)

LASALOCID E
$C_{35}H_{56}O_8$

A fourth constituent of the lasalocid complex isolated from the culture filtrate of *Streptomyces lasaliensis*, this antibiotic has been assigned the above structure on the basis of chemical correlations and spectroscopic data.

Westley et al., *J. Antibiotics* (Japan), **27**, 744 (1974)

LASPARTOMYCIN

This antibiotic has been obtained as a white powder with a purity of 72 per cent. It is produced by *Streptomyces viridochromogenes* var. *komabensis* strain M307-M5. It is produced by initially inoculating a sterile medium containing glucose, starch, soybean flour and inorganic salts with shaking at 27–29°C for 3 days. An inoculum of this medium was then used to inoculate flasks of the same medium and fermentation allowed to proceed for 10 days. The culture filtrate was assayed using the *Micrococcus flavus* cup method and the antibiotic isolated by adjusting the pH to 2·0 with dilute HCl, extracting with BuOH, washing with H_2O, adding H_2O and NaOH to pH 10·0. The aqueous fraction was then adjusted to pH 2·0 and extracted repeatedly with BuOH, the organic layer concentrated *in vacuo* and dried. The crude powder was then further purified by countercurrent distribution. Laspartomycin is a broad-spectrum antibacterial.

Umezawa et al., *U.S. Patent*, 3,639,582 (1972)
Umezawa et al., *Japanese Patent*, 7,205,717 (1972)

LATERIOMYCIN A
M.p. 202–206°C

Streptomyces griseoruber ATCC 17,919 produces two closely related antibiotics which may be isolated from the broth liquor and also from the mycelium. This antibiotic is obtained by extracting the broth into AcOEt at pH 7·0 followed by back extraction into 0·1M phosphate buffer at pH 2·5. The buffer is then re-extracted with AcOEt and chromatographed on silica gel. Lateriomycin A forms orange-red needles when recrystallized from AcOEt—CH_3OH.

Higashide et al., *U.S. Patent*, 3,655,878 (1972)

LATERIOMYCIN B
M.p. 234–236°C

Lateriomycin B is also produced by *Streptomyces griseoruber* ATCC 17,919 and is isolated by re-chromatographing the solvent phase following crystallization of the preceding antibiotic. It may be purified by recrystallizing from AcOEt—CH_3OH when it forms orange needles. It is active against a range of gram-positive bacteria.

Higashide et al., *U.S. Patent*, 3,655,878 (1972)

LATERIOMYCIN F
M.p. Indefinite

This antibiotic is obtained by cultivating *Streptomyces griseoruber* ATCC 17,919 in a common nutrient medium containing a small amount of a ferrous salt. When purified by dissolving the crude material in $(CH_3)_2CO$, filtering, concentrating, and adding Et_2O, it forms a red-orange amorphous powder. It is active against a number of gram-positive bacteria but has little activity against gram-negative organisms.

Takeda Chem. Indust., *French Patent*, 1,523,522 (1968)

LATERITIIN I
See Enniatin A

LATERITIIN II
$C_{26}H_{46}O_7N_2$
M.p. 125°C

This antibiotic is closely related to anniatin A and has been isolated from a species of *Fusarium* which is almost certainly a strain of *F. latericum*. It forms large, colourless crystals when purified by recrystallizing from EtOH, is very soluble in common organic solvents but only slightly soluble in H_2O. It is stable to heat and acids, but unstable under alkaline conditions. It has a similar activity to enniatin A *in vitro* with inhibition dilutions ($\times 1000$) as follows: *Bacillus subtilis* (3·0): *Mycobacterium phlei* I (19); *Myco. phlei* II (32); *Staphylococcus aureus* (4·0) and *Streptococcus pyogenes* (2·5). It also has a low toxicity *in vivo* when given intraperitoneally to mice.

Cook et al., *Nature*, **160**, 31 (1947)
Cook, Fox, Farmer, *ibid.*, **162**, 61 (1948)

LATEROSPORAMINE
Isolated from the culture broth of *Bacillus laterosporus* 340–19, this antibiotic is effective against gram-positive bacteria both *in vitro* and *in vivo*. It is a basic white powder for which the empirical formula $C_{17}H_{35}N_7O_4$ has been put forward. The structure has not yet been elucidated.

Shoji et al., *J. Antibiotics* (Japan), **29**, 390 (1976)

LATEROSPORIN A
M.p. Indefinite

One of two antibiotics elaborated by *Bacillus laterosporus*, the mixture is obtained by surface growth on a medium containing glucose and inorganic salts incubated at 37°C for 3–4 days, the final pH being 6·5–7·0 and the yield 1·0 unit/ml. The crude mixture from the culture filtrate is precipitated with picric acid and extracted with acidified EtOH in which this antibiotic is soluble, the pure compound being precipitated from dry Et_2O. Laterosporin A is a polypeptide, soluble in absolute EtOH and H_2O, the solubility in the latter decreasing from pH 2·0 to 9·0. It is insoluble in $CHCl_3$, Et_2O and amyl acetate and dialyses through a cellophane membrane. The antibiotic is assayed by cylinder plate with *Corynebacterium xerosis*, *Mycobacterium phlei* or *Staphylococcus aureus* as test organism, yielding an arbitrary standard 10 units/ml. The following inhibition concentrations (µg/ml) have been found *in vitro*: *Corynebacterium diphtheriae gravis* (0·12); *C. xerosis* (0·003–0·005); *Escherichia coli* (0·6); *Mycobacterium phlei* (0·004–0·0008); *Myco. Smegmatis* (10); *Myco. tuberculosis* (1·0); *Pseudomonas aeruginosa* (5·0–10); *Salmonella enteriditis* (1·2–2·5); *S. typhi* (0·6); *Staphylococcus aureus* (0·01) and *Streptococcus pyogenes* (0·03–0·12).

Barnes, *Brit. J. Exptl. Path.*, **30**, 100 (1949)

LATEROSPORIN B
M.p. Indefinite

Isolated from *Bacillus laterosporus* together with the preceding antibiotic, laterosporin B may be separated from the former by its insolubility in absolute EtOH. It is assayed in the same manner as laterosporin A giving an arbitrary standard of 12·5 units/ml. The antibiotic spectrum *in vitro* is identical with that given above for laterosporin A.

Barnes, *Brit. J. Exptl. Path.*, **30**, 100 (1949)

LAURUSIN
M.p. 254–255°C (*dec.*)

A variant of *Streptomyces lavendulae* elaborates this antibiotic when grown on a medium containing glycerol, cottonseed flour and inorganic salt at 27°C for 6 days with aeration. When purified by recrystallizing from H_2O laurusin forms colourless crystals and is laevorotatory with a specific rotation of $[\alpha]_D^{22} - 44°$ (c 1·0, 0·1N-HCl). The antibiotic has only weak activity against bacteria but inhibits the growth of *Xanthomonas oryzae* at a concentration of 0·75–1·0 µg/ml.

Sumiki et al., *Japanese Patent*, 21,757 (1967)

LAVENDULIN
$C_{49}H_{63}O_{18}N_{13}S_3$ (helianthate)
M.p. Indefinite

An antibiotic closely related to streptothricin, this compound is obtained from a variant of *Streptomyces lavendulae*. It is formed by surface growth on a medium containing beef extract, peptone, agar, glucose and molasses at pH 6·0 and incubated at 28°C for 6 days giving a yield of 200–400 *Escherichia coli* units; or by submerged growth in shaker flasks with a similar medium, the final yield in this case being 1000 *E. coli* units. It is isolated on 'Decalso' cation exchange resin and purified by dissolving in 85 per cent aqueous CH_3OH, passing through an alumina column and adding aqueous sodium helianthate when the crystalline addition compound is formed on refrigerating. The helianthate compound forms orange needles or triangular blades from aqueous CH_3OH, m.p. 212–220°C (*dec.*). The free base gives negative Molisch and Sakaguchi tests and positive biuret and Fehlings reactions and also decolourizes potassium permanganate solution. It is thermostable in neutral solution and dialyses through a cellophane membrane.

Lavendulin is normally assayed by a serial dilution streak test with *Escherichia coli* as the test organism; the helianthate compound having 0·3–0·5 µg/unit and the crude base 0·5–1·0 µg/unit. Kelner and Morton have determined the inhibition concentrations (units/ml) against a large number of organisms *in vitro*: *Aerobacter aerogenes* (0·5); *Bacillus anthracis* (4·0–8·0); *B. cereus* (64); *B. mesentericus* (0·5); *B. mycoides* (0·06–32); *B. subtilis* (0·03–6·0); *Corynebacterium diphtheriae* (4·0); *Diplococcus pneumoniae* (128); *Eberthella communior* (1·0); *Eb. typhi* (0·015–1·0); *Escherichia coli* (1·0); *Gaffkya tetragena* (0·015); *Klebsiella pneumoniae* (0·03); *Micrococcus auranticus* (0·000007); *Mycobacterium tuberculosis bovis* (6·0); *Neisseria catarrhalis* (0·06); *Proteus vulgaris* (2·0); *Pseudomonas aeruginosa* (128); *Salmonella enteriditis* (0·25); *S. paratyphi* (0·06); *Sarcina lutea* (0·5); *Serratia marcescens* (4·0); *Shigella dysenteriae* (2·0); *Sh. paradysenteriae* (2·0); *Staphylococcus aureus* (0·015); *Streptococcus alpha* (>128); *Strep. gamma* (128); *Strep. pyogenes* (128); *Trichoderma interdigitalis* (16) and *Vibrio comma* (0·25).

The activity of lavendulin is drastically reduced in the presence of saline. When given to mice intraperitoneally, 25 µg of the antibiotic afforded complete protection against experimental infection with *Klebsiella pneumoniae*. The LD_{100} in mice, given intraperitoneally, is 0·5 mg.

Kelner *et al.*, *J. Bact.*, **51**, 581 (1946)
Kelner, Morton, *ibid.*, **53**, 695 (1947)
Morton, *Proc. Soc. Exptl. Biol. Med.*, **64**, 327 (1947)
Junowicz-Kocholaty, Kocholaty, *J. Biol. Chem.*, **168**, 757 (1947)

LECANORIN A

This compound was isolated by Roques from *Lecanora esculenta*. The aqueous extract is stated to inhibit the germination of the seeds of *Lepidium sativa*. Little is known concerning the chemical and physical properties of this substance.

Roques, *Bull. soc. chim. biol.*, **31**, 15 (1949)

LANTICILLIN

See Procaine Penicillin G

LEUCEMOMYCIN

M.p. Indefinite

This antibiotic has been obtained in an impure form from *Streptomyces griseus* strains IMET JA 3963, IMET JA 5570, IMET JA 10086 and IMET JA 10431, cultured on a common nutrient medium containing glucose, soybean flour, inorganic salts and H_2O after prior incubation for 10–14 days on a medium consisting of sucrose, dextrin, urea, yeast extract, peptone and inorganic salts. After a period of 72 hours at 28°C a product was isolated containing 80 µg/ml of the antibiotic.

Leucemomycin has been shown to possess cancerostatic, mycoplasma bactericidal and virostatic properties.

Strauss, Fleck, Prauser, *East German Patent*, 100,493 (1973)

LEUCINOSTATIN

M.p. 131–136°C (*dec.*)

Penicillium lilacinum (FERM-P 1588) yields this peptide antibiotic when cultured with shaking at 27°C for 4 days in a medium consisting of sucrose, corn steep liquor and inorganic salts. The culture filtrate is adjusted to pH 2·0 and extracted with AcOEt and $CHCl_3$, the extract washed with 1 per cent aqueous sodium bicarbonate solution, concentrated under reduced pressure and the crude syrup purified by chromatography on silica gel and Sephadex LH-20, eluting with CH_3OH. The antibiotic is then crystallized from Et_3O-petroleum ether. Leucinostatin forms colourless crystals and is dextrorotatory with a specific rotation of $[\alpha]_D^{25} + 644°$ (c 0·5, CH_3OH). The ultraviolet spectrum in CH_3OH shows only an inflection at 220 nm. It is active against some gram-positive bacteria but is predominantly active against fungi. It is also cytotoxic to HeLa cells and has an inhibitory effect on Ehrlich subcutaneous solid tumours. The LD_{50} in mice is 1·6 mg/kg when administered intraperitoneally. It has a marked hypotensive effect on blood pressure in the rabbit but no effect upon epinephrine and acetylcholine responses.

The structure of the antibiotic is not yet known. Hydrolysis gives predominantly leucine indicative of its peptide character. It is soluble in the lower alcohols and esters, $CHCl_3$ and $(CH_3)_2CO$, slightly soluble in C_6H_6 and Et_2O and insoluble in H_2O, hexane, petroleum ether and cyclohexane. It gives a positive biuret reaction and a negative ninhydrin reaction, although the latter is positive after hydrolysis.

Arai *et al.*, *J. Antibiotics* (Japan), **26**, 157 (1973)
Arai, *Japanese Patent*, 7,441,594 (1974)

LEUCOMYCINS

Streptomyces kitasatoensis Hata elaborates an antibiotic complex, leucomycin, which has been separated into a large number of components, all of which are macrolide substances having antibacterial properties, particularly against such organisms as *Bacillus*, *Sarcina* and *Staphylococcus* species. The structure of most of the antibiotics have been elucidated and these are described below.

Watanabe, Fujii, Satake, *J. Biochem.*, **50**, 197 (1961)

LEUCOMYCIN A$_1$
$C_{40}H_{67}O_{14}N$
M.p. 135–138°C

This antibiotic forms colourless crystals from CHCl$_3$ and gives an ultraviolet spectrum having a single absorption maximum at 233 nm.

Watanabe, Fujii, Satake, *J. Biochem.*, **50**, 197 (1961)
Abe et al., *J. Chem. Soc., Japan*, **81**, 969 (1960)
Watanabe, *Bull. Chem. Soc., Japan*, **33**, 1100 (1960)
Watanabe et al., *Angew. Chem.*, **76**, 792 (1964)
Structure
  Satoshi et al., *J. Antibiotics* (Japan), **20A**, 234 (1967)
  Satakibara et al., *Japanese Patent*, 7,364,286 (1973)
Biological activity
  Iwata, Akiba, *J. Antibiotics* (Japan), **15A**, 258 (1962)

LEUCOMYCIN A$_2$
$C_{65}H_{111}O_{22}N$
M.p. 142–144°C

This is the most complex of all the leucomycins. It gives an ultraviolet spectrum virtually identical to that of the preceding antibiotic with a single absorption maximum at 231 nm.

Watanabe, Fujii, Satake, *J. Biochem.*, **50**, 197 (1961)

LEUCOMYCIN A$_3$

This component of the leucomycin complex has recently been demonstrated to be identical with josamycin (q.v.).

Omura et al., *J. Antibiotics* (Japan), **23**, 511 (1970)

LEUCOMYCIN A$_4$
$C_{41}H_{67}O_{15}N$
M.p. 126–127°C

Also present in the leucomycin complex elaborated by *Streptomyces kitasatoensis* Hata, this compound is readily obtained in a crystalline form. It has a specific rotation of $[\alpha]_D^{25} - 50 \cdot 0°$ (c 1·0, CHCl$_3$).

Satoshi et al., *J. Antibiotics* (Japan), **20A**, 234 (1967)

LEUCOMYCIN A$_5$
$C_{39}H_{65}O_{14}N$
M.p. 120–123°C

Leucomycin A_5 forms a white amorphous powder which cannot be obtained in the crystalline form. It is laevorotatory with a specific rotation of $[\alpha]_D^{25} - 52.0°$ (c 1·0, $CHCl_3$).

Satoshi et al., *J. Antibiotics* (Japan), **20A**, 234 (1967)
Sakakibara et al., *Japanese Patent*, 7,364,286 (1973)

LEUCOMYCIN A_6
$C_{40}H_{65}O_{15}N$
M.p. 135–137°C

This component of leucomycin complex forms colourless crystals and has a specific rotation of $[\alpha]_D^{25} - 56°$ (c 1·0, $CHCl_3$). The antibacterial activity is similar to that of the other leucomycins.

Satoshi et al., *J. Antibiotics* (Japan), **20A**, 234 (1967)

LEUCOMYCIN A_7
$C_{38}H_{63}O_{14}N$
M.p. Indefinite

A white amorphous powder, this antibiotic has no definite melting point and has not been obtained in a crystalline form. It has a specific rotation of $[\alpha]_D^{25} - 65°$ (c 1·3, $CHCl_3$).

Satoshi et al., *J. Antibiotics* (Japan), **20A**, 234 (1967)
Sakakibara et al., *Japanese Patent*, 7,364,286 (1973)

LEUCOMYCIN A_8
$C_{39}H_{63}O_{15}N$
M.p. 147–149°C

When crystallized from EtOH or $CHCl_3$, this antibiotic constituent of the leucomycin complex forms colourless needles. It has a specific rotation of $[\alpha]_D^{25} - 58.3°$ (c 1·8, $CHCl_3$).

Satoshi et al., *J. Antibiotics* (Japan), **20A**, 234 (1967)

LEUCOMYCIN A_9
$C_{37}H_{61}O_{14}N$
M.p. Indefinite

This antibiotic resembles leucomycin A_7 in being amorphous with no definite melting point. It is also laevorotatory with a specific rotation of $[\alpha]_D^{25} - 65 \cdot 1°$ (c 1·0, $CHCl_3$).

Satoshi et al., *J. Antibiotics* (Japan), **20A**, 234 (1967)
Sakakibara et al., *Japanese Patent*, 7,364,286 (1973)

LEUCOMYCIN B_1
$C_{35}H_{59}O_{13}N$
M.p. 214·5–216·5°C

This constituent of the antibiotic complex produced by *Streptomyces kitasatoensis* Hata forms colourless needles. It has an ultraviolet spectrum consisting of a single absorption maximum at 234 nm.

Watanabe, Fujii, Satake, *J. Biochem.*, **50**, 197 (1961)
Abe et al., *J. Chem. Soc., Japan*, **81**, 969 (1960)

LEUCOMYCIN B_2
$C_{38}H_{65}O_{16}N$
M.p. 214–216°C

A macrocyclic antibiotic obtained from the leucomycin complex, this compound forms colourless crystals when recrystallized from EtOH and gives an ultraviolet spectrum with an absorption maximum at 234 nm.

Abe et al., *J. Chem. Soc., Japan*, **81**, 969 (1960)
Watanabe, Fujii, Satake, *J. Biochem.*, **50**, 197 (1961)

LEUCOMYCIN B_3
$C_{34}H_{53}O_{13}N$
M.p. 216–217°C

A further macrolide antibiotic related to the above compounds and present in cultures of *Streptomyces kitasatoensis* Hata, the ultraviolet spectrum in EtOH is identical with that of the preceding substance with an absorption maximum at 234 nm.

Abe et al., *J. Chem. Soc., Japan*, **81**, 969 (1960)
Watanabe, Fujii, Satake, *J. Biochem.*, **50**, 197 (1961)

LEUCOMYCIN B_4
$C_{38}H_{59}O_{16}N$
M.p. 221–223°C

This macrocyclic antibiotic has also been described by Japanese workers and is present in cultures of *Streptomyces kitasatoensis* Hata. It forms colourless needles when purified by crystallization from EtOH and gives an ultraviolet spectrum with an absorption maximum at 233 nm.

Abe et al., *J. Chem. Soc., Japan*, **81**, 969 (1960)
Watanabe, Fujii, Satake, *J. Biochem.*, **50**, 197 (1961)

LEUCOMYCIN U
$C_{36}H_{59}O_{13}N$
M.p. Indefinite

Streptomyces kitasatoensis Hata also elaborates this macrocyclic antibiotic which has the structure given above. Omura and his colleagues have shown that there is no change in biological activity with any change in the allylic system in the molecule. The activity is markedly decreased if the aldehyde group is altered to a hydroxyl or thiosemicarbazone, but acetylation of the 4″-hydroxyl group gives a very large increase in the activity, the lower the degree of acetylation, the higher the activity.

Omura et al., *Progr. Antimicrob. Anticancer Chemother.*, **2**, 1043 (1970)
Sakakibara et al., *Japanese Patent*, 7,564,295 (1975)

LEUCOMYCIN V
$C_{34}H_{57}O_{12}N$
M.p. Indefinite

A further member of the leucomycin group of antibiotics, this substance is the deacetyl derivative of the preceding compound. It shows a similar tendency regarding the biological activity of its derivatives.

Omura et al., *Progr. Antimicrob. Anticancer. Chemother.*, **2**, 1043 (1970)
Sakakibara et al., *Japanese Patent*, 7,564.295 (1975)

LEUCYLNEGAMYCIN
$C_{15}H_{29}O_5N_5$

Negamycin-producing *Streptomyces* species elaborate this antibiotic, e.g. *S. purpeofuscus* and *S.* M89-C2 may be incubated in a common medium aerobically at pH 7·4 and 27°C for 94 hours and the leucylnegamycin and negamycin separated by chromatography on an Amberlite column and subsequently lyophilized. This antibiotic has an antimicrobial activity against a variety of organisms and from the evidence at present available appears to be a direct metabolic intermediate in the biosynthesis of negamycin.

Kondo *et al.*, *J. Antibiotics* (Japan), **24**, 732 (1971)
Umezawa, Maeda, Kondo, *Japanese Patent*, 7,318,488 (1973)

LEVOMYCETIN
$C_{11}H_{12}O_5N_2Cl_2$

A synthetic antibiotic substance, levomycetin is highly active against a large number of *Salmonella* strains isolated from patients suffering with food-poisoning. The antibiotic is also active against *Salmonella anatum* but not against *Shigella*. It has been shown to decrease the DNA level, oxygen uptake and inhibit the activities of a number of enzymes when incubated with an exudate from guinea pig abdominal cavity at 37°C for 1 hour. These inhibitory effects are more pronounced than those which have been observed with penicillin.

Tsyganenko, Balakliets, *Mikrobiol. Zh.*, **35**, 760 (1973)
Rachkovskaya *et al.*, *Antibiotiki*, **19**, 136 (1974)

LEVORIN
A polyene antibiotic, this substance is produced by the simultaneous cultivation of *Streptomyces levoris* and a yeast which may belong to the genus *Candida*, *Monilia* or *Saccharomyces*. A typical method given by Tsyganov and his colleagues is to ferment an aqueous medium of soya bean flour, corn meal and inorganic salts with *Saccharomyces cerevisiae* at 37°C for 36 hours with shaking and then add a 2-day culture of *Streptomyces levoris* and incubate the mixture for a further 6 hours when a product is obtained having 62,300 units of the antibiotic per ml of culture fluid.

Levorin is active against a number of pathogenic fungi.

Tsyganov *et al.*, *German Patent*, 2,108,501 (1972)
Ganov *et al.*, *British Patent*, 1,347,020 (1974)
Tsyganov *et al.*, *U.S. Patent*, 2,802,998 (1974)

LIBRAMYCIN A
A recently discovered antibiotic, libramycin is produced by culturing *Streptomyces* strain 79-192 on a medium containing glucose, starch, soybean flour, dry yeast, beef extract and inorganic salts at 27°C for 3 days. The antibiotic is active against gram-positive bacteria and fungi, particularly *Mycobacterium phlei* and *Xanthomonas oryzae*.

Yahagi *et al.*, *J. Antibiotics* (Japan), **27**, 143 (1974)

LICHENIFORMIN
M.p. Indefinite

An antibiotic derived from *Bacillus licheniformis*, licheniformin is obtained by surface growth on a medium containing inorganic salts and ammonium and sodium lactates. The culture is incubated at 37°C for 6 days, the yield being 400–600 *Mycobacterium phlei* units/ml. Isolation is carried out by acidifying the culture liquor with HCl to pH 2·5, boiling or autoclaving, centrifuging, adjusting the pH to 5·0 with sodium hydroxide and adsorbing the active material on activated carbon, washing the cake with H_2O and denatured EtOH and eluting with *N*-BuOH saturated with H_2O. Purification is done by adjusting the aqueous BuOH fraction to pH 6·0, forming the precipitated picrate by pouring into excess picric acid solution, decomposing with HCl, dissolving the gummy precipitate in CH_3OH and reprecipitating from $(CH_3)_2CO$.

Licheniformin is normally obtained as the hydrochloride which is an amorphous white powder, soluble in H_2O and CH_3OH, slightly soluble in EtOH and insoluble in $(CH_3)_2CO$ and non-polar organic solvents. It is stable in the dry state but gradually loses its activity in aqueous solution. The salt is laevorotatory with $[\alpha]_D - 37°$ (c 1·09, CH_3OH). It gives positive Sakaguchi and biuret tests and negative Molisch, ninhydrin and glucosamine tests. The antibiotic forms several salts and derivatives; the sulphate is a white powder, the helianthate forms small red needles, the oxalate and rufianate are amorphous solids, the picrate, picrolonate and flavianate are oily, semi-solid precipitates which cannot be crystallized and the rhodanilate is an oil.

Licheniformin is assayed by serial dilution with *Mycobacterium phlei* as the test organism incubated for 4 days at 37°C. The antibiotic is active against a number of organisms, typical inhibition dilutions ($\times 1,000,000$) being: *Actinobacillus lingieresi* ($>0·01$); *Bacillus anthracis* (0·2); *Brucella abortus* (0·32); *Corynebacterium diphtheriae* (1·25–12·5); *Coryne. equi* (5·0); *Coryne. renale* (40); *Diplococcus pneumoniae* (0·12–0·16); *Erysipelothrix rhusiopathiae* (0·005); *Escherichia coli* (0·01–0·08); *Mycobacterium phlei* (2·5–5·0); *Myco. tuberculosis* (0·16–0·64); *Pseudomonas pyocyanea* (0·04); *Salmonella paratyphi* (0·02); *Shigella dysenteriae* (0·04–0·16); *Staphylococcus aureus* (1·0); *Staph. pyogenes* (1·25–5·0); *Streptococcus viridans* (0·02) and *Vibrio comma* (0·02).

The antibiotic shows little activity *in vivo*, providing virtually no protection to mice infected with *Staphylococcus pyogenes* and only partial protection against *Streptococcus pyogenes*. It exerts a suppressive effect on tuberculosis in combination with sulphetrone in aerosol-infected mice.

A solution of the hydrochloride ($2·5–5·0 \times 10^3$ units/ml) has an LD_{50} of 7·5 mg (intraperitoneal), 5·0 mg (intravenous) and 10 mg (subcutaneous) when injected into mice. Kidney damage occurs when a dose of 6 mg is given subcutaneously for 5 weeks. Physiologically, licheniformin produces a steep drop in blood pressure in cats when given at a dose of 1–2 mg/kg, evidently due to a histamine effect. There is no action on the isolated guinea pig ileum while in human skin there is a typical 'triple-response' at a dilution of 1:100,000.

Callow, Hart, *Nature*, **157**, 334 (1946)
Hart, Hills, *Biochem. J.*, **41**, xxvii (1947)
Callow, Glover, *ibid.*, (1947)
Callow et al., *Brit. J. Exptl. Path.*, **28**, 418 (1947)

LIENOMYCIN
$C_{27-28}H_{49}O_8N$
M.p. Indefinite

Actinomyces diastatochromogenes var. *lienomycini* strain 478 yields this antibiotic which is obtained in the form of an amorphous white powder with no definite melting point. The ultraviolet spectrum in CH_3OH has absorption maxima at 318, 333 and 349 nm, typical of a pentaene structure. Lienomycin is soluble in aqueous alcohols, AcOH, pyridine, dimethylformamide and dilute acids and alkalies, insoluble in $CHCl_3$, $(CH_3)_2CO$, AcOEt, C_6H_6 and H_2O. It is unstable to changes in pH, exposure to light and storage at low temperatures. Both the antibiotic and its salts are active against gram-positive bacteria in concentrations of 1·0–9·0 μg/ml but the salts are degraded more rapidly than lienomycin itself.

Gauze et al., *Antibiotiki*, **16**, 387 (1971)
Brazhnikova et al. *ibid.*, **16**, 483 (1971)

LILACININ
M.p. 102–103°C

A peptide antibiotic, lilacinin has been isolated from cultures of *Penicillium lilacinum* grown in a medium containing glucose and corn steep liquor for 5 days at 28°C and pH 5·4. Lilacinin is obtained by extraction of the culture filtrate with AcOEt followed by chromatography and crystallization from aqueous CH_3OH. It forms colourless crystals and is laevorotatory with a specific rotation of $[\alpha]_D^{26} - 26°$ (CH_3OH). It has little activity against bacteria but is effective in inhibiting both *Cryptococcus neoformans* and *Trichophyton rubrum*.

Yamano, Yamamoto, Suide, *Japanese Patent*, 7,122,552 (1971)

LINCOMYCIN
$C_{18}H_{34}O_6N_2S$
M.p. Indefinite

This antibacterial antibiotic was first obtained from cultures of *Streptomyces lincolnensis* var. *lincolnensis* NRRL 2936 in common nutrient media but has since been isolated from similar cultures of *S. espinosus* NRRL

3890, *S. pseudogriseolus* chemovar *linmyceticus* NRRL 3985 and *S. variabilis liniabilis* NRRL 5618. From the last named organism it is produced without the simultaneous formation of lincomycin B which is otherwise a normal constituent of these fermentations. The antibiotic is usually isolated and employed as the crystalline hydrochloride.

Lincomycin is active against a number of bacteria, particularly *Staphylococcus aureus*. Mates has shown that 0·1 μg/ml of the antibiotic inhibits lipase production by *S. aureus* but does not affect the growth of the organism. Lincomycin also possesses a marked interaction with *d*-tubocurarine as demonstrated by Samuelson and his coworkers who have pointed out that patients being given the antibiotic in the recovery room must be closely observed for signs of respiratory depression. The antibiotic has a high tolerance level in humans, an infusion of 4800–8400 mg given daily to healthy subjects for 7 days shows no difference in volunteers receiving the antibiotic and those given a placebo.

Novak *et al.*, *Clin. Pharmacol. Ther.*, **12**, 793 (1971)
Visser, *U.S. Patent*, 3,674,647 (1972)
Visser, *German Patent*, 2,138,784 (1972)
Witz, *German Patent*, 2,141,588 (1972)
Argoudelis, Coats, Pyke, *German Patent*, 2,164,664 (1972)
Argoudelis, Coats, *German Patent*, 2,231,007 (1973)
Argoudelis, Coats, *Japanese Patent*, 7,442,891 (1974)
Argoudelis, Coats, *German Patent*, 2,338,899 (1974)
Mates, *Chemotherapy* (Basle), **21**, 293 (1975)
Walsh, Feierabend, Levine, *Life Sci.*, **16**, 1683 (1975)
Samuelson *et al.*, *Anesth. Analg.* (Cleveland), **54**, 103 (1975)

LIPIARMYCIN

$C_{52}H_{74}O_{19}Cl_2$
M.p. 173–175°C

A crystalline antibiotic, lipiarmycin is produced by *Actinoplanes deccanensis* ATCC 21,983 cultured under aerobic conditions in common nutrient media at 25–35°C. Recrystallization of the compound from Et_2O-petroleum ether gives a white crystalline material which gives positive Tollens, $FeCl_3$ and H_2SO_4 reactions but negative Millon, Maltol and Schiff tests. Lipiarmycin is active against a range of pathogenic bacteria, particularly *Bacillus subtilis*, *Escherichia coli* and *Staphylococcus aureus*. It inhibits RNA synthesis in *B. subtilis* at less than 1·0 μg/ml and DNA and protein synthesis at 100 μg/ml. Elongation of DNA chains is instantly blocked at the latter concentration.

Parenti, Pagani, Beretta, *J. Antibiotics* (Japan), **28**, 247 (1975)
Sergio *et al.*, *ibid.*, **28**, 543 (1975)
Coronelli *et al.*, *German Patent*, 2,455,230 (1975)

LITMOCIDIN

M.p. 144–146°C (*dec.*)

An antibiotic pigment derived from *Proactinomyces cyaneus* var. *antibioticus* (*Nocardia cyanea*), litmocidin is extracted from the agar culture with H_2O, acidified to pH 3·5 and then adsorbed on activated carbon. The carbon is then eluted with acid $(CH_3)_2CO$, concentrated to dryness *in vacuo*, the residue dissolved in EtOH and precipitated with H_2O. Litmocidin is stable and soluble in dilute alkalies, being a red pigment under acid conditions and blue in alkali.

The antibiotic is assayed by serial dilution with *Staphylococcus aureus*, the purified material having 4000 units/ml. It is very active against gram-positive bacteria and mycobacteria but has only a limited activity against gram-negative organisms. Typical inhibition dilutions ($\times$ 1000) are: *Eberthella typhi* (1·0); *Escherichia coli* (1·0); *Salmonella paratyphi* (1·0); *S. schottmuelleri* (1·0); *Shigella dysenteriae* (1·0); *Shig. paradysenteriae* (10); *Staphylococcus aureus* (1000–4000); *Streptococcus hemolyticus* (400–2000); *Strep. viridans* (500) and *Vibrio comma* (500–2000). The mode of activity has been shown to be both bactericidal and bacteriostatic and is unaffected by 10–30 per cent human serum. The LD_{50} in mice is 50 mg/kg when administered intraperitoneally. It has no action against *Micrococcus pyogenes* var. *aureus* in mice.

Gause, *J. Bact.*, **51**, 649 (1946)
Brashnikova, *ibid.*, **51**, 665 (1946)

LIVIDOMYCIN A

$C_{29}H_{55}O_{18}N_5$

Cultures of *Streptomyces lividus* yield a number of aminoglycosidic antibiotics including lividomycins A and B, paromomycin (q.v.) and a minor constituent antibiotic 2230-C. Separation and purification may be carried out by ion-exchange resin chromatography. The structure given above is based upon chemical degradative experiments and spectroscopic determinations.

Lividomycin A is a broad-spectrum antibiotic and tests carried out *in vitro* against 90 strains of pathogenic bacteria at pH 7·2 have shown that it has an activity equal to or greater than that of either kanamycin or neomycin (q.v.). It shows a high degree of activity against *Escherichia coli*, *Proteus* species, *Pseudomonas aeruginosa* and *Staphylococcus aureus*. It is active in the presence of serum and tested *in vivo* in mice, it exerts a protective effect against experimental infections with *Pseudomonas aeruginosa* and *Staphylococcus aureus*. When administered intramuscularly into laboratory animals, most of the antibiotic appeared within 8 hours in the urine but only about 2 per cent was recovered in this way on oral administration, indicative of poor absorption from the gut.

Some toxic effects have been noted with this antibiotic. Doses of 100 mg/kg given intravenously to dogs produced inhibition of the cervical ganglionic potential while larger doses brought about circulation abnormalities in the kidney and liver and a decrease in the blood pressure. Doses in excess of 250 mg/kg given intravenously to dogs also brought about depression of respiration and spontaneous motor activity, excessive salivation, vomiting and vasodilatation. A similar dose given intraperitoneally to rabbits caused a decrease in cochlear microphonic amplitude and in the same animals, 300 mg/kg/day given intramuscularly for 10 days produced microscopic changes in the kidneys, two out of six animals dying of nephrotoxicity on the ninth day of treatment.

Mori *et al.*, *J. Antibiotics* (Japan), **24**, 339 (1971)
Mori *et al.*, *ibid.*, **25**, 534 (1972)
Mori, *Oyo Yakuri*, **6**, 681 (1972)
Mori, Kakishita, Kato, *ibid.*, **6**, 813 (1972)
Tamura *et al.*, *ibid.*, **6**, 845 (1972)
Mori *et al.*, *ibid.*, **6**, 857 (1972)
Vitali, Ripa, Viticchi, *Ann. Sclavo.*, **15**, 329 (1973)

LIVIDOMYCIN B
$C_{23}H_{45}O_{13}N_5$

This aminoglycosidic antibiotic accompanies the preceding compound in cultures of *Streptomyces lividus*, from which it may be separated and purified by ion-exchange resin chromatography. It has an antibiotic spectrum similar to that of lividomycin A. A number of derivatives of this antibiotic have been prepared and shown to possess antibacterial properties, in particular the 1-(L-(−)-γ-amino-α-hydroxybutyryl derivative.

Mori *et al.*, *J. Antibiotics* (Japan), **24**, 339 (1971)
Mori *et al.*, *ibid.*, **25**, 534 (1972)
Oda *et al.*, *Japanese Patent*, 7,344,234 (1973)
Naito *et al.*, *U.S. Patent*, 3,808,198 (1974)

LL-N313ζ
$C_{16}H_{22}O_3$
M.p. 172–173°C

This antibiotic substance is derived from *Sporormia affinis* and forms colourless crystals when recrystallized from CH_3OH. It is laevorotatory with a specific rotation of $[\alpha]_D^{25}$ − 113° (c 1·0, CH_3OH). It possesses only a slight activity against bacteria but is active against a number of pathogenic fungi.

McGahren *et al.*, *J. Amer. Chem. Soc.*, **96**, 1616 (1974)

LL-Z1271α
$C_{17}H_{20}O_5$
M.p. 214–216°C

LL-Z127γ

This antifungal antibiotic is obtained from a species of *Acrostalagmus* and has been shown to be the methyl ether of antibiotic LL-Z1271γ. It forms colourless crystals from CH_3OH and is laevorotatory with a specific rotation of $[\alpha]_D - 203°$ (c 0·29, CH_3OH).

Ellestad, Evans, Kunstmann, *J. Amer. Chem. Soc.*, **91**, 2134 (1969)

LL-Z1271γ
$C_{16}H_{18}O_5$
M.p. 238–240°C

Also produced by an *Acrostalagmus* species, this antifungal antibiotic has the structure given above. It forms colourless crystals when purified by recrystallization from CH_3OH and gives an ultraviolet spectrum consisting of a single absorption maximum at 257 nm.

Ellestad, Evans, Kunstmann, *J. Amer. Chem. Soc.*, **91**, 2134 (1969)

LL-Z1272α
$C_{23}H_{31}O_3Cl$
M.p. 72·7–73°C

A number of closely related antibiotics have been obtained from an unclassified species of *Fusarium*. This substance forms colourless crystals from aqueous CH_3OH or a mixture of CH_3OH and *iso*octane. It gives an ultraviolet spectrum in CH_3OH having absorption maxima at 228, 293 and 345 nm. It has a marked activity against *Tetrahymena pyriformis*.

Ellestad, Evans, Kunstmann, *Tetrahedron*, **25**, 1323 (1969)

LL-Z1272β
$C_{23}H_{32}O_3$
M.p. 97·5°C

Also isolated from the same unclassified *Fusarium* species, this antibiotic forms colourless needles when crystallized from aqueous CH_3OH. The ultraviolet spectrum in CH_3OH has absorption maxima at 223 and 297 nm with shoulders at 233 and 340 nm. The structure has been shown to be 2:4-dihydroxy-6-methyl-3-(3:7:11-trimethyldodeca-2:6:10-trienyl) benzaldehyde. Like the preceding antibiotic it is active against *Tetrahymena pyriformis*.

Ellestad, Evans, Kunstmann, *Tetrahedron*, **25**, 1323 (1969)

LL-Z1272γ
$C_{23}H_{29}O_4Cl$
M.p. 172–173°C

A third antibiotic obtained from a species of *Fusarium*, this substance gives colourless crystals from $(CH_3)_2CO$-hexane. It is laevorotatory with a specific rotation of $[\alpha]_D^{25} - 31°$ (c 0·99, CH_3OH) and gives an ultraviolet spectrum in CH_3OH with absorption maxima at 230, 293 and 347 nm. Like all of this group of antibiotics, it exhibits anti-*Tetrahymena pyriformis* activity.

Ellestad, Evans, Kunstmann, *Tetrahedron*, **25**, 1323 (1969)

LL-Z1272β

$C_{23}H_{31}O_4Cl$
M.p. 129·5–130·5°C

This antibiotic accompanies the preceding substance and forms colourless crystals from $(CH_3)_2CO$-hexane. It is slightly dextrorotatory with a specific rotation of $[\alpha]_D^{25} + 6°$ (c 1·0, CH_3OH) and the ultraviolet spectrum in CH_3OH exhibits absorption maxima at 231, 293 and 346 nm. It is also active against *Tetrahymena pyriformis* and has the structure 1-(3-chloro-5-formyl-2:6-dihydroxy-4-methylphenyl)-3-methyl-5-(1:2:6-trimethyl-3-oxocyclohexyl)pent-2-ene.

Ellestad, Evans, Kunstmann, *Tetrahedron*, **25**, 1323 (1969)

LL-Z1272ε

$C_{23}H_{32}O_4$
M.p. 171·5–172·5°C

A further antifungal antibiotic isolated from an unclassified species of *Fusarium*, the structure of this substance is 1-(3-formyl-2:6-dihydroxy-4-methylphenyl)-3-methyl-5-(1:2:6-trimethyl-3-oxocyclohexyl)pent-2-ene. It gives colourless crystals when recrystallized from AcOEt-hexane and is dextrorotatory with a specific rotation of $[\alpha]_D^{25} + 60$ (c 0·93, CH_3OH). It gives an ultraviolet spectrum in CH_3OH with absorption maxima at 223 and 295 nm with shoulders at 233 and 340 nm. It also shows activity against *Tetrahymena pyriformis*.

Ellestad, Evans, Kunstmann, *Tetrahedron*, **25**, 1323 (1969)

LL-Z1272ζ

$C_{25}H_{31}O_6Cl$
M.p. 156·5–157°C

A sixth antibiotic found in cultures of an unclassified species of *Fusarium*. It forms colourless needles from $(CH_3)_2CO$-hexane, is laevorotatory with $[\alpha]_D^{25} - 15°$ (c 1·0, CH_3OH) and gives an ultraviolet spectrum in CH_3OH with absorption maxima at 239, 293 and 346 nm. It also exhibits anti-*Tetrahymena pyriformis* activity and has been shown by chemical and spectroscopic investigations to be 1-(3-acetoxy-1:2:6-trimethyl-5-oxocyclohexyl)-5-(3-chloro-5-formyl-2:6-dihydroxy-4-methylphenyl)-3-methylpenta-1:3-diene.

Ellestad, Evans, Kunstmann, *Tetrahedron*, **25**, 1323 (1969)

LOCABIOTAL
See Fusafungine

LOMONDOMYCIN
M.p. Indefinite
Cultivation of *Streptomyces lomondensis* var. *lomondensis* NRRL 3252 at 28°C with shaking in a medium containing cottonseed flour, glucose, dextrin and inorganic salts yields this antibiotic which has been obtained in a reasonably pure form together with the crystalline potassium salt. Lomondomycin is active against a wide range of organisms, typical minimum inhibition concentrations being: *Bacillus subtilis* (31); *Candida albicans* (1000); *Nocardia asteroides* (100); *Proteus vulgaris* (125) and *Staphylococcus aureus* (62).

Bergy, Johnson, *U.S. Patent*, 3,359,165 (1967)

LOMYCIN
See Griseomycin

LONGICATENAMYCIN
$C_{35}H_{55}N_8O_9Cl$
Streptomyces strain S-520 elaborates a very complex antibiotic mixture of cogeners which has not been completely separated. The major component has, however, been isolated and shown, from chemical and spectroscopic evidence, to have the macrocyclic structure given above.

Shiba, Mukunoki, *J. Antibiotics* (Japan), **28**, 561 (1975)

LONOMYCIN
$C_{44}H_{76}O_{14}$

A complex polyether antibiotic, lonomycin is elaborated by *Streptomyces ribosidificus* strain TM-481 when grown on a common nutrient medium. It has been isolated and purified as the crystalline sodium salt which forms colourless prisms having m.p. 188–9°C. The antibiotic is active against a range of gram-positive bacteria.

Omura *et al.*, *J. Antibiotics* (Japan), **29**, 15 (1976)

LUCENSOMYCIN (*Etruscomycin*)
$C_{36}H_{53}O_{13}N$
M.p. Indefinite
A polyene antibiotic isolated from cultures of *Streptomyces lucensis*, lucensomycin forms a microcrystalline powder and is dextrorotatory with $[\alpha]_D^{20}$ + 296° (pyridine) and + 50° (methanolic 0·1N-HCl). The ultraviolet spectrum has absorption maxima at 218, 278, 290, 303 and 318 nm. It is unstable beyond pH 6·0–8·0 and to light, air or heat. Lucensomycin is active against a range of pathogenic fungi and has LD_{50} in mice of 1263 mg/kg given orally.

Arcamone *et al.*, *Giorn. Microbiol.*, **4**, 119 (1957)
Arcamone, Perego, *Ann. Chim.* (Rome), **49**, 345 (1959)
Marini, Pennella, *Proc. Symp. Antibiotics Prague*, 148 (1959)
Arcamone *et al.*, *U.S. Patent*, 3,170,837 (1965)
Structure
Guadiano *et al.*, *Tetrahedron Lett.*, 3559, 3567 (1966)
Guadiano *et al.*, *Gazz. Chim. Ital.*, **96**, 1470 (1966)
Guadiano *et al.*, *Chem. Ind.* (Milan), **48**, 1327 (1966)
See also
Strom *et al.*, *Biophys. J.*, **13**, 568, 581 (1973)

LUNATOIC ACID A
$C_{21}H_{24}O_7$

The fungus *Cochliobolus lunata* elaborates two antibiotic carboxylic acids which have been isolated and characterized as their crystalline methyl esters. Lunatoic acid A methyl ester forms yellow needles with m.p. 109°C and a specific rotation of $[\alpha]_D^{26}$ − 208° (c 0·17, CHCl$_3$). It gives an ultraviolet spectrum in MeOH having absorption maxima at 240, 262, 348 and 530 nm. This antibiotic inhibits the growth of a number of strains of *Cochliobolus lunata* at concentrations of 3–12 ppm. It has no action against bacteria or fungi except *Piricularia oryzae* which is inhibited at concentrations of 45–50 ppm. The structure of lunatoic acid A has been established from chemical and spectroscopic evidence.

Nukina, Marumo, *Tetrahedron Lett.*, 2603 (1977)

LUNATOIC ACID B
$C_{21}H_{26}O_7$

Isolated as the methyl ester, a yellow amorphous powder with m.p. indefinite and a specific rotation of $[\alpha]_D^{26} + 201°$ (c 0·71, $CHCl_3$), this antibiotic has also been isolated from *Cochliobolus lunata*. It has a growth inhibitory action against a number of strains of *Cochliobolus lunata* and is also active against *Piricularia oryzae*.

Nukina, Marumo, *Tetrahedron Lett.*, 2603 (1977)

LUPULON
$C_{26}H_{38}O_4$
M.p. 92°C

Humulus lupus, the hop vine, possesses antibacterial properties which have been recognized for many years. Precise determinations of the properties of humulon (q.v.) and lupulon, the actual antibiotic agents, have been made only comparatively recently. Lupulon is isolated by extracting the ground hops with absolute CH_3OH, diluting the extract with aqueous 2 per cent sodium chloride and re-extracting with petroleum ether. Evaporation gives a syrup which deposits crystals on cooling for several hours. Alternatively, the hops may be ground with solid carbon dioxide, extracted with petroleum ether, the solution evaporated *in vacuo* to a syrup and crystallized at −15°C. It is purified by recrystallizing from 70 per cent EtOH. The antibiotic forms white crystals which become yellow and amorphous on standing. It is optically inactive, moderately soluble in CH_3OH, EtOH, hexane, *iso*octane and petroleum ether, slightly so in neutral or acid aqueous solution. The sodium salt is freely soluble in H_2O. In both acidic and alkaline solutions, lupulon is comparatively stable but it is readily oxidized in air, the oxidation being inhibited by ascorbic acid. The presence of unsaturation in the molecule is shown by its decolourizing potassium permanganate solution and its ease of catalytic hydrogenation to give the dihydro derivative.

Lupulon is assayed by several methods including cylinder plate, turbidimetric and serial dilution with *Sclerotina fructicola* spore germination. The antibiotic is less active than humulon, the following inhibition dilutions (× 1000) being given by Lewis and his colleagues: *Bacillus anthracis* (300); *B. cereus* var. *mycoides* (1000); *B. subtilis* (1000); *Corynebacterium diphtheriae gravis* (100); *Diplococcus pneumoniae* I (300); *Micrococcus lysodeikticus* (300); *M. pyogenes* var. *aureus* (500); *Mycobacterium phlei* (300); *Myco. tuberculosis hominis* (100); *Sarcina lutea* (100); *Streptococcus coelicolor* (50) and *Strp. fecalis* (500). It is also active *in vitro* against a number of fungi, Michener giving the following 50 per cent inhibition concentrations (μg/ml): *Alternaria citri* (900); *Aspergillus niger* (1600); *Aspergillus oryzae* (200); *Botrytis cinerea* (200); *Fusarium lycopersici* (300); *Penicillium digitatum* (250); *Pythium* spp. (500); *Rhizopus nigricans* (40); *Sclerotina fructicola* (40) and *Sclerotina bataticola* (80).

In the presence of serum there is a large reduction in activity against *Mycobacterium phlei*, no reduction against *Myco. tuberculosis* but almost complete loss of activity against *Staphylococcus aureus*. No synergism with other antitubercular agents was observed by Michener and his coworkers.

Lupulon shows some activity *in vivo* in mice treated for an experimentally induced disease with *Mycobacterium tuberculosis*, the antibiotic being given as a 1·5 per cent solution in cottonseed oil, administered intramuscularly for 30 days at a dose of 69 mg/kg each day. A similar protection was afforded by an oral administration of 150 mg/kg given twice a day for 30 days, the lupulon being given in this case as a 3 per cent solution in 6 per cent aqueous gum acacia.

The toxicity of lupulon is quite low. The LD_{50} in mice, given intramuscularly, is 600 mg/kg of the 1·5 per cent solution in cottonseed oil. When given orally, the LD_{50} is stated to be 1500 mg/kg given as a 5 per cent solution in 6 per cent aqueous gum acacia.

Walker, Parker, *J. Inst. Brewing*, **43**, 17 (1937)

Shinwell, *ibid.*, **43**, 111 (1937)
Michener, Snell, Jansen, *Arch. Biochem.*, **19**, 199 (1948)
Lewis *et al.*, *J. Clin. Invest.*, **28**, 916 (1949)
Chin, Chang, Anderson, *ibid.*, **28**, 909 (1949)
Michener, Anderson, *Science*, **110**, 68 (1949)
Chin *et al.*, *Proc. Soc. Exptl. Biol. Med.*, **70**, 158 (1949)
Salle, Jann, Ordanik, *ibid.*, **70**, 408 (1949)

LUTEOMYCIN
$C_{23}H_{29}O_9N$
M.p. 199–200°C (*dec.*)

This antibiotic has been obtained from *Streptomyces tanashiensis* (a mold related to *S. antibioticus* and *S. aureus*). It is extracted from the broth with organic solvents at pH 7·5–8·0 followed by back extraction with H_2O at pH 3·0 and chromatography on an alumina column, the latter being developed with CH_3OH or $(CH_3)_2CO$. Luteomycin is basic in nature and readily forms a hydrochloride which is freely soluble in $CHCl_3$, moderately so in H_2O, CH_3OH, EtOH, AcOEt and BuOEt, but insoluble in Et_2O, C_6H_6 or petroleum ether. The ultraviolet spectrum exhibits two absorption maxima at 270 and 430 nm. Luteomycin is comparatively unstable with a maximum stability under acid conditions.

The antibiotic is primarily active against mycobacteria and gram-positive bacteria, having only a limited activity against the Enterobacteriaceae although showing some activity against *Brucella* and *Hemophilus*. *In vivo* it has activity against *Brucella melitensis*, *Hemophilus pertussis* and the pneumococci. The LD_{50} in mice, both subcutaneous and intravenous, is approximately 10 mg/kg.

Hata *et al.*, *Arch. Exp. Med.*, **32**, 229 (1949)
Hata *et al.*, *J. Antibiotics* (Japan), **3**, 313 (1950)
Hata *et al.*, *ibid.*, **5**, 529 (1952)
Sano, *ibid.*, **5**, 535 (1952)

LYCOMARASMINE
$C_9H_{15}O_7N_3$
Dec. 227–229°C

A comparatively simple peptide antibiotic, this substance is elaborated by *Fusarium lycopersici* and has the structure given above. It forms colourless crystals which decompose without melting. It has a specific rotation of $[\alpha]_D^{20}$ − 42° to − 48° (H_2O at pH 7·0), is readily soluble in dilute acids and alkalies, but only sparingly so in H_2O. It is active against tomato-wilt in plants.

Plattner, Clauson-Kaas, *Helv. Chim. Acta*, **28**, 188 (1945)
Structure
Plattner, Clauson-Kaas, *Experientia*, **1**, 195 (1945)
Hardegger *et al.*, *Helv. Chim. Acta*, **46**, 60 (1963)

LYCOSPERSIN
See Bikaverin

LYMECYCLINE
$C_{29}H_{38}O_{10}N_4$
M.p. Indefinite

A semi-synthetic tetracycline antibiotic, lymecycline has the structure N-lysinomethyltetracycline and forms a white amorphous powder. The sodium salt has been prepared and gives an ultraviolet spectrum in H_2O with a single absorption maximum at 376 nm. It is active against a range of gram-positive and some gram-negative bacteria.

Blackwood *et al.*, *U.S. Patent*, 3,042,716 (1962)
Lauria, Logemann, *German Patent*, 1,134,071 (1962)
Tubaro, Raffaldoni, *Boll. Chim. Farm.*, **100**, 9 (1961)

LYMPHOMYCIN
M.p. Indefinite

An antitumour antibiotic, lymphomycin has been obtained from cultures of *Streptomyces* strain S-66. It is precipitated from the culture broth by ammonium sulphate, indicative of its protein-like nature and has a molecular weight of approximately 11,000. It is black and amorphous and has been shown to contain valine as an N-terminal aminoacid. There are no nucleic acids or carbohydrates in the molecule. Lymphomycin is cytotoxic to Burkitt lymphoma and to human lymphoblastoid cells as well as peritoneal macrophages. It has no inhibitory effects, however, on human eperdermoid HeLa carcinoma. A dose of 80 mg/kg per day for 6 days has proved lethal to tumour-bearing mice given intraperitoneally, but half this dose is not toxic.

Ishida et al., Progr. Antimicrob. Anticancer Chemother., **1**, 93 (1969)

LYSOCELLIN
$C_{34}H_{60}O_{10}$
M.p. Indefinite
An amorphous antibiotic, this compound has been obtained from cultures of *Streptomyces cacaoi* var. *asoensis*. The sodium salt is crystalline, m.p. 158–160°C; $[\alpha]_D^{25} + 11 \cdot 5°$ (c 1·0, CH_3OH) and insoluble in H_2O. The silver salt has also been prepared in a crystalline form, melting above 123°C. Lysocellin is active against gram-positive bacteria, mycobacteria and fungi. It has proved effective in the treatment of coccidial infections in poultry.

Ebata et al., J. Antibiotics (in press)
Structure
Otaka et al., Chem. Commun., 92 (1975)

M

MACARBOMYCIN

A number of antibiotics have been obtained from cultures of *Streptomyces phaeochromogenes* by precipitation at pH 3·0 and separated by chromatography on a DEZE-cellulose column. Macarbomycin gives an ultraviolet spectrum in H_2O with a single absorption maximum at 257–258 nm. Chemical analysis indicates the presence of phosphorus in the molecule. The antibiotic is active against gram-positive bacteria but has only a limited activity against gram-negative organisms. It is active against a resistant strain of *Staphylococcus aureus* FDA209P and also against the episome-carrying strain of *Escherichia coli* K-12 ML3966, more so than against the parent strain *E. coli* K-12 W3630.

Takahashi et al., *J. Antibiotics* (Japan), **26**, 542 (1973)

MACARBOMYCIN 1_a

A minor constituent of the culture broth of *Streptomyces phaeochromogenes*, the ultraviolet spectrum of this antibiotic is H_2O shows no characteristic absorptions. It is active against gram-positive bacteria and more active against gram-negative bacteria than the preceding substance. It shows the same effect against strains of *Escherichia coli* as macarbomycin.

Takahashi et al., *J. Antibiotics* (Japan), **26**, 542 (1973)

MACARBOMYCIN 1_b

A further minor component found in the broth of *Streptomyces phaeochromogenes*, this antibiotic has a similar biological activity to macarbomycin but is only about a tenth as active.

Takahashi et al., *J. Antibiotics* (Japan), **26**, 542 (1973)

MACARBOMYCIN II

Streptomyces phaeochromogenes elaborates this minor antibiotic which closely resembles the preceding substances. The ultraviolet spectrum in H_2O shows a weak absorption maximum at 255–259 nm. It has a high degree of activity against gram-positive bacteria including the resistant strain of *Staphylococcus aureus* FDA209P. Like the other members of this group it is appreciably more active against the episome-carrying strain of *Escherichia coli* K-12 ML3933 than against the parent strain *E. coli* K-12 W3630.

Takahashi et al., *J. Antibiotics* (Japan), **26**, 542 (1973)

MACARBOMYCIN III

A fourth minor antibiotic obtained from the culture broth of *Streptomyces phaeochromogenes*, this substance is separated from the accompanying antibiotics by DEAE-cellulose column chromatography. The ultraviolet spectrum in H_2O is almost identical with that of macarbomycin itself with a strong absorption maximum at 257–258 nm. The antibiotic spectrum is similar to those of the other members of the group but it is about a quarter as active as macarbomycin itself.

Takahashi et al., *J. Antibiotics* (Japan), **26**, 542 (1973)

MACRASIDEMYCIN

An anticancer antibiotic, macrasidemycin has been obtained by the fermentation of *Streptomyces* strain M590-G2 aerobically on a medium of glucose, starch, soybean powder and inorganic salts at 27–29°C and pH 7·2 for 5 days. When given intraperitoneally at a dose of 78 micrograms/kg/day for 10 days the antibiotic completely controlled Ehlich ascites tumour in mice.

Umezawa et al., *Japanese Patent*, 75 126,893 (1975)

MACROMOMYCIN

M.p. Indefinite

Streptomyces macromomyceticus elaborates this antibiotic when cultivated under submerged aerobic conditions in a nutrient medium at 27°C for 4 days. The antibiotic, which has a molecular weight of about 15,000 is precipitated from the culture filtrate and separated by dialysis against H_2O from the low molecular weight impurities. Macromomycin is active in inhibiting the growth of *Bacillus subtilis*, *Sarcina lutea*, *Staphylococcus aureus*, Ehrlich ascites tumour, leukemia L-120 and sarcoma 180.

Umezawa et al., *U.S. Patent*, 3,595,954 (1971)

MAGMAMYCIN
See Carbomycin

MAGNESIDIN
$C_{28}H_{36}O_8N_2Mg$ + $C_{32}H_{44}O_8N_2Mg$
M.p. Indefinite

A novel magnesium-containing antibiotic, this compound is an equivalent mixture of the magnesium salts of 1-acetyl-3-n-hexanoyl-5-ethylidenetetraamino acid and 1-acetyl-3-n-octanoyl-5-ethylidenetetraamino acid. It is obtained by culturing *Pseudomonas magnesiorubra* ATCC 21,856 in a medium containing glucose, peptone, starch, yeast extract, magnesium sulphate and sodium chloride in H_2O at pH 7·4 and 28°C for 24–30 hours. It may be extracted from the filtrate with organic solvents and forms colourless crystals which are insoluble in H_2O but soluble in common organic solvents. When heated, the crystals begin to shrink at 123°C, soften at 150°C and are then unchanged up to 300°C.

Magnesidin is active against gram-positive bacteria and its use has been suggested as a preventative of food spoilage by bacterial spores. It is moderately non-toxic, the LD_{50} in mice being 50 mg/kg when given intraperitoneally and 1000 mg/kg when administered orally or subcutaneously.

Gandhi *et al.*, *J. Antibiotics* (Japan), **26**, 797 (1973)
Nazareth *et al.*, *German Patent*, 2,352,448 (1975)

MAGNOPEPTIN
This polypeptide antibiotic is produced by *Streptomyces kagoshimanus* when freshly isolated from soil and grown in a common medium for 3 days at 27°C. The antibiotic is isolated by adjusting the broth to pH 3·6, filtering, extracting the cake with 70 per cent aqueous $(CH_3)_2CO$ at pH 7·0, evaporating the solvent and re-extracting the residue with BuOH. Purification is carried out by chromatography on alumina and then Sephadex G-50. Magnopeptin is insoluble in H_2O at pH 3·0–4·0 and has a molecular weight of approximately 49,000. It inhibits the growth of *Mucor rouxii* and *Piricularia oryzae*.

Shirato *et al.*, *Japanese Patent*, 7,142,960 (1971)

MALEIMYCIN
$C_7H_7O_3N$

Streptomyces showdoensis produces this simple antibiotic. The structure, as 3-aza-6-hydroxybicyclo[3.3.0.]oct-$\Delta(1,5)$-ene-2:4-dione, has been established by means of proton and carbon-13 NMR spectroscopy. The antibiotic is active against *Escherichia coli*, *Staphylococcus aureus* and leukemia L-1210 cells and also twenty times more active against *Mycobacterium phlei* than showdomycin (q.v.). It has been demonstrated that the mode of biosynthesis of the maleimide ring in this antibiotic differs from the biosynthesis of showdomycin, even though both compounds are synthesized at the same time by the same organism and both contain the maleimide ring.

Elstner *et al.*, *Biochemistry*, **12**, 4992 (1973)
Elstner *et al.*, *Proc. Int. Conf. Stable Isotop. Chem. Biol. Med.*, **1st**, 89 (1973)
Synthesis
Singh, Weinreb, *Tetrahedron*, **32**, 2379 (1976)

MANNOSIDOSTREPTOMYCIN (*Streptomycin B*)
$C_{27}H_{49}O_{17}N_7$
M.p. 178–179°C (*dec.*)

Certain cultures of *Streptomyces griseus* contain this glycosidic antibiotic where it occurs with streptomycin (q.v.), being separated from the latter by chromatography over acid-washed alumina. The compound is dextrorotatory with a specific rotation of $[\alpha]_D^{25}$ + 47° (c 1·0, H_2O) and forms a trihydrochloride, m.p. 190–200°C (*dec.*); $[\alpha]_D^{25}$ − 48° (c 1·35, H_2O) and a crystalline reineckate which crystallizes from H_2O as the dihydrate, m.p. 178°C (*dec.*). The antibiotic covers the same biological spectrum as streptomycin but is approximately six times less active on a weight basis. The LD_{50} in mice is 250 mg/kg when administered intravenously.

Fried, Titus, *J. Biol. Chem.*, **168**, 391 (1942)
Fried, Titus, *J. Amer. Chem. Soc.*, **70**, 3615 (1948)
Fried, Staveley, *ibid.*, **71**, 135 (1949)
Fried, Staveley, *ibid.*, **74**, 5461 (1952)

MARASMIC ACID
$C_{16}H_{26}O_4$
M.p. 174–175°C (*in vacuo*)

Marasmus conigenus elaborates this antibiotic which is obtained by surface growth on a medium consisting of corn steep liquor and beechwood shavings incubated for approximately 1 month. At the end of this period a yield of 256–512 *Staphylococcus aureus* units/ml is produced. Marasmic acid is isolated by acidifying the culture filtrate with HCl to pH 2·0, extracting with $CHCl_3$, concentrating *in vacuo*, washing with phosphate buffer at pH 5·8, evaporating to dryness *in vacuo*, extracting the residue with 2 per cent sodium bicarbonate after dissolving in Et_2O, acidifying the alkaline extract, re-extracting with Et_2O and crystallizing slowly by evaporation. It is finally purified by recrystallization from aqueous EtOH, Et_2O or $(CH_3)_2CO$.

Marasmic acid forms large white needles, soluble in EtOH, $(CH_3)_2CO$, Et_2O, $CHCl_3$ and H_2O, insoluble in hexane. It is dextrorotatory with a specific rotation of $[\alpha]_D^{25} + 176°$ (c 1·4, $(CH_3)_2CO$) and gives an ultraviolet spectrum in EtOH with absorption maxima at 241 and 316 nm. It gives a 2:4-dinitrophenylhydrazone as orange crystals with m.p. 136–138°C.

Assay of the antibiotic may be carried out by serial dilution with *Staphylococcus aureus* as test organism or by the determination of the antiluminescent activity with *Photobacterium fischeri*. The activity against *Staph. aureus* is decreased significantly by human blood.

Kavanagh and his colleagues have measured the following inhibition concentrations (μg/ml): *Bacillus mycoides* (1·0); *B. subtilis* (1·0); *Escherichia coli* (64); *Klebsiella pneumoniae* (128); *Mycobacterium smegmatis* (32); *Photobacterium fischeri* (0·016); *Pseudomonas aeruginosa* (250) and *Staphylococcus aureus* (2·0). The antibiotic is also active against a number of fungi, similar inhibition concentrations being: *Aspergillus niger* (32); *Chaetomium globosum* (64); *Gliomastix convoluta* (250); *Memnoniella echinata* (64); *Myrothecium verrucaria* (64); *Penicillium notatum* (32); *Saccharomyces cerevisae* (32); *Stemphylium consortiale* (128) and *Trichoderma mentagrophytes* (4·0).

Wilkins, *Trans. Brit. Mycol. Soc.*, **28**, 110 (1945)
Kavanagh, Hervey, Robbins, *Proc. Nat. Acad. Sci.*, **35**, 343 (1949)

MARCELLOMYCIN
$C_{42}H_{55}NO_{17}$

The bohemic acid complex isolated from the culture filtrate of *Actinosporangium* species ATCC 31,127 has been shown to consist primarily of two major components, marcellomycin and musettamycin (q.v.). Marcellomycin has the structure given above which is based upon chemical and spectroscopic data. It is particularly effective against straphylococci, strepococci and inhibits a number of transplanted rodent leukemias and carcinosarcomas *in vivo*. The acute LD_{50} in mice is 6·35–10·56 mg/kg.

Nettleton *et al.*, *J. Antibiotics* (Japan), **30**, 525 (1977)
Nettleton *et al.*, *U.S. Patent*, 4,039,736 (1977)

MARIDOMYCIN I
$C_{42}H_{69}O_{16}N$

A strain of *Streptomyces hygroscopicus* No. B-5050, yields a number of similar macrocyclic antibiotics, the maridomycins. The compounds are isolated from the culture broth with organic solvents and separated and purified by adsorption on silica gel or partition chromatography. The structure of this antibiotic has been determined primarily from the mass spectral data. The antibiotic is active against gram-positive bacteria, rickettsia and some large viruses, but not against gram-negative bacteria.

Muroi *et al.*, *Experientia*, **28**, 878 (1972)
Ono *et al.*, *J. Antibiotics* (Japan), **26**, 191 (1973)
Muroi *et al.*, *ibid.*, **26**, 199 (1973)
Ono, Harada, Kishi, *ibid.*, **27**, 442 (1974)
Structure
Muroi *et al.*, *Experientia*, **28**, 129 (1972)

MARIDOMYCIN II
$C_{42}H_{69}O_{16}N$

Isolated from the culture filtrate of *Streptomyces hygroscopicus* B-5050, this isomer of the preceding antibiotic has the structure given above which is based upon the infrared and NMR evidence from a series of chemical transformations. Hydrolysis furnishes the sugars mycaminose and 4-O-*iso*valerylmycarose. Oxidation of the antibiotic yields carbomycin (q.v.). The antibiotic is active against gram-positive bacteria and rickettsia.

Moroi *et al.*, *Experientia*, **28**, 878 (1972)

MARIDOMYCIN III
$C_{41}H_{67}O_{16}N$

A further macrocyclic antibiotic elaborated by *Streptomyces hygroscopicus*, this compound has the structure given above. It has an antibiotic spectrum similar to that of the other member of this group.

Muroi *et al.*, *Experientia*, **28**, 129 (1972)

MARIDOMYCIN IV
$C_{40}H_{65}O_{16}N$

Streptomyces hygroscopicus also yields this antibiotic which has been shown to have the above structure based primarily upon mass spectral data. It is active against gram-positive bacteria and some rickettsia.

Muroi et al., *Experientia*, **28**, 129 (1972)

MARIDOMYCIN V
$C_{40}H_{65}O_{16}N$

A positional isomer of the preceding antibiotic, maridomycin V is also obtained from cultures of *Streptomyces hygroscopicus*. The structure has been established from the mass spectral fragmentation pattern.

Muroi et al., *Experientia*, **28**, 129 (1972)

MARIDOMYCIN VI
$C_{39}H_{63}O_{16}N$

This component of the antibiotic complex elaborated by *Streptomyces hygroscopicus* is separated from the accompanying compounds by silica gel chromatography. It has an antibiotic spectrum identical to those of the other maridomycins.

Muroi et al., *Experientia*, **28**, 129 (1972)

MARIMYCIN
Streptomyces mariensis yields this antibiotic when grown on a common nutrient medium. The culture filtrate is treated with zinc chloride and the resulting precipitate extracted with Na_2HPO_4 and further precipitated with MeOH or EtOH. Marimycin is active as a leucocyte increasing agent.

Soeda, *Japanese Patent*, 74 18,236 (1974)

MATROMYCIN
See Oleandomycin

MECILLINAM
$C_{15}H_{23}O_3N_3S$
M.p. Indefinite

A recently prepared semi-synthetic β-lactam antibiotic, mecillinam is particularly useful in medicine in that it has a high degree of activity against gram-negative organisms and maintains a high serum level for a period when given intravenously. It is, however, only poorly absorbed from the gastrointestinal tract. If required to be given orally, it must be used in the form of its pivaloyloxymethyl ester (pivmecillinam) which is not only well absorbed but hydrolyzed enzymatically to mecillinam quite rapidly in the body. The absorption of pivmecillinam is not affected by the presence of food in the stomach.

Matsuhashi et al., *J. Bact.*, **117**, 578 (1974)
Roholt, Nielsen, Kristensen, *Chemotherapy*, **21**, 146 (1975)

MEDERMYCIN
$C_{24}H_{29}NO_8$

An antibiotic obtained from the cultures of an unclassified *Streptomyces* species, this substance has been shown to possess both antitumour and antibacterial activity.

Takano et al., *J. Antibiotics* (Japan), **29**, 765 (1976)

MEGALOMYCIN A
$C_{44}H_{80}O_{25}N_2$

Micromonospora inositola MK-41 (ATCC 21,773) elaborates an antibiotic complex consisting of a number of macrocyclic polyether compounds when

MEGALOMYCIN C₁
$C_{48}H_{82}O_{17}N_2$

Megalomycin C$_1$ has been shown to be diacetylmegalomycin A, the structure being based upon chemical analysis and mass spectral data. It has an antibiotic spectrum similar to that of the other members of this group.

Nara *et al.*, *German Patent*, 2,301,080 (1973)
Janet, Mallams, Vernay, *J. Chem. Soc., Perkin I*, 1389 (1973)

aerobically grown on a common nutrient medium at 30°C and pH 7·0 for 5 days. The complex is isolated by extraction with CHCl$_3$ followed by chromatographic separation on an alumina column. The structure of megalomycin A has been determined by chemical and spectroscopic methods. The antibiotic is active against a number of gram-positive, gram-negative bacteria and fungi.

Nara *et al.*, *German Patent*, 2,301,080 (1973)
Janet, Mallams, Vernay, *J. Chem. Soc., Perkin I*, 1389 (1973)

MEGALOMYCIN B
$C_{46}H_{82}O_{16}N_2$

This component of megalomycin, obtained from cultures of *Micromonospora inositola* MK-41 is the acetyl derivative of the preceding antibiotic. It also possesses activity against gram-positive, gram-negative bacteria and fungi.

Nara *et al.*, *German Patent*, 2,301,080 (1973)
Janet, Mallams, Vernay, *J. Chem. Soc., Perkins I*, 1389 (1973)

MEGALOMYCIN C₂
$C_{49}H_{84}O_{17}N_2$

A further macrocyclic polyether antibiotic obtained from cultures of *Micromonospora inositola* MK-41, megalomycin C$_2$ has the structure given above which is based mainly upon the mass spectral fragmentation pattern. It is active against a number of bacteria and fungi.

Nara *et al.*, *German Patent*, 2,301,080 (1973)
Janet, Mallams, Vernay, *J. Chem. Soc., Perkin I*, 1389 (1973)

MELANOSPORIN
$C_{56-63}H_{105-117}O_{20-22}N_3$
M.p. 132–134°C

An extremely complex antibiotic elaborated by *Streptomyces melanosporus*, the structure of this compound is still unknown and the empirical formula is, as yet, somewhat uncertain. It forms an amorphous white powder which possesses a sharp melting point. It is dextrorotatory with a specific rotation of $[\alpha]_D^{20} + 30°$ (c 1·57, CH_3OH).

Arcamone et al., *Giorn. microbiol.*, **7**, 207 (1959)

MELINACIDIN
This antibiotic compound has been obtained from cultures of *Acrostalagmus cinnabarinus* var. *melinacidinus*. The substance is a white crystalline material which is a mixture of a number of closely related antibiotics, apparently belonging to the 3:6-epidithiodiketo piperazine class. The mixture inhibited the growth of a number of gram-positive bacteria *in vitro* but is highly toxic and has no effect upon experimental bacterial infections in mice at non-toxic doses. It also inhibited the growth of L-1210 and KB leukemia cells when cultured in tissue.

Argoudelis, Reusser, *J. Antibiotics* (Japan), **24**, 383 (1971)

MEPICYCLINE
$C_{29}H_{38}O_9N_4$
Dec. 162–163°C

A semi-synthetic antibiotic of the tetracycline class, mepicycline forms a yellow crystalline powder which decomposes without melting. It is laevorotatory with a specific rotation of $[\alpha]_D^{20} - 195°$ (c 0·5, H_2O) and $[\alpha]_D^{20} - 175°$ (c 0·5, CH_3OH). The ultraviolet spectrum in 0·2 N-HCl has two absorption maxima at 286 and 355 nm. Mepicycline is readily soluble in H_2O, CH_3OH and formamide, slightly so in EtOH and *iso*PrOH and virtually insoluble in $CHCl_3$, C_6H_6 and Et_2O. The crystals are sensitive to heat and exposure to air and light.

Mepicycline is a broad-spectrum antibiotic and is more active than tetracycline, an activity of 1 g of this antibiotic being equivalent to 756 g of tetracycline hydrochloride. The LD_{50} in mice is given as 188 mg/kg when administered intravenously.

Pedrazzoli et al., *Boll. Chim. Farm.*, **98**, 516 (1959)
Gradnik et al., *Pharm. acta Helv.*, **35**, 529 (1960)
Gradnik et al., *British Patent*, 888,968 (1963)

METACYCLINE
See Methacycline

METAMPICILLIN
$C_{17}H_{19}O_4N_3S$

This semi-synthetic penicillin has proved to be more resistant than ampicillin (q.v.) to penicillinase both *in vitro* and *in vivo*. It is active against both gram-positive and gram-negative bacteria but not against *Candida albicans*. Metampicillin has an excellent effect against bacteria causing maxillofacial infections and is also useful for the prophylaxis of surgical infections.

Pizzoni, *Minerva Stomatol*, **18**, 159 (1969)
Gradnik, Fleischmann, *Farmaco, Ed. Prat.*, **26**, 186 (1971)

METHACYCLINE (*Metacycline*)
$C_{22}H_{22}O_8N_2$
M.p. 205°C (*dec.*)

Also a semi-synthetic antibiotic belonging to the tetracycline group, this compound has the structure 6-methylene-5-hydroxytetracycline. It is normally obtained as the crystalline hydrochloride (*Londomycin*, *Rondomycin*) which crystallizes as the hemihydrate or with 0·5 mole of CH_3OH from a mixture of CH_3OH-Et_2O-$(CH_3)_2CO$-HCl, decomposing at 222°C.

This salt has found some use in medicine as a broad-spectrum antimicrobial.

Blackwood et al., J. Amer. Chem. Soc., **83**, 2773 (1961)
Blackwood et al., ibid., **85**, 3943 (1963)
Chas. Pfizer & Co., U.S. Patent, 3,026,354 (1962)

METHICILLIN (Belfacillin, Celbenin, Dimocillin, Staphcillin)
$C_{17}H_{20}O_6N_2S$

Methicillin is a semi-synthetic antibiotic of the penicillin group which is normally employed as the crystalline sodium salt. The antibiotic is an antibacterial having a low toxicity. It is highly active against *Staphylococcus* species although resistant strains of *Staph. aureus* and *Staph. epidermidis* have been encountered in patients receiving both this antibiotic and others. Increased levels of blood serum alanine aminotransferase and aspartate aminotransferase together with elevated values of the bromsulphalein test have been found in children receiving therapeutic treatment with this antibiotic. In rats, helatic ultrastructure damage has been found but these are reversible resulting in a near-normal state following discontinuation of the drug.

Doyle et al., J. Chem. Soc., 1457 (1962)
Doyle et al., U.S. Patent, 2,951,839 (1960)
Glombitza, Annalen, **673**, 166 (1964)
Bentley, Contrib. Microbiol. Immunol., **650** (1973)
Hewitt, Sanderson, J. Med. Microbiol., **6**, 223 (1974)
Dobosz-Latalska, Ann. Univ. Mariae Curie-Sklodowska, **29D**, 35 (1974)
Ayliffe, Andrews, Williams, Lancet, **1** (7857), 573 (1974)
Shchekotova, Antibiotiki, **20**, 311 (1975)

4-METHOXY-2:2′-DIPYRIDYL-6-syn-ALDOXIME (Caerulomycin)
M.p. 175°C
$C_{12}H_{11}O_3N_2$

Isolated from *Streptomyces caerulens*, this antibiotic forms colourless needles when recrystallized from EtOH. With $FeCl_3$ it gives a characteristic red colour. The methyl ether forms colourless crystals, m.p. 90°C and gives an ultraviolet spectrum with an absorption maximum at 240 nm and an inflexion at 273 nm. The acetyl derivative also forms colourless needles from aqueous EtOH, m.p. 102°C. The ultraviolet spectrum of this compound has an absorption maximum at 237 nm and an inflexion at 263, 281 and 292 nm.

Structure
  Divekar, Read, Can. J. Chem., **45**, 1215 (1967)
Synthesis
  Ranganathan, Singh, Divekar, ibid., **47**, 165 (1969)

2-METHYL-L-ARGININE
$C_7H_{16}N_4O_2$

A simple arginine derivative isolated from the culture broth of *Streptomyces* sp. nov., this antibiotic has the structure shown above based upon chemical and spectroscopic data. It exhibits both antibacterial and antifungal activity.

Maehr et al., J. Antibiotics (Japan), **29**, 213 (1976)
Synthesis
  Maehr, Yarmchuk, Leach, J. Antibiotics (Japan), **29**, 221 (1976)

α-METHYLBIOTIN
$C_{11}H_{18}O_3N_2S$
M.p. 186–188°C

Streptomyces lycidus produces this antimetabolite antibiotic, the structure of which has been established by chemical methods and confirmed by synthesis. It forms colourless crystals when recrystallized from aqueous EtOH.

Martin, Hanka, Reineke, Tetrahedron Lett., 3791 (1971)

α-METHYLDETHIOBIOTIN
$C_{11}H_{20}O_3N_2$
M.p. 161–162.5°C

A second antimetabolite antibiotic elaborated by *Streptomyces lycidus*, this compound crystallizes from $(CH_3)_2CO$ as colourless plates.

Martin, Hanka, Reineke, *Tetrahedron Lett.*, 3791 (1971)

METHYLENOMYCIN A
$C_9H_{10}O_4$
M.p. 115°C (*dec.*)

A simple antibiotic isolated from *Streptomyces violaceoruber* strain No. 2416, this compound is extracted from the culture filtrate with organic solvents and crystallized from $CHCl_3$ when it forms colourless crystals. It is dextrorotatory with a specific rotation of $[\alpha]_D^{20} + 42.3°$ (c 1.0, $CHCl_3$). The structure has been shown by chemical and spectroscopic methods to be 2,3-epoxy-2:3-dimethyl-5-methylene-4-oxocyclopentane-1-carboxylic acid. The antibiotic is active against both gram-positive and gram-negative bacteria, particularly *Proteus* species.

Haneishi *et al.*, *J. Antibiotics* (Japan), **27**, 386, 393 (1974)

METHYLENOMYCIN B
$C_8H_{10}O_2$

A second antibiotic obtained from the culture filtrate of *Streptomyces violaceoruber* strain No. 2416, this compound is a colourless oil which has the structure 2,3-epoxy-2:3-dimethyl-5-methylenecyclopentane. It is also active against gram-positive and gram-negative bacteria, especially *Proteus* species.

Haneishi *et al.*, *J. Antibiotics* (Japan), **27**, 386, 393 (1974)

9-METHYLSTREPTINIDONE
$C_{17}H_{25}NO_4$

The culture filtrate of an unidentified species of *Streptomyces* yields this antibiotic which has the structure given above. It possesses antiviral activity, inhibiting the growth of Newcastle disease virus, poliovirus and vesicular stomatitis virus. The acute LD_{50} in mice is 280 mg/kg given intraperitoneally.

Saito *et al.*, *J. Antibiotics* (Japan), **27**, 206 (1974)

METHYMYCIN
$C_{25}H_{43}O_7N$
M.p. 195.5–197°C

Methymycin is a macrocyclic antibiotic first isolated from cultures of a streptomycete found in soil near Oswego, New York State, U.S.A. It has subsequently been obtained from cultures of *Streptomyces venezuelae*. The antibiotic forms colourless prisms from absolute EtOH and is dextrorotatory with specific rotations of $[\alpha]_D^{22} + 61°$ (c 0.7, CH_3OH) and $[\alpha]_D^{22} + 74°$ (c 1.1, $CHCl_3$). The ultraviolet spectrum in CH_3OH has two absorption maxima at 223 and 322 nm. It is soluble in CH_3OH, $(CH_3)_2CO$,

$CHCl_3$ and dilute acids, moderately soluble in Et_2O and EtOH and insoluble in hexane and H_2O. Methymycin is active against gram-positive bacteria, somewhat less so against gram-negative organisms.

Donin et al., *Antibiotics Annual*, **1**, 179 (1953–54)
Dutcher et al., *U.S. Patent*, 2,916,483 (1959)
Structure
Djerassi, Zderic, *J. Amer. Chem. Soc.*, **78**, 6390 (1956)
Biosynthesis
Birch et al., *J. Chem. Soc.*, 5274 (1964)
Partial synthesis
Masaume et al., *J. Amer. Chem. Soc.*, **97**, 3512 (1975)

MICROCIN A

An unclassified species of *Micromonospora* elaborates two closely related antibiotics. The broth filtrate is extracted with AcOEt at pH 2·0 followed by back extraction of the AcOEt fraction with phosphate buffer at pH 7·0. The microcin A is found in the AcOEt fraction whereas the buffer containing the accompanying microcin B (q.v.). This particular antibiotic forms a neutral red-violet powder which is soluble in H_2O. It is active against a wide range of both gram-positive and gram-negative bacteria and fungi. The LD_{50} in mice is about 625 mg/kg when given intravenously.

Taira, Fujii, *J. Antibiotics* (Japan), **5**, 185 (1952)

MICROCIN B

This antibiotic accompanies the preceding compound from which it is separated by partition between AcOEt and phosphate buffer. It forms a yellowish-red powder which is only slightly soluble in H_2O. Its biological activity and toxicity are very similar to those of microcin A.

Taira, Fujii, *J. Antibiotics* (Japan), **5**, 185 (1952)

MICROCOCCIN

M.p. 220–223°C

Micrococcin is produced by a species of *Micrococcus* resembling *M. varians*. It is obtained by surface growth on a medium containing meat extract, peptone and sodium chloride incubated for 3 days at 37°C, the final pH being 8·4–8·6. The antibiotic is isolated by adsorbing the activity of the culture filtrate on activated carbon, washing with EtOH and eluting with pyridine. The eluate is evaporated *in vacuo*, the residue dissolved in EtOH and precipitated with Et_2O. Purification of the crude material is carried out by dissolving in $CHCl_3$, chromatographing over alumina, eluting with EtOH and evaporating to dryness. Micrococcin is a creamy amorphous powder which is soluble in $CHCl_3$, EtOH, $(CH_3)_2CO$, pyridine glacial AcOH and propylene glycol. It is only slightly soluble in H_2O and insoluble in C_6H_6, Et_2O, glycerin, amyl acetate and vegetable oils. It dialyses through a cellophane membrane and is dextrorotatory with a specific rotation of $[\alpha]_D^{20} + 50°$ to $75°$ (c 1·0, EtOH). The solution gives a blue fluorescence under ultraviolet light and has an ultraviolet spectrum exhibiting a single absorption maximum at 345 nm. Micrococcin is thermostable but unstable in alkalies. It gives a negative ninhydrin reaction.

The antibiotic is assayed by the cylinder plate method and serial dilution on an agar slant with *Bacillus subtilis* as the test organism. The inhibition concentrations (µg/ml) which have been measured *in vitro* are: *Bacillus anthracis* (0·1); *B. subtilis* (0·016); *Corynebacterium diphtheriae gravis* (0·1); *Coryne. diphtheriae mitis* (0·1); *Coryne. xerosis* (0·016); *Clostridium sporogenes* (6·25); *Cl. welchii* (3·13); *Escherichia coli* (>1000); *Mycobacterium tuberculosis* (6·25); *Proteus vulgaris* (>1000); *Pseudomonas aeruginosa* (>1000); *Staphylococcus albus* (0·1); *Streptomyces* spp. (0·1); *Vibrio comma* (0·1). Resistant strains of *Staphylococcus aureus* have been encountered but there is no cross-resistance with penicillin.

Su, *Brit. J. Exptl. Path.*, **29**, 473 (1948)

MICROMONOSPORIN

Certain species of *Micromonospora* have been examined by Waksman and his colleagues and two antibiotics having the same name have been isolated. By precipitation of the culture filtrate with ammonium sulphate and dialysation of the precipitates against H_2O, a complex antibiotic is obtained, the structure of which consists of a protein in association with a carbohydrate, neither of which have been identified. This material does not dialyse through collodion, is adsorbed on activated carbon and eluted by H_2O, buffers and common organic solvents, and is inactivated at pH below 3·0 and above 9·0. It gives a positive Molisch test and negative tests with naphthoresorcinol, orcinol and phloroglucinol. It is not digested by either pepsin or trypsin. This antibiotic has no activity against gram-negative bacteria *in vitro* but is active against gram-positive bacteria, the following inhibition concentrations (units/mg × 1000) having been determined: *Bacillus mycoides* (80); *B. subtilis* (800); *Sarcina lutea* (300) and *Staphylococcus aureus* (30).

The second antibiotic, also described as micromonosporin, is obtained from the culture mycelium and is believed to be a quinone. It gives an orange to red colour with dilute potassium hydroxide but no change of colour with alcoholic $FeCl_3$ solution. It also has no activity against gram-negative bacteria and is less active against gram-positive organisms than the more complex compound described above. Typical inhibition concentrations (units/mg × 1000) are: *Bacillus mycoides* (200); *B. subtilis* (20,000); *Sarcina lutea* (6000) and *Staphylococcus aureus* (200).

Waksman, Geiger, Bugie, *J. Bact.*, **53**, 355 (1947)

MIHARAMYCIN A
$C_{22}H_{38}O_{10}N_{10}$

Streptomyces miharaensis (ATCC 19,440) elaborates two closely related antibiotics when grown aerobically under submerged culture conditions on a nutrient medium at 25–35°C and pH 7·0 for 3 days. Isolation is carried out by the use of cation-exchange resins, activated carbon of alumina and fractionation with Dowex 1-X2. Miharamycin A is obtained as the crystalline dihydrochloride, m.p. 210–214°C (*dec.*). This salt is laevorotatory with a specific rotation of $[\alpha]_D^{24} - 59°$ (c 1·0, H_2O). It is active against *Piricularia oryzae* and *Pseudomonas tabaci*. The LD_{50} in mice is 10–15 mg/kg when given intravenously.

Niida *et al.*, *Japanese Patent*, 7,134,198 (1971)

MIHARAMYCIN B
$C_{21}H_{36}O_{11}N_{10}$

Also isolated from cultures of *Streptomyces miharaensis* (ATCC 19,440), this antibiotic is normally obtained as the monohydrochloride with m.p. 215–218°C (*dec.*). It is laevorotatory with a specific rotation of $[\alpha]_D^{24} - 63°$ (c 1·0, H_2O). The antibiotic spectrum is identical with that of the preceding antibiotic.

Niida *et al.*, *Japanese Patent*, 7,134,198 (1971)

MIKAMYCIN A
$C_{31}H_{39}O_9N_3$
Dec. 178°C

Cultures of *Streptomyces mitakaensis*, isolated from soil near Mitaka City, Japan, yield an antibiotic mixture from which two crystalline antibiotics have so far been isolated, although others are probably present as minor constituents. Mikamycin A forms colourless crystals from AcOEt which decompose without melting. It gives an ultraviolet spectrum with absorption maxima at 226 and 270 nm. When hydrolysed with dilute alkalies it furnishes an acid, mikamycinine. The structure shows that it belongs to the polypeptide class of antibiotics. The compound is active against gram-positive bacteria. Both of the major components exhibit synergistic action *in vitro* and *in vivo*.

Arai *et al.*, *J. Antibiotics* (Japan), **9A**, 193 (1956)
Arai *et al.*, *ibid.*, **11A**, 14 (1958)
Arai, Okabe, *ibid.*, **11A**, 21 (1958)
Okabe, *ibid.*, **12A**, 89 (1959)
Tanaka *et al.*, *ibid.*, **12A**, 290 (1959)
Watanabe, *ibid.*, **13A**, 62 (1960)
Kanegafuchi Chem. Co., *French Patent*, 1,349,946 (1964)
Watanabe, *U.S. Patent*, 3,137,640 (1964)

MIKAMYCIN B
$C_{45}H_{54}O_{10}N_8$
M.p. 160°C (*dec.* 262–263°)

The second major component of mikamycin, obtained from cultures of *Streptomyces mitakaensis*, this antibiotic crystallizes as the monohydrate which melts at 160°C. The anhydrous form, obtained by drying the hydrate at 150°C *in vacuo* for 16 hours, decomposes at 262–263°C. The antibiotic is laevorotatory with a specific rotation of $[\alpha]_D^{20} - 60·3°$ (c 1·0, CH_3OH) and gives an ultraviolet spectrum in CH_3OH with absorption maxima at 209, 260 and 305 nm. It is readily soluble in CH_3OH, EtOH, $(CH_3)_2CO$, $CHCl_3$, hexane, C_6H_6 and butyl acetate, insoluble in H_2O and petroleum ether. It is stable under neutral and acid conditions, but unstable in alkalies. It has found some use as an antimicrobial.

Watanabe et al., *J. Antibiotics* (Japan), **12A**, 112 (1959)
Watanabe et al., *ibid.*, **13A**, 291, 293 (1960)
Structure
Watanabe et al., *J. Antibiotics* (Japan), **13A**, 291 (1960)
Watanabe, *ibid.*, **14A**, 14 (1961)

MILBEMYCINS

Streptomyces strain B-41-146 yields an antibiotic complex when cultured on a common nutrient medium which consists of at least thirteen components; milbemycins α1 to α10, β1, β2 and β3. The structures of the last three constituents have been determined (q.v.). The antibiotics are active against gram-positive and some gram-negative bacteria.

Mishima et al., *Tetrahedron Lett.*, 771 (1975)

MILBEMYCIN β_1
$C_{32}H_{48}O_7$

This component of the milbemycin complex has been shown to have the structure given above based upon chemical analysis and spectroscopic data.

Mishima et al., *Tetrahedron Lett.*, 711 (1975)

MILBEMYCIN β_2
$C_{33}H_{50}O_7$
The structure of this constituent of the antibiotic complex elaborated by *Streptomyces* strain B-41-146 has been established from chemical examination and a study of the infrared, NMR, mass and X-ray spectra.

Mishima et al., *Tetrahedron Lett.*, 711 (1975)

MILBEMYCIN β_3
$C_{31}H_{42}O_5$

This constituent of the milbemycin complex isolated from cultures of *Streptomyces* strain B-41-146 has the above structure based upon chemical and spectroscopic evidence.

Mishima et al., *Tetrahedron Lett.*, 711 (1975)

MIMOSAMYCIN
$C_{12}H_{11}NO_4$

A simple antibiotic isolated together with the chlorocarcins (q.v.) from cultures of *Streptomyces lavendulae* No. 314, this compound is primarily active against *Mycobacteria*.

Arai et al., *J. Antibiotics* (Japan), **29**, 398 (1976)

MINIMYCIN
$C_9H_{11}O_7N$

One of a large number of antibiotics derived from *Streptomyces hygroscopicus*, this simple compound is extracted from the culture broth with organic solvents and purified by column chromatography. The structure has been established from the mass spectrum and the 100 MHz NMR spectrum. It is active against both gram-positive and gram-negative bacteria and also exhibits marked antitumour activity against transplantable tumours.

Kusakabe et al., *J. Antibiotics* (Japan), **25**, 44 (1972)
Sasaki et al., *ibid.*, **25**, 151 (1972)

MINOCYCLINE
$C_{23}H_{27}O_7N_3$
M.p. Indefinite

A semi-synthetic antibiotic of the tetracycline class, this substance is an amorphous yellow-orange powder which is laevorotatory having a specific rotation of $[\alpha]_D^{25} - 166°$ (c 0·524, 0·1 N-HCl). The structure is 6-demethyl-6-deoxy-7-dimethylaminotetracycline. Minocycline is effective against staphylococci which are resistant to tetracycline, particularly such strains of *Staphylococcus aureus* isolated from hospital patients. It also possesses the advantage that considerably lower inhibitory concentrations are required and for this reason it has been proposed as a useful antibiotic in the treatment of minor infections. It has also been shown to have a longer half-life in man than most of the other tetracyclines and is more rapidly absorbed and has greater lipophilic properties which may account for the observed highly favourable ratios of ·tissue to serum concentrations. Kuck has demonstrated that minocycline is the most active of the tetracyclines against strains of *Fusobacterium necrophorum* in mice, tetracycline itself being relatively ineffective. The antibiotic has also proved active against *Plasmodium berghei*, *Escherichia coli*, *Klebsiella pneumoniae* and *Candida albicans*. It is also active against other species of *Candida*, an unusual effect since these organisms are, in general, quite resistant to antibacterial antibiotics.

Martell, Boothe, *J. Med. Chem.*, **10**, 44 (1967)
Church, Schaub, Weiss, *J. Org. Chem.*, **36**, 723 (1971)
Schmid, *Med. Welt.*, **24**, 2073 (1973)
McDonald et al., *Clin. Pharmacol. Ther.*, **14**, 852 (1973)
Leigh, Simmons, *Lancet*, **7**(7864), 1006 (1974)
Waterworth, *J. Clin. Pathol.*, **27**, 269 (1974)
Kaddu, Warhurst, Peters, *Ann. Trop. Med. Parasitol.*, **68**, 41 (1974)
Kuck, *Antimicrobial Agents & Chemotherapy*, **7**, 421 (1975)

MINOSAMINOMYCIN
$C_{25}H_{46}O_{10}N_8$
M.p. 225–260°C (dec.)

Streptomyces aureomonopodiales MA 514-A1 produces this antibiotic, the full structure of which is not yet known. The organism is cultured aerobically on a medium containing glucose, starch, soybean flour, yeast extract and inorganic salts at pH 7·4 and 27°C for 113 hours. Isolation is carried out by adsorbing the activity of the culture filtrate on Amberlite IRC-50 at pH 8·6 and eluted with 1 N-HCl. The eluate is then neutralized, adsorbed on activated carbon, eluted with 50 per cent CH_3OH containing 0·05 N-HCl, the active fraction concentrated under reduced pressure to give a crude preparation of the hydrochloride. The base antibiotic is a white, amorphous powder which decomposes over a wide range of temperature and is dextrorotatory with a specific rotation of $[\alpha]_D^{22} + 30°$ (H_2O). It is soluble in H_2O but insoluble in almost all inorganic acids and organic solvents. Hydrolysis furnishes a myo-inosamine, $C_6H_{13}O_5N$. Minosaminomycin is active against gram-positive bacteria and is comparatively non-toxic, the LD_{50} in mice being 50–100 mg/kg when administered intravenously.

Hamada et al., *J. Antibiotics* (Japan), **27**, 81 (1974)
Umezawa et al., *Japanese Patent*, 7,536,695 (1975)

MIRAMYCIN

An uncharacterized antibiotic obtained from *Streptomyces mirabilis*, no details have been reported concerning the method of extraction and the structure is unknown. It is stated to be thermostable and active against both gram-positive and gram-negative bacteria. It is also said to be non-toxic.

Ruschmann, *Die Pharmazie*, **7**, 542, 639, 823 (1952)

MITHRAMYCIN
$C_{52}H_{76}O_{24}$

Cultivation of *Streptomyces argillaceus* or *S. plicatus* produces an antibiotic complex, mithramycin, which consists of between 85–98 per cent mithramycin A (having the structure given above) and 15–20 per cent of mithramycins B and C. The organism is cultivated under aerobic conditions in a common nutrient medium at 24–30°C and the complex isolated from the culture filtrate by acidification and extraction with methyl-*iso*butyl ketone. Concentration of the extract is followed by chromatography on an acid-washed alumina column and development with $CHCl_3$—CH_3OH.

Both mithramycin A and B exhibit inhibition of mammary adenocarcinoma CA-755. Mithramycin C has a similar effect but requires higher doses. When tested *in vitro*, mithramycin A caused a biphasic effect on ADP-induced aggregation of human blood platelets, the effect being enhanced at low doses of the order of 10 µg/ml but variable at higher doses of more than 50 µg/ml. Within the dose range where such aggregation occurs, the antibiotic increased the uptake of calcium by the platelets but did not affect the blood clotting time nor the ionic calcium concentration. In growing rabbits, mithramycin A had no effect upon bone formation or resorption although there was a slight increase in phosphate-induced soft-tissue calcification and a decrease in bone resorption when increased by phosphate supplementation in adult rabbits. At the dosage levels where bone resorption was affected, hepatorenal degeneration and dysfunction were also observed.

Sobin et al., *U.S. Patent*, 3,646,194 (1972)
Robins, Jowsey, *J. Lab. Clin. Med.*, **82**, 576 (1973)
Chao, Tullis, *Thromb. Diath. Haemorrh.*, **29**, 712 (1973)
Bradley, Adams, *Antimicrobial Agents & Chemotherapy*, **7**, 322 (1975)

MITOMYCIN A
$C_{16}H_{19}O_6N_3$
Dec. 159–161°C

An antibiotic complex, mitomycin, was first obtained from cultures of *Streptomyces caespitosus* (syn. *S. griseovinaceseus*) and later from *S. verticillatus*. Chromatographic studies have resulted in the isolation and characterization of at least four constituents, namely mitomycins A, B and C and porfiromycin (q.v.).

Mitomycin A forms reddish-violet crystals when purified by recrystallization from $(CH_3)_2CO$—CCl_4 and is soluble in H_2O and most organic solvents but insoluble in xylene, CCl_4, ligroin, cyclohexane, CS_2 and petroleum ether. The ultraviolet and visible spectra exhibit absorption maxima at 215, 318 and 530 nm. Mitomycin A possesses antitumour properties and is comparatively toxic with LD_{50} in mice of 2 mg/kg when administered intravenously.

Hata et al., J. Antibiotics (Japan), **9A**, 141 (1956)
Yamamoto, Umezawa, Japanese Patent, 2898 (1956)
Kenkyusho, British Patent, 830,874 (1960)
Gourevitch et al., U.S. Patent, 3,042,582 (1962)
Webb et al., J. Amer. Chem. Soc., **84**, 3185, 3187 (1962)
Hornemann, Cloyd, J. Chem. Soc., **D**, 301 (1971)

MITOMYCIN B
$C_{16}H_{19}O_6N_3$
Dec. 182–184°C

A second component of the mitomycin complex elaborated by *Streptomyces caespitosus* and *S. verticillatus*, this compound forms violet needles when crystallized from $(CH_3)_2CO$—CCl_4. It gives an ultraviolet spectrum in H_2O with absorption maxima at 220, 320 and 550 nm in the visible spectrum. The antibiotic is soluble in H_2O and many organic solvents, but insoluble in xylene, CCl_4, ligroin, petroleum ether, CS_2, C_6H_6, toluene, nitrobenzene, cyclohexane and trichloroethylene. It is slightly less toxic than the preceding antibiotic with LD_{50} in mice of 10 mg/kg given intravenously. It is also an antitumour antibiotic.

Hata et al., J. Antibiotics (Japan), **9A**, 141 (1956)
Yamamoto, Umezawa, Japanese Patent, 2898 (1956)
Kenkyusho, British Patent, 830,874 (1960)
Gourevitch et al., U.S. Patent, 3,042,582 (1962)
Webb et al., J. Amer. Chem. Soc., **84**, 3185, 3187 (1962)
Hornemann, Cloyd, J. Chem. Soc., **D**, 301 (1971)

MITOMYCIN C
$C_{15}H_{18}O_5N_4$
M.p. >360°C

Mitomycin C is the most extensively studied of the components of the complex elaborated by *Streptomyces caespitosus* and *S. verticillatus*. It forms blue-violet crystals which do not melt below 360°C and gives an ultraviolet and visible spectrum with absorption maxima at 216, 360 and 560 nm. It is soluble in H_2O, CH_3OH, $(CH_3)_2CO$, cyclohexanone and butyl acetate, slightly soluble in CCl_4, C_6H_6, Et_2O, and insoluble in petroleum ether. It is an antineoplastic agent and has LD_{50} in mice of 5 mg/kg given intravenously.

Mitomycin C is an antitumour agent and also has antineoplastic properties. It is active against Ehrlich ascitic tumour in mice and caused regression of small, young Yoshida sarcomas in rat livers on intravascular injection into either the portal vein or the hepatic artery. In rats having large, well-developed tumours, however, only the arterial route proved effective. Numerous studies on the treatment of sarcomas with this antibiotic have been carried out.

Hata et al., J. Antibiotics (Japan), **9A**, 141 (1956)
Yamamoto, Umezawa, Japanese Patent, 2898 (1956)
Kenkyusho, British Patent, 830,874 (1960)
Gourevitch et al., U.S. Patent, 3,042,582 (1962)
Webb et al., J. Amer. Chem. Soc., **84**, 3185, 3187 (1962)
Hornemann, Cloyd, J. Chem. Soc., D, 301 (1971)
Fujimoto et al., Jap. J. Surg., **1**, 72 (1971)
Lai, Wei, Sheng Wu K'o Hsueh, **1**, 37 (1972)
Bempong, Trower, J. Hered., **64**, 324 (1973)
Ehling, Neuhaeuser, Lab. Anim. Drug Test., Symp. Int. Comm. Lab. 5th 1972, 331 (1973)
Levy, Proc. West. Pharmacol. Soc., **16**, 262 (1973)
Morad, Jonasson, Lindsten, Hereditas, **74**, 273 (1973)
Orstavik, Acta Pathol. Microbiol. Scand., **81B**, 711 (1973)
Ichihashi et al., Nagoya J. Med. Sci., **36**, 63 (1974)

Orstavik, *Acta Pathol. Microbiol. Scand.*, **82B**, 270 (1974)
Buecher, Yarwood, Hansen, *Proc. Soc. Exp. Biol. Med.*, **146**, 299 (1974)
Shimamura *et al.*, *J. Med. Microbiol.*, **7**, 277 (1974)
Lee, *Kalullik Taehak Uihakpu Nonmumjip.*, **27**, 219 (1974)

MOCIMYCIN
See Antibiotic MYC-8003

MOENOMYCIN
M.p. Indefinite
This antibiotic, obtained by cultivation of *Streptomyces bambergiensis* (ATCC 13,879), *S. ederensis* (ATCC 15,304), *S. geysiriensis* (ATCC 15,303) or *S. ghanaensis* (ATCC 14,672) in an aqueous nutrient medium under aerobic submerged conditions. It may be extracted by organic solvents and purified by chromatography on an alumina column. Moenomycin is an acid polysaccharide which contains a lipid portion and phosphate ester groups and has a molecular weight of between 68,000 and 70,000. It forms a white amorphous powder with no definite melting point. The antibiotic has a high activity against staphylococci which are resistant to most other antibiotics. It is comparatively non-toxic, the LD_{50} for mice being greater than 2000 mg/kg when given intraperitoneally, orally or subcutaneously.

Lindner, Wallhaeusser, *U.S. Patent*, 3,674,866 (1972)

MOLDIN
Streptomyces phaeochromogenes furnishes this antibiotic. The extraction of the broth or mycelium with AcOEt is followed by concentration *in vacuo* to a syrup which is then washed with aqueous petroleum ether and the residue is then dissolved in EtOH and precipitated with H_2O. Moldin is soluble in AcOEt or EtOH but only slightly soluble in Et_2O, C_6H_6 or petroleum ether. It is active against *Candida*, *Cryptococcus neoformans*, *Histoplasma capsulatum* and *Trichophyton*. The LD_{50} in mice is about 10 mg/kg when administered intraperitoneally.

Maeda *et al.*, *J. Antibiotics* (Japan), **5A**, 465 (1952)
Maeda *et al.*, *Japan. J. Med. Sci. Biol.*, **5**, 327 (1952)

MONAMYCIN A
$C_{33}H_{55}O_8N_7$
M.p. 119–121°C
Streptomyces jamaicensis produces a group of antibiotics, all of which are macrocyclic polypeptides. This particular component may be purified by precipitation from *n*-pentane when it forms an amorphous white solid.

Hassall, Magnus, *Nature*, **184**, 1223 (1959)
Bevan *et al.*, *Experientia*, **26**, 122 (1970)
Bevan *et al.*, *J. Chem. Soc.*, C, 514 (1971)
Hassall *et al.*, *ibid.*, 526 (1971)

MONAMYCIN B₁
$C_{33}H_{55}O_8N_7$

A positional isomer of the preceding antibiotic, this substance has also been obtained from *Streptomyces jamaicensis*.

Bevan *et al.*, *J. Chem. Soc.*, C, 514 (1971)
Hassell *et al.*, *ibid.*, 526 (1971)

MONAMYCIN B₂
$C_{33}H_{55}O_8N_7$
A third member of the group of antibiotics isolated from *Streptomyces jamaicensis*, this isomer is present only in small amounts.

Monamycin B₃

Bevan et al., *J. Chem. Soc., C*, 514 (1971)
Hassell et al., *ibid.*, 526 (1971)

MONAMYCIN B₃
$C_{33}H_{55}O_8N_7$

This antibiotic is a fourth positional isomer of this group of antibiotics obtained from *Streptomyces jamaicensis*.

Bevan et al., *J. Chem. Soc., C*, 415 (1971)
Hassell et al., *ibid.*, 526 (1971)

MONAMYCIN C
$C_{34}H_{57}O_8N_7$
M.p. 112–114°C

This antibiotic from *Streptomyces jamaicensis* crystallizes as colourless plates from CHCl₃-pentane which contains CHCl₃ of crystallization and have the melting point given above. The compound has a specific rotation of $[\alpha]_D^{30} - 44 \cdot 2°$ (c 0·24, CHCl₃).

Bevan et al., *J. Chem. Soc., C*, 514 (1971)
Hassell et al., *ibid.*, 526 (1971)

MONAMYCIN D₁
$C_{34}H_{57}O_8N_7$

This isomer of the preceding antibiotic also occurs in the culture of *Streptomyces jamaicensis*. The structure has been determined by chemical and spectroscopic methods.

Bevan et al., *J. Chem. Soc., C*, 514 (1971)
Hassell et al., *ibid.*, 526 (1971)

MONAMYCIN D₂
$C_{34}H_{57}O_8N_7$

A third positional isomer of monamycin C, the structure of this antibiotic is based upon chemical analysis and spectroscopic techniques.

MONAMYCIN E
$C_{35}H_{59}O_8N_7$

One of two isomeric antibiotics found in the cultures of *Streptomyces jamaicensis*, this substance is the methyl analogue of monamycin C (q.v.).

Bevan *et al.*, *J. Chem. Soc.*, C, 514 (1971)
Hassell *et al.*, *ibid.*, 526 (1971)

MONAMYCIN F
$C_{35}H_{59}O_8N_7$

Streptomyces jamaicensis also elaborates this antibiotic which has been shown to possess the structure given above.

Bevan *et al.*, *J. Chem. Soc.*, C, 514 (1971)
Hassell *et al.*, *ibid.*, 526 (1961)

MONAMYCIN G₁
$C_{33}H_{54}O_8N_7Cl$
A chlorine-containing antibiotic from *Streptomyces jamaicensis*, this compound has been shown to have the given structure which is based upon chemical and spectroscopic evidence.

Bevan *et al.*, *J. Chem. Soc.*, C, 514 (1971)
Hassell *et al.*, *ibid.*, 526 (1971)

MONAMYCIN G₂
$C_{33}H_{54}O_8N_7Cl$

An isomer of monamycin G₁, this antibiotic from *Streptomyces jamaicensis* has the structure given above. It occurs only in small amounts in the antibiotic complex.

Bevan *et al.*, *J. Chem. Soc.*, C, 514 (1971)
Hassell *et al.*, *ibid.*, 526 (1971)

MONAMYCIN G₃
$C_{33}H_{54}O_8N_7Cl$
A further isomer of the two preceding antibiotics also elaborated by *Streptomyces jamaicensis*. It occurs as a minor constituent of the complex.

Bevan *et al.*, *J. Chem. Soc.*, C, 514 (1971)
Hassell *et al.*, *ibid.*, 526 (1971)

Momamycin H₁

MONAMYCIN H₁
$C_{34}H_{56}O_8N_7Cl$

This antibiotic from *Streptomyces jamaicensis* is the methyl derivative of monamycin G₁ (q.v.).

Bevan et al., *J. Chem. Soc., C*, 514 (1971)
Hassell et al., *ibid.*, 526 (1971)

MONAMYCIN H₂
$C_{34}H_{56}O_8N_7Cl$

An isomer of the preceding antibiotic, this compound has also been isolated, in small quantities, from the culture of *Streptomyces jamaicensis*.

Bevan et al., *J. Chem. Soc., C*, 514 (1971)
Hassell et al., *ibid.*, 526 (1971)

MONAMYCIN I
$C_{35}H_{58}O_8N_7Cl$
M.p. 110–113°C

This antibiotic from *Streptomyces jamaicensis* forms colourless crystals when recrystallized from CHCl₃-pentane. It is laevorotatory with a specific rotation of $[\alpha]_D^{25} - 64\cdot3°$ (c 0·3, CHCl₃).

Bevan et al., *J. Chem. Soc., C*, 514 (1971)
Hassell et al., *ibid.*, 526 (1971)

MONENSIN (*Monensic acid*)
$C_{36}H_{62}O_{11}$
M.p. 103–105°C

A strain of *Streptomyces cinnamonensis* yields a group of closely-related acidic compounds which are biologically active. These are purified by solvent extraction followed by chromatography on activated carbon or silica gel and crystallization. The principal component is monensin which forms colourless needles of the monohydrate. It has a specific rotation of $[\alpha]_D^{20} + 47\cdot7°$ (CH₃OH) and that of the monosodium salt is $+ 57\cdot3°$ (CH₃OH). Monensin is slightly soluble in H₂O, more so in hydrocarbons and freely soluble in common organic solvents. It has a moderate *in vitro* activity against gram-positive bacteria, certain mycobacteria and is cytotoxic to HeLa cells and murine clone NCTC 1742 cells. It is also an effective treatment for coccidiosis in chickens.

Haney et al., *Antimicrobial Agents & Chemotherapy*, 349 (1967)

MONOMYCIN A
See Paromomycin

MORACIN A
$C_{16}H_{14}O_5$
M.p. 83–85°C

A plant antibiotic, this substance has been isolated, together with moracin B, from the extract of diseased mulberry plants (*Morus alba*). It is a phyoalexin and forms colourless crystals giving an ultraviolet spectrum with absorption maxima at 217, 304, 313, 326 nm in EtOH. It has been characterized as the diacetate with m.p. 126–127°C. Moracin A has antifungal activity and the following minimal concentrations (micrograms/litre) causing 100 per cent inhibition of spore formation have been determined—*Cochliobolus miyabeanus* (12–25), *Diaportha nomurai* (6–12), *Fusarium lateritium* f. sp. *mori* (25–49), *F. roseum* (6–12) and *Stigminia mori* (6–12).

Takasugi *et al.*, *Tetrahedron Lett.*, 797 (1978)

MORACIN B
$C_{16}H_{14}O_5$
M.p. 184–185°C

A further phytoalexin isolated from diseased mulberry plants, this antibiotic forms colourless crystals and gives an ultraviolet spectrum in EtOH having absorption maxima at 218, 285, 294, 325 and 337 nm. It possesses similar antifungal properties to the preceding compound with minimal concentrations (micrograms/litre) causing 100 per cent inhibition of spore formation of—*Cochliobolus miyabeanus* (49), *Diaportha nomurai* (12), *Fusarium lateritium* f. sp. *mori* (49), *F. roseum* (12–25) and *Stigminia mori* (12–25).

Takasugi *et al.*, *Tetrahedron Lett.*, 797 (1978)

MORONAL
See Nystatin

MORPHOCYCLINE
$C_{27}H_{33}O_9N_3$

A semi-synthetic tetracycline antibiotic, morphocycline is active against gram-positive and gram-negative organisms. A dose of 5 mg/kg given intravenously twice daily for 7 days to rabbits decreases the arterial blood pressure, respiration, pulse rate and causes alterations in the electrocardiogram. It has no effect, however, upon the urinary system.

Kanorskii, Koroleva, Svetukhin, *Antibiotiki*, **19**, 465 (1974)
Aleutskii, Berger, *ibid.*, **20**, 467 (1975)

MOROYAMYCIN A
$C_{18}H_{30}O_{10}N_{18}$
Dec. 170°C

Streptomyces species 3525 (FERM-P 1152) and its mutant strains produce an antibiotic complex, moroyamycin, when cultivated on common media at 27°C and pH 7·4 for 36 hours. The activity of the culture filtrate is adsorbed on activated carbon and eluted with CH_3OH, $(CH_3)_2CO$ or EtON. Further purification by column chromatography on a cation exchange resin, activated carbon or cellulose, separates the complex into three components, moroyamycins A, B and C. This antibiotic is soluble in H_2O, slightly soluble in AcOH and CH_3OH and insoluble in C_6H_6, AcOEt, $(CH_3)_2CO$ and hexane. It is active against gram-positive and gram-negative bacteria at a concentration of less than 50 µg/ml and is lethal against tick larvae (96·2 and 95 per cent) at a concentration of 50 and 25 µg/ml respectively.

Sakagami, *Japanese Patent*, 7,382,090 (1973)

MOROYAMYCIN B
$C_{26}H_{42}O_{10}N_{16}$
Dec. 169°C

Also produced by *Streptomyces* No. 3525 (FERM-P 1152), this antibiotic forms a white microcrystalline powder which decomposes without melting. It has a similar range of solubilities to those of the preceding compound and is equally effective against gram-positive and gram-negative bacteria and tick larvae. The LD_{50} in mice is 10–20 mg/kg when given intravenously and greater than 300 mg/kg when administered orally.

Sakagami, *Japanese Patent*, 7,382,090 (1973)

MOROYAMYCIN C
$C_9H_{16}O_8N_4$
M.p. Indefinite

A further antibiotic isolated from cultures of *Streptomyces* No. 3525 (FERM-P 1152), this substance is isolated as a white amorphous powder with no definite melting point. It is less active against bacteria and tick larvae than the two accompanying antibiotics.

Sakagami, *Japanese Patent*, 7,382,090 (1973)

MUCONOMYCIN A
See Verrucarin A

MYCONOMYCIN B
$C_{27}H_{32}O_8$
Dec. 235°C

A cytostatic antibiotic isolated from cultures of *Myrothecium verrucaria*, this compound crystallizes from Et_2O as colourless needles. It is dextrorotatory with $[\alpha]_D^{19} + 54°$ (c 1·0, C_6H_6). The ultraviolet spectrum exhibits absorption maxima at 220·5 and 261 nm.

Vittimberga, *J. Org. Chem.*, **28**, 1786 (1963)
Vittimberge, Vittimberga, *ibid.*, **30**, 746 (1965)

MULTHIOMYCIN
M.p. Indefinite

This antibiotic has been obtained by cultivating *Streptomyces antibioticus* 8446-CC1 on a medium containing dextrin, dried yeast and inorganic salts at 27°C for four days. The antibiotic is extracted from the cells with CH_3OH followed by back extraction with AcOEt, or from the culture filtrate with BuOH or C_6H_6. A product having a purity of approximately 60 per cent has been obtained in this manner. The antibiotic is active primarily against gram-positive bacteria.

Tanaka *et al.*, *Japanese Patent*, 7,329,157 (1973)

MUSARIN
$C_{35}H_{60}O_{14}N_2$
M.p. Indefinite

Isolated from a species of *Streptomyces* (Meredith's actinomycete), this antibiotic is named after the banana plant, *Musa sapientum*, and not after the organism which elaborates it. The antibiotic is highly active against a parasitic fungus, *Fusarium oxysporum* var. *cubense* which attacks this particular plant. It is produced by both surface and submerged growth and is present in both the broth and the mycelium. When the broth is acidified to pH 4·0 with phosphoric acid it forms a precipitate. The filtrate is then extracted with neutral phosphate buffer, back extracted with BuOH, concentrated *in vacuo*, the residue dissolved in CH_3OH and then precipitated with Et_2O. Musarin is a pale yellow powder which is unstable and decomposes at 170°C. It is acidic in nature, soluble in EtOH and aqueous $(CH_3)_2CO$, insoluble in H_2O or $(CH_3)_2CO$. The sodium salt, however, is soluble in H_2O and the lower aliphatic alcohols, but insoluble in Et_2O and $(CH_3)_2CO$. The antibiotic is stable in the form of its sodium or potassium salts. The sodium salt is dextrorotatory with a specific rotation of $[\alpha]_D^{20} + 38·7° \pm 2·7°$ (c 0·736, CH_3OH) and gives an ultraviolet spectrum consisting of two absorption maxima at 240 and 267 nm.

Musarin is assayed by a number of methods including cylinder plate, serial dilution, agar-plate dilution, agar-well plate and inhibition of spore germination, all with *Fusarium oxysporum* var. *lateritum* as the test organism. With a concentration of 80–100 units/mg, the following growth inhibition dilutions ($\times 10,000$) for bacteria have been determined by Arnstein and his coworkers: *Bacillus subtilis* (10); *Escherichia coli* ($>0·5$); *Mycobacterium phlei* (10); *Staphylococcus aureus* (50) and *Streptococcus pyogenes* (2·5). The same workers have determined spore germination inhibition dilutions ($\times 10,000$) for a larger number of fungi: *Alternaria* spp. (40); *Aspergillus niger* (10); *Aspergillus parasiticus* (5·0); *Botrytis cinerea* (40); *Ceratostomella paradoxa* (40); *Corticium solani* (80); *Fusarium oxyspora* var. *cubense* (10); *F. oxysporum* var. *culmorum* (10); *F. oxysporum* var. *latericum* (10); *F. oxysporum* var. *lini* (5·0); *Melanospora destruens* (40); *Penicillium notatum*

(5·0); *Rhizopus stolonifer* (5·0); *Sclerotinia fructigena* (80); *Verticillium albo-astrum* (80) and *Vert. dahliae* (80).

Thaysen, Butlin, *Nature*, **156**, 781 (1945)
Meredith, *Phytopath*, **33**, 403 (1943)
Meredith, *ibid.*, **34**, 426 (1944)
Thaysen, Morris, *Nature*, **159**, 100 (1947)
Arnstein, Cook, Lacey, *J. Gen. Microbiol.*, **2**, 111 (1948)

MUSETTAMYCIN
$C_{36}H_{45}NO_{14}$

A constituent of the bohemic acid complex isolated from cultures of *Actinosporangium* species ATCC 31,127, this antibiotic has been assigned the structure given above from chemical analysis and a study of the infrared, NMR and mass spectra. Like the accompanying marcellomycin (q.v.), it is especially effective against staphylococci, streptococci and inhibits various transplanted rodent leukemias and carcinosarcomas *in vivo*. The acute LD_{50} in mice is 9·8–21·12 mg/kg.

Nettleton *et al.*, *J. Antibiotics* (Japan), **30**, 525 (1977)
Nettleton *et al.*, *U.S. Patent*, 4,039,736 (1977)

MUTALOMYCIN
$C_{40}H_{70}O_{12}$

A polyether antibiotic, mutalomycin has been obtained fr m cultures of *Streptomyces mutabilis* NRRL 8081 grown on a common nutrient medium. It is normally purified and isolated as the sodium salt. Mutalomycin is active against gram positive bacteria and *Eimeria tenella*. The structure given above has been determined from chemical correlations and a study of the infrared, NMR and mass spectra.

Fehr, King, Kuhn, *J. Antibiotics* (Japan), **30**, 903 (1977)

MUTAMICIN 1
$C_{19}H_{37}N_5O_8$

A mutant strain of *Micromonospora inyouensis* (which produces sisomicin on the addition of 2-deoxystreptamine to the culture medium) also produces a further series of antibiotics, the mutamicins, in the presence of analogues of 2 deoxystreptamine. Addition of streptamine itself in place of 2-deoxystreptamine yields the mutamicin 1 complex which has been separated into three components by column and thin layer chromatography. Mutamicin 1 has the structure shown above based upon chemical and spectroscopic evidence. It possesses broad spectrum activity similar to, or slightly less than, that of sisomicin. It does, however, exhibit significant activity against gentamicin-sisomicin-adenylating strains of bacteria.

Tegta *et al.*, *J. Antibiotics* (Japan), **27**, 917 (1974)

MUTAMICIN 1a
$C_{20}H_{37}N_5O_9$

Mutamicin 1b

A component of the mutamicin 1 complex produced by a mutant strain of *Micromonospora inyouensis* in the presence of added streptamine, this antibiotic has the above structure which has been established from chemical correlations with sisomicin and spectroscopic data. It has a broad spectrum activity similar to that of mutamicin 1.

Tegta *et al.*, *J. Antibiotics* (Japan), **27**, 917 (1974)

MUTAMICIN 1b
$C_{18}H_{35}N_5O_8$

The third constituent of the mutamicin 1 complex isolated from a mutant strain of *Micromonospora inyouensis* grown in the presence of streptamine, mutamicin 1b has the structure given above which has been elucidated from chemical and spectroscopic data and comparison with that of sisomicin. It is a broad spectrum antibiotic which is effective against gentamicin-sisomicin adenylating strains of bacteria.

Tegta *et al.*, *J. Antibiotics* (Japan), **27**, 917 (1974)

MUTAMICIN 2
$C_{19}H_{37}N_5O_6$

Two structurally similar antibiotics, mutamicins 2 and 2a are obtained when the mutant strain of *Micromonospora inyouensis* is cultured in the presence of added 2,5-dideoxystreptamine. They have been separated and purified by column and thin layer chromatography. Mutamicin 2 has the above structure based upon chemical and spectroscopic evidence. It has a similar broad spectrum activity to the members of the mutamicin 1 complex but differs from them in having a favourable effect against gentamicin-sisomicin-acetylating bacterial strains.

Tegta *et al.*, *J. Antibiotics* (Japan), **27**, 917 (1974)

MUTAMICIN 2a
$C_{18}H_{36}N_4O_9$

A second component of the mutamicin 2 mixture produced by a mutant strain of *Micromonospora inyouensis*, this substance has been shown to have the structure given above which has been deduced from chemical correlations and a study of the infrared, NMR and mass spectra. It has a similar antibiotic activity to the preceding substance and is also effective against gentamicin-sisomicin-acetylating strains of bacteria.

Tegta *et al.*, *J. Antibiotics* (Japan), **27**, 917 (1974)

3-O-(α-L-MYCAROSYL)-8-HYDROXYERYTHRONOLIDE B
$C_{28}H_{50}O_{11}$

This substance has been prepared by the cultivation of *Streptomyces erythreus* NRRL 3887 with added 8-hydroxyerythronolide B. It has been extracted from the culture filtrate with AcOEt and purified by chromatography on a silica gel column. A dose of 200 mg/kg given orally reduced experimentally induced fever in mice by 70 per cent within an hour.

Martin, U.S. Patent, 3,684,794 (1972)
Martin, U.S. Patent, 3,740,425 (1973)

MYCELIANAMIDE
$C_{22}H_{28}O_5N_2$
M.p. 170–172°C (dec.)

An antibiotic isolated from *Penicillium griseofulvum*, mycelianamide is obtained by surface culture on a medium containing glucose and inorganic salts and incubated, with shaking, for 35 days at 25°C. Ammonium tartrate is normally added as a source of nitrogen. The mycelium is powdered after washing with H_2O and drying *in vacuo*, extracted with Et_2O and the solvent evaporated slowly. The crude material thus obtained is extracted with boiling C_6H_6, cooled, crystallized and then recrystallized from AcOEt.

Mycelianamide forms shiny leaflets when pure and is laevorotatory with $[\alpha]_{5461}^{19}$ − 217° and $[\alpha]_{5790}^{19}$ − 182° (c 0·8688, $CHCl_3$). It is soluble in dioxan and $(CH_3)_2CO$, sparingly so in $CHCl_3$, EtOH, C_6H_6, Et_2O and glacial AcOH, insoluble in HCl and dilute sodium bicarbonate solution. It is stable to heat and forms insoluble salts with heavy metals, gives a negative Millon, biuret and muroxide test and does not form a methiodide or picrate. Oxford and Raistrick have suggested that it is the amide of o-mecelyl-N-pyruvyl-β-ketotyrosine.

Mycelianamide is not active against gram-negative bacteria but inhibits the growth of *Bacillus anthracis*, *Staphylococcus albus*, *Staph. aureus*, *Streptococcus pyogenes* and *Strep. viridans* at a dilution of 1:20,000–50,000.

Anslow, Raistrick, *Biochem. J.*, **25**, 39 (1931)
Oxford, Raistrick, Simonart, *ibid.*, **29**, 1002 (1935)
Oxford, Raistrick, Simonart, *ibid.*, **33**, 240 (1939)
Oxford, Raistrick, *ibid.*, **42**, 323 (1948)
Structure
Birch et al., *J. Chem. Soc.*, 3717 (1956)
Configuration
Gallena et al., *Gazz. Chim. Ital.*, **94**, 1301 (1964)

MYCELIN
An antibiotic obtained from *Streptomyces roseoflavus*, this substance is extracted from the mycelium with CH_3OH followed by concentration *in vacuo* and precipitation of the inactive materials with EtOH and barium hydroxide which leaves the crude mycelin in solution. The substance is then further purified by chromatography on an alumina column. Mycelin crystallizes as colourless prisms from $(CH_3)_2CO$ and is soluble in $CHCl_3$, CH_3OH, EtOH, BuOH, C_6H_6 and $(CH_3)_2CO$ but insoluble in H_2O, Et_2O and petroleum ether. It is a stable compound which contains no nitrogen or sulphur, being active against filamentous fungi but not against bacteria. No data has been given regarding its toxicity.

Aiso et al., *J. Antibiotics* (Japan), **5**, 217 (1952)

MYCETIN
This antibiotic has been described by Russian workers who have isolated it from *Streptomyces violaceus*. The material is extracted from the dried, powdered agar culture with either equal parts of EtOH and CH_2Cl_2 or a mixture of $CHCl_3$ and C_6H_6. Following evaporation of the solvent the substance is then dissolved in EtOH. Mycetin is said to be a deep violet-coloured compound although it is not yet known whether the pure antibiotic is so intensely coloured. Mycetin is active against gram-positive bacteria, micrococci, streptococci, corynebacteria and spore-forming organisms, but not against gram-negative bacteria. It has only a limited activity *in vivo* and both pus and proteins lower the activity.

Krassilnikov, Koreniako, *Mikrobiologia*, **8**, 673 (1939)
Fainschmidt, Koreniako, *Biokhimiya*, **9**, 147 (1944)
Krassilnikov, Koreniako, *Mikrobiologia*, **14**, 80 (1945)

MACOBACIDIN
See Actithiazic Acid

MYCOBACILLIN
$C_{65}H_{85}O_{30}N_{13}$
M.p. 235–240°C

```
Asp—Ala—Asp—Pro—Asp—Glu
                            |
                            Tyr
                            |
Glu—Leu—Asp—Ser—Tyr—Asp
```

This antibiotic substance has been isolated from the culture filtrates of *Bacillus subtilis*. It forms colourless crystals and gives an ultraviolet spectrum in a mixture of AcOH-*n*-BuOH—H_2O-95 per cent EtOH with a single absorption maximum at 277 nm. Mycobacillin has been shown to be a cyclin polypeptide having the above structure which is based primarily upon a study of the hydrolysis products. It consists of seven aminoacids, alanine, aspartic acid, glutamic acid, leucine, proline, serine and tyrosine. Mycobacillin is active against gram-positive and gram-negative bacteria.

Majumdar, Bose, *Nature*, **181**, 134 (1958)
Majumdar, Bose, *Biochem. J.*, **74**, 596 (1960)
Configuration
Banerjee, Bose, *Nature*, **200**, 471 (1963)

MYCOCIDIN

A species of *Aspergillus* elaborates this antibiotic which is produced by surface growth on a Czapek-Dox medium and incubated for 14 days at 35°C. Mycocidin is isolated by acidifying the filtrate to pH 1·5, extracting with Et_2O, shaking the ethereal fraction with sodium hydroxide solution and neutralizing the aqueous phase with dilute HCl. The antibiotic is insoluble in acid solution, the precipitate however dissolving in Et_2O, H_2O, AcOEt and alkalies.

Mycocidin is assayed by serial dilution with *Mycobacterium tuberculosis hominis* as the test organism. The crude extract inhibits *M. tuberculosis hominis in vitro* in Long's medium, while *in vivo* experiments show that when tubercle bacilli are treated with the antibiotic prior to injection into guinea pigs, no infection is caused.

Gerber, Gross, *Science*, **101**, 616 (1945)
Gerber, Gross, *ibid.*, **103**, 167 (1946)

MYCOINE

Vonkennel and his colleagues have reported the presence of a class of antibiotic substances termed 'mycoines' derived from a number of fungi, e.g. *Achorion, Actinomycetes, Aspergillus, Cephalosporium, Fusarium* and *Microsporum*. These bactericidal substances have not been examined since their discovery and little is known of them.

Vonkennel, Kimmig, Lembke, *Klin. Wochenschr.*, **22**, 321 (1943)

MYCOLUTEIN

$C_{22}H_{24}O_6N$?
M.p. 157–185°C
An unidentified species of *Streptomyces* produces this antifungal antibiotic which crystallizes from CH_3OH—C_6H_6 as bright yellow tabular crystals. It is dextrorotatory with a specific rotation of $[\alpha]_D^{25} + 54°$ (c 1·0, $CHCl_3$). The ultraviolet spectrum in $CHCl_3$ has absorption maxima at 254 and 345 nm. Mycolutein is soluble in $(CH_3)_2CO$, $CHCl_3$, C_6H_6, AcOH, dioxan, pyridine and the lower alcohols, but insolubel in H_2O. It is unstable in dilute alkalies being readily decomposed under these conditions.

Mycolutein is active against *Candida albicans, Candida tropicalis* and *Geotrichum* species in agar at a concentration of 1·0 µg/ml. Mice tolerate a dose of 0·1 mg/20 g mouse but 0·5 mg/20 g mouse is lethal.

Schmitz, Woodside, *Antibiotics & Chemotherapy*, **5**, 652 (1955)

MYCOMYCIN

$C_{13}H_{10}O_2$
M.p. 75°C

$HC\equiv C-C\equiv C-CH=CH-CH=CH-CH=CH-CH_2-COOH$

Nocardia acidophilus elaborates this antibiotic which is a highly unsaturated fatty acid that decomposes explosively at its melting point. It is produced on a 'Tryptone'-starch medium and is obtained by extraction with Et_2O or amyl acetate. Mycomycin is laevorotatory having a specific rotation of $[\alpha]_D^{25} - 130°$ (c 1·0, EtOH).

The antibiotic is assayed by serial dilution with *Bacillus subtilis* as the test organism. It is active against bacteria, mycobacteria and fungi, a crude extract inhibiting *Bacillus subtilis* at a dilution of 1:7000 and a virulent strain of *Mycobacterium tuberculosis* at 1:5000. It has no activity, however, *in vivo*. No reliable data are available concerning its toxicity although it has been stated that crude concentrates are non-toxic to mice. An absoprtion curve is shown by erytheocytes over a 24-hour period.

Johnson, Burdon, *J. Bact.*, **54**, 281 (1947)
Johnson, *Soc. Amer. Bacteriologists*, 68 (1949)
Celmer, Solomons, *J. Amer. Chem. Soc.*, **74**, 1870 (1952)
Jenkins, *Trans. 11th Conf. Chemotherapy of Tuberculosis*, 309 (1952)

MYCOPHENOLIC ACID

$C_{17}H_{20}O_6$

This antibiotic is believed to be the first to have been obtained in a crystalline form by Gosio in 1896. It is produced by *Penicillium brevi-compactum* and *P. stoloniferum*. The antibiotic may be produced by surface growth on a Raulin-Thom medium incubated for 34 days at 24°C or on a Czapek-Dox medium with corn steep liquor, Isolation is carried out by evaporating the culture filtrate *in vacuo* and extracting with Et_2O. The crude material is purified by crystallizing from $(CH_3)_2CO$—$CHCl_3$ or from boiling H_2O.

Mycophenolic acid is normally assayed by cylinder plate with *Staphylococcus aureus* as test organism. It has no activity against *Bacillus acoidcae*, *B. tumefaciens*, *Leuconostoc* species, *Pseudomonas marginalis* and *Ps. syringae*, but does inhibit a large number of the *Ectothrix*, *Endodermophyton*, *Endothrix*, *Epidermophyton*, *Favus* and *Microsporum* species together with certain fungi which are pathogenic to plants at dilutions of 1:5000–8000. Gulliver and Florey and his coworkers have measured inhibition dilutions ($\times$ 1000) for a number of bacteria and fungi as follows: *Actinomyces scabies* (5·0–10); *Bacillus subtilis* (20); *Claviceps purpurea* (20); *Corynebacterium diphtheriae* ($>$4·0); *Coryne. michiganense* (320); *Coryne. sepedonicum* (160); *Coryne. xerosis* (4·0); *Escherichia coli* ($>$1·0); *Phytophthora erythroseptica* (20); *Rhizoctinia crocorum* (20); *Salmonella typhi* ($>$1·0); *Stereum purpureum* (80); *Staphylococcus aureus* (1·0–6·4); *Streptococcus pyogenes* ($>$1·0); *Verticillium dahliae* (20) and *Xanthomonas begoniae* (10).

Abraham has demonstrated that when *Staphylococcus aureus* is grown in heart broth, mycophenolic acid hinders either the synthesis or the utilization of some growth intermediate which results in an increased lag phase in the growth of the organism. This bacterium, however, soon acquires a resistance to the antibiotic when serially transferred on media containing it.

Mycophenolic acid is comparatively toxic to mice. The lethal dose is 40 mg given orally or 10 mg given intravenously. However, when administered subcutaneously, 10 mg was tolerated. An ointment containing the antibiotic produces no reaction on human skin.

Alsberg, Black, *U.S.D.A., Bur. Plant Industry*, Bulletin 270 (1913)
Clutterbuck *et al.*, *Biochem. J.*, **26**, 1441 (1932)
Clutterbuck, Raistrick, *ibid.*, **27**, 654 (1933)
Wilkins, Harris, *Brit. J. Exptl. Path.*, **24**, 141 (1943)
Abraham, *Biochem. J.*, **39**, 398 (1945)
Florey, *Brit. M. J.*, **4427**, 635 (1945)
Gilliver, *Ann. Bot.*, **10**, 271 (1946)
Florey *et al.*, *Lancet*, **1**, 46 (1946)
Birkinshaw, Bracken, Morgan, *Biochem. J.*, **42**, xxxix (1948)

MYCORRHIZIN A
$C_{14}H_{15}O_4Cl$
M.p. 163–165°C

A bright yellow crystalline antibiotic, mycorrhizin A is produced, together with chloromycorrhizin A, by culturing a fungus D37 found on the roots of *Monotropa hypopitys* in a medium containing asparagine, thiamine hydrochloride and inorganic salts at 28–30°C and pH 5·8 for 11 days. The culture filtrate is extracted with AcOEt and chromatographed to separate and purify the two antibiotics. Mycorrhizin A crystallizes from $CHCl_3$-hexane and is dextrorotatory with a specific rotation of $[\alpha]_D^{25}$ + 33·3° (c 1·89, EtOH) and gives an ultraviolet spectrum in EtOH consisting of two absorption maxima at 229 and 298 nm. It is active against the root rot fungus *Fomes annosus*.

Trofast, Wickberg, *Tetrahedron*, **33**, 875 (1977)

MYCOSTATIN
See Nystatin

MYCOSUBTILIN
M.p. 256–257°C

An antifungal antibiotic, derived from *Bacillus subtilis* and obtained by submerged growth on a medium containing beet molasses, diammonium phosphate and a trace of manganous sulphate, incubated for 5 days to 25°C. Mycosubtilin is isolated by acidifying the culture liquor to pH 2·5 with HCl, centrifuging and extracting the bacterial cells with EtOH, adding the extract to H_2O when the active material is then precipitated. Extraction of the precipitate with EtOH is followed by evaporation to dryness, dissolving the residue in pyridine, precipitating with a large volume of H_2O and cooling. The crude material is then purified by recrystallization from pyridine and 70 per cent EtOH giving a potency of 700 *Trichophyton* sp. units/mg.

Mycosubtilin forms white crystals, soluble in dilute sodium hydroxide solution, pyridine and 70 per cent EtOH, but insoluble in all other common solvents. It gives an ultraviolet spectrum in aqueous EtOH with a single absorption maximum at 277 nm. It does not react with 2:4-dinitrophenylhydrazine or reduce Fehling's solution, but gives positive ninhydrin and Millon reactions.

The antibiotic is assayed by streak plate with *Trichophyton* species. It is inactive against bacteria *in vitro* with the exception of *Micrococcus lysodeikticus* which is inhibited by 0·001 mg/ml. Walton and Woodruff have shown that a large number of fungi are inhibited at the following concentrations (µg/ml): *Acharion schoenleinii* (5·0); *Aspergillus niger* (>20); *Chaetomium bostrychodes* (5·0); *Epidermophyton inguinale* (5·0); *Fusarium moniliforme* (7·5); *Microsporum audouini* (5·0); *Microsporum lanosum* (10); *Minor flavus* (>20); *Nematospora coryli* (7·5); *Penicillium notatum* (7·5); *Rhizopus javanicus takela* (>20); *Sclerotinia fructicola* (2·5); *Trichoderma* spp. (>20); *Trichophyton* spp. (1·5) and *Ustilago zeae* (1·6). In addition, the following yeasts are also inhibited: *Candida guilliermondi* (>20); *Debaryomyces gruetzii* (>20); *Dipodescus uninuceatus* (3·75); *Hansenula anomala* (3·75); *Mycoderma valida* (7·5); *Rhodotorula rubra* (5·0); *Saccharomyces carlsbergensis* (7·5); *Sporobolmyces roseus* (5·0); *Torulopsis delbruckii* (3·75); *Torula cremoris* (5·0) and *Zygopichia californica* (>20). The antibiotic is completely antagonized by 10 per cent horse serum.

When tested *in vivo* in mice, a dose of 0·25 mg given subcutaneously was tolerated while twice this dose proved lethal.

Michener, Snell, *A.A.A.S. Bot. Soc. Amer.*, San Diego, Calif. (1947)
Walton, Woodruff, *J. Clin. Invest.*, **28**, 924 (1949)

MYDECAMYCIN
See Antibiotic SF-837

MYRIOCIN
This antifungal antibiotic has been isolated from the thermophilic ascomycete *Myriococcum albomyces*. The antibiotic is present in both the culture filtrate and the mycelium from which it may be isolated by conventional methods. Myriocin forms colourless needles from EtOH and possesses a high degree of activity against yeasts and dermatophytes *in vitro*. The toxicity, however, appears to be too high for therapeutic purposes.

Kluepfel et al., *J. Antibiotics* (Japan), **25**, 109 (1972)

MYROPROZINE
See Pimaricin

MYRORIDIN I
Myrothecium species 285F elaborates two closely related peptide antibiotics which have been obtained by extraction of the culture filtrate and separation and purification of the crude extract by column chromatography. This component has a molecular weight of approximately 1300. It is not active against bacteria but effective against yeasts.

Kondo, *Tohoku J. Exp. Med.*, **122**, 403 (1977)

MYRORIDIN II
A further peptide antibiotic isolated from the culture filtrate of *Myrothecium* species 285F, this substance has a molecular weight of about 1200 and is active against yeasts but not against bacteria.

Kondo, *Tohoku J. Exp. Med.*, **122**, 403 (1977)

MYRTUCUMMULONE A
$C_{38}H_{52}O_{10}$

An antibiotic substance isolated from the leaves of *Myrtus communis*, this compound has the structure shown above which has been established from chemical and spectroscopic data. It has no effect *in vitro* against gram-negative bacteria but has been shown to be as effective against gram-positive bacteria as streptomycin and the penicillins.

Rotstein, Lifshitz, *Antimicrobial Agents & Chemotherapy*, **6**, 539 (1974)

MYXIN 3C
$C_{13}H_{10}O_4N_2$
M.p. 120–130°C

A potent broad-spectrum antibiotic, myxin 3C has been obtained from cultures of *Sporangium* strain 3C, a myxobacter isolated from soil. The pure compound forms red needles when crystallized from $(CH_3)_2CO$ and has a strongly exothermic reaction at 140–149°C and may explode on heating. It is stable in solution between pH 5·0–9·0 at room temperature and also at 70°C in solution except in phosphate buffer. The ultraviolet and visible spectra in 0·1 N-HCl have absorption maxima at 283, 340 and 505 nm. Myxin 3C is active in inhibiting a range of gram-positive and gram-negative bacteria, fungi and yeasts.

Peterson et al., *Can. J. Microbiol.*, **12**, 231 (1966)
Structure
Edwards, Gillespie, *Tetrahedron Lett.*, 4867 (1966)
Synthesis
Weigele, Leimgruber, *Tetrahedron Lett.*, 715 (1967)
See also
Rachlin, *Chem. Engr.*, Sept. 4, 1967

N

NAFCILLIN
$C_{21}H_{22}O_5N_2S$

A semi-synthetic antibiotic of the penicillin class, this substance is active mainly against gram-positive bacteria. Experiments in a canine model have established a direct method for the determination of the uptake, storage and elimination of this, and other, antibiotics, by the liver and kidney.

Barza et al., J. Infect. Diseases, **131** (Suppl), S86 (1975)

NANAOMYCIN A
$C_{16}H_{14}O_6$
M.p. 178–180°C

Cultures of *Streptomyces rosa* produce two closely related antibodies. This compound crystallizes from EtOH as orange needles. It is laevorotatory with a specific rotation of $[\alpha]_D^{26} - 27.5°$ (c 1.0, MeOH). It is active against gram-positive bacteria.

Omura et al., J. Antibiotics (Japan), **27**, 363 (1974)
Tanaka et al., J. Antibiotics (Japan), **28**, 925 (1975)

NANOMYCIN B
$C_{16}H_{16}O_7$
M.p. Indefinite

A second antibiotic isolated from cultures of *Streptomyces rosa*, nanomycin B forms an orange-red powder with no definite melting point. Like the preceding antibiotic it is laevorotatory with a specific rotation of $[\alpha]_D^{26} - 74.5°$ (c 1.0 CH_3OH) and is active against gram-positive bacteria.

Omura et al., J. Antibiotics (Japan), **27**, 363 (1974)
Tanaka et al., J. Antibiotics (Japan), **28**, 925 (1975)

NANAOMYCIN C
$C_{16}H_{15}NO_5$

A amide of nanomycin A, this antibiotic has been isolated from cultures of *Streptomyces rosa* var. *notoensis*. The structure has been elucidated from chemical correlations and a study of the infrared, NMR and mass spectra. It is active against gram-positive bacteria, fungi, and particularly against *Mycoplasma gallisepticum*.

Tanaka et al., J. Antibiotics (Japan), **28**, 925 (1975)

α-NAPHTHOCYCLINONE
$C_{33}H_{30}O_{15}$
M.p. 188–192°C (*dec.*)

One of three antibiotic pigments isolated from cultures of *Streptomyces arenae*. This compound crystallizes from EtOH as orange crystals. The structure has been elucidated by chemical and spectroscopic methods. α-Naphthocyclinone possesses only weakly antibiotic properties.

Zeeck, Mardin, *Annalen*, 1063 (1974)

β-NAPHTHOCYCLINONE
$C_{35}H_{32}O_{14}$
M.p. 183°C (*dec.*)

A second antibiotic obtained from *Streptomyces arenae*, this compound forms red needles when purified by chromatography and recrystallization from EtOH. It is laevorotatory with a specific rotation of $[\alpha]_D^{20} - 783°$. The structure differs from that of the preceding antibiotic only in the nature of the quinoid side-chain.

Zeeck, Mardin, *Annalen*, 1100 (1974)

γ-NAPHTHOCYCLINONE
$C_{35}H_{30}O_{14}$
M.p. 272–275°C (*dec.*)

Streptomyces arenae also produces this antibiotic pigment which forms red plates when crystallized from EtOH. It is strongly laevorotatory having a specific rotation of $[\alpha]_D^{20} - 977°$. The polycyclic structure is very similar to those of the two accompanying antibiotics.

Zeeck, Mardin, *Annalen*, 1100 (1974)

NAPHTHYRIDINOMYCIN
$C_{21}H_{27}O_6N_3$
M.p. 108–110°C (*dec.*)

This naphthyridine antibiotic is elaborated by *Streptomyces* strain NRRL 8034. It may be extracted from the culture filtrate with organic solvents and forms red crystals. Naphthyridinomycin is dextrorotatory with a specific rotation of $[\alpha]_D^{25} + 69.4°$ (c 1.0, $CHCl_3$).

Sygusch *et al.*, *Tetrahedron Lett.*, 4021 (1974)
Revised structure
Sygusch *et al.*, *Tetrahedron Lett.*, 170 (1975)
Kluepfel, Sehgal, Vezina, *U.S. Patent*, 4,003,902 (1977)

NARAMYCIN A
See Actidione

NARASIN
$C_{43}H_{72}O_{11}$

A polyether antibiotic isolated from cultures of *Streptomyces aureofaciens*, this substance is purified by extraction of the culture filtrate with an organic solvent followed by silica gel chromatography. It is effective *in vitro* against gram-positive bacteria, anaerobic bacteria and fungi. Tests have shown it to be active in the protection of chickens against coccidial infections.

Berg, Hamill, *J. Antibiotics* (Japan), **31**, 1 (1978)

NARBOMYCIN
$C_{28}H_{47}O_7N$
M.p. 113·5–115°C

Narbomycin has been isolated from *Streptomyces narbonensis*, a mold found in soil near Cannes, France. It forms colourless crystals when purified by recrystallization from Et_2O-petroleum ether and is dextrorotatory with a specific rotation of $[\alpha]_D^{20} + 68·5°$ (c 1·35, $CHCl_3$). The ultraviolet spectrum in absolute EtOH has absorption maxima at 225 and 286 nm.

Narbomycin has a high activity against gram-positive organisms *in vitro*, but is inactive *in vivo*. It is relatively non-toxic, the LD_{50} in mice being 500 mg/kg when administered subcutaneously.

Corbaz *et al.*, *Helv. Chim. Acta*, **38**, 935 (1955)
Structure
Prelog *et al.*, *Helv. Chim. Acta*, **45**, 4 (1962)

NATAMYCIN
See Pimaricin

NEAMINE (*Neomycin A*)
$C_{12}H_{26}O_6N_4$
Dec. 225–226°C

Neamine is one of the degradation products of neomycins B and C although there is some evidence that it may also be produced in small quantities by *Streptomyces fradiae*. It is a basic substance, forming colourless crystals from H_2O or aqueous EtOH, and is dextrorotatory with a specific rotation of $[\alpha]_D^{25} + 112·8°$ (c 1·0, H_2O). It is soluble in H_2O and may be separated from the neomycins by paper chromatography and countercurrent distribution. It forms a tetrahydrochloride as an amorphous powder which decomposes at 250–260°C and has a specific rotation of $[\alpha]_D^{25} + 83°$ (c 1·0, H_2O). The N-acetyl derivative forms colourless crystals from CH_3OH with m.p. 334–336°C and $[\alpha]_D^{25} + 87°$ (c 1·0, H_2O).

Neamine possesses very little antibiotic activity being primarily active against gram-positive bacteria. It is comparatively non-toxic, the LD_{50} in mice being 1250 mg/kg (subcutaneous) and 320 mg/kg when given intravenously. It has not found any use in medicine.

Peck *et al.*, *J. Amer. Chem. Soc.*, **71**, 2590 (1949)
Dutcher *et al.*, *ibid.*, **73**, 1384 (1951)
Leach, Teeters, *ibid.*, **73**, 2794 (1951)
Peck *et al.*, *ibid.*, **75**, 1018 (1953)
Peck, Hoffhine, Folkers, *U.S. Patent*, 2,691,675 (1954)
Structure
Carter *et al.*, *J. Amer. Chem. Soc.*, **83**, 3723 (1961)
Hichens, Rinehart, *ibid.*, **85**, 1547 (1963)
Synthesis
Umezawa *et al.*, *J. Antibiotics* (Japan), **20A**, 53 (1967)

NEBRAMYCIN
This antibiotic complex is produced by growing *Streptomyces tenebrarius* ATCC 17920 under aerobic submerged conditions in a medium containing dextrose, soybean grits and inorganic salts at 27°C for 5 days. Nebramycin is isolated by adsorption on a cationic exchange resin and elution with EtOH or by precipitation as the insoluble salts of alkylsulphoacetic acids. So far, the

NEGAMYCIN
$C_9H_{20}O_4N_4$

An aminoacid, this antibiotic has an action similar to that of most aminoglycosidic antibiotics including streptomycin and kanamycin, causing inhibition of protein synthesis and misreading of the genetic code. Minimum inhibition concentrations (μg/ml) determined on 0·5 per cent peptone agar are: *Escherichia coli* K-12 (3·1); *E. coli* K-12 ML1629 (1·6); *Klebsiella pneumoniae* (3·1); *Pseudomonas aeruginosa* A3 (6·3); *Ps. aeruginosa* No. 12 (6·3); *Salmonella typhi* T-63 (3·1); *Shigella sonnei* (6·3) and *Staphylococcus aureus* FDA 209P (12·5).

Mizuno, Nitta, Umezawa, *J. Antibiotics* (Japan), **23**, 581, 589 (1970)
Kondo *et al.*, *J. Amer. Chem. Soc.*, **93**, 6305 (1971)
Shibahara *et al.*, *ibid.*, **94**, 4553 (1972)

NEMOTIN
$C_{11}H_8O_2$

An antibiotic produced by a number of *Basidiomycetes*, e.g. *Poria corticola* (Fries) Cooke and *P. tenuis* (Schwein.) Cooke, this substance has so far only been isolated in solution, being unstable in the condensed phase. It rapidly undergoes polymerization forming a gum or brittle glassy laquer which are only slightly active. It is moderately soluble in organic solvents and only sparingly so in H_2O. Nemotin is dextrorotatory with a specific rotation of $[\alpha]_D^{17} + 380°$ (c 0·3, H_2O). It exhibits activity *in vitro* against *Mycobacterium tuberculosis*. Solutions of this antibiotic should be handled with care since it may cause severe dermatitis.

Anchel *et al.*, *Arch. Biochem.*, **25**, 208 (1950)
Kavanagh *et al.*, *Proc. Nat. Acad. Sci.*, **36**, 1 (1950)
Structure
Bu'Lock *et al.*, *J. Chem. Soc.*, 4270 (1955)

NEOANTIMYCIN
$C_{36}H_{46}O_{12}N_1$
M.p. 121–122°C (*dec.*)

A macrocyclic antibiotic produced by *Streptoverticillium orinoci*, this substance forms colourless crystals from a mixture of AcOEt and *n*-hexane. Neoantimycin has a specific rotation of $[\alpha]_D^{25} + 58·3°$ (c 1·0, $CHCl_3$). It gives an ultraviolet spectrum with absorption maxima at 227 and 319 nm in EtOH solution, with $FeCl_3$ solution it yields a deep violet colour. One phenolic hydroxyl group is present in the molecule and the methyl ether is obtained as yellow crystals from AcOEt-hexane, m.p. 108–110°C; $[\alpha]_D^{25} + 2·01°$ (c 1·0, CCl_4). The ultraviolet spectrum of this derivative in EtOH has a single absorption maximum at 293 nm.

Caglioti *et al.*, *Tetrahedron*, **25**, 2193 (1969)

NEOCARCINOSTATIN
M.p. Indefinite

Neocarcinostatin is produced by the submerged, aerobic culture of *Streptomyces carcinostaticus* var. *neocarcinostaticus* ATCC 15,944 and 15,945 in a medium containing defatted soybean meal, glucose, urea and inorganic salts. The antibiotic has not been obtained in a completely pure form, that which has been isolated being a white amorphous powder with no definite melting point. Neocarcinostatin is a potent antitumour antibiotic. A dose of 0·8 mg/kg given daily for 6 days, 24 hours after mice were infected with 4 ± 10^6 sarcoma 180 ascites tumour cells cured the animals, while doses of 0·2–3·2 mg/kg prolonged the lives of mice with leukemia SN-36. The acute toxicity in mice is given as 30 mg/kg.

Kudo, Chihara, *Hakko Kogaku Zasshi*, **45**, 712 (1967)
Ishida, *German Patent*, 1,252,365 (1967)

complex has been separated into eight components including apramycin, 6″-O-carbamoylkanamycin B and 6″-O-carbamoyl-tobramycin.

Thompson, Stark, Higgens, *U.S. Patent*, 3,691,279 (1972)
Koch, Davis, Rhoades, *J. Antibiotics* (Japan), **26**, 745 (1973)

NEOMACARBOMYCIN I$_a$

This culture filtrate of *Streptomyces phaeochromogenes* yields crude neomacarbomycin which has been separated into three components by silica gel chromatography and ion exchange resin. This antibiotic forms a white powder with no definite melting point and is weakly acidic. It has been shown to contain phosphorus and gives glucose and glucosamine on acid hydrolysis. It is active against a range of gram-positive bacteria.

Umezawa, Maeda, Fukatsu, *Japanese Patent*, 7,400,493 (1974)

NEOMACARBOMYCIN I$_b$

A further amorphous antibiotic isolated from the antibiotic complex elaborated by *Streptomyces phaeochromogenes*. This compound is also weakly acidic, contains phosphorus and on acid hydrolysis yields glucose, glucosamine and glycine. It has an antibiotic spectrum similar to that of the preceding compound.

Umezawa, Maeda, Fukatsu, *Japanese Patent*, 7,400,493 (1974)

NEOMACABOMYCIN II

A third antibiotic which may be separated from the crude neomacarbomycin derived from *Streptomyces phaeochromogenes*, this compound forms an amorphous white powder having a composition similar to that of neomacarbomycin I$_a$.

Umezawa, Maeda, Fukatsu, *Japanese Patent*, 7,400,493 (1974)

NEOMETHYMYCIN
$C_{25}H_{43}O_7N$
M.p. 156–158°C

Neomethymycin is a macrocyclic antibiotic which accompanies methymycin (q.v.), being found in the mother liquors from the culture of *Streptomyces venezuelae*. The structure differs from that of methymycin only in the position of one hydroxyl group. The antibiotic forms colourless crystals from Et$_2$O-hexane and is dextrorotatory with a specific rotation of $[\alpha]_D^{25} + 93°$. It gives an ultraviolet spectrum having a single absorption maximum at 227 nm. When crystallized from various solvents, it solvates readily, e.g. the solvate from CH$_2$Cl$_2$ forms large crystals with m.p. 154–156°C and and $[\alpha]_D + 66°$ (c 1·0, EtOH). It is soluble in EtOH, CHCl$_3$, (CH$_3$)$_2$CO, C$_6$H$_6$, AcOEt and Et$_2$O, but virtually insoluble in hexane and aliphatic hydrocarbons. It is slightly soluble in H$_2$O and dibutyl ether. It has found some use as an experimental antimicrobial.

Djerassi, Halpern, *J. Amer. Chem. Soc.*, **79**, 2022 (1957)
Djerassi, Halpern, *Tetrahedron*, **3**, 255 (1958)
Djerassi, Halpern, *ibid.*, **4**, 369 (1958)
Dutcher *et al.*, *U.S Patent*, 2,916,486 (1959)
Djerassi, Halpern, *Angew. Chem.* **69**, 519 (1967)

NEOMYCIN A
See Neamine

NEOMYCIN B (*Actilin, Enterfram, Framycetin, Soframycin*)
$C_{23}H_{46}O_{13}N_6$
M.p. Indefinite

An amorphous antibiotic first obtained from cultures of *Streptomyces fradiae* and subsequently from other *Streptomyces* species including *S. coeruleoprunus* and also from *Micromonospora* species 69–683, noemycin B is isolated by adsorption of the activity from the culture broth on activated carbon followed by elution with acidified EtOH. This antibiotic is separated from the accompanying neomycin C by chromatography over alumina. It is a basic glycosidic white powder with no definite melting point, has a specific rotation of $[\alpha]_D^{25} + 83°$ (c 1·0, 0·2 N-H_2SO_4). Hydrolysis with dilute acids furnishes a mixture of neamine (q.v.), D-ribose and a diaminohexose. It gives no typical absorptions in the ultraviolet.

Neomycin B is not active against fungi but is active against gram-positive and gram-negative bacteria, mycobacteria and actinomycetes. It does not diffuse in agar as rapidly as neomycin C but is more potent by dilution assay (290 units/mg against 153 units/mg). It is comparatively non-toxic, the LD_{50} in mice being 220 mg/kg when given subcutaneously. In medicine it has found use in the treatment of bacterial infections of the eye and skin and also for the sterilization of the intestine. When tested in chickens, therapeutic doses of the sulphate inhibited the contractile activity of the crop and stomach and later stimulated the contractile activity.

Waksman, Lechevalier, *Science,* **109**, 305 (1949)
Waksman *et al., J. Clin. Invest.,* **28**, 934 (1949)
Swart *et al., ibid.,* **28**, 1045 (1949)
Peck *et al., J. Amer. Chem. Soc.,* **71**, 2590 (1949)
Regna, Murphy, *ibid.,* **72**, 1045 (1950)
Dutcher *et al., ibid.,* **73**, 1384 (1951)
Hamre *et al., Antibiotics & Chemotherapy,* **2**, 135 (1952)
Peck *et al., J. Amer. Chem. Soc.,* **75**, 1018 (1953)
Ford *et al., ibid.,* **77**, 5311 (1955)
Rinehart *et al., ibid.,* **79**, 4567, 4568 (1957)
Rinehart *et al., ibid.,* **80**, 6461, 6463 (1958)
Structure
Rinehart *et al., J. Amer. Chem. Soc.,* **82**, 2970 (1960)
Rinehart *et al., ibid.,* **84**, 3216, 3218 (1962)
Hichens, Rinehart., *ibid.,* **85**, 1547 (1963)
See also
Wagman *et al., J. Antibiotics* (Japan), **26**, 732 (1973)
Gol'tsgaker, *Sb. Rab. Leningr. Vet. Inst.,* **33**, 39 (1973)
Preobrazhenskya *et al., Antibiotiki,* **19**, 411 (1974)

NEOMYCIN B GLUCOSIDE
$C_{29}H_{57}O_{18}N_6$

This antibiotic derivative of neomycin B is produced by culturing *Streptomyces fradiae* 3535 on a medium containing 6–9 per cent glucose under aerobic conditions at 30°C for 6 days. The antibiotic is present to the extent of approximately 50 per cent. It has a similar antibiotic spectrum to that of the preceding compound.

Perlman, Cowan, *J. Antibiotics* (Japan), **27**, 637 (1974)

NEOMYCIN C
$C_{23}H_{46}O_{13}N_6$
M.p. Indefinite

A further amorphous component of the neomycin complex produced by *Streptomyces fradiae*. Neomycin C is dextrorotatory with a specific rotation of $[\alpha]_D^{25} + 121°$ (c 1·0, 0·2 N-H_2SO_4). On acid hydrolysis it yields neamine (q.v.) and neobiosamine C, a disaccharide composed of neosamine C and D-ribose. It is soluble in H_2O, CH_3OH and acidified lower alcohols, virtually insoluble in organic solvents. The antibiotic finds use in medicine as a broad-spectrum antimicrobial having negligible gastro-intestinal absorption and is employed principally for the supression of intestinal bacteria and topical therapy, being used normally as the sulphate, the usual dose being 1 g given orally. It has a number of side-effects including nephrotoxic and ototoxic effects which sometimes occur with parenteral use. It also has a use in veterinary medicine for the treatment of enteric, systemic and reproductive infections, together with local infections of the ear, eye and skin due to a wide variety of gram-positive and gram-negative organisms.

Waksman, Lechevalier, *Science*, **109**, 305 (1949)
Waksman *et al.*, *J. Clin. Invest.*, **28**, 934 (1949)
Swart *et al.*, *ibid.*, **28**, 1045 (1949)
Peck *et al.*, *J. Amer. Chem. Soc.*, **71**, 2590 (1949)
Regna, Murphy, *ibid.*, **72**, 1045 (1950)
Dutcher *et al.*, *ibid.*, **73**, 1384 (1951)
Hamre *et al.*, *Antibiotics & Chemotherapy*, **2**, 135 (1952)
Peck *et al.*, *J. Amer. Chem. Soc.*, **75**, 1018 (1953)
Ford *et al.*, *ibid.*, **77**, 5311 (1955)
Rinehart *et al.*, *ibid.*, **79**, 4567, 4568 (1957)
Rinehart *et al.*, *ibid.*, **80**, 6461, 6463 (1958)
Structure
Rinehart, Woo, *J. Amer. Chem. Soc.*, **80**, 6463 (1958)
Rinehart *et al.*, *ibid.*, **84**, 3216, 3218 (1962)

NEOMYCIN D
See Paromamine

NEOMYCIN E
See Paromomycin I

NEOMYCIN F
See Paromomycin II

NEONOCARDIN
An antibiotic obtained from *Nocardia kuroishi*, this compound has been shown to differ from other known antibiotics by means of paper chromatography. It is highly active against *Bacillus anthracis*, *Escherichia coli* and *Micrococcus pyogenes* var. *aureus* but shows little activity against *Bacillus subtilis* or *Pseudomonas aeruginosa*. No data are available concerning the toxicity of this antibiotic.

Uesaka, *J. Antibiotics* (Japan), **3C**, 27 (1950)
Uesaka, *ibid.*, **5**, 75 (1952)
Uesaka, *ibid.*, **5**, 170 (1952)

NEOSCHIZOPHYLLANE
This antibiotic has been obtained from cultures of *Schizophyllum commune*. It has been isolated from the culture fluid by extraction with polar solvents followed by column chromatography. Neoschizophyllane is a polysaccharide and possesses antitumour activity. It is also effective against a range of gram-positive bacteria.

Kamasuka *et al.*, *German Patent*, 2,648,834 (1977)

NEOTELOMYCIN
$C_{59}H_{77}O_{19}N_{13}$

A polypeptide antibiotic isolated from a number of *Streptomyces* species, this compound is active against a number of gram-positive and gram-negative bacteria, minimum inhibition concentrations being *Bacillus megaterium* (0·3 μg/ml), *Escherichia coli* (> 500 μg/ml) and *Staphylococcus aureus* (6·0–10 μg/ml). Neotelomycin significantly inhibited the activities of glucose dehydrogenase, citric dehydrogenase and succinic dehydrogenase when incubated with a sensitive strain of *B. megaterium*. This effect was much less pronounced in the case of *E. coli* B and *S. aureus* 209 cells. It also showed a high lytic effect when added to a suspension of *B. megaterium* cells at a concentration of 2·5–30 μg/ml and it appears that the bacterial cytoplasmic membranes are destroyed, thereby accounting for the antimicrobial activity of the antibiotic.

Petrykina *et al.*, *Antibiotiki*, **18**, 986, 1098 (1973)

NEOTHRAMYCIN A
$C_{13}H_{14}N_2O_4$

An unclassified species of *Streptomyces* yields two structurally similar antibiotics of the anthramycin group when cultures on a common nutrient medium. They have been separated and purified by column and thin layer chromatography. This substance is active against gram-positive bacteria and also exhibits antitumour activity.

Takeuchi *et al.*, *J. Antibiotics* (Japan), **29**, 93 (1976)

NEOTHRAMYCIN B
$C_{13}H_{14}N_2O_4$

A further anthramycin type antibiotic isolated from cultures of an unclassified species of *Streptomyces*, this substance possesses a similar antibacterial and antitumour activity to that of the preceding antibiotic.

Takeuchi *et al.*, *J. Antibiotics* (Japan), **29**, 93 (1976)

NEOTHRICIN
$C_{16}H_{35-37}O_{11}N_7$

This antibiotic has recently been obtained by culturing *Streptomyces lavendulae* IN-309-T in a common medium and treating the culture filtrate with Amberlite IRC-50 to yield the trihydrochloride. This salt is soluble in H_2O and is active against *Shigella dysenteriae, Staphylococcus aureus* and *Xanthomonas oryzae*. A dose of 300 mg/kg, given intraperitoneally to mice was tolerated.

Omi *et al.*, *Japanese Patent*, 7,128,832 (1971)

NETILMICIN
$C_{21}H_{41}N_5O_7$

A semi-synthetic antibiotic aminoglycoside produced from sisomicin, this substance has antibiotic properties similar to gentamicin. It is active against gram-negative bacteria to a greater extent than gentamicin and also effective against staphylococci and streptococci. It is active against pencillin G-susceptible and resistant strains of Staphylococcus aureus and is more active than gentamicin, sisomicin, amikacin or tobramycin against *Serratia marcescens* and the Enterobacteriaceae. Experiments have shown that more than 90 per cent of clinical gram-negative bacterial isolates are inhibited at a concentration of 1·56 micrograms/millilitre.

Phillips, Smith, Shannon, *Antimicrobial Agents & Chemotherapy*, **11**, 402 (1977)
Stewart, Bodey, LeBlanc, *ibid.*, **11**, 1017 (1977)

NETROPSIN
$C_{32}H_{48}O_4N_{18}$

Produced by *Streptomyces netropsis*, this antibiotic is normally obtained as the crystalline sulphate by the following procedure. The broth is acidified with phosphoric acid to pH 2·0 and then filtered on Super-Cel, the filtrate being brought to pH 6·5 with NaOH and the addition of ammonium oxalate, the precipitate being filtered off. HCl is then used to adjust the broth to pH 5·5 and the dye Orange II is added. The dye precipitate is then filtered and washed with distilled H_2O before being air-dried. The cake of material is suspended in an 80:20 mixture of $(CH_3)_2CO$ and CH_3OH and a 50 per cent solution of trimethylamine sulphate in CH_3OH is added. The precipitate is then filtered, washed with CH_3OH—$(CH_3)_2CO$ and extracted with distilled H_2O to give a solution of netropsin sulphate which contains 485 streptomycin units/mg.

Netropsin sulphate has a m.p. 224–225°C and is more soluble in hot H_2O than in cold. It is insoluble in all organic solvents. The ultraviolet spectrum of the sulphate has absorption maxima at 236 and 296 nm at pH 5·5. The antibiotic exhibits an inhibitory effect upon the growth of several gram-positive and gram-negative organisms and is also effective against the black carpet beetle and clothes moth larvae. When administered to mice it has been found to possess no activity against the viruses of poliomyelitis, influenza, feline pneumonia and Western equine encephalomyelitis. The LD_{50} in mice is 70 mg/kg when given subcutaneously and 17 mg/kg when administered intravenously.

Finlay, Sobin, *J. Amer. Chem. Soc.*, **73**, 341 (1951)
Finlay, Sobin, *U.S. Patent*, 2,586,762 (1952)
Schabel *et al.*, *Proc. Soc. Exptl. Biol. Med.*, **83**, 1 (1953)

NEUTRAMYCIN

$C_{34}H_{54}O_{14}$
M.p. 222–223°C

First isolated from a variant strain of *Streptomyces rimosus*, this macrolide antibiotic is obtained in higher yields from *S. luteoverticillatus* and forms colourless crystals from EtOH. It gives an ultraviolet spectrum having an absorption maximum at 216 nm and a shoulder at 240 nm. The structure given above has been determined by chemical and spectroscopic methods.

Lefemine *et al.*, *Antimicrobial Agents & Chemotherapy*, **41**, 137 (1963)
Kunstmann, Mitscher, Porter, *U.S. Patent*, 3,549,502 (1970)
Structure
Kuntsmann, Mitscher, *Experientia*, **21**, 372 (1965)
Mitscher, Kuntsmann, *ibid.*, **25**, 12 (1969)

NIGERICIN

$C_{39}H_{69}O_{11}$
M.p. 246–254°C

This complex antibiotic has been obtained from the culture of an unidentified species of *Streptomyces*. The substance may be obtained from the broth by extraction with several solvents including AcOEt, Et$_2$O, BuOH and butyl acetate or by adsorption on charcoal followed by elution with EtOH. It is an organic acid which crystallizes from EtOH as long, colourless needles. The sodium salt has also been prepared. The antibiotic is soluble in CH$_3$OH, EtOH and BuOH and slightly soluble in H$_2$O. It has been found to be quite stable at pH 7·0 for 2 hours at 100°C.

Nigericin is active against gram-positive bacteria, mycobacteria and some fungi, e.g. *Candida albicans* and *Trichoderma mentagrophytes*. It is only slightly active against gram-negative organisms and its biological activity is inhibited by the presence of potassium ions. The LD$_{50}$ in mice is 2·5 mg/kg when given intraperitoneally. Owing to its high toxicity it has found no use in medicine.

Harned *et al.*, *Antibiotics & Chemotherapy*, **1**, 594 (1951)

NIKKOMYCIN

$C_{20}H_{25}N_5O_{10}$

An antibiotic isolated from cultures of *Streptomyces tendae* TVE 901, this substance has been assigned the above structure on the basis of chemical and spectroscopic evidence. It is prepared by culturing the organism on a medium of mannitol and soybean meal at 27°C for 78 hours. Nikkomycin is useful in the control of *Botrytis cinerea* and *Uromyces phaseoli*.

Daehn *et al.*, *German Patent*, 2,537,028 (1977)

NILEMYCIN

A peptide antibiotic, nilemycin has been isolated from cultures of *Streptomyces parvullus nilenensis*. It is soluble in organic solvents and on acid hydrolysis it furnishes aspartic acid, lysine, serine, phenylalanine, tyrosine, valine and a mixture of tetra-, penta- and hexadecenoic acids.

Shim, Dewader, Mourad, *Antibiotica*, **12**, 5 (1974)

NIPHYMICINE

An antibiotic having antimycotic activity, niphymicine is produced by aerobic cultivation of *Streptomyces hygroscopicus* in a medium containing glucose, soybean flour and inorganic salts at 25–30°C for 70–80 hours. After separation of the biomass, this is dried, deoiled twice with butyl acetate and extracted with 65 per cent EtOH. The ethanol is then distilled off under reduced pressure leaving an aqueous suspension. The precipitate is then separated to yield a product which contains 1000 μg/mg of the antibiotic.

Georgieva *et al.*, *French Patent*, 1,604,171 (1971)

NITRAMINOACETIC ACID
$C_2H_4O_4N_2$
M.p. 106°C

$$O_2N-N(H)-CH_2COOH$$

This simple antibiotic substance has been isolated from cultures of *Streptomyces noursei* 8054-MC$_3$. It is active against a number of bacteria, inhibiting the growth of *Escherichia coli*, *Pseudomonas tabaci* and *Xanthomonas oryzae* at concentrations of 0·18, 0·78 and 25 μg/ml respectively. It has no inhibitory action against *Bacillus subtilis*, *Salmonella enteritidis* and *Shigella sonnei* at 100 μg/ml, nor was it active against fungi or yeasts. The LD_{50} in mice were 32 mg/kg (intravenous), 40 mg/kg (oral) and 43 mg/kg (intraperitoneal.)

Miyazaki *et al.*, *J. Antibiotics* (Japan), **21**, 279 (1968)

D-*threo*-1-(p-NITROPHENYL)-2-PROPIONAMIDO-1:3-PROPANEDIOL
$C_{12}H_{16}O_5N_2$

Japanese workers have prepared this antibiotic by the aerobic fermentation of carbohydrates by *Arthrobacter oxamicetus* var. *propiophenicolus* ATCC 21,814 at pH 7·0 and 28°C. The antibiotic is active against gram-positive and some gram-negative bacteria but is less active *in vivo* in mice than chloramphenicol. It is significantly less toxic, however, with LD_{50} of 2000 mg/kg on intravenous administration, compared with 280 mg/kg for chloramphenicol.

Kawaguchi *et al.*, *German Patent*, 2,343,798 (1974)

NITROSPORIN
$C_{20}H_{26}O_6N_2$

An antibiotic isolated from *Streptomyces fasciculus* (*S. nitrosporeus*), nitrosporin closely resembles proactinomycin. It is obtained by adsorption on activated carbon followed by elution with acidified $(CH_3)_2CO$ or by adsorption on a cation exchange resin and elution with dilute acid. The antibiotic is soluble in EtOH and AcOEt, slightly so in Et_2O and CH_2Cl_2 and insoluble in H_2O although the solubility is quite high in dilute acids. It possesses only a limited stability.

Nitrosporin is mainly active against gram-positive bacteria, showing only a limited activity against gram-negative organisms and no activity at all against mycobacteria. The LD_{50} in mice is 16 mg/kg when administered intravenously.

Umezawa, Takeuchi, *J. Antibiotics* (Japan), **5**, 270 (1952)

NOCAMYCIN
$C_{26}H_{33}NO_9$
M.p. 147–149°C

Nocardiopsis syringae elaborates this antibiotic which forms colourless crystals when purified by chromatography and crystallization. It is laevorotatory having a specific rotation of $[\alpha]_D^{20} - 50°$ ($CHCl_3$) and gives an ultraviolet spectrum having absorption maxima at 235 and 348 nm. Nocamycin has antitumour activity.

Brazhnikova *et al.*, *Antibiotiki*, **22**, 486 (1977)

NOCARDAMIN
$C_{27}H_{43}O_9N_6$
M.p. 192–195°C

A macrocyclic antibiotic, nocardamin has been isolated from cultures of *Actinomyces buchanan* and from a *Nocardia* species closely resembling *N. flavescens* obtained from old honeycombs. The original formulae of $C_8H_{16}O_2N_2$ and $C_9H_{14}O_3N_2$ have been revised to that given above. The antibiotic is obtained by extraction of the broth with BuOH followed by concentration *in vacuo*, extraction of the residue with hot H_2O and cooling when the antibiotic crystallizes as pale reddish needles. It is optically inactive, has no basic properties, and is soluble in boiling CH_3OH, slightly soluble in hot H_2O.

Nocardamin is active only against mycobacteria, showing no activity against bacteria or fungi. The mode of action of the antibiotic is bacteriostatic; only in high concentrations is it bactericidal. The activity against *Mycobacterium tuberculosis in vitro* is markedly decreased by serum. No data are available regarding its toxicity.

Stoll, Renz, Brack, *Helv. Chim. Acta*, **34**, 862 (1951)
Stoll *et al.*, *Pathol. Bakt.*, **14**, 225 (1951)

NOCARDIANIN
$C_{66}H_{100}O_{15}N_{18}$
M.p. 228–235°C (*dec.*)

A complex antibiotic, nocardianin has been isolated from a species of *Nocardia*. It is extracted from the mycelium with Et_2O and chromatographed on an alumina column with $CHCl_3$—EtOH. When purified by recrystallization from CH_3OH it forms deep red prisms and is laevorotatory with a specific rotation of $[\alpha]_D^{25} - 223°$ (c 0·3, CH_3OH). It is freely soluble in pyridine, $CHCl_3$ and glacial AcOH, moderately so in CH_3OH and $(CH_3)_2CO$, slightly soluble in Et_2O and H_2O and insoluble in CS_2, CCl_4 and petroleum ether. The ultraviolet spectrum in CH_3OH exhibits a single absorption maximum at 440 nm. It is an unstable substance and yields no aminoacids on hydrolysis. Although active against gram-positive bacteria, it shows no activity against gram-negative bacteria or mycobacteria.

Bick, Jann, Gram, *Antibiotics & Chemotherapy*, **21** 255 (1952)

NOCARDICIN A
$C_{23}H_{24}N_4O_9$

Nocardia uniformis subsp. *tsuyamanensis* ATCC 21806 yields a number of antibiotics which have been separated by chromatographic methods. This antibiotic forms colourless crystals and has been isolated and characterized as the sodium salt with m.p. 234–235°C and a specific rotation of $[\alpha]_D - 135·0°$ (H_2O). It is monocyclic β-lactam antibiotic and is moderately active *in vitro* against gram-positive bacteria. It exhibits a broad spectrum activity against gram-negative organisms, particularly against *Proteus* and *Pseudomonas* species. Tests have shown that it possesses a low toxicity in experimental animals.

Aoki *et al.*, *J. Antibiotics* (Japan), **29**, 492 (1976)
Structure
Hashimoto, Komori, Kamiya, *J. Amer. Chem. Soc.*, **98**, 3023 (1976)

NOCARDICIN B
$C_{23}H_{24}N_4O_9$
M.p. 262–264°C (*dec.*)

A further monocyclic-lactam antibiotic isolated from cultures of *Nocardia uniformis* subsp. *tsuyamanensis* ATCC 21806, this substance forms colourless crystals. It gives a sodium salt as colourless needles with m.p. 258–260°C (*dec.*) having a specific rotation of $[\alpha]_D - 162·0°$ (H_2O). The structure is stereoisomeric with that of the preceding antibiotic at the oxime group. It has an antibiotic activity similar to that of nocardicin A.

Aoki *et al.*, *J. Antibiotics* (Japan), **29**, 492 (1976)
Structure
Hashimoto, Komori, Kamiya, *J. Amer. Chem. Soc.*, **98**, 3023 (1976)

NOCARDICIN C
$C_{23}H_{28}N_4O_7$

Nocardia uniformis subsp. *tsuyamanensis* ATCC 21806 yields a number of structurally similar antibiotics which have been separated and purified by chromatographic methods. This antibiotic has the structure given above which has been established from chemical and spectroscopic evidence. It is particularly active in inhibiting the growth of *Pseudomonas aeruginosa*.

Hosoda *et al.*, *Agr. Biol. Chem.*, **41**, 2013 (1977)

NOCARDICIN D
$C_{23}H_{25}N_3O_8$

A diketonic antibiotic, this substance has been isolated from cultures of *Nocardia uniformis* subsp. *tsuyamanensis* ATCC 21806 and its structure elucidated from chemical correlations and a study of the infrared, NMR and mass spectra. It has an antibiotic activity similar to those of the other nocardicins.

Hosoda *et al.*, *Agr. Biol. Chem.*, **41**, 2013 (1977)

NOCARDICIN E
$C_{19}H_{19}N_3O_6$
M.p. 228–231°C (*dec.*)

A further antibiotic obtained from cultures of *Nocardia uniformis* subsp. *tsuyamanensis* ATCC 21806, this substance has the syn-oxime structure determined from chemical and spectroscopic data. It is inhibitory against *Pseudomonas aeruginosa* at a concentration of 125 micrograms/millilitre.

Hosoda *et al.*, *Agr. Biol. Chem.*, **41**, 2013 (1977)
Hosoda, Aoki, Imanaka, *German Patent*, 2,651,655 (1977)

NOCARDICIN F
$C_{19}H_{19}N_3O_6$
M.p. 230–231°C (*dec.*)

Nocardia uniformis subsp. *tsuyamanensis* ATCC 21806 also elaborates this antibiotic which is the anti-oxime form of nocardicin E. It is particularly active against *Pseudomonas aeruginosa*, having an inhibitory concentration of 100 micrograms/millilitre.

Hosoda *et al.*, *Agr. Biol. Chem.*, **41**, 2013 (1977)
Hosoda, Aoki, Imanaka, *German Patent*, 2,651,655 (1977)

NOCARDICIN G
$C_{19}H_{21}N_3O_5$

This antibiotic has also been isolated from the culture broth of *Nocardia uniformis* subsp. *tsuyamanensis* ATCC 21806 and shown to have the structure given above. It is active against a number of bacteria, especially *Pseudomonas aeruginosa*.

Hosoda *et al.*, *Agr. Biol. Chem.*, **41**, 2013 (1977)

NOCARDIN
Produced by *Nocardia coeliaca*, this antibiotic is obtained by extraction of the mycelium with a mixture of Et_2O and 95 per cent EtOH or by adsorption on activated carbon from the culture filtrate and elution with acidified EtOH or a mixture of Et_2O and 95 per cent EtOH. So far, the antibiotic has not been obtained in the pure state. The crude preparation is thermostable and soluble in H_2O.

Nocardin is active both *in vitro* and *in vivo* against *Mycobacterium tuberculosis* and in mice it has about one-tenth of the activity of streptomycin.

The filtrate of *N. coeliaca* also show a high degree of activity *in vitro* against *Micrococcus pyogenes* var. *aureus* and *Bacillus anthracis* and, to a somewhat lesser extent, against *Escherichia coli* and *Bacillus subtilis*. The crude nocardin appears to be appreciably more toxic than streptomycin.

Emmart, Kissling, Stark, *J. Bact.*, **57**, 509 (1949)
Levaditi, Henry, *Produits Pharm.*, **4**, 11 (1949)

NOFORMICIN
$C_8H_{15}ON_5$

A *Nocardia* antibiotic, noformicin has been obtained from *Nocardia formica*. Two isomeric forms of the substance are possible but only that which is obtained from the culture filtrate is biologically active. The dihydrochloride forms colourless crystals with m.p. 265°C (*dec.*); the sulphate crystallizes from aqueous CH_3OH, decomposing at 263°C and the picrate forms small yellow needles which decompose at 261–262°C. When hydrolysed, the antibiotic forms ammonia, glutamic acid and a variety of other bases. The structure has been established by chemical methods. Noformicin is soluble in H_2O and moderately so in common organic solvents. So far, its use has been limited to that of an experimental antiviral agent.

Harris, Woodruff, *Antibiotics Annual*, 609 (1953–54)
Gray, *Phytopath*, **45**, 281 (1955)
Peck, Schafer, Wolf, *U.S. Patent*, 2,804,463 (1957)

NOGALAMYCIN
M.p. 195–196°C (*dec.*)

This antibiotic is produced by a number of *Streptomyces* species and is obtained from the filtered broth by extraction with AcOEt and purified by repeated extraction with dilute acid, neutralized, and re-extracted with AcOEt. It is finally purified by chromatography on silica gel in CH_3OH—$CHCl_3$ and recrystallization from CH_3OH when it forms an orange-red solid. Acid hydrolysis furnishes nogalarol, $C_{29}H_{31}O_{13}N$, m.p. 220°C (*dec.*), nogalorene, $C_{29}H_{27}O_{11}N$, decomposing at 230°C, having a specific rotation of $[\alpha]_D^{25} + 843°$ ($CHCl_3$) and nogalose, $C_{10}H_{20}O_5$, m.p. 115–121°C and with a specific rotation of $[\alpha]_D^{25} - 10.6°$ (CH_3OH).

The antibiotic itself is strongly dextrorotatory with a specific rotation of $[\alpha]_D^{25} + 479°$ (c 1·0, $CHCl_3$). The ultraviolet spectrum in EtOH has absorption maxima at 236, 258, 292, 390 and 480 nm, shifted to 240, 259, 290 and 553 nm in alkaline EtOH solution.

Bhuyan, Dietz, *Antimicrobial Agents & Chemotherapy*, 836 (1965)
Bhuyan *et al.*, *U.S. Patent*, 3,183,157 (1965)
Wiley *et al.*, *Tetrahedron Lett.*, 663 (1968)

NOJIRIMYCIN
$C_6H_{13}O_5N$
M.p. 126–130°C (*dec.*)

A simple antibiotic, nojirimycin is elaborated by several species of *Streptomyces*. It forms colourless crystals and is dextrorotatory, the specific rotation falling from $[\alpha]_D^{24} + 100°$ to $+ 73.5°$ over a period of 20 hours. The structure of 2:3:4:5-tetrahydroxy-6-hydroxymethyl-piperidine, has been confirmed by synthesis. Nojirimycin is active primarily against gram-positive bacteria.

Inouye *et al.*, *Tetrahedron*, **24**, 2125 (1968)

NONACTIN
$C_{40}H_{64}O_{12}$
M.p. 148°C

A macrocyclic antibiotic, nonactine has been isolated from *Streptomyces* species which also produce actidione (q.v.). The antibiotic forms colourless needles when recrystallized from CH_3OH and is optically inactive in $CHCl_3$. The ultraviolet spectrum in CH_3OH exhibits a weak maximum at 264 nm. Hydrolysis furnishes nonactinic acid, $C_{10}H_{18}O_4$, a colourless liquid with b.p. 120°C/0·01 mm which is also optically inactive. Nonactin is extremely unreactive towards chemical compounds and microbes.

Corbaz et al., *Helv. Chim. Acta*, **38**, 1445 (1955)
Dominguez et al., *ibid.*, **45**, 129 (1962)
Beck et al., *ibid.*, **45**, 620 (1962)
Gerlach, Prelog, *Annalen*, **669**, 121 (1963)

NORCYCLINE
See Sencycline

NORPLICACETIN
$C_{24}H_{33}N_5O_7$

This antibiotic has been obtained from *Streptomyces plicatus* when the organism is cultured in a medium comprising sucrose, soybean meal, corn steep liquor, molasses and inorganic salts at 28°C for 118 hours with agitation. The antibiotic is extracted from the culture filtrate with BuOH and purified by column chromatography. It is active against gram-positive bacteria and *Mycobacteria*.

Evans, Weare, *J. Antibiotics* (Japan), **30**, 604 (1977)

NOSIHEPTIDE
$C_{51}H_{43}N_{13}O_{11}S_6$

A complex thiostrepton antibiotic, nosiheptide has been isolated from cultures of *Streptomyces actuosus*. The structure has been elucidated from chemical and spectroscopic evidence and confirmed by X-ray analysis, the crystals being tetragonal with space group I4 and cell constants a = b = 36·05 and c = 11·44 Å with Z = 8. Nosiheptide is highly active *in vitro* against gram-positive bacteria but has a much lower activity against gram-negative organisms.

Pagano et al., *Antibiotics Ann.*, 554 (1956)
Structure
Pranje et al., *Nature*, **265** (5990), 189 (1977)

NOTATIN
See Penatin

NOVALICHIN
M.p. Indefinite

Paecilomyces fusisporous ATCC 24148 elaborates this antibiotic. The optimum conditions for production of the compound have been found to be incubation of Czapek medium enriched with yeast extract and sucrose at 29–30°C and pH 4·5 for 13–17 days followed by inoculation of the medium with the organism and stationary aeration. Novalichin forms a yellow amorphous powder and is active against filamentous fungi and yeasts, particularly plant pathogens, e.g. *Candida albicans* and *Ceratostomella paradoxa*. It has no activity against gram-positive or gram-negative bacteria.

Gabriel *et al.*, *J. Philips. Med. Assoc.*, **42**, 299 (1973)
Tumangan, Santos, Gabriel, *Acta Manilana.*, **11A**, 19 (1973)

NOVENAMINE
$C_{19}H_{24}O_9N_2$

An enzymic cleavage product of novobiocin (q.v.), this antibiotic is obtained by incubating *Arthrobacter* species N18 (NRRL B-3652) on a medium containing glucose, enzymically-degraded casein and inorganic salts at 28°C and pH 6·8–7·8, centrifuging the cells, suspending in H_2O and adding the sodium salt of novobiocin. Following incubation under nitrogen for 20 hours, the cells are centrifuged and the cell-free solution treated with 6N-HCl, washed with CH_2Cl_2 and freeze-dried. The antibiotic is active against gram-positive bacteria.

Sebek, Hoeksema, *German Patent*, 2,026,687 (1970)

NOVOBIOCIN
$C_{31}H_{36}O_{11}N_2$
M.p. 152–156°C (*dec.*); 174–178°C

A glycosidic antibiotic, novobiocin has been isolated from various species of *Streptomyces* including *S. niceus*, *S. niveas* and *S. spheroides*. In the literature it has been described under a variety of pseudonyms, e.g. Albamycin, Biotexin, Cardelmycin, Cathocin, Cathomycin, Inamycin, Spheromycin, Streptonivicin, Vulcamycin and Vulkamycin. When recrystallized from $(CH_3)_2CO$ it forms pale yellow orthorhombic crystals which are sensitive to light. Two crystal modifications have been obtained, that having the higher melting point being only rarely encountered. Novobiocin is laevorotatory with a specific rotation of $[\alpha]_D^{24} - 63°$ (c 1·0, EtOH) and gives an ultraviolet spectrum in alkaline EtOH with an absorption maximum at 306 nm which is shifted to 330 nm in acid EtOH. It is soluble in aqueous solutions above pH 7·5 but almost insoluble under more acid conditions. It is also soluble in AcOEt, amyl acetate, $(CH_3)_2CO$ and the lower alcohols. Two sodium salts are known, the acid sodium salt which is crystalline, m.p. 210–215°C; $[\alpha]_D^{25} - 34°$ (c 1·08, H_2O) and the disodium salt which forms an amorphous white powder with no definite melting point.

The antibiotic is active against gram-positive organisms and is used in medicine as an antimicrobial, the normal dose being between 250 and 500 mg given orally. Side effects are jaundice, skin rashes and blood dyscrasias. Novobiocin also finds use in veterinary work, particularly against infections caused by *Staphylococcus aureus* either in primary infections such as septicemia or in secondary complications, e.g. feline panleukopenia and distemper. Here, it is normally used where the disease has proved resistant to other antibiotics at a dose of 10–30 mg given intramuscularly.

Kaczka *et al.*, *J. Amer. Chem. Soc.*, **77**, 6404 (1955)
Hinman *et al.*, *ibid.*, **78**, 1072 (1956)
Shunk *et al.*, *ibid.*, **78**, 1770, 2655, 5454 (1956)
Hinman *et al.*, *ibid.*, **79**, 3789 (1957)
Weiss *et al.*, *Antibiotics & Chemotherapy*, **7**, 374 (1957)
Vaterlaus *et al.*, *Experientia*, **19**, 383 (1963)
Structure
    Hoeksema *et al.*, *J. Amer. Chem. Soc.*, **78**, 2019 (1956)
    Walton *et al.*, *ibid.*, **82**, 1489 (1960)
Conformation
    Golding, Richards, *Chem. Ind.* (London), 1081 (1963)
Synthesis
    Stammer, *U.S. Patent*, 2,925,411 (1960)
    Walton, Spencer, *U.S. Patent*, 2,966,484 (1960)
    Vaterlaus *et al.*, *Helv. Chim. Acta*, **47**, 390 (1964)

NUCLEOCIDIN
$C_{11}H_{16}O_8N_6S$
M.p. Indefinite

This antibiotic obtained from cultures of *Streptomyces calvus* is said to be a glycoside of adenine in which sulphamic acid is present as an ester of the carbohydrate moeity. The antibiotic is characterized as the crystalline picrate, m.p. 143–144°C.

Waller et al., *J. Amer. Chem. Soc.*, **79**, 1911 (1957)
Thomas et al., *U.S. Patent*, 2,914,525 (1959)

NUDIC ACID A
$C_{14}H_{20}O_3$?
M.p. 123–125°C

A species of *Basidiomycete*, *Tricholoma nudum*, produces a number of antibiotic substances of which two have been examined in detail. Nudic acid A forms large colourless needles or plates when purified by recrystallization from *n*-hexane. It is optically inactive in EtOH and is readily soluble in the common organic solvents, slightly soluble in H_2O and dissolves freely in sodium carbonate and sodium hydroxide solutions.

Heatley, *Antibiotics*, Vol. I, Ed. Florey et al., Oxford University Press (1949)

NUDIC ACID B
See Diatretyne II

NYBOMYCIN
$C_{16}H_{14}O_4N_2$
M.p. 325–330°C

Nybomycin has been isolated from streptomycete A 717, isolated from a sample of soil from Missouri. It is purified by recrystallization from AcOH when it forms colourless needles which sublime at 250°C/15 mm. The antibiotic is optically inactive and gives an ultraviolet spectrum with absorption maxima at 266 and 285 nm. It is only slightly soluble in H_2O, alkalies and common organic solvents but dissolves readily in concentrated mineral acids. It forms a crystalline acetate, m.p. 236–237°C and a succinate which is virtually insoluble in H_2O.

Nybomycin is active against gram-positive bacteria and also possesses antiphage properties. It is comparatively non-toxic, 250 mg/kg of a suspension in peanut oil given intraperitoneally being tolerated by mice.

Strelitz, *Proc. Nat. Acad. Sci.*, **41**, 620 (1955)
Eble et al., *Antibiotics & Chemotherapy*, **8**, 627 (1958)
Brock, Sokolski, *ibid.*, **8**, 631 (1958)
Structure
Rinehart, Renfroe, *J. Amer. Chem. Soc.*, **83**, 3729 (1961)

NYPHIMYCIN
M.p. Indefinite

An antibiotic elaborated by *Streptomyces hygroscopicus* strains NRRL 2751 and 2752 cultivated under submerged aerobic conditions in aqueous nutrient media for 2–4 days at 26–32°C. The compound is extracted from the myceluim by conventional techniques and has a bacteriostatic activity of 800–1000 units/ml. Nyphimycin is insoluble in H_2O and inhibits the development of Ehrlich carcinoma cells and also inactivtes herpes virus.

DSO Farmakhim, *British Patent*, 1,254,721 (1971)

NYSTATIN (*Fungicidin, Moronal, Mycostatin, Nystan*)
$C_{46}H_{83}O_{18}N$
Dec. 160°C

Streptomyces noussei produces a polyene antibiotic complex which possesses marked antifungal properties. Nystatin forms a pale yellow powder which begins to decompose at 160°C without melting. It gives an ultraviolet spectrum in EtOH with absorption maxima at 290, 307 and 322 nm and has the following specific rotations: $[\alpha]_D^{25} + 21°$ (pyridine); $[\alpha]_D^{25} - 10°$ (glacial AcOH); $[\alpha]_D^{25} - 7°$ (0·1 N-HCl in CH_3OH) and $[\alpha]_D^{25} + 12°$ (dimethylformamide). It is insoluble in H_2O, soluble in dimethylformamide, CH_3OH, EtOH and propylene glycol. In solution, and as a suspension in H_2O, it rapidly begins to lose its activity although aqueous suspensions are stable at 100°C for 10 minutes at pH 7·0. Light, oxygen and heat accelerate decomposition of this substance. Nystatin has been shown to be a complex mixture of dienes and tetraenes, one component of which has the probable structure given above.

Nystatin is active against fungi and yeasts but not against bacteria or viruses. It is not inactivated by either blood or serum. The LD_{50} in mice is about 200 mg/kg when administered intraperitoneally. In medicine it has found some use as an antimonial for oral or topical administration. Side effects include skin irritation and diarrhoea.

Hazen, Brown, *Science*, **112**, 423 (1950)
Hazen, Brown, *Proc. Soc. Exptl. Biol. Med.*, **76**, 93 (1951)
Dutcher, Walter, Wintersteiner, *Congr. intern. biochem. Resumes communs. 3° Congr. Brussels*, 1 (1951)
Raubitscheck, Acker, Waksman, *Antibiotics & Chemotherapy*, **2**, 179 (1952)
Cohen, Webb, *Arch. Pediatrics*, **69**, 414 (1952)
Dutcher *et al.*, *Antibiotics Annual*, **191** (1953–54)
Walter, Dutcher, Wintersteiner, *J. Amer. Chem. Soc.*, **79**, 5076 (1957)
Birch *et al.*, *Tetrahedron Lett.*, 1491 (1964)

OBTUSIN

An antibiotic derived from a species of *Basidiomycete*, little is yet known concerning its chemical, biological and physical characteristics.

Robbins, Kavanagh, Hervey, *J. N.Y. Bot. Gardens*, **46**, 130 (1945)

OLEANDOMYCIN (*Amimycin, Landomycin, Matromycin, Romicil*)
$C_{35}H_{61}O_{12}N$
M.p. 110°C (*dec.*)

This macrocyclic antibiotic has been isolated from *Streptomyces antibioticus* ATCC 11891. It is normally obtained as an amorphous white powder although a crystalline form, obtained from EtOH, has been described which decomposes at the melting point given above. It is laevorotatory with a specific rotation of $[\alpha]_D^{25} - 65°$ (c 1·0, CH_3OH) and gives an ultraviolet spectrum in CH_3OH with an absorption maximum at 286–289 nm. Oleandomycin is readily soluble in CH_3OH, EtOH, BuOH and $(CH_3)_2CO$, moderately so in H_2O and dilute acids, insoluble in CCl_4, hexane and dibutyl ether. The hydrochloride crystallizes from AcOEt as long, colourless needles, m.p. 134–135°C and has a specific rotation of $[\alpha]_D^{25} - 54°$ (c 1·0, CH_3OH). The three hydroxyl groups may be acetylated to give the triacetate (Euramycin) which forms colourless crystals from *iso*PrOH, decomposing at 176°C and having $[\alpha]_D^{25} - 23°$ (CH_3OH). The antibiotic is normally used as the hydrochloride which forms a number of crystalline hydrates and has LD_{50} in mice of 15 mg/20 g mouse when administered intravenously.

Oleandomycin finds some use in medicine as an antimicrobial, the normal dose being 200 mg given intramuscularly.

Sobin, English, Celmer, *Antibiotics Annual*, 87 (1954–55)
Celmer, Murai, *ibid.*, 476 (1957–1958)
Els, Celmer, Murai, *J. Amer. Chem. Soc.*, **80**, 3777 (1958)
Celmer, *Antibiotics Annual*, 277 (1958–1959)
Hochstein *et al.*, *J. Amer. Chem. Soc.*, **82**, 3225 (1960)
Celmer, *ibid.*, **87**, 1797 (1965)
Popov, Dzhezhev, *Gig. Sanit.*, 83 (1973)
Soifer *et al.*, *Antibiotiki*, **18**, 11 (1973)
Kleiner *et al.*, *Soviet Patent*, 145,720 (1973)

3-O-OLENDROSYL-5-O-DESOSAMINYL ERYTHRONOLIDE A OXIME
$C_{36}H_{66}N_2O_{13}$

A semi-synthetic macrocyclic antibiotic produced from erythronolide A oxime by *Streptomyces antibioticus* ATCC 11891, this substance has been found to possess a lower antibiotic activity than erythronolide A oxime but has the advantage of being more stable in the presence of acid.

Lemahieu *et al.*, *J. Antibiotics* (Japan), **29**, 728 (1976)

OLEFICIN
$C_{34}H_{47}O_9N$
M.p. Indefinite

Streptomyces strain A-461, related to *S. parvullus*, elaborates this antibiotic which has the above polyene structure based upon degradation and spectroscopic studies. The original formula of $C_{38}H_{55}O_{10}N$ has been revised to that given above. The organism is cultured in a medium containing glucose, soybean flour, corn steep liquor, casamino acid and inorganic salts at pH 3·0 in a shaken culture. Oleficin is a dark red-black solid with no definite melting point. It is soluble in CH_3OH, moderately soluble in C_6H_6, $(CH_3)_2CO$ and AcOEt, slightly soluble in CCl_4 and insoluble in H_2O and petroleum ether.

Oleficin is active against gram-positive bacteria but not against fungi or yeasts. It is also effective in mice against Yoshida sarcoma when given subcutaneously. The LD_{50} in mice is 40 mg/kg given subcutaneously.

Gyimesi *et al.*, *Hung. Teljes*, 423 (1970)
Gyimesi *et al.*, *J. Antibiotics* (Japan), **24**, 277 (1971)
Structure
Horvath, Gyimesi, Mehesfalvi-Vajna, *Tetrahedron Lett.*, 3643 (1973)

OLEOMORPHOCYCLINE
$C_{62}H_{94}O_{21}N_4$
M.p. Indefinite

A macrocyclic, semi-synthetic antibiotic, oleomorphocycline is active against *Brucella abortus*, *B. melitensis* and *B. suis in vitro* and, *in vivo*, against *B. melitensis*. When given at a dose of 10–15 mg/day intramuscularly to mice infected with the latter organism it rendered 90–95 per cent of the animals free of the bacterium after 15 days. Under these conditions, the drug is found in the blood, intestine, liver, kidneys, lung, spleen, stomach and muscles 3–12 hours after injection. When applied in the form of an aerosol it is located only in the blood and lungs.

Surdzhiiska, Bessarabov, *Mater. Vses. Nauch. Soveshch. Konf. Vses. Nauch.-Issled. Tekhnol. Inst. Ptitsevod*, No. 5, 365 (1972)
Kutyreva, Uraleva, *Probl. Osobo Opasnykh Infekts.*, 97 (1974)

OLIGOMYCIN A
$C_{45}H_{74}O_{11}$
M.p. 140–141°C; 150–151°C

One of a number of antifungal antibiotics obtained from *Streptomyces diastatochromogenes*, this compound exists in two crystal modifications with the above melting points when crystallized from a mixture of Et_2O and light petroleum. The lower melting modification forms slender needles whereas the other exists as hexagonal plates. The antibiotic has a specific rotation of $[\alpha]_D^{23} - 54·5°$ (c 4·4, dioxan). It is readily soluble in $(CH_3)_2CO$, EtOH, AcOH and Et_2O, sparingly so in C_6H_6 and almost insoluble in H_2O and petroleum ether. The diacetate crystallizes from CCl_4-light petroleum with m.p. 112–113°C and $[\alpha]_D^{24} - 86·1°$ (c 1·74, EtOH). The original formula of $C_{24}H_{40}O_6$ has been revised to that given above.

Masamune *et al.*, *J. Amer. Chem. Soc.*, **80**, 6092 (1958)
Revised formula
Chamberlain, Gorman, Agtarap, *Biochem. Biophys. Res. Commun.*, **34**, 448 (1969)
Prouty, Schnoes, Strong, *ibid.*, **34**, 511 (1969)

OLIGOMYCIN B
$C_{45}H_{72}O_{12}$
M.p. 160–161°C

Also obtained from cultures of *Streptomyces diastatochromogenes*, this antifungal antibiotic forms colourless platelets when crystallized from CH_3OH. It has a specific rotation of $[\alpha]_D^{23\cdot5} - 49\cdot5°$ (c 1·03, CH_3OH) and is freely soluble in $(CH_3)_2CO$, Et_2O and C_6H_6, less so in AcOH and EtOH and only slightly soluble in H_2O or light petroleum. The diacetate forms colourless crystals, m.p. 135·5–136·5°C; $[\alpha]_D^{25} - 66\cdot6°$ (c 0·63, dioxan). Like the preceding antibiotic, the empirical formula for this compound has recently been revised.

Masamune et al., *J. Amer. Chem. Soc.*, **80**, 6092 (1958)
Revised formula
Chamberlain, Gorman, Agterap, *Biochem. Biophys. Res. Commun.*, 34 (1969)
Prouty, Schnoes, Strong, *ibid.*, **34**, 511 (1969)

OLIGOMYCIN C
$C_{28}H_{46}O_6$
M.p. 198–200°C
A third antifungal antibiotic isolated from cultures of *Streptomyces diastatochromogenes*, this substance crystallizes from Et_2O-light petroleum as colourless rods. It is laevorotatory with a specific rotation of $[\alpha]_D^{23} - 80\cdot7°$ (c 3·7, dioxan) and dissolves freely in AcOH, $(CH_3)_2CO$, EtOH and Et_2O, less so in C_6H_6 and is virtually insoluble in H_2O or light petroleum.

Masamune et al., *J. Amer. Chem. Soc.*, **80**, 6092 (1958)

OLIVOMYCIN
This antibiotic is elaborated by *Streptomyces olivoreticuli* grown on common nutrient media. Karpov and his colleagues have demonstrated from radioactive tracer studies, adding methionine-methyl-^{14}C to the medium, that the radioactivity is in the glucoside intermediate of the antibiotic.

Karpov et al., *Antibiotiki*, **17**, 693 (1972)

OOSPOREIN (*Chaetomidin*)
$C_{14}H_{10}O_8$
M.p. 290–295°C

Oosporein has been isolated from a number of species, e.g. *Acremonium* species, *Beauveria bassiana*, *Chaetomium aureus* Chivers and *Oospora colorans* van Beyma. It is a dimeric quinone and forms bronze-coloured plates when crystallized from aqueous CH_3OH. The ultraviolet spectrum in EtOH has two absorption maxima at 216 and 287 nm. The antibiotic has been characterized as the tetramethyl ether which forms orange needles from aqueous CH_3OH, m.p. 123°C, giving an ultraviolet spectrum in EtOH with adsorption maxima at 285·5 and 394 nm, and the tetraacetate, yellow needles from EtOH, m.p. 190°C, with an ultraviolet spectrum in EtOH consisting of a single absorption maximum at 262 nm.

Kögl, van Wessem, *Rev. Trav. Chim.*, **63**, 5 (1944)
Lloyd et al., *J. Chem. Soc.*, 2163 (1955)
Divekar et al., *Can. J. Chem.*, **37**, 2097 (1959)
Vining et al., *Can. J. Microbiol.*, **8**, 931 (1962)
See also
Smith, Thompson, *Tetrahedron*, **10**, 148 (1960)

OPHIOCORIN
$C_{21}H_{22}N_2O_8$
An antibiotic produced by culturing *Cordyceps ophiglossoides* strain TU276 in submerged culture in a medium consisting of glycerol, soybean meal at 27°C. The fermentation medium is acidified and the antibiotic extracted with BuOH and purified by column chromatography on DEAE-Sephadex and cellulose. Ophiocorin is effective against a small range of fungi but is not active against bacteria. It has a limited use since the antifungal action is antagonized by ammonium and nitrate ions and certain aminoacids.

Kneifel et al., *Arch. Microbiol.*, **113**, 121 (1977)

ORACILLIN
See Penicillin V

ORIENTOMYCIN
See Oxamycin

ORYZACHLORIN
$C_{23}H_{31}O_8N_2S_2Cl$
M.p. 210°C (*dec.*)
This antibiotic from *Aspergillus oryzae* has recently been described by Japanese workers. Little is yet known concerning its structure and biological activity.

Kato et al., *Japanese Patent*, 7,200,035 (1972)

ORYZACIDIN
$C_8H_{13}O_5N$
Dec. 162–163°C
Produced by a strain of *Aspergillus oryzae*, this antibiotic forms colourless hygroscopic needles which decompose before melting. It is laevorotatory with with a specific rotation of $[\alpha]_D^{13.5} - 133°$ and is readily soluble in H_2O, CH_3OH, EtOH, *iso*PrOH and hot $(CH_3)_2CO$, slightly soluble in BuOH AcOEt, and virtually insoluble in $(CH_3)_2CO$, Et_2O, $CHCl_3$ and CCl_4. It is active against gram-positive bacteria.

Shimoda, *J. Agr. Chem. Soc., Japan*, **25**, 254 (1951)
Shimoda, *Japanese Patent*, 1594 (1952)

ORYZACIDIN A
$C_{22}H_{34}O_{12}N_4$
M.p. 231°C
This antibiotic has been isolated from cultures of a *Streptomyces* species and forms an amorphous orange powder. It is readily soluble in most organic solvents but insoluble in H_2O, hexane, $(CH_3)_2CO$, CS_2, *iso*propyl ether and petroleum ether. The ultraviolet spectrum in EtOH has a single absorption maximum at 243 nm.

Shimoda, *Japanese Patent*, 13,198 (1965)

ORYZOXYMYCIN
$C_{10}H_{13}O_5N$

Streptomyces venezuelae var. *oryzoxymyceticus*, freshly isolated from soil, elaborates this antibiotic. The organism is grown in a medium containing sucrose and inorganic salts at 27°C for 3 days and the antibiotic isolated from the culture filtrate by ion exchange resin treatment. Oryzoxymycin is dextrorotatory with a specific rotation of $[\alpha]_D^{22} + 349°$ (c 1·0, H_2O). The structure given above has been established from chemical and spectroscopic evidence. The antibiotic is active against *Xanthomonas oryzae* but other plant pathogenic fungi appear to be insensitive to it. It is relatively non-toxic, the LD_{50} in mice being 50–100 mg/kg when administered intravenously. Hashimoto and his colleagues have recently determined the absolute configuration of the antibiotic.

Hashimoto *et al., J. Antibiotics* (Japan), **21**, 653 (1968)
Hashimoto *et al., ibid.*, **25**, 350 (1972)
Umezawa *et al., Japanese Patent*, 7,140,759 (1971)
Absolute configuration
Hashimoto *et al., J. Antibiotics* (Japan), **27**, 86 (1974)

OSTREOGRYCIN (*E129 Complex*)
A group of antibiotics has been isolated from a soil organism *Streptomyces ostreogriseus* which, by a combination of fractional precipitation, counter-current distribution and chromatographic analysis, has been separated into six individual members, ostreogrycins A, B, B_1, B_2, B_3 and G. Structurally, these fall into two groups, A and G forming one and B, B_1, B_2 and B_3 the other. When tested individually, these antibiotics possess only a low activity but they show a strong synergism with mixtures of the two groups, or of individuals from each group having a marked activity against gram-positive bacteria. The properties of the individual members are described below.

Ball *et al., Biochem. J.*, **68**, 24P (1958)
Bessell *et al., ibid.*, **68**, 24P (1958)

OSTREOGRYCIN A (*Staphylomycin M, Antibiotic PA 114A*)
$C_{28}H_{35}O_7N_3$
M.p. 203–205°C

The pure antibiotic crystallizes from AcOEt as colourless laths and is laevorotatory with a specific rotation of $[\alpha]_D^{20} - 218°$ (c 0·34, EtOH). The ultraviolet spectrum in 95 per cent EtOH has an absorption maximum at 228 nm and an inflexion at 272 nm; in 6*N*-ethanolic HCl the absorption maximum is at 303 nm and in 0·2*N*-ethanolic NaOH it is shifted to 293 nm. The structure given has been confirmed by high resolution mass spectrometry of the fully reduced compound and NMR examination of the antibiotic itself.

Structure
Delpierre *et al., J. Chem. Soc.*, C, 1653 (1966)
Kingston, Lord Todd, Williams, *ibid.*, 1669 (1966)

OSTREOGRYCIN B$_1$
See Vernamycin B$_\gamma$

OSTREOGRYCIN B$_2$
See Vernamycin B$_\beta$

OSTREOGRYCIN B$_3$
$C_{45}H_{54}O_{11}N_8$
M.p. 215°C

A polypeptide antibiotic, ostreogrycin B$_3$ occurs as a minor constituent of the ostreogrycin complex isolated from *Streptomyces ostreogriseus*. It has a specific rotation of $[\alpha]_D^{25} - 57°$ (c 1·0, CH$_3$OH). The structure has been established from chemical degradation and spectroscopic investigation.

Cox *et al.*, *Chem. Commun.*, 1623 (1970)

OXACILLIN
$C_{19}H_{19}O_5N_3S$

A somewhat unstable antibiotic of the pencillanic type, oxacillin is normally prepared as the crystalline sodium salt which has m.p. 188°C (*dec.*) and a specific rotation of $[\alpha]_D^{20} + 201°$ (c 1·0, H$_2$O). The structure is 6-(5-methyl-3-phenyl-1-*iso*xazolecarboxamido)penicillanic acid. The antibiotic is resistant to penicillinase and is useful in medicine and vetinary work in the treatment of diseases produced by penicillin-resistant gram-positive organisms. The normal dose for humans is 0·5–1·0 g given orally. Side effects which have been observed include pruritus, rashes and gastrointestinal disturbances. The antibacterial activity persists in the serum for 2–3 hours, the rapid decrease in this level thereafter being due to its urinary excretion.

Doyle *et al.*, *Nature*, 1183 (1961)
Doyle, Nayler, *U.S. Patent*, 2,996,501 (1962)
Gilain, Stadtsbaeder, *Ann. Inst. Pasteur, Paris*, **120**, 599 (1971)
Windorfer, *Monatsschr. Kinderheilk.*, **121**, 469 (1973)
Sadowski, Tubylewicz, *Pol. Tyg. Lek.*, **29**, 355 (1974)

OXAMICETIN
$C_{29}H_{42}O_{10}N_6$
M.p. 176–179°C

A recently discovered antibiotic, this substance has been isolated from the fermentation broth of *Arthrobacter oxamicetus*. It forms colourless crystals and is characterized as the hydrochloride, m.p. 205–210°C (*dec.*); $[\alpha]_D^{25} + 66°$ (c 0·4, H$_2$O). The antibiotic possesses antitubercular and antileukemic properties similar to those of amicetin (q.v.).

Konishi *et al.*, *J. Antibiotics* (Japan), **26**, 752, 757 (1973)

OXAMYCIN (*Cycloserine, Orientomycin*)
$C_3H_6O_2N_2$
M.p. 156°C (*dec.*)

A simple antibiotic isolated from *Streptomyces garyphalus S. lavendulae, S. nagasakiensis* and *S. orchidaceus*, oxamycin forms colourless crystals from EtOH. It has $[\alpha]_{5461}^{25} + 137°$ (c 5·0, 2N-NaOH). The structure has been established as D-4-amino-3-*iso*xazolidone.

Harris *et al., Antibiotics & Chemotherapy*, **5**, 183 (1955)
Harned, Hidy, la Baw, *ibid.*, **5**, 204 (1955)
Stammer *et al., J. Amer. Chem. Soc.*, **79**, 3236 (1957)

OXAZINOMYCIN
$C_9H_{11}O_7N$
M.p. 164–166°C

A new antibiotic produced by *Streptomyces tanesashiensis* when freshly isolated from soil. The organism is cultured, after a 7-day preculture, on a medium containing glucose, peptone and yeast extract. The antibiotic has been purified by filtration of the broth, column chromatography on silica gel and activated carbon and recrystallization from CH_3OH. It is dextrorotatory with a specific rotation of $[\alpha]_D^{20} + 19·7°$ (c 1·0, H_2O) and is soluble in H_2O, CH_3OH, EtOH and BuOH, insoluble in hexane, C_6H_6, $(CH_3)_2CO$, AcOEt and $CHCl_3$. The minimum inhibition concentration against some strains of *Staphylococcus aureus* was 1·56–12·5 µg/ml but greater than 500 µg/ml against *Candida albicans, Escherichia coli, Mycobacterium smegmatis, Proteus vulgaris, Pseudomonas aeruginosa* and *Trichophyton interdigitale*. When administered to mice with ascites tumour at a dose of 1·25 mg/kg it prolonged the survival period.

Haneishi *et al., Japanese Patent*, 7,316,198 (1973)

OXOTOMAYCIN
$C_{15}H_{16}O_4N_2$

An antitumour antibiotic, oxotomaymycin is elaborated by *Streptomyces achromogenes*. The structure has been established from chemical and spectroscopic data.

Kariyone, Yazawa, Kohsaka, *Chem. Pharm. Bull.*, **19**, 2289 (1971)

OXYPYRROLNITRIN
$C_{10}H_6O_3N_2Cl_2$
M.p. 215–216°C (*dec.*)

Pseudomonas pyrrolnitrica and other pyrrolnitrin-producing species of *Pseudomonas* elaborate this antibiotic. The organism is cultivated, with aeration, on a medium containing glycerol, dry yeast, corn steep liquor and inorganic salts at 30°C for 3 days. The cells are then extracted with $(CH_3)_2CO$, the extract evaporated *in vacuo*, dissolved in Et_2O and shaken with 5 per cent NaOH, leaving the antibiotic in the ethereal layer. This is chromatographed to give the pure compound. Oxypyrrolnitrin inhibits the growth of *Trichophyton asteroides* at a concentration of 20 µg/ml.

Hattor, Hashimoto, Ohasi, *Japanese Patent*, 7,029,432 (1970)

OXYTETRACYCLINE
See Terramycin

P

PACTAMYCIN
$C_{28}H_{38}O_8N_4$
M.p. Indefinite

An antibiotic obtained from *Streptomyces pactum*, pactamycin forms an amorphous powder with no definite melting point. It has a specific rotation of $[\alpha]_D^{24} + 79°$ (c 1·0, EtOH) and gives an ultraviolet spectrum in EtOH with absorption maxima at 239, 313 and 356 nm with a shoulder at 264 nm. Cheung et al. have demonstrated that in the presence of this antibiotic there was a marked reduction in polymethionine synthesis in rabbit reticulocyte ribosomes in the presence of poly r(A-U-G) messenger and peptide initiation factors, accompanied by a concomitant increase in the synthesis of met–met and met–val dipeptide. From the observations it appeared that the latter dipeptide was synthesized in response to endogenous hemoglobin messenger.

Argoudelis, Jahnke, Fox, *Antimicrobial Agents & Chemotherapy*, 191 (1961)
Cheung, Stewart, Gupta, *Biochem. Biophys. Res. Commun.*, **54**, 1092 (1973)

PAECILOMYCEROL
$C_{27}H_{40}O_4$
M.p. 193–194°C

Paecilomyces elegans elaborates this antibiotic which forms colourless needles from CH_3OH. The ultraviolet spectrum in CH_3OH consists of a single absorption maximum at 293 nm. The antibiotic is obtained by culturing the organism, with shaking and aeration, in an aqueous medium containing glucose, peptone, yeast extract and inorganic salts at 26·5°C for 4 days.

Kato et al., *J. Antibiotics* (Japan), **22A**, 419 (1969)
Tamura et al., *Japanese Patent*, 7,200,040 (1972)

PAPULACANDIN A
$C_{47}H_{66}O_{16}$
A minor constituent of an antibiotic complex produced by the culture of *Papularia sphaerosperma* on a common nutrient medium. The antibiotic has been separated from the accompanying substances by chromatographic techniques and is active against *Candida albicans* and a number of other yeasts.

Traxler, Grunger, Auden, *J. Antibiotics* (Japan), **30**, 289 (1977)

PAPULACANDIN B
$C_{47}H_{64}O_{17}$
The main component of papulacandin isolated from cultures of *Papularia spaerosperma*, this antibiotic has an antiyeast activity, particularly against *Candida albicans*. The structure has not yet been fully established.

Traxler, Grunger, Auden, *J. Antibiotics* (Japan), **30**, 289 (1977)

PAPULACANDIN C
$C_{47}H_{64}O_{17}$
A third constituent of the antibiotic complex produced by culturing *Papularia sphaerosperma* on a common nutrient medium, this substance has an activity similar to that of the two preceding antibiotics. The structure is not known.

Traxler, Grunger, Auden, *J. Antibiotics* (Japan), **30**, 289 (1977)

PAPULACANDIN D
$C_{31}H_{42}O_{10}$
Paularia sphaerosperma also elaborates this complex antibiotic when grown on a common nutrient medium. It has been separated from the accompanying antibiotics by column and thin layer chromatography and is effective against *Candida albicans* and certain other yeasts.

Traxler, Grunger, Auden, *J. Antibiotics* (Japan), **30**, 289 (1977)

PAPULACANDIN E

This antibiotic obtained from the papulacandin complex from the fermentation broth of *Papularia sphaerosperma* is present only in small quantities and has not yet been extensively investigated.

Traxler, Grunger, Auden, *J. Antibiotics* (Japan), **30**, 289 (1977)

PAROMAMINE
$C_{11}H_{25}N_3O_7$

An antibiotic produced by *Streptomyces rimosus* forma *paromomycinus*, this compound has the structure given above based upon chemical and spectroscopic evidence. It is dextrorotatory having a specific rotation of $[\alpha]_D^{26} + 114°$ (c 1·35, H_2O) and has been characterized as the trihydrochloride which crystallizes as the hemihydrate and the N,N,N-triacetate which forms colourless crystals having a specific rotation of $[\alpha]_D^{25} + 108°$ (c 1·0, H_2O). It has an antibiotic activity similar to that of the paromomycins.

Haskell, French, Bartz, *J. Amer. Chem. Soc.*, **81**, 3480, 3482 (1959)
Hessler *et al.*, *J. Antibiotics* (Japan), **23**, 464 (1970)
Synthesis
Umezawa, Koto, *J. Antibiotics* (Japan), **19**, 88 (1966)
Umezawa *et al.*, *ibid.*, **25**, 530 (1972)

PAROMOMYCIN (*Catenulin, Hydroxymycin, Monomycin A*)
$C_{23}H_{45}O_{14}N_5$
M.p. Indefinite

A glycosidic antibiotic, paromomycin has been isolated from cultures of *Streptomyces catenulae* and *S. rimosus* forma *paromomycinus*. It forms an amorphous white powder with no definite melting point and is dextrorotatory with a specific rotation of $[\alpha]_D^{25} + 64°$ (c 1·0, H_2O). A further preparation of paromoycin from *S. microsporeus* has been described by Ezaki *et al.* who cultured the organism in a medium consisting of millet honey, soybean flour, wheat embryos and sodium chloride at 30°C for 2 days. The specific rotation given for this material was $[\alpha]_D^{25} + 61°$ (c 0·5, H_2O). Paromomycin is soluble in H_2O, moderately soluble in CH_3OH but only sparingly so in absolute EtOH. The hydrochloride has a specific rotation of $[\alpha]_D^{25} + 56·5°$ (c 1·0, H_2O) and is more soluble in hot H_2O than in cold. The sulphate has also been prepared with $[\alpha]_D^{25} + 50·5°$ (c 1·5, H_2O). Paromomycin has been shown to be identical with catenulin, hydroxymycin and monomycin A and may be identical with zygomycin A. It has been used in medicine as an antimicrobial. It is comparatively non-toxic, the LD_{50} in mice being 156 mg/kg (intravenous), > 650 mg/kg (subcutaneous) and > 1625 mg/kg (oral).

Haskell *et al.*, *J. Amer. Chem. Soc.*, **81**, 3480, 3482 (1959)
Haskell, French, Bartz, *Belgium Patent*, 547,976 (1959)
Frohardt *et al.*, *U.S. Patent*, 2,916, 485 (1959)
Davisson, Finlay, *U.S. Patent*, 2,895,876 (1959)
Coffey *et al.*, *Antibiotics & Chemotherapy*, **9**, 730 (1959)
Schillings, Schaffner, *Antimicrobial Agents & Chemotherapy*, 274 (1961)
Rinehart *et al.*, *J. Amer. Chem. Soc.*, **84**, 3218 (1962)
Hichens, Rinehart, *ibid.*, **85**, 1547 (1963)
Konstantinova, Brazhnikova, *Antibiotiki*, **10**, 34 (1965)
Ezaki *et al.*, *Japanese Patent*, 7,036,158 (1970)
Endo, *J. Antibiotics* (Japan), **27**, 141 (1974)

PARTRICIN

A polyene antibiotic, partricin has been obtained by culturing a new strain of *Streptomyces aureofaciens* under submerged aerobic conditions in a medium containing glucose, soybean flour and inorganic salts at 23–30°C for 3 days. The compound was isolated by adjusting the mycelium to pH 1·8–2·0, filtering, suspending the moist mycelium in BuOH, adjusting the pH to 9·5–10 with ammonium hydroxide, filtering, concentration the BuOH fraction *in vacuo* and cooling rapidly when the antibiotic is precipitated. The precipitate is finally washed with BuOH and petroleum ether. Partricin has little activity against gram-positive or gram-negative bacteria but has marked antifungal and antiprotozoal activities, inhibiting the growth of *Saccharomyces cerevisiae* at a dilution of 1·25–2·5 µg/ml. It has a low toxicity with LD_{50} in mice of approximately 2000 mg/kg given orally.

Bruzzese, Ferrari, *U.S. Patent*, 3,773,925 (1973)

PARTRICIN METHYL ETHER

This semi-synthetic polyene antibiotic has been prepared by treating the preceding antibiotic with diazomethane in $(CH_3)_2SO$. It has no activity against bacteria but is active against several pathogenic and saprophytic fungi and some protozoa. Minimum inhibitory concentrations which have been determined (µg/ml) are: *Candida albicans* (0·05) and *Trichomonas vaginalis* (2·0). The mammalian toxicity is low, the LD_{50} in mice being greater than 2000 mg/kg when administered orally.

Bruzzese *et al.*, *Experientia*, **28**, 1515 (1972)
Bruzzese, Ferrari, *German Patent*, 2,154,436 (197)

PARVULINE A

Streptomyces parvullus, when fermented on a common medium, produces an antibiotic complex, parvuline, of unknown structure. It consists of at least three components, parvulines A, B and C, of which the first predominates. Hydrolysis experiments have shown that parvuline A consists of aspartic acid, glycine, proline, valine, pipecolic acid and α, γ-diaminobutyric acid in the ratios of 4:3:1:2:1:2, together with an unidentified aminoacid and C_{11-13} fatty acids. The antibiotic is active against *Staphylococcus aureus* in 6·0 µc/ml concentration and *Streptococcus fecalis* in 50µg/ml concentration. It is relatively non-toxic with LD_{50} in white mice of 300 mg/kg given intraperitoneally.

Toth-Sarudy *et al.*, *Hung. Teljes*, 422 (1970)

PARVULINE B

A minor component of the antibiotic complex produced by *Streptomyces parvullus*, this antibiotic contains aspartic acid, glycine, proline, valine, pipecolic acid and α,γ-diaminobutyric acid in the ratios of 4:2:1:1:1:1 as well as the previously mentioned unidentified aminoacid and C_{11-13} fatty acids. The biological activity and toxicity are similar to those given for parvuline A.

Toth-Sarudy *et al.*, *Hung. Teljes*, 422 (1970)

PARVULINE C

A further minor constituent of parvuline, isolated from cultures of *Streptomyces parvullus*, this substance consists of aspartic acid, glycine, proline, pipecolic acid and α,γ-diaminobutyric acid in the ratios of 4:1:1:2:2, together with the unidentified aminoacid and C_{11-13} fatty acids. It has a similar activity to *Staphylococcus aureus* and *Streptococcus fecalis* and toxicity in white mice as the preceding antibiotics.

Toth-Sarudy *et al.*, *Hung. Teljes*, 422 (1970)

PEARLMYCIN

$C_{16}H_{32}O$
B.p. Indefinite

A colourless oily antibiotic, pearlmycin has been obtained by culturing *Botryotrichum piluliferum* FERM-P 1647 with agitation in a medium of potato extract and 2 per cent glucose. The culture filtrate is concentrated to dryness, extracted with Et_2O and the extract chromatographed on thin layer silica gel. Pearlmycin has been characterized as the acetate which forms colourless crystals with m.p. 26°C. It is a broad spectrum antibiotic active against gram-positive, gram-negative and acidophilic bacteria. It is particularly effective against *Piricularia oryzae*.

Nishimura *et al.*, *Japanese Patent*, 74 81,596 (1974)

PECILOSIN (*Variotin*)

$C_{17}H_{25}O_3N$
B.p. Indefinite

A somewhat unstable antibiotic derived from *Paecilomyces varioti* Bainier var. *antibioticus*, this compound is a neutral oil having an ester-like odour.

It has no definite boiling or decomposition point but forms a monohydrate as colourless crystals, m.p. 41·5–42·5°C. The free antibiotic is laevorotatory with a specific rotation of $[\alpha]_D^{29} - 5·68°$ (c 1·0, CH_3OH). It is readily soluble in most organic solvents but only slightly soluble in H_2O, petroleum ether and ligroin. The solution in CH_3OH gives an ultraviolet spectrum consisting of two absorption maxima at 318 and 324 nm. Pecilosin is moderately stable in organic colvents but unstable in a dessicator or under alkaline conditions. It has found limited use as an antifungal agent.

Takeuchi et al., *J. Antibiotics* (Japan), **12A**, 109 (1959)
Sumiki et al., *British Patent*, 866,425 (1961)
Takeuchi et al., *J. Antibiotics* (Japan), **17A**, 267 (1964)
Takeuchi, Yonehara, *Tetrahedron Lett.*, 5197 (1966)

PENAMECILLIN
$C_{19}H_{22}O_6N_2S$
M.p. 106–108°C

A semi-synthetic antibiotic of the penicillin type, this compound forms colourless crystals from EtOH-isoPrOH. It is dextrorotatory with a specific rotation of $[\alpha]_D^{20} + 154°$. The structure is the hydroxymethyl ester acetate of penicillin G (q.v.). Penamecillin behaved similarly to penicillin V when administered orally to infants with mild respiratory infections with regard to antibacterial activity, excretion and resorption. The maximum level attained in the blood (approximately 2·5 µg/ml) after 1·5 hours was found to be highly effective *in vitro* against *Streptococcus hemolyticus* and also effective against *Micrococcus tetragenes* and *Pneumococcus* strains isolated from patients. Some resistance to the antibiotic was developed by less sensitive strains of *Staphylococcus aureus* incubated in a medium containing penamecillin. The antibiotic is not inactivated by gastric acid and the normal dose for humans in 350 mg.

Jansen, Russell, *J. Chem. Soc.*, 2127 (1965)
Jansen, Russell, *British Patent*, 1,003,479 (1965)
Ivady et al., *Acta Paediat.* (Budapest), **13**, 215 (1972)

PENATIN (*Corylophylin, Notatin, Penicillin A, Penicillin B*)
M.p. Indefinite

Derived primarily from *Penicillium notatum*, this antibiotic also occurs in cultures of *P. corylophylum* and *P. resticulosum*. It is obtained by surface growth on various media and may be isolated by a number of methods including precipitation with phosphotungstic acid; concentrating the filtrate *in vacuo*, chilling and adding $(CH_3)_2CO$, separating the precipitate, dissolving in H_2O and reprecipitating from cold $(CH_3)_2CO$; and by precipitating the activity of the culture filtrate with tannic acid followed by extraction with $(CH_3)_2CO$. Purification may be carried out by dialyzing against distilled H_2O, by precipitating with Reinecke's salt, decomposing with AcOH and subsequently precipitating from cold $(CH_3)_2CO$, and by chromatography on alumina and eluting with phosphate buffer at pH 5·0. The antibiotic is a flavoprotein and has a molecular weight of about 152,000 (ultracentrifuge). It forms a pale yellow or buff-coloured amorphous powder which is soluble in H_2O, insoluble in common organic solvents and does not dialyse through a cellophane membrane. It is laevorotatory with $[\alpha]_D^{22} - 4·8°$ (c 0·0125, H_2O) and gives an ultraviolet spectrum with absorption maxima at 280, 375 and 465 nm. In solution, it is unstable below and above pH 2·0–8·0 and gives positive reactions for protein. From solution it is precipitated by flavianic, phosphomolybdic, phosphotungstic, rufianic, tannic, trichloroacetic and tungstic acids.

Penatin is assayed by serial dilution with *Staphylococcus aureus* or by agar streak with *Escherichia coli*. Coulthard et al. and Kocholaty have determined the following inhibition dilutions ($\pm$ 1,000,000) *in vitro*: *Aerobacter aerogenes* (25); *Bacillus anthracis* (10–25); *B. brevis* (42); *B. mycoides* (25); *B. subtilis* (25); *Brucella abortus* (10–25); *Clostridium diphtheriae* (42); *Cl. histolyticum* (42); *Diplococcus pneumoniae* (12·5–100); *Gaffkya tetragena* (250); *Klebsiella pneumoniae* (0·1–1·0); *Neisseria catarrhalis* (250); *Proteus vulgaris* (100–1000); *Pseudomonas aeruginosa* (42); *Salmonella cholera-suis* (0·01–0·1); *S. enteriditis* (10); *S. paratyphi* (25–100); *S. schottmuelleri* (10); *S. typhimurium* (10); *Shigella sonnei* (1·0); *Staphylococcus albus* (125); *Staph. aureus* (42–125); *Streptomyces lavendulae* (42).

Inhibition concentrations (ppm) have also been measured by Roberts and his colleagues: *Aerobacter aerogenes* (1·6–3·2); *Bacillus subtilis* (12·8); *Brucella abortus* (6·4); *Br. melitensis* (12·8); *Br. suis* (12·8); *Eberella typhi* (12·8); *Escherichia coli* (0·8–3·2); *Diplococcus pneumoniae* (0·8); *Proteus vulgaris* (12·8); *Salmonella enteriditis* (6·4); *S. paratyphi* (12·8); *S. schottmuelleri* (3·2); *Staphylococcus aureus* (51·2) and *Vibrio comma* (12·8).

Penatin has a bacteriostatic action and its activity appears to be due to the production of hydrogen peroxide formed by reason of its enzymatic action upon glucose.

When tested *in vivo*, penatin gave no protection to mice against *Staphy-*

lococcus aureus, *Streptococcus hemolyticus* and *Salmonella* infections. In guinea pigs, however, repeated small doses of the antibiotic given subcutaneously, brought about a gain in weight in animals infected with *Brucella abortus*.

Penatin is comparatively toxic. The LD_{50} in mice has been given as 3 mg/kg (intraperitoneal), 50 mg/kg (oral) and 4·5 mg/kg (subcutaneous). When administered subcutaneously, the antibiotic causes adhesions, local edema, swelling and subcutaneous hemorrhage. The toxicity appears to increase in step with the potency of the preparation.

Coulthard, Michaelis, Short, *British Patent*, 552,619 (1941)
Skrimshire, *British Patent*, 561,175 (1942)
Kocholaty, *J. Bact.*, **44**, 143 (1942)
Kocholaty, *ibid.*, **44**, 469 (1942)
Coulthard et al., *Nature*, **150**, 634 (1942)
Roberts et al., *J. Biol. Chem.*, **147**, 47 (1943)
Van Bruggen et al., *ibid.*, **148**, 365 (1943)
Birkinshaw, Raistrick, *ibid.*, **148**, 459 (1943)
Levaditi et al., *Compt. rend. soc. biol.*, **137**, 359 (1943)
Penau et al., *ibid.*, **137**, 592 (1943)
Kocholaty, *Science*, **97**, 186 (1943)
Anderson, *J. Bact.*, **46**, 110 (1943)
Kocholaty, *ibid.*, **46**, 313 (1943)
Kocholaty, *Arch. Biochem.*, **2**, 73 (1943)
Schales, *ibid.*, **2**, 487 (1943)
Waksman, Horning, *Mycologia*, **35**, 47 (1943)
Levaditi et al., *Compt. rend. soc. biol.*, **138**, 5 (1944)
Coulthard et al., *Biochem. J.*, **39**, 24 (1945)
Carr, *Nature*, **155**, 202 (1945)
Levaditi, Vaisman, *Compt. rend. soc. biol.*, **139**, 1041 (1945)
Broom et al., *Brit. J. Pharmacol. Chemotherapy*, **1–2**, 225 (1946–1947)
Keilin, Hartree, *Biochem. J.*, **42**, 221 (1948)
Cecil, Ogston, *ibid.*, **42**, 227 (1948)
Keilin, Hartree, *ibid.*, **42**, 230 (1948)

PENICIDIN

M.p. Indefinite

Penicidin has been obtained from an unclassified species of *Penicillium* grown by surface culture on a modified Czapek-Dox medium for 5 days at 20°C. The culture filtrate is concentrated *in vacuo*, the pH adjusted to 7·0 and extracted with Et_2O. The ethereal extract is then shaken with H_2O, the pH adjusted to 4·0 with dilute H_2SO_4, the aqueous extract neutralized, extracted further with Et_2O, the ethereal fraction evaporated *in vacuo* and petroleum ether added when the crude product separates as a yellow oil.

Penicidin is stable in aqueous solution between pH 3·0 and 7·8 and is thermostable when neutral. It is unstable under highly alkaline conditions. The antibiotic is soluble in Et_2O, EtOH, $CHCl_3$, C_6H_6 and dilute mineral acids, insoluble in petroleum ether. It readily dialyses through a cellophane membrane. It gives negative biuret, Millon and Molisch reactions and dissolves in sodium hydroxide solution giving a yellow solution which shows a yellow fluorescence under ultraviolet light.

The antibiotic is active against both gram-positive and gram-negative bacteria and inhibits *Eberella typhi* at a concentration of 1:100,000.

Atkinson, *Austral. J. Exptl. Biol. Med. Sci.*, **20**, 287 (1942)

PENICILLIC ACID

$C_8H_{10}O_4$

M.p. 64–65°C; 86–87°C

Penicillic acid was first obtained from *Penicillium puberulum* and *P. stoloniferum* by Alsberg and Black in 1913. It has subsequently been isolated from *Aspergillus melleus*, *A. ochraceus*, *A. quercinus*, *A. sulphureus*, *Penicillium cyclopium*, *P. suavolens*, *P. thomii* and by synthesis. *Aspergillus ochraceus* is normally grown on a Czapek-Dox medium with corn-steep liquor whereas *Penicillium cyclopium* and *P. puberulum* are grown by surface culture on a medium containing glucose, tartaric acid, diammonium tartrate and inorganic salts incubated for 23 days at 24°C. Isolation is carried out by several methods including evaporating the culture filtrate *in vacuo*, acidifying and extracting with Et_2O; acidifying the filtrate to pH 2·0, extracting with Et_2O and removing the solvent *in vacuo* and adsorbing the activity on activated carbon at pH 7·0, eluting with CH_3OH and evaporating *in vacuo* when a crystalline material is obtained. The crude material may be purified by recrystallizing from 50 per cent CH_3OH or by sublimation at 75°C in a high vacuum.

When crystallized from H_2O, the monohydrate is obtained, the anhydrous form being isolated by crystallizing from petroleum ether. Both forms are obtained as large colourless crystals or hexagonal plates which are freely soluble in EtOH, Et_2O, $CHCl_3$, C_6H_6 and H_2O, but insoluble in petroleum ether. The antibiotic gives an orange colour when heated with $FeCl_3$ solution.

Penicillic acid is assayed by serial dilution with *Escherichia coli* or *Staphylococcus aureus* as the test organism. Oxford has determined the following inhibition dilutions ($\times 10,000$) *in vitro*: *Bacillus anthracis* (10); *Eberella typhi* (3·3); *Escherichia coli* (50); *Proteus vulgaris* (5·0); *Salmonella paratyphi* (3·3); *S. typhimurium* (3·3); *Shigella dysenteriae* (5·0–10); *Staphylococcus albus* (10); *Staph. aureus* (> 2·0–5·0); *S. citreus* (> 2·0); *Streptococcus viridans* (> 1·2) and *Vibrio comma* (10). The antibiotic is antagonized by amines, aminoacids, nutrient broth and peptones.

The LD_{50} in mice is 5·0 mg/kg (intravenous); 12 mg/kg (oral) and 2·2 mg/kg (subcutaneous).

Alsberg, Black, *U.S. Dept. Agric. Bur. Plant. Ind.*, Bull. 270 (1913)
Birkinshaw, Oxford, Raistrick, *Biochem. J.*, **30**, 394 (1936)
Oxford, *ibid.*, **36**, 438 (1942)
Oxford, Raistrick, Smith, *Chem. Ind.*, **61**, 22 (1942)
Oxford, *ibid.*, **61**, 48 (1942)
Karow, Woodruff, Foster, *Arch. Biochem.*, **5**, 279 (1944)
Raphael, *Nature*, **160**, 261 (1947)
Gill-Carey, *Brit. J. Exptl. Path*, **30**, 119 (1949)
Burton, *Nature*, **165**, 274 (1950)

PENICILLIN A
See Penatin

PENICILLIN B
See Penatin

PENICILLIN AT
See Penicillin O

PENICILLIN BT
$C_{14}H_{22}O_4N_2S_2$
M.p. Indefinite

A semi-synthetic penicillin, this antibiotic has been characterized as the procaine salt which forms colourless needles from EtOH with m.p. 110°C. It is active against a range of gram-positive bacteria.

Behrens *et al.*, *J. Biol. Chem.*, **175**, 793 (1948)
Rhodehamel, *U.S Patent*, 2,528,175 (1950)
Umezawa, *Chem. Abstr.*, **45**, 9128 (1951)
Behrens *et al.*, *U.S. Patent*, 2,623,876 (1952)

PENICILLIN F
See 2-Pentenylpenicillin

PENICILLIN G
See Benzylpenicillin

PENICILLIN KPN
$C_{13}H_{20}N_2O_5S$

A penicillin antibiotic, this substance has been isolated from cultures of *Penicillium carneus*. The antibiotic is obtained by adsorbing the culture filtrate on activated carbon and ion-exchange resins and purifying by silica gel column chromatography. The structure has been shown to be 6-(5-hydroxy-*n*-valeramido)-penicillanic acid by spectroscopic methods and comparison with the authentic specimen prepared synthetically.

Kitano *et al.*, *Hakko Kogaku Zasshi*, **54**, 705 (1976)

PENICILLIN N (*Adicillin, Cephalosporin N, Synnematin B*)
$C_{14}H_{21}O_6N_3S$
M.p. Indefinite

This penicillin antibiotic is produced by a number of organisms, e.g. *Penicillium chrysogenum*, *Actinomyces cinereorectus* nova, *Cephalosporium* species found in sewage outpours and *Paecilomyces persicimus*. The antibiotic is soluble in H_2O and may be characterized as the barium salt which forms an amorphous white powder and is dextrorotatory with a specific rotation of $[\alpha]_D^{20} + 187°$ (c. 0·6, H_2O). This salt is readily soluble in H_2O, sparingly so in CH_3OH and virtually insoluble in EtOH. An aqueous solution kept at 37°C and pH 2·7 for 2 hours shows a gradual loss of activity and an increase in dextrorotation. Penicillin N is active against *Diplococcus pneumoniae, Proteus vulgaris, Salmonella typhimurium* and *Sarcina lutea* but shows little activity against *Bacillus subtilis* or *Staphylococcus aureus*. It has a lower toxicity than penicillin G and is excreted more slowly.

Gottshall *et al., Proc. Soc. Exptl. Biol. Med.*, **76**, 307 (1951)
Abraham *et al., Nature*, **171**, 343 (1953)
Abraham *et al., ibid.*, **176**, 551 (1955)
Miller *et al., U.S. Patent*, 2,831,797 (1958)
Goodall, Sutcliffe, *U.S. Patent*, 2,899,425 (1959)
Pisano *et al., Antibiotics Annual*, **41**, 48 (1960)
Flynn *et al., J. Amer. Chem. Soc.*, **84**, 4594 (1962)
Chugasova, Terekhova, Fedorova, *Antibiotiki*, **19**, 195 (1974)
Structure
Abraham, Newton, *Biochem. J.*, **58**, 103 (1954)

PENICILLIN O (*Penicillin AT*)

$C_{13}H_{18}O_4N_2S_2$

A further penicillin type antibiotic, this substance forms a white powder and is normally employed as the potassium or sodium salt, both of which may be purified by recrystallization from $(CH_3)_2CO$. Other salts which have been used in medicine are the procaine and 2-chloroprocaine derivatives, the latter forming slender needles from hot H_2O with m.p. 79–81°C. Penicillin O and its salts are used as antimicrobials in medicine. Side effects include allergic reactions but these are generally rarer than with penicillin G.

Behrens *et al., J. Biol. Chem.*, **175**, 793 (1948)
Rhodehamel Jr., *U.S. Patent*, 2,528,175 (1950)
Behrens *et al., U.S. Patent*, 2,623,876 (1952)
Ford *et al., Antibiotics & Chemotherapy*, **3**, 1149 (1953)
Ford, *U.S. Patent*, 2,647,894 (1953)
Paleckova, Slechta, *Chem. Abstr.*, **50**, 17309 (1956)

PENICILLIN RIT 2214

$C_{13}H_{19}N_3O_6S_2$

Normally isolated as the ammonium salt, this antibiotic is produced by *Acremonium chrysogenum* ATCC 20389 in the presence of L-S-carboxymethylcysteine. The substance is extracted by adsorption on activated carbon followed by successive column chromatography on ion-exchange resins. It has been purified by column chromatography on cellulose. Proof of the above structure has been provided by spectroscopic examination and semi-synthesis. It exhibits antibiotic activity typical of the penicillins.

Troonen, Roelants, Boon, *J. Antibiotics* (Japan), **29**, 1258 (1976)

PENICILLIN S

$C_{14}H_{18}O_4N_2S_2Cl$

Obtained by fermenting a penicillin-producing mould in a culture medium in the presence of α-chlorocrotylmercaptoacetic acid, this antibiotic is normally isolated as the crystalline potassium salt which forms colourless needles from $(CH_3)_2CO$. It possesses a disagreeable odour and taste. The bioassay gives a figure of 1900 units/mg. It is mainly active against gram-positive bacteria.

Ford *et al., J. Amer. Chem. Soc.*, **70**, 3522 (1948)
Ford *et al., Antibiotics & Chemotherapy*, **3**, 1149 (1953)

PENICILLIN V (*Eskacillin V, Fenacilin, Oracillin, Phenopenicillin, Stabicillin, V-Cillin, Vebecillin*)

$C_{16}H_{18}O_5N_2S$
Dec. 120–128°C

A penicillin type antibiotic, penicillin V is produced by the addition of 2-phenoxyethanol to the culture medium of the *Penicillium* organism, using yeast autozylate as a nitrogen source. The antibiotic forms colourless crystals which decompose on heating. Penicillin V is stable in air up to 37°C and is soluble in H_2O and polar organic solvents but virtually insoluble in petroleum ether and vegetable oils. The ultraviolet spectrum in H_2O shows two absorption maxima at 268 and 274 nm. The D-form is biologically active, the corresponding L-form possessing very little activity. The DL-form has been prepared but is only half as active as D-penicillin V.

Penicillin V is used in medicine as an antimicrobial being resistant to inactivation by gastric acid. The normal oral dose is 125–250 mg and the side effects which have been observed include allergic reactions and diarrhoea. The antibiotic has been registered under a variety of trade-names other than those given above, including Acipen-V, Distaquaine V, Fenospen, Fenoxypen, Meropenin, Oratren, Ospen, Pen-Oral, Pen-Vee and V-Cil.

Brandl, Giovannini, Margreiter, *Wien. med. Wochschr*, 602 (1953)
Parker, Cox, Richards, *J. Pharm. Pharmacol*, **7**, 683 (1953)
Brandl, Margreiter, *Österr. Chem.-Ztg.*, **55**, 11 (1954)
Weiss *et al.*, *Antibiotics & Chemotherapy*, **7**, 374 (1957)
Glambitza, *Annalen*, **673**, 166 (1964)
Total synthesis
Sheehan, Henery-Logan, *J. Amer. Chem. Soc.*, **79**, 1262 (1957)
Sheehan, Henery-Logan, *ibid.*, **81**, 3089 (1959)
Sheehan, Henery-Logan, *ibid.*, **84**, 2983 (1962)

PENICILLIN V POTASSIUM SALT (*Alphacillin, Beromycin, Isocillin*)
$C_{16}H_{17}O_5N_2SK$

This derivative of the preceding antibiotic forms colourless crystals and is soluble in H_2O. It is dextrorotatory with $[\alpha]_D^{25} + 223°$ (c 0·2, H_2O). The biological activity and toxicity are similar to those of the base antibiotic. This antibiotic has also been registered under the following trade-names: Apsin VK, Aracil, Beromycin 400, Calciopen K, Distakaps V-K, Distaquaine V-K, DQV-K, Icipen, Ispenoral, Oracil-VK, Orapen, Pedipen, Pencompren, Pen-Vee K, Penkival, Sumapen VK and V-Cil-K.

Brandl, Giovannini, Margreiter, *Wein. med. Wochschr.*, 602 (1953)
Parker, Cox, Richards, *J. Pharm. Parmacol.*, **7**, 683 (1953)
Brandl, Margreiter, *Österr. Chem.-Ztg.*, **55**, 11 (1954)
Glambitza, *Annalen*, **673**, 166 (1964)

PENICILLIN I
See Pentenylpenicillin

PENICILLIN II
See Benzylpenicillin

PENIMEPICYCLINE
$C_{16}H_{18}O_5N_2S.C_{29}H_{38}O_9N_4$
Dec. 144°C

Penimepicycline is a compound of penicillin V with mepicycline. It forms a yellowish-white crystalline powder which decomposes above 144°C. The antibiotic is sensitive to light and air and is thermolabile. It is laevorotatory with a specific rotation of $[\alpha]_D^{20} - 50·5°$ (c 2·0, CH_3OH) and is freely soluble in H_2O. Penimepicycline has found some use in medicine as an antimicrobial. It is known under a number of trade-names including Criseocil, Geotricyn, Mepenicycline, Olimpen, Penetracyne and Peniltetra.

Pedrazzoli *et al.*, *Boll. Chim. Farm.*, **98**, 516 (1959)
Gradnik *et al.*, *Pharm. Acta Helv.*, **35**, 529 (1960)
Gradnik, Pedrazzoli, *British Patent*, 897,826 (1962)

PENSTEMIDE
$C_{21}H_{30}O_{10}.H_2O$

A plant antibiotic, this iridoid glucoside has been isolated from the flowers, fruit, leaves and stems of *Penstemon deutus*. It is the major component of the extract and has been shown to have the structure given above relating it to plumericin. It gives an ultraviolet spectrum consisting of a single absorption maximum at 214 nm. Penstemide is active against P-388 lymphocytic leukemia.

Jolad *et al.*, *Tetrahedron Lett.*, 4119 (1976)

PENTACIDIN
A methylpentaene antibiotic, pentacidin has been isolated from cultures of a

strain of *Streptomyces hygroscopicus* obtained from Caucasian soil. It is active against a range of gram-positive and some gram-negative bacteria.

Frolova et al., *Antibiotiki*, **20**, 198 (1975)

PENTALENOLACTONE (*Antibiotic PA-132*)
$C_{15}H_{16}O_5$
M.p. 61–62°C

A strain of *Streptomyces*, species 8403-MC$_1$, elaborates this antibiotic which forms colourless crystals. It has a specific rotation of $[\alpha]_D^{23} - 172°$ (c 1·0, CH$_3$OH) and gives an ultraviolet spectrum in CH$_3$OH having a single absorption maximum at 218·5 nm. This substance is extremely hygroscopic. Catalytic hydrogenation furnishes the tetrahydro derivative as colourless needles, m.p. 107–108·5°C.

Takeuchi, Ogawa, Yonehara, *Tetrahedron Lett.*, 2737 (1969)

PENTAMYCIN
See Lagosin

PENTENOMYCIN I
$C_6H_8O_4$
M.p. Indefinite

Streptomyces eurythermus MCRL 0739 yields two closely related antibiotics when cultured on a common nutrient medium at 26–28°C for 42 hours. This antibiotic is an amorphous, hygroscopic powder with no definite melting point. It is laevorotatory with a specific rotation of $[\alpha]_D^{21} - 32°$ (c 0·3, EtOH) and has the structure (4S,5S)-4:5-dihydroxy-5-hydroxymethyl-cyclopent-2-en-1-one.

Pentenomycin I exhibits a moderate activity against both gram-positive and gram-negative bacteria *in vitro*. When tested *in vivo*, a dose of 50 mg/kg administered intraperitoneally protected mice against *Staphylococcus aureus*. It is comparatively non-toxic, mice surviving more than 24 days without abnormal symptoms after intravenous administration of 400 mg/kg.

Umino et al., *J. Antibiotics* (Japan), **26**, 506 (1973)
Umino et al., *Chem. Pharm. Bull.*, **22**, 1233 (1974)
Crystal structure
Date et al., *Chem. Pharm. Bull.*, **22**, 1963 (1974)

PENTENOMYCIN II
$C_9H_{10}O_5$
M.p. Indefinite

A second antibiotic isolated from cultures of *Streptomyces* strain MCRL 0738, this compound has been shown to be the 4-acetyl derivative of pentenomycin I. It is also an amorphous, hygroscopic powder having no definite melting point and is laevorotatory with a specific rotation of $[\alpha]_D^{28} - 55°$ (c 1·45, CH$_3$OH). The antibiotic is active against both gram-positive and gram-negative bacteria and 150 mg/kg given intraperitoneally to mice caused no symptoms, the animals surviving for more than 24 days.

Umino et al., *J. Antibiotics* (Japan), **26**, 506 (1973)
Umino et al., *Chem. Pharm. Bull.*, **22**, 1233 (1974)
Crystal structure
Date et al., *Chem. Pharm. Bull.*, **22**, 1963 (1974)

2-PENTENYLPENICILLIN (*Penicillin F, Penicillin I*)
$C_{14}H_{20}O_4N_2S$

This antibiotic is produced by certain strains of *Penicillium chrysogenum* and *P. notatum* and is separated from the accompanying penicillins and purified by partition chromatography. It is normally prepared as the sodium salt which forms a sesquihydrate and a trihydrate. The anhydrous form has m.p. 204–205°C (*dec.*) and $[\alpha]_D^{25} + 316°$ (c 0·88, H$_2$O). There are no characteristic absorption maxima in the ultraviolet spectrum in H_2O apart from the typical penicillin cut-off absorption below 260 nm, 2-pentenylpenicillin, as the sodium salt, is freely soluble in H_2O, isotonic saline solution and in glucose solutions. In the latter, however, it is rapidly inactivated, as it is in EtOH and other primary alcohols. The antibiotic is active against gram-positive and some gram-negative bacteria.

Boon, Carrington, *Chemistry of Penicillin*, Princeton, (1949)
Wintersteiner, Adler, *U.S. Patent*, 2,485,227 (1949)

2-n-PENTYL-4-QUINOLINOL
$C_{14}H_{17}NO$

A simple antibiotic substance isolated from cultures of a marine *Pseudonomad*, this compound has the structure given above based upon chemical and spectroscopic examination. It is active against a number of bacteria and yeasts including *Staphylococcus aureus*, *Vibrio anquillarum*, *V. harveyi* and *Candida albicans*.

Wratten *et al.*, *Antimicrobial Agents & Chemotherapy*, **11**, 411 (1977)

PEPTHIOMYCIN A
M.p. Indefinite
Streptomyces roseospinous, freshly isolated from soil, elaborates two sulphur-containing polypeptide antibiotics which are obtained by filtering the broth at pH 3·5 and extracting the residue with CH_3OH. Separation of the two components was accomplished by chromatography of the extract on an alumina column. Pepthiomycin A is dextrorotatory with a specific rotation of $[\alpha]_D^{20} + 35°$ (dimethylformamide) and gives an ultraviolet spectrum in CH_3OH with an absorption maximum at 230 nm. It is insoluble in H_2O and is active against resistant strains of *Staphylococcus aureus* and *Xanthomonas oryzae*. It is comparatively non-toxic with LD_{50} in mice greater than 250 mg/kg when given intraperitoneally.

Umezawa *et al.*, *Japanese Patent*, 7,140,760 (1971)

PEPTHIOMYCIN B
M.p. indefinite
This sulphur-containing polypeptide antibiotic is separated from the mixture obtained from cultures of *Streptomyces roseospinous* by chromatography on an alumina column. It forms an amorphous powder and is laevorotatory with a specific rotation of $[\alpha]_D^{20} - 30°$ (dimethylformamide). The ultraviolet spectrum in CH_3OH has a single absorption maximum at 246 nm. It has a similar biological activity and toxicity to those of the preceding antibiotic.

Umezawa *et al.*, *Japanese Patent*, 7,140,760 (1971)

PERIMYCIN A (*Fungimycin NC-1968, Aminomycin*)
$C_{57}H_{86}N_2O_{16}$

Streptomyces coelicolor var. *aminophilus* NRRL 2390 yields three closely related macrocyclic polyene antibiotics which have been isolated by extraction of the culture broth followed by column and thin layer chromatography. Perimycin A is the major constituent of the antibiotic mixture and has the structure given above based upon chemical and spectroscopic examination. It is active against a variety of yeasts but unlike other macrocyclic polyene antibiotics it induces specific changes in the permeability of the yeast plasma membrane which results in the loss of potassium ions from the cells.

Woolridge, *British Patent*, 828,792
Borowski *et al.*, *Antimicrobial Agents Ann*, 1960, Plenum Press, 532 (1961)
Structure
Kolodziejeyk *et al.*, *Tetrahedron Lett.*, 3603 (1976)

PERIMYCIN B
This minor constituent of the antibiotic complex produced by *Streptomyces coelicolor* var. *aminophilus* NRRL 2390 has a similar effect upon the permeability of yeast plasma membrane. It belongs to the macrocyclic polyene

group of antibiotics but the complete structure has not yet been reported.

Woolridge, *British Patent*, 828,792
Borowski *et al.*, *Antimicrobial Agents Ann.*, 1960, Plenum Press, 532 (1961)

PERIMYCIN C
A third component of the antibiotic complex isolated from the culture filtrate of *Streptomyces coelicolor* var. *aminophilus* NRRL 2390, this antibiotic occurs only in small quantities and its structure has not been elucidated. Its action on the permeability of the yeast plasma membrane is similar to that of the two preceding antibiotics.

Woolridge, *British Patent*, 828,792
Borowski *et al.*, *Antimicrobial Agents Ann.*, 1960, Plenum Press, 532 (1961)

PHACIDIN
$C_{16}H_{22}O_5$
M.p. 118–121°C

This antibiotic substance has been isolated from cultures of *Potebniamyces balsamicola* var. *boycei*. The culture filtrate is extracted with C_6H_6 and the extract chromatographed to yield the pure compound as yellowish crystals when recrystallized from either aqueous $(CH_3)_2CO$ or C_6H_6-hexane. Phacidin inhibits the growth of a wide variety of fungi.

Poulton, Williams, McMullan, *Tetrahedron Lett.*, 2611 (1974)
Funk, McMullan, *Can. J. Microbiol.*, **20**, 422 (1974)

PHAEOFACIN
An antibiotic produced by *Streptomyces phaeofaciens*, phaeofacin is extracted from the mycelium or the broth with AcOEt, the extract concentrated *in vacuo* to form a syrup which is then dissolved in $(CH_3)_2CO$ and on cooling yields a precipitate of the antibiotic. Phaeofacin is soluble in AcOEt, EtOH, $(CH_3)_2CO$ and C_6H_6, slightly so in Et_2O and petroleum ether and insoluble in H_2O. It is active against *Achorion gypseum*, *Cryptococcus neoformans*, *Histoplasma capsulatum*, *Torula utilis* and Trichophyton at dilutions of 0·7–6·0 µg/ml. In mice, the LD_{50} is approximately 200 mg/kg when administered intraperitoneally. So far, it has found no use in medicine.

Maeda *et al.*, *J. Antibiotics* (Japan), **5A**, 465 (1952)
Maeda *et al.*, *J. Med. Sci. Biol.*, **5**, 327 (1952)

PHAGOLESSIN A-58
Produced by an unnamed *Streptomyces* species A-58, this antibiotic is precipitated from the culture medium with phosphotungstic acid, followed by extraction with 80 per cent CH_3OH at pH 3·0 and purified by chromatography on alumina. Phagolessin A-58 is a pale yellow powder which is hygroscopic but stable at −10°C for at least 1 year. It is readily soluble in H_2O, dilute acids and CH_3OH, less soluble in EtOH and insoluble in Et_2O, $(CH_3)_2CO$ or C_6H_6. It has a maximum stability at pH 3·0, being stable for 15 minutes at 100°C but at pH 9·0 an immediate irreversible inactivation occurs.

Phagolessin A-58 inhibits *Klebsiella pneumoniae* at a concentration of 3 µg/ml but other organisms have been found to be more resistant although certain bacteria and mycobacteria are moderately sensitive. It has phagocidal activity against bacterial viruses and may be employed to eradicate phage from phage-infected strains of *Streptomyces griseus*. The LD_{100} in mice when given intraperitoneally is less than 31 mg/kg.

Asheshov, Strelitz, Hall, *Antibiotics & Chemotherapy*, **2**, 361, 366 (1952)

PHAGOPEDIN SIGMA
See Fumagillin

PHALAMYCIN
M.p. Indefinite
This antibiotic has been obtained from a variant of *Streptomyces noursei*. It forms an amorphous powder or long hexagonal plates having no definite melting point and contains nitrogen. It is readily soluble in the lower alcohols, esters, $(CH_3)_2CO$ and $CHCl_3$, but only slightly soluble in Et_2O, C_6H_6 and H_2O. It is almost certainly neutral in reaction and relatively stable over the pH range from 2·5–7·0. The ninhydrin, biuret, Molisch and Sakaguchi tests are all negative. The ultraviolet spectrum exhibits a slight inflexion between 293 and 316 nm.

Phalamycin is active *in vitro* against a range of saprophytic and pathogenic gram-positive bacteria including *Mycobacterium tuberculosis* and pathogenic *Nocardia* species. It is, however, inactive against fungi and gram-negative bacteria. In mice it shows a marked activity against *Streptococcus hemolyticus*, affording protection when infected with ten times the lethal dose of this organism. The LD_{50} in mice is greater than 29 mg/kg when administered intraperitoneally and greater than 115·7 mg/kg when given subcutaneously.

Brown, Hazen, *Antibiotics & Chemotherapy*, **3**, 818 (1953)
Brown, *N.Y. State Dept Health, Ann. Rep. Div. Labs & Research*, 18 (1956)
Kelley, Brown, *ibid.*, 91 (1964)

PHENBENICILLIN
$C_{22}H_{22}O_5N_2S$

A semi-synthetic antibiotic, this substance is normally obtained as the crystalline potassium salt (Penspek) which forms colourless crystals with m.p. 88–95°C and decomposing at 120–125°C. It is active against a number of gram-positive bacteria.

Beecham Research Laboratories, *British Patent*, 877,120 (1962)

PHENETHICILLIN
$C_{17}H_{20}O_5N_2S$
Dec. 238–239°C (potassium salt)

A further semi-synthetic antibiotic based upon the penicillin structure, phenethicillin is normally employed as the potassium salt. The D-form of this salt forms colourless crystals from $(CH_3)_2CO$, m.p. 234–235°C and $[\alpha]_D^{20} + 252°$ (c 1·0, H_2O); the L-form, colourless crystals from aqueous BuOH, m.p. 238–239°C (*dec.*), $[\alpha]_D^{24} + 218°$ (c 0·01, H_2O) and the DL-form, m.p. 230–232°C (*dec.*). The latter is significantly less hygroscopic than benzylpenicillin sodium salt. This antibiotic has been employed in medicine as an antimicrobial.

Perron *et al.*, *Antibiotics Annual*, 107 (1959–1960)
Perron *et al.*, *J. Amer. Chem. Soc.*, **82**, 3934 (1960)
Glombitza, *Annalen*, **673**, 166 (1964)

PHENECIN (*Phoenicin*)
$C_{14}H_{10}O_6$
M.p. 230–231°C

The antibiotic activity of this compound obtained from *Penicillium phoeniceum* and *P. rubrum* was first discovered by Burton in 1949 although it had earlier been described by Friedheim in 1933 who designated it as a respiratory pigment. It is obtained by surface growth on a medium containing glucose, peptone and malt extract incubated for 8 days at 35°C. Isolation is carried out by acidifying the culture filtrate with HCl, extracting with $CHCl_3$ and shaking the chloroform extract with sodium bicarbonate solution to give a violet extract. The material is purified by chromatographing the $CHCl_3$ solution over alumina. Phenicin forms yellowish-brown crystals which are soluble in $CHCl_3$, AcOH and warm EtOH slightly soluble in H_2O. It is a dibasic organic acid, the structure, as 2:2'-dihydroxy-4:4'-dimethylbiphenyl-3:6:3':6'-diquinone, having been confirmed by synthesis.

Phenicin is active *in vitro* against *Corynebacterium xerosis*, *Mycobacterium phlei* and *Staphylococcus aureus*. It exhibits little activity *in vivo*.

Friedheim, *Compt. rend. soc. biol.*, **112**, 1030 (1933)
Friedheim, *Helv. Chim. Acta*, **21**, 1464 (1938)
Posternak, *ibid.*, **21**, 1326 (1938)
Posternak, *Chem. Abstr.*, **33**, 8596 (1939)
Burton, *Brit. J. Exptl. Path.*, **30**, 151 (1949)
Charollais *et al.*, *Arch. Sci.* (Geneva), **16**, 474 (1963)
Synthesis
Posternak, *Helv. Chim. Acta*, **26**, 2031 (1943)
Musso, Beecken, *Chem. Ber.*, **92**, 1416 (1959)

PHENOMYCIN
M.p. Indefinite
An antitumour antibiotic elaborated by *Streptomyces fervens* var. *phenomyceticus* freshly isolated from soil. The culture in a common medium is shake-cultured at 27–29°C for 5 days, the culture filtrate treated with Amberlite IRC-50 and the material purified on Sephadex G-25 and CM-cellulose. Phenomycin is a basic peptide compound which has a molecular

weight between 2500 and 10,000. The ultraviolet spectrum has a single absorption maximum at 278 nm. The antibiotic has no activity against bacteria but the growth of Ehrlich ascites sarcoma in mice was 100 per cent inhibited by a dose of 0·3 µg/mouse/day.

Umezawa, Nakamura, *Japanese Patent*, 7,137,877 (1971)

PHENOPENICILLIN
See Penicillin V

5-PHENYLPHENOXYMETHYLPENICILLIN
$C_{22}H_{22}O_5N_2S$

A further synthetic antibiotic, this substance has been prepared by the cycloaddition of azidoacetyl chloride to benzyl-D-5:5-dimethyl-2-phenyl-2-thiazoline-4-carboxylate, followed by reduction, acylation, isomerization and hydrogenolysis, yielding the antibiotic as the potassium salt. This antibiotic is also active against gram-positive and some gram-negative bacteria, the minimum inhibitory concentration against *Staphylococcus aureus* being 37 µg/ml.

Vanderhaeghe, Thomis, *J. Med. Chem.*, **18**, 486 (1975)

PHLEBIAKAURANOL
$C_{21}H_{34}O_7$
M.p. 208–213°C

Phlebia strigosozonata elaborates two closely related kaurene type antibiotics which are present both in the culture filtrate and the mycelium. The two compounds are separated and purified by countercurrent distribution and crystallization. This antibiotic crystallizes from CH_3OH as colourless crystals, the structure having been determined by X-ray diffraction methods. It is active against *Staphylococcus aureus* at a dilution of 16 µg/ml.

McMorris, Anchel, *Tetrahedron*, **23**, 3985 (1963)
Structure
Lisy, Clardy, *Chem. Commun.*, 406 (1975)

PHLEBIANORKAURANOL
$C_{19}H_{28}O_5$
M.p. 218–228°C

A second kaurane type antibiotic isolated from the mycelium and culture filtrate of *Phelbia strigosozonata*, this compound crystallizes from AcOEt as colourless crystals. The structure of this antibiotic has also been determined by X-ray crystallography. Like the preceding compound it is active against *Staphylococcus aureus* at a dilution of 16 µg/ml.

McMorris, Anchel, *Tetrahedron*, **23**, 3985 (1963)
Structure
Lisy, Clardy, *Chem. Commun.*, 406 (1975)

PHLEOMYCIN
M.p. Indefinite
An antiviral antibiotic isolated from cultures of a *Streptomyces* species, this compound has been shown to be active in blocking the synthesis of infectious simian papovavirus SV 40 in primary green monkey kidney cells. It has no effect, however, on the synthesis of SV 40 tumour antigen but a moderate effect upon the synthesis of a simian adenovirus, SV 15. It inhibits the multiplication of vaccinia virus but has considerably less effect against viruses of the herpes group. This differential effect of the antibiotic appears to depend on the content of thymine and adenine in the viral DNA.

Tevethia, Rapp, *Cancer. Res.*, **29**, 912 (1969)

PHOENICIN
See Phenecin

PHOLIPOMYCIN
Streptomyces lividoclavatus elaborates this antibiotic which is formed primarily in the solid residue of the culture medium. It has been isolated by extraction of the mycelial cake with MeOH and finally purified by ion-exchange and silica gel chromatography. Chemical investigation has shown that it belongs to the phosphoglycolipid group of antibiotics. Although principally active against gram-positive bacteria, including clinically isolated resistant bacteria, pholipomycin differs from other phosphoglycolipid antibiotics in being active against a range of gram-negative bacteria. Mice were protected against infection with *Staphylococcus aureus* and the antibiotic proved to be non-toxic with LD_{50} of 600 mg/kg when administered intravenously. Given orally, pholipomycin has shown some promise as a growth promoter in pigs and chickens.

Arai *et al.*, *J. Antibiotics* (Japan), **30**, 1049 (1977)
Torikata *et al.*, *ibid.*, **30**, 1060 (1977)

PHOMALACTONE
$C_8H_{11}O_3$
M.p. Indefinite

A simple antibiotic derived from *Phoma minispora* isolated from soil, this antibiotic is prepared by shake culture in a common nutrient medium at 24°C for 7 days. The culture filtrate is extracted at pH 5·0 with AcOEt and the extract chromatographed on alumina to give the purified crystalline compound. Phomalactone is dextrorotatory with a specific rotation of $[\alpha]_D^{22} + 179°$ (CHCl$_3$). It is readily soluble in H$_2$O and only sparingly so in Et$_2$O. The antibiotic is moderately effective against *Pseudomonas* and *Trichophyton* species.

Yamano *et al.*, *Japanese Patent*, 7,132,800 (1971)

L-(N⁵-PHOSPHONO)METHIONINE-S-SULPHOXIMINYL-ALANYL-L-ALANINE
A comparatively new antibiotic, this substance has been isolated from the fermentation broth of an unclassified species of *Streptomyces*. The antibiotic is active against *Bacillus subtilis* and a number of *Serratia* species. However, the activity is reversed upon the addition of L-glutamine to the medium.

Preuss *et al.*, *J. Antibiotics* (Japan), **26**, 261 (1973)

PHOSPHONOMYCIN
See 1,2-Epoxypropylphosphonic acid

PHTHIOCOL
$C_{11}H_8O_3$
M.p. 173–174°C

Phthiocol is obtained from *Mycobacterium tuberculosis* and was first isolated in 1933 by Anderson and Newman although its antibiotic properties were not recognised until 1946 by Lichstein and Van de Sand. The antibiotic is obtained by extracting the culture with (CH$_3$)$_2$CO followed by saponification of the (CH$_3$)$_2$CO extract and re-extraction with Et$_2$O. Phthiocol forms light yellow prisms when recrystallized from Et$_2$O which are soluble in organic solvents but insoluble in H$_2$O and petroleum ether. The structure has been established as 2-methyl-3-hydroxy-1:4-naphthoquinone.

The antibiotic is active against a number of bacteria, typical inhibition concentrations expressed as per cent, being: *Bacillus anthracis* (0·02); *Corynebacterium diphtheriae* (0·05); *Diplococcus pneumoniae* (0·02); *Eberthella typhi* (0·1); *Escherichia coli* (0·05); *Neisseria catarrhalis* (0·1); *Pseudomonas aeruginosa* (0·1); *Shigella paradysenteriae* (0·05); *Staphylococcus aureus* (0·05); *Streptococcus pyogenes* (0·02) and *Strep. salivarius* (0·05).

Anderson, Newman, *J. Biol. Chem.*, **103**, 197 (1933)
Lichstein, Van de Sand, *J. Bact.*, **52**, 145 (1946)

PICROMYCIN (*Pikramycin*)
$C_{25}H_{43}O_7N$
M.p. 169·5–170°C

A somewhat unstable antibiotic, similar to the proactinomycins (q.v.), picromycin was first isolated from cultures of *Actinomyces* species and later from *Streptomyces felleus*. It has been extracted from the latter culture with Et_2O under slightly alkaline conditions and further purified by solvent fractionation and chromatography on an alumina column. It is a white powder which may be obtained as small, rectangular plates from CH_3OH, having an intensely bitter taste and an alkaline reaction. The antibiotic is very soluble in C_6H_6, $CHCl_3$, $(CH_3)_2CO$ and AcOEt, moderately soluble in Et_2O and cold CH_3OH, slightly so in CS_2, H_2O and petroleum ether. It gives no typical ultraviolet spectrum.

The specific rotations measured are $[\alpha]_D^{24} + 8\cdot 2°$ (EtOH), $[\alpha]_D^{20} - 33\cdot 5°$ (c 2·07, $CHCl_3$) and $[\alpha]_D^{24} - 50\cdot 2°$ (c 6·3, $CHCl_3$).

Picromycin is active against certain gram-positive bacteria but has only a limited activity against *Mycobacterium tuberculosis* and very little against *Escherichia coli*, and other gram-negative bacteria. It is somewhat toxic to mammals, the LD_{50} in mice being 150 mg/kg when given intravenously. It has a beneficial effect upon some bacterial skin infections.

Brockmann, Henkel, *Naturwiss.*, **37**, 138 (1950)
Suhren, *Med. Klin.* (Munich), **46**, 722 (1951)
Brockmann, Henkel, *Chem. Ber.*, **84**, 284 (1951)
Brockmann, Genth, Stufe, *Ber.*, **85**, 426 (1952)
Brockmann, Bohne, *U. S. Patent*, 2,693,433 (1954)
Structure
  Brockmann, Oster, *Chem. Ber.*, **90**, 605 (1957)
  Anliker, Gubler, *Helv. Chim. Acta*, **40**, 119, 1768 (1957)
Stereochemistry
  Djerassi, Halpern, *J. Amer. Chem. Soc.*, **79**, 3926 (1957)
See also
  Maezawa et al., *J. Antibiotics* (Japan), **26**, 771 (1973)

PIKRAMYCIN
See Picromycin

PIMAFUGIN
See Pimaricin

PIMARICIN (*Myprozine, Natamycin, Pimafucin, Tennecetin*)
$C_{33}H_{47}O_{13}N$
Dec. 200°C

A macrocyclic antiniotic, pimaricin is produced by *Streptomyces chattanoogensis* and *S. natalensis*. It is an organic acid and forms colourless crystals from aqueous CH_3OH which decompose at the melting point. In the dry state, the antibiotic is quite stable although sensitive to light. It gives an ultraviolet spectrum with absorption maxima at 279, 290, 303 and 318 nm. Pimaricin is moderately soluble in diethylene glycol, propylene glycol, formamide and dimethylformamide, slightly soluble in CH_3OH and H_2O and insoluble in the higher alcohols, ethers, esters, hydrocarbons, dioxan, ketones, cyclohexanol and vegetable oils. It may be characterized as the N-acetyl derivative, m.p. 200°C, which is dextrorotatory with a specific rotation of $[\alpha]_D^{25} + 230°$. Acid hydrolysis of the antibiotic furnishes mycosamine.

Pimaricin is virtually inactive against gram-positive and gram-negative bacteria but is active against a number of pathogenic fungi, particularly *Candida albicans*.

Struyk et al., *Antibiotics Annual*, 878 (1957–1958)
Patrick et al., *J. Amer. Chem. Soc.*, **80**, 6688, 6689 (1958)
American Cyanamid, *British Patent*, 846,933 (1960)
Divekar et al., *Antibiotics & Chemotherapy*, **11**, 377 (1961)
Ceder et al., *Chimie*, **17**, 352 (1963)
Ceder et al., *Acta Chem. Scand.*, **18**, 77 (1964)
Structure
  Golding et al., *Tetrahedron Lett.*, 3551 (1966)
  Gaudiano et al., *Chim. Ind.* (Milan), **48**, 1327 (1966)
Revised structure
  Ceder, Hensson, Rapp, *Tetrahedron*, **33**, 2703 (1977)

PIOMYCIN A
This antibiotic has been obtained by culturing *Streptomyces piomogenus*

FERM-P 240 in a nutrient medium for 120–144 hours at 27°C with aeration. The active constituent is adsorbed on an ion-exchange resin, eluted with 0·2N H_2SO_4, adsorbed on activated carbon, desorbed with 70 per cent MeOH, concentrated and precipitated from EtOH-AcOEt. It is then purified by silica gel chromatography. Piomycin A is active against gram-positive bacteria.

Okamoto, Matsuoka, *Japanese Patent*, 75 20,158 (1975)

PIPERACILLIN (*Antibiotic T-1220*)
$C_{23}H_{26}N_5O_7SNa$

A new semi-synthetic antibiotic, piperacillin has the structure given above. It shows an appreciably higher activity against *Klebsiella pneumoniae* and *Pseudomonas* species than other antibiotics of this group but has a lower activity against *Straphylococcus aureus* than ampicillin. It is resistant to the penicillinase from *Pseudomonas aeruginosa* and the activity is only moderately influenced by the size of the inoculum. Piperacillin exhibits a synergistic effect against clinically isolated strains of *Pseudomonas aeruginosa* and *Sarcina marcescens in vitro* when used with gentamicin. When rats were given 250–1000 mg/kg subcutaneously for 11 days beginning at the seventh day of gestation no significant teratogenicity was observed. A dose of 2000 mg/kg given intravenously to beagle dogs over a period of six months resulted in increased megakaryocytes in the spleen and the number of red cells, Hb and hematocrit values decreased. In this test lacrimation, salivation, emesis, intestinal intonation and an increase in the heart rate were noted immediately after injection but these effects were all moderate following repeated administration of the dose.

Koike *et al.*, *Chemotherapy* (Tokyo), **25**, 765 (1977)
Saikawa *et al.*, *ibid.*, **25**, 789, 797 (1977)
Jones *et al.*, *J. Antibiotics* (Japan), **30**, 1107 (1977)
Toxicity tests
Takai *et al.*, *Chemotherapy* (Tokyo), **25**, 884, 915, 928, 934 (1977)

PIRBENICILLIN
$C_{24}H_{26}O_5N_6S$

A semi-synthetic antibiotic, pirbenicillin is a broad-spectrum antibiotic which is active *in vitro* and *in vivo* against a range of gram-positive and gram-negative bacteria and also against experimental infection after parenteral administration to mice. It possesses a three to four-fold potency advantage over carnebicillin (q.v.) against *Pseudomonas aeruginosa* both *in vitro* and *in vivo*. Pirbenicillin also has a greater stability than carbenicillin in serum and does not inactivate gentamicin as rapidly. When used against *Escherichia coli*, *Citrobacter*, *Serratia* and *Enterobacter* isolates its activity is comparable to that of carbenicillin but it is more active against gram-positive bacteria especially *Streptococcus faecalis*. The intrinsic activity of pirbenicillin against ampicillin-resistant *Escherichia coli* is said to be intermediate between that of ampicillin and carbenicillin, but it is less active than either against indole-positive *Proteus* species.

Bodley, Rodriguez, Weaver, *Antimicrobial Agents & Chemotherapy*, **9**, 668 (1976)
Retsema, English, Lynch, *ibid.*, **9**, 975 (1976)
Wise, Andrews, *J. Antimicrob. Chemother.*, **3**, 175 (1977)
Greenwood *et al.*, *ibid.*, **3**, 185 (1977)

PIVAMPICILLIN
$C_{22}H_{28}O_6N_3S$

A semi-synthetic antibiotic, this compound is pivaloyloxymethyl-D-α-aminobenzylpenicillinate and is normally used in medicine as the hydrochloride. Pivampicillin is active against numerous strains of *Escherichia coli* and *Staphylococcus*, the activity being similar to that of ampicillin (q.v.)

against both types of organism. The antibiotic is rapidly hydrolysed *in vitro* by enzymes present in the blood and tissues from various species, to form ampicillin and when administered orally is absorbed extremely well and hydrolysed, thereby giving rise to much higher blood and tissue concentrations of ampicillin than similar oral doses of ampicillin itself. When given to mice experimentally infected with β-lactamase-producing strains of *Escherichia coli*, the protective action of this antibiotic is better than that of ampicillin. Hubmann and Ritzerfeld have also shown that 210 mg/kg/day given orally to rats with acute ascending pyelonephritis caused by *Escherichia coli* was as effective as 450 mg of ampicillin in decreasing the bacterial count in renal parenchyma and urine.

Von Daehne *et al.*, *Antimicrobial Agents & Chemotherapy*, 431 (1970)
Garaci, Ravagnan, D'Antonio, *Antibiotica*, **10**, 5 (1972)
Nishimura *et al.*, *Chemotherapy* (Tokyo), **22**, 505 (1974)
Simon *et al.*, *Deut. Med. Wochenschr.*, **99**, 137 (1974)
Kawahara, Inage, *Sankyo Kenkyusho Nempo*, **26**, 140 (1974)
Hubmann, Ritzerfeld, *Arzneim-Forsch.*, **25**, 168 (1975)

PLANOMYCIN
See Fervenulin

PLATENOCIDIN
Streptomyces platensis yields this antibiotic which has been isolated from the fermentation broth filtrate by adsorption on an ion-exchange resin followed by elution with 1N-ammonium hydroxide and subsequent chromatography. Both acid and alkaline hydrolysis furnishes 5-hydroxymethyluracil. Platenocidin has an inhibitory activity against a variety of yeasts but none against bacteria. No toxic symptoms have been found with mice injected intraperitoneally with doses of 10 mg/mouse.

Honke *et al.*, *J. Antibiotics* (Japan), **30**, 439 (1977)

PLEOCIDIN
An antibiotic related to streptothricin (q.v.), pleocidin is produced by an organism resembling *Streptomyces lavendulae*. It is purified by chromatography on Norit A using CH_3OH as a developer. The antibiotic is a white, basic, hygroscopic powder having no definite melting point and has a maximum stability between pH 4·0 and 6·0. It is a broad spectrum antibiotic being active against both gram-positive and gram-negative bacteria, fungi and mycobacteria. The LD_{50} in mice is 3 mg/kg when administered intraperitoneally and it shows no rabbit's eye toxicity. Although not in general use, it is possible that pleocidin may find some application as a topical antibiotic.

Charney, Roberts, Fisher, *Antibiotics & Chemotherapy*, **2**, 307 (1952)
Fisher, Charney, *ibid.*, **2**, 311 (1952)

PLEOCIDIN A
This antibiotic closely resembles the preceding compound from which it may be separated by reason of the greater solubility of the helianthate. Its chemical, physical and biological properties are virtually identical to those of pleocidin.

Charney, Roberts, Fisher, *Antibiotics & Chemotherapy*, **2**, 307 (1952)
Fisher, Charney, *ibid.*, **2**, 311 (1952)

PLEOMYCIN
$C_{14}H_{12}O_8$
M.p. 235°C
Streptomyces pleofaciens elaborates this antibiotic which is an organic acid, forming colourless rectangular plates when crystallized from EtOH or AcOEt. It sublimes at 200°C, at atmospheric pressure, without any loss of activity. The ultraviolet spectrum in 0·13M phosphate buffer at pH 7·0 has absorption maxima at 270 and 330–340 nm. It is freely soluble in CH_3OH, EtOH, AcOEt, Et_2O and C_6H_6. Pleomycin forms H_2O-soluble alkali salts and is active against gram-positive and gram-negative bacteria and some fungi but is highly toxic to mammals.

Machlowitz *et al.*, *Antibiotics Annual*, 806 (1954–1955)

PLEURIN
One of six antibiotics derived from an unclassified *Basidiomycete*, little is known about this compound which has not been extensively studied since its discovery.

Robbins, Kavanagh, Hervey, *J. N.Y. Bot. Gardens*, **46**, 130 (1945)

PLEUROMUTILIN (*Drosophilin B*)
$C_{22}H_{34}O_5$
M.p. 170–171°C
An antibiotic elaborated by *Drosophila substrata*, *Pleurotus mutilus* (Fr.) Sacc. and *P. passeckerianus* Pilat, pleuromutilin forms colourless crystals from EtOH—Et_2O or AcOEt-Skellysolve B. The antibiotic is dextrorotatory with a specific rotation of $[\alpha]_D^{24}$ + 20° (c 3·0, EtOH) and gives an

ultraviolet spectrum in 95 per cent EtOH consisting of a single absorption maximum at 290 nm. Pleuromutilin is soluble in CH_3OH, EtOH, $CHCl_3$ and AcOEt. A number of crystalline derivatives have been prepared including the diacetate, m.p. 145·5°C, di-(3,5-dintrobenzoyl), m.p. 249–250°C and the hydrazone, m.p. 94°C.

Pleuromutilin is active mainly against gram-positive bacteria. The LD_{50} in mice is 60 mg/kg but it has been shown that repeated contact with the solid antibiotic or solutions of it can cause mild urticaria in susceptible strains.

Kavanagh, Hervey, Robbins, *Proc. Nat. Acad. Sci.*, **37**, 570 (1951)
Kavanagh, Hervey, Robbins, *ibid.*, **38**, 555 (1952)
Anchel, *J. Biol. Chem.*, **199**, 133 (1952)
Arigoni, *Gazzetta*, **92**, 884 (1962)
Birch et al., *Chem & Ind.* (London), 374 (1963)

PLEUROTIN
$C_{20}H_{22}O_5$
M.p. 200–215°C (dec.)

Pleurotus griseus elaborates this antibiotic which is obtained by surface growth on beechwood shavings in a medium containing corn steep liquor, glucose and inorganic salts incubated for a month at 25°C. The activity of the culture liquor may be adsorbed by activated carbon and the cake dried in air and then eluted with $CHCl_3$. The crude material is purified by recrystallization from Et_2O—$CHCl_3$. Pleurotin forms yellow needles by rapid evaporation of the solvent and amber crystals when crystallized slowly. It is soluble in $(CH_3)_2CO$, $CHCl_3$ and CH_3OH, slightly so in H_2O, insoluble in mineral acids and petroleum ether. It is laevorotatory with a specific rotation of $[\alpha]_D^{23} - 20°$ (c 0·59, $CHCl_3$) and gives an ultraviolet spectrum with a single absorption maximum at 250 nm.

Pleurotin is assayed by serial dilution with *Staphylococcus aureus* as the test organism. Kavanagh and his coworkers have determined the following inhibition concentrations (μg/ml) *in vitro*: *Bacillus mycoides* (1·6–3·0); *B. subtilis* (0·2); *Escherichia coli* (500); *Klebsiella pneumoniae* (500); *Mycobacterium phlei* (> 32); *Myco. smegmatis* (32); *Myco. tuberculosis* H234 (> 100); *Photobacterium fischeri* (6·0) and *Staphylococcus aureus* (0·8).

The antibiotic is comparatively non-toxic. A dose of 24 mg/kg administered intravenously to mice was tolerated. Owing to the limited solubility in H_2O, it was not possible to administer larger doses.

Robbins, Kavanagh, Hervey, *Proc. Nat. Acad. Sci.*, **33**, 171 (1947)
Kavanagh, *Arch. Biochem.*, **15**, 95 (1947)
Kavanagh, *J. Bact.*, **54**, 761 (1947)

PLICATIN (*Amicetin B*)
$C_{25}H_{35}O_7N_5$
M.p. 182–184°C

An aminosugar nucleoside antibiotic, plicatin is obtained from cultures of *Streptomyces plicatus*. It forms colourless needles when purified by recrystallizing from aqueous CH_3OH. Plicatin is dextrorotatory having a specific rotation of $[\alpha]_D^{26} + 181°$ (c 2·7, CH_3OH). The structure given above has been confirmed by the total synthesis of the antibiotic. The antibiotic is active against gram-positive bacteria.

Haskell et al., *J. Amer. Chem. Soc.*, **80**, 743 (1958)
Total synthesis
Stevens et al., *J. Amer. Chem. Soc.*, **94**, 3280 (1972)

PLUMBAGIN
$C_{11}H_8O_3$
M.p. 78–79°C

This antibiotic substance is a plant product isolated from the roots of *Plumbago europaea*, *P. rosea* and *P. zeylonica*. It may also be obtained by synthesis from acetylsuccinic ester and *m*-toluyl chloride. Plumbagin forms orange-yellow crystals which are freely soluble in organic solvents but only slightly so in H_2O. The constitution as 2-methyl-5-hydroxy-1:4-naphthoquinone shows it to be a position isomer of phthiocol (q.v.).

Saint-Rat and his colleagues have determined inhibition dilutions ($\times$ 1000) *in vitro* against a number of organisms, e.g. *Bacillus subtilis* ($>$ 0·3); *Eberthella typhi* (1·0–5·0); *Escherichia coli* (1·0–5·0); *Mycobacterium tuberculosis* (5·0–10); *Pneumococcus* spp. (10–50); *Staphylococcus* spp. (10–50); and *Streptococcus hemolyticus* (10–50). The antibiotic also inhibits *Coccidioides immitis*, *Ctenomyces radians*, *Histoplasma capsulatum*, *Phialophora verrucosa* and *Trichophyton ferrugineum* at a dilution of 1:50,000.

Some encouraging results have been obtained with plumbagin *in vivo* for treatment of *Staphylococcus* infections causing acne and furuncles, the antibiotic being given intravenously. It has a very low toxicity *in vivo* although there is a lethal action on the respiratory system in frogs, rats and guinea pigs.

Saint-Rat, Luteran, *Compt. rend. acad. sci.*, **224**, 1587 (1943)
Saint-Rat, Olivier, Shouteau, *Bull. Acad. Med.*, **130**, 57 (1946)
Blanchon, Saint-Rat, Bonet-Mawry, *ibid.*, **132**, 125 (1948)
Synthesis
Fieser, Dunn, *J. Amer. Chem. Soc.*, **58**, 572 (1936)

PLURALLIN

M.p. Indefinite

A strain of *Streptomyces pluricolorescens* yields this glycoprotein antibiotic which has a molecular weight of between 30,000 and 60,000 as determined by chromatography. The organism is cultivated on a medium containing a source of nitrogen, e.g. soybean flour, under aerobic submerged conditions. Plurallin is active against a number of bacteria, inhibiting the growth of *Corynebacterium xerosis*, *Mycobacterium phlei* and *Sarcina lutea*.

Umezawa *et al.*, *U.S. Patent*, 3,655,877 (1972)

POLYETHERIN A

$C_{42-43}H_{72-74}O_{12}$
M.p. 183·5–185°C

A complex antibiotic, polyetherin A has been isolated from cultures of *Streptomyces hygroscopicus* strain E-749. It forms colourless needles and is dextrorotatory with a specific rotation of $[\alpha]_D^{24} + 36·2°$ (c 0·842, $CHCl_3$). Polyetherin A shows no characteristic absorption in the ultraviolet and generally behaves as a lipophilic acid, probably being a polycyclic polyether. The antibiotic has been shown to be active against gram-positive bacteria, mycobacteria and a number of phytopathogenic fungi at concentrations of 0·5–5·0 µg/ml.

Shoji *et al.*, *J. Antibiotics* (Japan), **21**, 402 (1968)

POLYMYXINS

Bacillus polymyxa elaborates a complex of closely related polypeptide antibiotics initially separated into five components, polymyxina A, B, C, D and E, but subsequent work has shown that most of these are heterogeneous and a much larger number of constituents of the complex have now been isolated and characterized, these being detailed below. Polymyxin A has been shown to be identical with aerosporin isolated from cultures of *Bacillus aerosporus*.

Polymyxin B is the component generally used clinically. It is active against most gram-negative bacilli except *Proteus* species and is particularly effective against *Escherichia coli*, *Enterobacter*, *Klebsiella* and *Pseudomonas aeruginosa*. Other sensitive gram-negative organisms include *Hemophilus influenzae*, *Bordetella pertussis*, *Shigella* and *Salmonella*. It is inactive against *Neisseria gonorrhoeae*, *N. meningitidis*, gram-positive bacteria and fungi. Classical *Vibrio* cholerae is sensitive to the antibiotic but the *eltor* biotype is resistant.

Those bacteria susceptible to polymyxin B do not readily acquire resistance but when resistance occurs *in vitro* there is complete cross-resistance between polymyxin B and colistin (q.v.).

Polymyxin B is used intramuscularly, or preferably intravenously, in the treatment of systemic and urinary tract infection by suceptible organisms, particularly *Pseudomonas aeruginosa*. It is also applied topically in the treatment of skin and eye infections. Meningitis has been successfully treated by intrathecal injections of the antibiotic.

Toxic effects associated with polymyxin B includes dizziness, ataxia and sensory disturbances of the face and extremities following parenteral administration. Dose related nephrotoxicity can also develop but these symptoms are normally reversed on withdrawal of the drug.

Ainsworth, Brown, Brownlee, *Nature,* **160**, 263 (1947)
Brownlee, *Ann. N.Y. Acad. Sci.,* **51**, 875 (1949)
Vogler, Studer, *Experientia,* **22**, 345 (1966)
Hoeprich, *Med. Clins. N. Amer.,* **54**, 257 (1970)
Geelhoed, Ketcham, *J. Surg. Oncol.,* **5**, 265 (1973)
Geelhoed, Ketcham, *J. Amer. med. Assoc.,* **226**, 1627 (1973)
Cooperstock, *Antimicrobial. Agents & Chemotherapy,* **6**, 422 (1974)

Toxic effects
Lindesmith *et al., Ann. intern. Med.,* **68**, 318 (1968)
Lindesmith *et al., J. Amer. med. Assoc.,* **203**, A215 (1968)
Rodriguez *et al., Clin, Pharmac. Ther.,* **11**, 106 (1970)
Rosenow, *Ann. intern. Med.,* **77**, 977 (1972)

POLYMYXIN A (*Aerosporin*)

This antibiotic has been shown to consist of at least two components, polymyxins A_1 and A_2.

POLYMYXIN A_1
$C_{53}H_{100}O_{13}N_{16}$

```
        CH3
        |
        CH2
        |
   H3CCH                              Dbu—D-Leu—Thr
        |                             |          |
   (CH2)4—CO—Dbu—Thr—D-Dbu—Dbu        |
                              |       |
                              Thr—D-Dbu—Dbu
```

A complex polypeptide antibiotic, the structure of this substance has been determined primarily from a study of the hydrolysis products which include L-α,γ-diaminobutyric acid, D-leucine, L-threonine and D-6-methyloctanoic acid. Polymyxin A_1 is a potent antimicrobial agent.

Structure
Wilkinson, Lowe, *Nature,* **212**, 311 (1966)

POLYMYXIN A_2
$C_{52}H_{98}O_{13}N_{16}$

```
   CH(CH3)2                           Dbu—D-Leu—Thr
        |                             |          |
   (CH2)4CO—Dbu—Thr—D-Dbu—Dbu
                              |
                              Thr—D-Dbu—Dbu
```

This antibiotic possesses a structure similar to that of the preceding compound. Acid hydrolysis furnishes L-α,γ-diaminobutyric acid, D-leucine, L-threonine and *iso*-octanoic acid. It has a similar antimicrobial effect to polymyxin A_1.

Structure
Wilkinson, Lowe, *Nature,* **212**, 311 (1966)

POLYMYXIN B_1
$C_{56}H_{98}O_{13}N_{16}$

```
        CH3
        |
        CH2
        |
   H3CCH                              Dbu—D-Phe—Leu
        |                             |          |
   (CH2)4CO—Dbu—Thr—Dbu—Dbu
                              |
                              Thr—D-Dbu—Dbu
```

A further polypeptide antibiotic isolated from cultures of *Bacillus polymyxa* and separated from the accompanying compounds by chromatography and countercurrent distribution methods, this antibiotic yields L-α,γ-diaminobutyric acid, D-leucine, L-threonine, L-phenylalanine and D-6-methyloctanoic acid on hydrolysis. It has been shown to increase the respiration and decrease the blood pressure in rabbits. Experiments have also shown that it may be clinically useful in antagonizing heparin, and that the latter may also decrease the toxicity of the antibiotic.

Hausmann, Craig, *J. Amer. Chem. Soc.,* **76**, 4892 (1954)
Hausmann, *ibid.,* **78**, 3663 (1956)
Biserte, Dautrevaux, *Bull. soc. chim. biol.,* **39**, 795 (1957)
Wilkinson, Lowe, *Nature,* **200**, 1008 (1963)
Wilkinson, Lowe, *ibid.,* **202**, 1211 (1964)
Volger *et al., Experientia,* **20**, 365 (1964)
Onishi, *Shikoku Igaku Zasshi,* **30**, 350, 379 (1974)

Synthesis
Volger *et al., Helv. Chim. Acta,* **48**, 1161 (1965)

POLYMYXIN B_2
$C_{55}H_{96}O_{13}N_{16}$

```
   CH(CH3)2                           Dbu—D-Phe—Leu
        |                             |          |
   (CH2)4CO—Dbu—Thr—Dbu—Dbu
                              |
                              Thr—D-Dbu—Dbu
```

Structurally, this polypeptide antibiotic closely resembles the preceding compound. Hydrolysis furnishes L-α,γ-diaminobutyric acid, D-leucine, L-phenylalanine, L-threonine and *iso*-octanoic acid. It possesses similar antimicrobial and antiheparin activity to polymyxin B_1.

Hausmann, Craig, *J. Amer. Chem. Soc.*, **76**, 4892 (1954)
Hausmann, *ibid.*, **78**, 3663 (1956)
Biserte, Dautrevaux, *Bull. soc. chim. biol.*, **39**, 795 (1957)
Wilkinson, Lowe, *Nature*, **200**, 1008 (1963)
Structure
Wilkinson, Lowe, *Nature*, **204**, 185, 993 (1964)

POLYMYXIN D_1
$C_{49}H_{92}O_{14}N_{16}$
M.p. Indefinite

```
        CH(CH3)2                    Dbu—Leu—Thr
                                    |
(CH2)5CO—Dbu—Thr—D-Ser—Dbu
                                    |
                                    Thr—Dbu—Dbu
```

This polypeptide antibiotic, isolated from cultures of *Bacillus polymyxa*, has a structure closely resembling that of polymyxin A_1 but with D-serine replacing 2:4-diaminobutyric acid in the side chain. The structure has been elucidated from a study of the hydrolysis products.

Structure
Hayashi, Suketa, Tsukamoto, *Experientia*, **22**, 354 (1966)

POLYMYXIN D_2
$C_{49}H_{92}O_{14}N_{16}$
M.p. Indefinite

```
        CH3
        |
        CH2
        |
   H3CCH                            Dbu—Leu—Thr
                                    |
   (CH2)4CO—Dbu—Thr—D-Ser—Dbu
                                    |
                                    Thr—Dbu—Dbu
```

The original polymyxin D obtained by cultivating *Bacillus polymyxa* in a common nutrient medium has been shown by chromatography and countercurrent distribution to consist of two components. This particular antibiotic is an isomer of the preceding compound and yields 6-methyl-octanoic acid on hydrolysis. It possesses a similar antibiotic activity to the other polymyxins and also shows some activity against *Brucella bronchisepta*.

Structure
Hayashi *et al.*, *Experientia*, **22**, 354 (1966)

POLYMYXIN E_1

```
        CH3
        |
        CH2
        |
   H3CCH                            Dbu—Thr—Leu
                                    |
   (CH2)4CO—Dbu—Thr—Dbu—Dbu
                                    |
                                    Thr—Dbu—Dbu
```

This polypeptide antibiotic obtained from cultures of *Bacillus polymyxa* has been shown to be identical with coliston (q.v.).

POLYMYXIN E_2
M.p. Indefinite

```
        CH(CH3)2                    Dbu—Thr—Leu
                                    |
   (CH2)5CO—Dbu—Thr—Dbu—Dbu
                                    |
                                    Thr—Dbu—Dbu
```

A further polypeptide antibiotic, polymyxin E_2 has been separated from polymyxin E_1 by countercurrent distribution techniques. Hydrolysis furnishes D-leucine, L-threonine, L-α,γ-diaminobutyric acid and *iso*-octanoic acid. It is active against a number of gram-positive bacteria.

Wilkinson, Lowe, *Nature*, **200**, 1008 (1963)

POLYMYXIN F

This polymyxin has been isolated from cultures of *Bacillus circulans* ATCC 31228. Hydrolysis experiments have shown 2,4-diaminobutyric acid, serine, threonine, isoleucine and leucine to be present in molar ratios of 5:1:1:1:2. Since the hydrolyzate also contains octanoic, isooctanois and 6-methyl-octanoic acids, it is believed that polymyxin F is a mixture of at least three components corresponding to these three acids. The antibiotic activity is similar to that of polymyxin B_1.

Parker *et al.*, *J. Antibiotics* (Japan), **30**, 767 (1977)

POLYMYXIN M
This antibiotic which is produced by *Bacillus polymyxa* var. Ross under a variety of cultivation conditions is almost certainly identical with the original polymyxin A. It is formed when the organism is grown in a medium containing L-valine or ammonium salts as the nitrogen source. The lysine analogue of this antibiotic has recently been prepared synthetically and shown to possess antibacterial activity against *Brucella bronchiseptica*.

Nefelova *et al.*, *Antibiotiki.*, **16**, 250 (1971)
Morozova, Oksenoit, Lysogorskaya, *Khim. Prir. Soedin*, **11**, 280 (1975)

POLYMYXIN P$_1$
When *Bacillus polymyxa* strain T-39 is cultured in a medium consisting of yeast extract, corn meal, starch and inorganic salts at pH 2·0 and 27–30°C for 3 days it furnishes two new polymyxins P$_1$ and P$_2$. These are separated by countercurrent distribution. Polymyxin P$_1$ forms a white, amorphous powder with no definite melting point and is active in inhibiting the growth of a range of gram-positive bacteria.

Kimura, *Japanese Patent*, 7,227,038 (1972)

POLYMYXIN P$_2$
M.p. Indefinite
This component of the polymyxin P complex isolated from cultures of *Bacillus polymyxa* T-39 is also a white, amorphous powder. It has a similar inhibitory action to that of the preceding antibiotic.

Kimura, *Japanese Patent*, 7,227,038 (1972)

POLYMYXIN S$_1$
A further polymyxin, this antibiotic has been isolated from cultures of *Bacillus polymyxa* strain RS-6. It is a strongly basic amorphous white powder and has been characterized as the hydrochloride which is soluble in both H$_2$O and MeOH. It is particularly effective against gram-negative bacteria *in vitro* and *in vivo*.

Shoji *et al.*, *J. Antibiotics* (Japan), **30**, 1029 (1977)

POLYMYXIN T$_1$
This member of the polymyxin class of antibiotics has been obtained from cultures of *Bacillus polymyxa* strain E-12. Like the preceding substance it is a strongly basic amorphous white powder forming a hydrochloride which is soluble in H$_2$O and MeOH. It has an antibiotic activity against gram-negative bacteria *in vitro* and *in vivo* as polymyxin S$_1$.

Shoji *et al.*, *J. Antibiotics* (Japan), **30**, 1029 (1977)

POLYOXINS
A large number of antifungal antibiotics have been isolated from cultures of *Streptomyces cacaoi* var. *asoensis* and *S. piomogenus*. All have very similar structure and are particularly active against *Alternaria kikuchiana*, *Ophiobolus miyabeanus* and *Piricularia oryzae*. In general, they exhibit a low toxicity in mice. The structures, outlined below, of the individual antibiotics have been determined by chemical and spectroscopic methods.

POLYOXIN A
$C_{23}H_{32}O_{14}N_6$
M.p. Indefinite

This component of the antibiotic complex has been isolated from *Streptomyces cacaoi* var. *asoensis*. It forms a white powder and is laevorotatory with a specific rotation of $[\alpha]_D^{20} - 30°$ (c 1·02, H$_2$O). Mild hydrolysis furnishes polyoxin C, polyoximic acid, polyoxamic acid, 5-hydroxymethyluracil, ammonia and carbon dioxide.

Isono, Suzuki, *Tetrahedron Lett.*, 1133 (1968)

POLYOXIN B
$C_{17}H_{25}O_{13}N_5$
M.p. Indefinite
Also formed in cultures of *Streptomyces cacaoi* var. *asoensis*, this antibiotic has the structure given above. It has a specific rotation of $[\alpha]_D^{20} + 34°$

(c 1·03, H₂O). It is an amphoteric compound and on hydrolysis yields the same products as polyoxin A except that no polyoximic acid is formed.

Isono, Suzuki, *Tetrahedron Lett.*, 1133 (1968)

POLYOXIN C
$C_{11}H_{15}O_8N_3$
M.p. Indefinite

A further antibiotic isolated from cultures of *Streptomyces cacaoi* var. *asoensis*, this compound is also obtained by mild hydrolysis of polyoxins A and B. Hydrogenolysis over platinum yields the deoxy derivative, m.p. 240–244°C; $[\alpha]_D^{22}$ + 8·7° (c 0·2, H₂O).

Isono, Suzuki, *Agr. Biol. Chem.*, **32**, 1193 (1968)

POLYOXIN D
$C_{17}H_{23}O_{14}N_5$
Dec. > 190°C

One of a number of antifungal antibiotics produced by *Streptomyces cacaoi* var. *asoensis*. Polyoxin D forms a microcrystalline powder which decomposes above 190°C. It is dextrorotatory having a specific rotation of $[\alpha]_D^{20}$ + 30° (c 1·0, H₂O) and gives an ultraviolet spectrum with absorption maxima at 218 and 276 in 0·05 N-HCl and a single absorption maximum at 271 nm in 0·05 N-NaOH. The antibiotic is active against a number of saprophytic and pathogenic fungi.

Suzuki et al., *Agr. Biol. Chem.*, **30**, 817 (1966)
Isono et al., *ibid.*, **31**, 190 (1967)
Structure
Isono, Asahi, Suzuki, *J. Amer. Chem. Soc.*, **91**, 7490 (1969)

POLYOXIN E
$C_{17}H_{23}O_{13}N_5$
Dec. > 180°C

Also produced by *Streptomyces cacaoi* var. *asoensis*, this antibiotic has a specific rotation of $[\alpha]_D^{20}$ + 19° (c 1·0, H₂O) and has ultraviolet spectra in acid and alkali which are identical with those of the preceding compound. The antifungal properties are also similar to those of polyoxin D.

POLYMYXIN E₁
See Colistin A

POLYOXIN F
$C_{23}H_{30}O_{16}N_6$
Dec. > 190°C

A further antifungal antibiotic isolated from cultures of *Streptomyces cacaoi* var. *asoensis*, this substance is an amorphous powder which decomposes above 190°C. It is laevorotatory with $[\alpha]_D^{20} - 18°$ (c 1·0, H₂O) and gives an ultraviolet spectrum in 0·05 N-HCl with an absorption maximum at 276 nm and a shoulder at 215 nm. In 0·05 N-NaOH there is a single absorption maximum at 271 nm.

Suzuki *et al.*, *Agr. Biol. Chem.*, **30**, 817 (1966)
Isono *et al.*, *ibid.*, **31**, 190 (1967)
Structure
Isono, Asahi, Suzuki, *J. Amer. Chem. Soc.*, **91**, 7490 (1969)

POLYOXIN G
$C_{17}H_{25}O_{12}N_5$
Dec. > 190°C

This antifungal antibiotic produced by *Streptomyces cacaoi* var. *asoensis* is also an amorphous white powder which decomposes without melting. It has a specific rotation of $[\alpha]_D^{20} + 37°$ (c 1·0, H₂O) and gives an ultraviolet spectrum in 0·05 N-HCl with an absorption maximum at 262 nm and in 0·05 N-NaOH an absorption maximum at 264 nm.

Suzuki *et al.*, *Agr. Biol. Chem.*, **30**, 817 (1966)
Isono *et al.*, *ibid.*, **31**, 190 (1967)
Structure
Isono, Asahi, Suzuki, *J. Amer. Chem. Soc.*, **91**, 7490 (1969)

POLYOXIN H
$C_{23}H_{32}O_{13}N_6$
M.p. Indefinite

Streptomyces cacaoi var. *asoensis* yields this antifungal antibiotic which crystallizes as colourless needles. It has a specific rotation of $[\alpha]_D^{20} - 38°$ (c 1·0, H₂O). The ultraviolet spectrum in 0·05 N-HCl has a single absorption maximum at 265 nm and in 0·05 N-NaOH at 266 nm.

POLYOXIN I
$C_{17}H_{22}O_9N_4$
M.p. Indefinite

An amorphous antifungal antibiotic, also produced by *Streptomyces cacaoi* var. *asoensis*, this substance is laevorotatory with a specific rotation of $[\alpha]_D^{20} - 35°$ (c 1·0, H_2O) and has an ultraviolet spectrum with an absorption maximum at 262·5 nm in 0·05 N-HCl and one at 264 nm in 0·05 N-NaOH.

Isono *et al.*, *Agr. Biol. Chem.*, **31**, 190 (1967)
Structure
Isono, Asahi, Suzuki, *J. Amer. Chem. Soc.*, **91**, 7490 (1969)

POLYOXIN J
$C_{17}H_{25}O_{12}N_5$
M.p. Indefinite

An antifungal antibiotic closely resembling polyoxin E (q.v.), this compound is also elaborated by *Streptomyces cacaoi* var. *asoensis*. It has a specific rotation of $[\alpha]_D^{22} + 31·7°$ (c 1·0, H_2O). In 0·05 N-HCl the absorption maximum in the ultraviolet spectrum occurs at 264 nm, and in 0·05 N-NaOH at 267 nm.

Isono, Kobinata, Suzuki, *Agr. Biol. Chem.*, **32**, 792 (1968)
Structure
Isono, Asahi, Suzuki, *J. Amer. Chem. Soc.*, **91**, 7490 (1969)
Synthesis
Kuzuhara, Ohrui, Emoto, *Tetrahedron Lett.*, 5055 (1973)

POLYOXIN K
$C_{22}H_{30}O_{13}N_6$
M.p. Indefinite

This antifungal antibiotic elaborated by *Streptomyces cacaoi* var. *asoensis* has a structure identical to that of polyoxin F but minus a carboxylic acid group. It has a specific rotation of $[\alpha]_D^{22} - 16·5°$ (c 1·0, H_2O) and gives an ultraviolet spectrum in 0·05 N-HCl with an absorption maximum at 259 nm and in 0·05 N-NaOH at 262 nm.

Isono, Kobinata, Suzuki, *Agr. Biol. Chem.*, **32**, 792 (1968)
Structure
Isono, Asahi, Suzuki, *J. Amer. Chem. Soc.*, **91**, 7490 (1969)

POLYOXIN L
$C_{16}H_{23}O_{12}N_5$

Also isolated from *Streptomyces cacaoi* var. *asoensis*, this antibiotic has antifungal properties. It is dextrorotatory with a specific rotation of $[\alpha]_D^{22} + 34·4°$ (c 1·0, H_2O) and gives an ultraviolet spectrum in 0·05 N-HCl with an absorption maximum at 259 nm and in 0·05 N-NaOH at 262 nm.

Isono, Kobinata, Suzuki, *Agr. Biol. Chem.*, **32**, 792 (1968)
Structure
Isono, Asahi, Suzuki, *J. Amer. Chem. Soc.*, **91**, 7490 (1969)

POLYOXIN M
$C_{16}H_{23}O_{11}N_5$
M.p. Indefinite

This polyoxin antibiotic has been isolated from cultures of *Streptomyces cacaoi* var. *asoensis* and also from *S. piomogenus*. It may also be obtained by treatment of polyoxin D with sodium bisulphite followed by column chromatography. Like all of this group of antibiotics it is active against *Alternaria kikuchiana*, *Ophiobolus miyabeanus* and *Piricularis oryzae*.

Shibuya *et al.*, *Agr. Biol. Chem.*, **36**, 1229 (1972)
Suzuki *et al.*, *Japanese Patent*, 7,223,596

POLYOXIN N
M.p. Indefinite

Streptomyces piomogenus elaborates polyoxins N and O which may be separated by chromatography on powdered cellulose, eluting with a mixture of BuOH—AcOH—H_2O. Polyoxin N is a potent antifungal antibiotic, active against *Alternaria kikuchiana*, *Ophiobolus miyabeanus* and *Piricularia oryzae*. It has a low toxicity in mice.

Suzuki *et al.*, *Japanese Patent*, 7,223,596 (1972)

POLYOXIN O
M.p. Indefinite
Isolated together with the preceding antibiotic from cultures of *Streptomyces piomogenus*, polyoxin O has a similar antifungal activity and toxicity.

Suzuki *et al.*, *Japanese Patent*, 7,223,596 (1972)

POLYPEPTIN
$C_{56}H_{96}O_{13}N_{12}$
M.p. 176°C

Bacillus krzemieniewski elaborates this antibiotic which forms colourless crystals from EtOH. It was originally believed to be identical with circulin (q.v.) but this view is no longer held. Acid hydrolysis yields three moles of L-α,γ-diaminobutyric acid, two moles of L-leucine and one mole each of L-isoleucine, D-phenylalanine, L-threonine and D-valine. Polypeptin may be characterized as the sulphate which is laevorotatory with a specific rotation of $[\alpha]_D^{20}$ − 93·3° (c 3·0, 70 per cent *iso*PrOH). The antibiotic is active against a number of gram-positive bacteria.

Howell, *J. Biol. Chem.*, **186**, 863 (1950)
Hausmann, Craig, *ibid.*, **198**, 405 (1952)

POLYPORIN
An antibiotic first described by Bose, polyporin is obtained from *Polystictus sanguineus* by surface growth on a Czapek-Dox medium with 1 per cent peptone, incubated for 14 days at 22–32°C. Polyporin has acidic properties and is thermostable, but heating with acids or alkalies decomposes the compound. It is insoluble in H_2O but freely soluble in most common organic solvents. It is not inactivated by pepsin or gastric juice.

Polyporin is assayed by cylinder plate or the disc method using *Escherichia coli*, *Staphylococcus aureus* or *Streptococcus pyogenes* as the test organism. The antibiotic is active *in vitro* against *Eberella typhi*, *Escherichia coli*, *Salmonella paratyphi*, *S. schottmuelleri*, *Shigella paradysenteriae*, *Staphylococcus aureus*, *Streptococcus pyogenes*, *Strep. viridans* and *Vibrio comma*.

Some encouraging results have been obtained with the antibiotic *in vivo*, the crude compound being effective against infections caused by *Staphylococcus aureus*, *Streptococcus pyogenes* and *Strep. viridans*. Preliminary clinical trials have also been carried out by oral administration and polyporin has been found to be effective against cholera, paratyphoid and typhoid infections. Bose has shown, however, that it neutralizes typhoid vaccine. Polyporin is remarkably non-toxic. When administered intramuscularly in humans there is no hemolytic or pyrogenic effect and it has no irritating effect upon ulcers, open wounds or the conjunctiva.

Bose, *Curr. Sci.*, **13**, 233 (1944)
Bose, *Nature*, **156**, 171 (1945)
Bose, *J. Ind. Med. Assoc.*, **14**, 214 (1945)
Bose, *Nature*, **158**, 292 (1946)

PORFIROMYCIN
$C_{16}H_{20}O_5N_4$
Dec. 201–201·5°C

Porfiromycin was first isolated from the culture broth of *Streptomyces ardus* and later from *S. verticillatus*. When recrystallized from CH_3OH it forms dark purple triclinic crystals which decompose without melting. The antibiotic is dextrorotatory with specific rotations of $[\alpha]_D^{25} + 242° \pm 100°$ (c 0·045, CH_3OH) and $[\alpha]_D^{25} + 275° \pm 55°$ (c 0·1, CH_3OH). The ultraviolet spectrum in H_2O has absorption maxima at 217 and 364 nm with a shoulder at 248 nm. Porfiromycin is moderately soluble in polar organic solvents, slightly soluble in H_2O and insoluble in hydrocarbons. It has found a limited use in medicine as an antimicrobial.

Herr *et al.*, *Antimicrobial Agents Annual*, 23, Plenum Press, New York (1961)
Webb *et al.*, *J. Amer. Chem. Soc.*, **84**, 3185, 3187 (1962)
Bohonos *et al.*, *U.S. Patent*, 3,219,530 (1965)

PORICIN
M.p. Indefinite
An antitumour antibiotic, poricin has been obtained from an aqueous extract of the mycelium of a basidiomycete *Poria corticola*. It forms a white amorphous powder when purified by precipitation with EtOH followed by a number of chromatographic stages. Poricin would appear to be an acidic protein which is active in inhibiting a number of tumours. It is, however, highly toxic and the toxicity of the crude material is not reduced by further purification.

Ruelius *et al.*, *Arch. Biochem. Biophys.*, **125**, 126 (1968)

PORTAMYCIN
See Streptolydigin

PRASINOMYCINS
A group of antibiotics have been isolated from cultures of *Streptomyces prasinus*, obtained from soil from Colorado. The organism is cultured on a medium containing glucose, soybean flour and inorganic salts at 25°C for 7 days on a rotary shaker. The mycelium cake is adjusted to pH 2·0, filtered, extracted with CH_3OH, neutralized, the CH_3OH evaporated and the residue extracted with $CHCl_3$, concentrated *in vacuo* and precipitated with $(CH_3)_2CO$ giving a light tan-coloured powder. Assay against *Staphylococcus aureus* by tube dilution gives a minimum inhibition concentration of 0·15 µg/ml. Separation by partition paper chromatography and countercurrent distribution gives five components of which three have been characterized, viz, Prasinomycin A, m.p. 166–169°C (*dec.*); $[\alpha]_D + 0·8°$ (H_2O), prasinomycin B, m.p. 167–170°C (*dec.*); $[\alpha]_D + 2·8°(H_2O)$ and prasinomycin C, m.p. 178–180°C (*dec.*); $[\alpha]_D + 4·4°$ (H_2O). The ultraviolet spectra of all three are virtually identical with absorption maxima at 244–246 and 256–257 nm. All have high molecular weights of 30,800 to 32,000 as determined in the ultracentrifuge in buffer solution. The prasinomycins, individually and as the complex, are active *in vitro* against gram-positive bacteria and *Mycobacterium tuberculosis bovis* B.C.G. but have little activity against gram-negative bacteria, fungi or yeasts. They are active *in vivo* giving a prolonged protective effect in mice when administered subcutaneously and there is no cross resistance with the penicillins or tetracyclines. The major antibacterial effect of these antibiotics is due to inhibition of cell wall biosynthesis by the relevant organisms.

Weisenborn *et al.*, *Nature*, 1092 (1967)
Laskin *et al.*, *Antimicrobial Agents & Chemotherapy*, 251 (1967)

PREMCILLIN
See Procaine Penicillin G

PRENOMYCIN
M.p. Indefinite

Prenomycin is a recently discovered phosphorus-containing antibiotic which has been obtained by culturing *Streptomyces ambofaciens* after two pre-incubation stages in a medium containing soybean flour, distillers' solubles, corn meal, lactose, corn steep liquor, sodium citrate and inorganic salts with aeration. The cell mass is extracted with CH_3OH and the extract chromatographed on Sephadex G-25. The antibiotic is active against a range of gram-positive and some gram-negative organisms.

Martinez Mata, Stapley, *U.S. Patent*, 3,891,753 (1975)

PRIMOCARCIN
$C_{10}H_{16}O_3N_2$
M.p. 130–131°C

An antineoplastic antimicrobial antibiotic, primocarcin has been isolated from cultures of *Nocardia fukaya*. The structure, 5-acetamido-4-oxo-5-hexenamide, has been confirmed by synthesis. Primocarcin forms colourless needles when crystallized from hot CH_3OH. The ultraviolet spectrum in H_2O has an absorption maximum at 235 nm while in 0·1 *N*-NaOH, there are two maxima at 215 and 347 nm. The antibiotic is soluble in H_2O, the lower alcohols, pyridine and $(CH_3)_2CO$, slightly soluble in other organic solvents. Hydrogenation gives the dihydro derivative, m.p. 137–141°C and the tetrahydro compound, m.p. 183°C. The LD_{50} in mice is 200 mg/kg (intravenous) and 55·5 mg/kg (intraperitoneal).

Isono, Suzuki, *J. Antibiotics* (Japan), **15A**, 77 (1962)
Structure
Isono, *J. Antibiotics* (Japan), **15A**, 80 (1962)
Synthesis
Bowman *et al.*, *J. Chem. Soc.*, 470 (1965)

PRIMYCIN
$C_{55}H_{102}O_{17}N_2^+ \cdot 0·5\ SO_4^{2-}$
Dec. 166–168°C

A highly complex macrolide antibiotic, this substance is derived from an actinomycete found in the intestinal tract of *Galeria melonella* (wax moth).

The earlier formula of $C_{19}H_{37}O_7N$ has been drastically modified following the elucidation of the structure of this compound. Primycin forms colourless crystals from CH_3OH—BuOH which decompose without melting. It is moderately soluble in CH_3OH, less so in the higher alcohols and only slightly soluble in H_2O, AcOH and pyridine.

Primycin is a wide-spectrum antibiotic and also has some virucidal activity. It is, however, highly toxic to mammals although its use has been proposed for tropical application.

Valyi-Nagy, Uri, Szilagyi, *Nature*, **174**, 1105 (1954)
Szilagyi *et al.*, *ibid.*, **193**, 243 (1962)
Structure
Aberhart *et al.*, *J. Chem. Soc., Perkin I*, 816 (1974)
Fehr *et al.*, *ibid.*, 836 (1974)

PRISTINAMYCIN
$C_{45}H_{54}O_{10}N_7$
M.p. Indefinite

A cyclic polypeptide antibiotic elaborated by a strain of *Streptomyces*, the structure of pristinamycin has been established as that given above by chemical and spectroscopic methods. The antibiotic is active against a number of gram-positive and gram-negative bacteria, particularly *Staphylococcus aureus*. Resistant strains of the latter have been encountered but such resistance is lost following several passages on a medium free of the antibiotic. Castro *et al.* have shown that these resistant strains are cross-resistant to erythromycin (q.v.) but not vice versa. Neither heat nor treatment with acridine dyes has any effect upon this resistance.

Mancy *et al., French Patent*, 1,301,857 (1962)
Castro *et al., Antibiotica*, **7**, 163 (1969)

PROACTINOMYCIN

An antibiotic material isolated by Gardner and Chain from *Nocardia gardneri* (*Proactinomyces*), this substance has since been separated into three components, proactinomycins A, B and C by countercurrent distribution. The properties of the individual antibodies are described below. The complex is obtained by surface growth on a glucose agar medium which is incubated for 2 days when glucose broth is then added and fermentation continued for a further 2 days at 25°C. The material is isolated by acidifying the culture liquor to pH 5·0 with dilute HCl and extracting with Et_2O to remove impurities. The remaining culture liquor is then adjusted to pH 10, extracted with Et_2O and the ethereal fraction shaken with H_2O at pH 4·0, the aqueous extract being concentrated *in vacuo* and freeze-dried.

The mixture thus obtained forms an amorphous white powder which is soluble in C_6H_6, CCl_4, Et_2O and amyl acetate. It is precipitated from solution by picric, picrolonic and reinecke acids. It is normally assayed by serial dilution with *Staphylococcus aureus*, the following inhibition dilutions ($\times 1000$) for the impure antibiotic having been determined by Gardner and Chain and by Florey *et al. Corynebacterium diphtheriae* (512–2048); *Coryne. hofmanni* (512–2048); *Escherichia coli* ($> 1\cdot0$–$2\cdot0$); *Neisseria meningitidis* (500–800); *Pseudomonas aeruginosa* ($> 2\cdot0$); *Salmonella enteriditis* (32–160); *S. paratyphi* ($> 2\cdot0$); *S. typhi* ($> 1\cdot0$); *Shigella dysenteriae* ($> 2\cdot0$); *Staphylococcus aureus* (32–640); *Streptococcus pneumoniae* (200–1500); *Strep. pyogenes* (160–640); *Strep. viridans* (256) and *Vibrio comma* (6·0). The antibiotic is inactive against fungi and *Endameba histolytica* but inhibits both *Leishmania donovani* and *Trypanosoma equiperdum*.

When tested *in vivo* with mice, the crude antibiotic affords partial protection against experimental infections with *Streptococcus pyogenes* when administered either orally or intraperitoneally. Repeated doses produce chronic toxicity in mice, possibly associated with liver damage.

Gardner, Chain, *Brit. J. Exptl. Path.*, **23**, 123 (1942)
Florey, Jennings, Sanders, *ibid.*, **26**, 337 (1945)
Abraham, *ibid.*, **26**, 349 (1945)
Marston, *ibid.*, **30**, 398 (1949)
Marston, Florey, *ibid.*, **30**, 407 (1949)

PROACTINOMYCIN A

$C_{27}H_{47}O_8N$
M.p. 168–169°C

This component of proactinomycin is resolved from the basic mixture by countercurrent distribution. It forms colourless crystals which are soluble in EtOH, $(CH_3)_2CO$, Et_2O, $CHCl_3$ and C_6H_6. It is only slightly soluble in H_2O. The ultraviolet spectrum in Et_2O has an absorption maximum at 260 nm. In solution it is stable over the pH range from 2·0 to 8·0. Although active against gram-positive bacteria it shows only a limited activity against gram-negative bacteria and affords little protection to mice infected with *Streptococcus pneumoniae*. The LD_{50} when given intravenously in mice is 150 mg/kg.

Marston, *Brit. J. Exptl. Path.*, **30**, 398 (1949)
Marston, Florey, *ibid.*, **30**, 407 (1949)

PROACTINOMYCIN B

$C_{28}H_{49}O_8N$
M.p. 83–87°C

Also present in the antibiotic complex from *Nocardia gardneri*, this antibiotic resembles the preceding compound in its chemical and physical properties. It is less active against gram-positive bacteria on a weight basis than either proactinomycin A or C and has a toxicity of LD_{50} in mice of 120 mg/kg when given intravenously.

Gardner, Chain, *Brit. J. Exptl. Path.*, **23**, 120 (1942)
Marston, *ibid.*, **30**, 398 (1949)
Marston, Florey, *ibid.*, **30**, 407 (1949)

PROACTINOMYCIN C

$C_{24}H_{41}O_6N$
M.p. Indefinite

The third component of the antibiotic complex isolated from *Nocardia gardneri* and purified by countercurrent distribution, proactinomycin C has a biological activity against gram-positive bacteria very similar to that of proactinomycin A. It is somewhat more toxic than either of the two preceding antibiotics, the LD_{50} in mice being 80 mg/kg on intraveous injection.

Gardner, Chain, *Brit. J. Exptl. Path.*, **23**, 120 (1942)
Marston, *ibid.*, **30**, 398 (1949)
Marston, Florey, *ibid.*, **30**, 407 (1949)

PROCAINE PENICILLIN G (*Afsillin, Aquacillin, Cyticillin, Hydracillin, Ilcocillin P, Ladercillin, Lenticillin, Premocillin*)

$C_{29}H_{38}O_6N_4S$
M.p. 106–110°C (dec.)

A semi-synthetic antibiotic, this compound is prepared by the reaction of penicillin G with 2-(diethylamino)ethyl *p*-aminobenzoate. It forms monoclinic hemimorphic crystals from aqueous CH_3OH and is soluble in H_2O, CH_3OH and $CHCl_3$. It is not significantly affected by exposure to light or air. Acids, alkalies, alkali hydroxides and oxidizing agents, however, rapidly inactivate it. The penicillin potency is approximately 1000 units/mg. The LD_{50} in mice is 70 mg/kg when given intravenously. Procaine penicillin G is used in medicine as an antimicrobial although allergic side reactions may occur. In veterinary medicine, it finds a use in the treatment of infections caused by certain clostridia, erysipelothrix, staphylococci and streptococci.

Ruskin, *U.S. Patent*, 2,676,961 (1954)
Sumner, Grenfell, *U.S. Patent*, 2,725,336 (1955)
Bardolph, *U.S. Patent*, 2,739,962 (1956)
Weiss *et al.*, *Antibiotics & Chemotherapy*, **7**, 374 (1957)
Crystal structure
Rose, *Anal. Chem.*, **27**, 1841 (1955)

PRODIGIOSIN

$C_{20}H_{25}ON_3$

Two compounds of this name have been described in the literature. One is a red pigment derived from *Serratia marcescens* (*Chromobacterium prodigiosum*) by Wrede and Rothaus. When examined *in vitro*, however, it proved to be completely inactive against ten representative species of bacteria at a concentration of 0·005–0·1 per cent.

The second compound, also isolated from *Serratia marcescens*, is colourless, thermostable and soluble in H_2O. Lichstein and Van de Sand have demonstrated that this compound has a bacteriostatic activity against a number of organisms including *Bacillus subtilis*, *Corynebacterium diphtheriae* and *Staphylococcus aureus*.

Wrede, Hettche, *Chem. Ber.*, **62**, 2678 (1929)
Lasseur, Georges, *Trav. Lab. Microbiol. Nancy*, **9**, 47 (1936)
Lasseur, Melcion, *ibid.*, **13**, 192 (1944)
Wrede, Rothaus, *Zeit. f. physiol. Chem.*, **226**, 95 (1945)
Lichstein, Van de Sand, *J. Bact.*, **52**, 145 (1946)
Synthesis
Wasserman *et al.*, *J. Amer. Chem. Soc.*, **82**, 506 (1960)
Rapoport, Holden, *ibid*, **82**, 5510 (1960)
Rapoport, Holden, *ibid.*, **84**, 635 (1962)
Castro *et al.*, *J. Org. Chem.*, **28**, 857 (1963)
Morgan, Tanner, *J. Chem. Soc.*, 3305 (1955)
Kalesperis, Prahlad, Lynch, *Can. J. Microbiol.*, **21**, 213 (1975)

PROPACIN
See Thiamphenicol

N-PROPIONYLHOLOTHIN

$C_8H_8N_2O_2S_2$

A derivative of holothin, this antibiotic has been isolated from cultures of a mutant strain of *Streptomyces* P6621-7N-49. It occurs with holothin and has been separated from the extract with BuOH followed by thin layer chromatography.

Okamura *et al.*, *J. Antibiotics* (Japan), **30**, 334 (1977)

PROPIONYLMARIDOMYCIN I

$C_{46}H_{75}O_{17}N$

The semi-synthetic antibiotic propionylmaridomycin has been shown by Ohkubo to consist of six components which are all closely related aminoglycosidic macrolide compounds. Most of the biological studies have been

Propionylmaridomycin II

carried out using propionylmaridomycin III which is the major component of the complex (see propionylmaridomycin III).

Ohkubo, *Chemotherapy* (Tokyo), **21**, 907 (1973)

PROPIONYLMARIDOMYCIN II
$C_{45}H_{73}O_{17}N$

This minor component of the propionylmaridomycin complex differs in structure from the preceding antibiotic only in having an acetoxy group in the macrolide moiety in place of the propoxy group.

Ohkubo, *Chemotherapy* (Tokyo), **21**, 907 (1973)

PROPIONYLMARIDOMYCIN III
$C_{44}H_{71}O_{17}N$

The major component isolated from propionylmaridomycin complex, this antibiotic is active against a large number of bacteria. It inhibits the growth of anaerobic organisms, e.g. *Bacteroides*, *Peptococcus* and *Peptostreptococcus* freshly isolated from clinical materials at a concentration of 12·5 µg/ml but has no action against *Fusobacterium* even at a concentration of 500 µg/ml. It also shows a high activity against *Mycoplasma pneumoniae*, *Sarcina lutea* and *Staphylococcus aureus*. Hara and his colleagues have found that the antibiotic is metabolized in the blood to maridomycin, 4″-deacylmaridomycin and other unidentified metabolites. From these observations it appears that maridomycin is the active form of this antibiotic.

Ohkuno, *Chemotherapy* (Tokyo), **21**, 907 (1973)
Matsuzawa, *ibid*, **21**, 920 (1973)
Nakazawa, *ibid.*, **21**, 932 (1973)
Fugono, Kita, Maeda, *ibid.*, **21**, 989 (1973)
Fukaya *et al.*, *ibid.*, **21**, 1020 (1973)
Okubo *et al*, *ibid.*, **21**, 1035 (1973)
Hara *et al.*, *ibid.*, **21**, 1060, 1068 (1973)

PROPIONYLMARIDOMYCIN IV
$C_{43}H_{69}O_{17}N$

Propionylmaridomycin V

A further minor constituent of the propionylmaridomycin complex, the structure of this antibiotic has been determined by chemical degradation and spectroscopic studies.

Ohkuno, *Chemotherpy* (Tokyo), **21**, 907 (1973)

PROPIONYLMARIDOMYCIN V
$C_{43}H_{69}O_{17}N$

A positional isomer of the preceding antibiotic, this substance has been isolated from the propionylmaridomycin complex by chromatography and countercurrent distribution. The structure has been determined from chemical and spectroscopic studies.

Ohkuno, *Chemotherapy* (Tokyo), **21**, 907 (1973)

PROPIONYLMARIDOMYCIN VI
$C_{41}H_{67}O_{17}N$

3-O-propionyl-5-O-mycaminosyl platenolide II

The propionylmaridomycin complex also yields this minor component when subjected to chromatography and countercurrent distribution. The structure has been established chemically and spectroscopically.

Ohkuno, *Chemotherapy* (Tokyo), **21**, 907 (1973)

3-O-PROPIONYL-5-O-MYCAMINOSYL PLATENOLIDE I
$C_{31}H_{50}NO_{10}$

Streptomyces platensis subsp. *malvinus* MCRL 0388 elaborates this macrocyclic antibiotic which occurs in the culture broth of blocked mutants of this species. It has been obtained and purified by extraction of the culture filtrate with an organic solvent followed by column chromatography. The antibiotic is effective against a range of gram-positive bacteria.

Furumai, Suzuki, *J. Antibiotics* (Japan), **28**, 775 (1975)

3-O-PROPIONYL-5-O-MYCAMINOSYL PLATENOLIDE II
$C_{31}H_{52}NO_{10}$

A second antibiotic isolated from the culture filtrate of blocked mutants of *Streptomyces platensis* subsp. *malvinus* MCRL 0399, this substance is a dihydro derivative of the preceding antibiotic. It has the structure given above and is active against gram-positive bacteria.

Furumai, Suzuki, *J. Antibiotics* (Japan), **28**, 775 (1975)

PROPICILLIN
$C_{18}H_{22}O_5N_2S$

A semi-synthetic antibiotic, propicillin is normally employed as the potassium salt under the names of Brocillin and Ultrapen. This salt decomposes at 195–197°C. It has antibiotic properties similar to phenbenicillin and phenathicillin (q.v.).

Perron *et al.*, *J. Amer. Chem. Soc.*, **82**, 3934 (1960)
Beecham Research Laboratories, *British Patent*, 877,120 (1962)
Glombitza, *Annalen*, **673**, 166 (1964)

PROTICIN
$C_{31}H_{44}O_7NaP$
M.p. Indefinite

An antibiotic isolated from *Bacillus licheniformis* var. *mesentericus*, ATCC 21,552, this substance contains both sodium and phosphorous in the molecule. It yields a colourless, amorphous powder with no definite melting point and has a specific rotation of $[\alpha]_D^{22} - 78°$ (c 0.35, EtOH). Proticin is active against *Escherichia coli*, *Proteus mirabilis* and *Streptococcus hemolyticus*, somewhat less active against *Mycobacterium tuberculosis*, *Salmonella* and *Shigella* species. The LD_{50} in mice is > 150 mg/kg given intraveneously and > 1000 mg/kg when administered subcutaneously.

Präve, Sukatsch, Vertesy, *J. Antibiotics* (Japan), **25**, 1 (1972)
Vertesy, *ibid.*, **25**, 4 (1972)
Nesemann *et al.*, *Naturwiss.*, **59**, 81 (1972)
Vertesy, Präve, Sukatsch, *German Patent*, 2,035,812 (1972)
Farbwerke Hoechst A.-G., *British Patent*, 1,350,271 (1974)

PROTOANEMONIN
See Anemonin

PROTOSTREPTOVARICIN I
$C_{36}H_{47}NO_9$
M.p. 270–271°C

Further examination of the streptovaricin complex isolated from cultures of *Streptomyces spectabilis* has resulted in the isolation of a series of antibiotics, protostreptovaricins I–V which have been separated and purified by chromatographic methods. This substance forms colourless crystals and is dextrorotatory with a specific rotation of $[\alpha]_D^{25} + 703°$ (c 0.202 CHCl$_3$). It has been shown to inhibit Rauscher leukemia virus RNA-dependent DNA polymerase to the extent of 69 per cent. The structure has been elucidated by chemical and spectroscopic techniques.

Kakinuma, Rinehart, *J. Antibiotics* (Japan), **27**, 733 (1974)
Rinehart *et al.*, *Biochemistry*, **13**, 861 (1974)
Prabhakar *et al.*, *J. Amer. Chem. Soc.*, **98**, 870 (1976)

PROTOSTREPTOVARICIN II
$C_{37}H_{49}NO_9$
M.p. 151–161°C

A further component of the streptovaricin complex obtained from cultures of *Streptomyces spectabilis*, this antibiotic yields colourless crystals and has a specific rotation of $[\alpha]_D^{25} + 241°$ (c 0.315, CHCl$_3$). It has the structure shown above and inhibits Rauscher leukemia virus RNA-dependent DNA polymerase to the extent of 66 per cent.

Kakinuma, Rinehart, *J. Antibiotics* (Japan), **27**, 733 (1974)
Rinehart *et al.*, *Biochemistry*, **13**, 861 (1974)
Prabhaker *et al.*, *J. Amer. Chem Soc.*, **98**, 870 (1976)

PROTOSTREPTOVARICIN III
$C_{36}H_{47}NO_{10}$
M.p. 135–137°C

A minor component of the streptovaricin complex, this antibiotic forms colourless crystals and is dextrorotatory having a specific rotation of $[\alpha]_D^{24}$ + 286° (c. 0·206, $CHCl_3$). It is a hydroxy derivative of protostreptovaricin I, having the above structure which is based upon chemical examination and the infrared, NMR and mass spectra.

Kakinuma, Rinehart, *J. Antibiotics* (Japan), **27**, 733 (1974)
Rinehart *et al.*, *Biochemistry*, **13**, 861 (1974)
Prabhakar *et al.*, *J. Amer. Chem. Soc.*, **98**, 870 (1976)

PROTOSTREPTOVARICIN IV
$C_{37}H_{49}NO_{10}$
M.p. 140–142°C

Also present in the streptovaricin complex of antibiotics isolated from cultures of *Streptomyces spectabilis*, this substance has been obtained as colourless crystals and has a specific rotation of $[\alpha]_D^{24}$ + 302° (c 0·281, $CHCl_3$). The structure has been determined primarily from spectroscopic data.

Kakinuma, Rinehart, *J. Antibiotics* (Japan), **27**, 733 (1974)
Rinehart *et al.*, *Biochemistry*, **13**, 861 (1974)
Prabhakar *et al.*, *J. Amer. Chem. Soc.*, **98**, 870 (1976)

PROTOSTREPTOVARICIN V
$C_{35}H_{45}NO_9$
M.p. 160–162°C

A further minor component of the streptovaricin complex, this antibiotic yields colourless crystals and is strongly dextrorotatory with a specific rotation of $[\alpha]_D^{25}$ + 490°C (c 0·145, $CHCl_3$). It has been assigned the above structure on the basis of chemical and spectroscopic evidence.

Kakinuma, Rinehart, *J. Antibiotics* (Japan), **27**, 733 (1974)
Rinehart *et al.*, *Biochemistry*, **13**, 861 (1974)
Prabhakar *et al.*, *J. Amer. Chem. Soc.*, **98**, 870 (1976)

PRUMYCIN
$C_8H_{17}O_4N_3$

A simple antibiotic, prumycin has been isolated from *Streptomyces kagawaensis* (ATCC 21,811), isolated from soil. The antibiotic was obtained from the fermentation broth by ion-exchange adsorption and gel-filtration. The structure has been determined as the 5-D-alanyl derivative of 2:5-diamino-2:5-dideoxypentose. Prumycin may be characterized as the dihydrochloride which forms colourless needles with m.p. 195°C (*dec.*) and a specific rotation of $[\alpha]_D^{25}$ + 68° to + 155·2° (c 1·0, H_2O) varying between these values over a period of 5 hours. The N:N'-diacetyl derivative, m.p. 180°C (dec.); $[\alpha]_D^{25} + 52°$ (c 0·41, H$_2$O) and the tetraacetyl derivative with a specific rotation of $[\alpha]_D^{25} + 33°$ (c 0·21, CH$_3$OH) have also been prepared.

Prumycin has no activity against most bacteria and yeasts but is mainly active against phytopathogenic fungi, e.g. *Botrytis fabae* and *Sclerotinia sclerotiorum*. Mice tolerate an oral administration of 500 mg/kg with no toxic reactions.

Hata et al., *J. Antibiotics* (Japan), **24**, 900 (1971)
Omura et al., *J. Chem. Soc., Chem. Commun.*, 633 (1972)
Omura et al., *Agr. Biol. Chem.*, **37**, 2805 (1973)

PSEUDOMONIC ACID A
C$_{26}$H$_{44}$O$_9$

An antibiotic produced by *Pseudomonas fluorescens*, pseudomonic acid is characterized as the methyl ester which forms colourless needles when recrystallized from C$_6$H$_6$-light petroleum, m.p. 76·5–78°C; $[\alpha]_D^{24} - 9°$ (c 1·5, CHCl$_3$). This ester gives an ultraviolet spectrum having a single absorption maximum at 221·5 nm in EtOH.

Fuller et al., *Nature*, **234**, 416 (1971)

PSEUDOMONIC ACID B
C$_{26}$H$_{44}$O$_{10}$

A minor constituent of the antibiotic extract of the culture filtrate of *Pseudomonas fluorescens* NCIB 10586, grown in submerged culture, this antibiotic is a hydroxy derivative of pseudomonic acid A. It has been isolated as the methyl ester which is an optically inactive, colourless oil giving an ultraviolet spectrum in ethanol having a single absorption maximum at 221 nm.

Fuller et al., *Nature*, **234**, 416 (1971)
Chain, Fellows, *Chem. Commun.*, 847 (1974)
Structure
Chain, Mellows, *J. Chem. Soc., Perkin I*, 318 (1977)

PSICOFURANINE (*Angustmycin C*)
C$_{11}$H$_{15}$O$_5$N$_5$
Dec. 212–214°C

Streptomyces hygroscopicus var. *decoyicus* elaborates this antibiotic which has the structure 6-amino-9-D-psicofuranosylpurine. It forms colourless crystals from EtOH and is laevorotatory with a specific rotation of $[\alpha]_D^{25} - 68°$ (c 1·0; dimethylformamide). The ultraviolet spectrum in 0·01 N-HCl has an absorption maximum at 259 nm which is slightly shifted to 261 nm in 0·01 N-NaOH. The antibiotic is moderately soluble in H$_2$O, CH$_3$OH and EtOH, slightly soluble in BuOH and AcOEt. Psicofuranine is active against a number of gram-positive and gram-negative bacteria and also exhibits antitumour activity. It inhibits the conversion of xanthosine-5'-phosphate to guanosine-5'-phosphate.

Yüntsen, *J. Antibiotics* (Japan), **11A**, 244 (1958)
Hoeksema et al., *Antibiotics & Chemotherapy*, **9**, 419 (1959)
Slechta, *Biochem. Pharmacol.*, **5**, 96 (1960)
Structure
Schroeder, Hoeksema, *J. Amer. Chem. Soc.*, **81**, 1767 (1959)
Garrett, *ibid.*, **82**, 827 (1960)
Synthesis
Farkas, Sorm, *Collect. Czech. Chem. Commun.*, **28**, 882 (1963)
Biosynthesis
Sugimori, Suhadolnik, *J. Amer. Chem. Soc.*, **87**, 1136 (1965)

PTERYGOSPERMIN

An uncharacterized antibiotic substance, pterygospermin is obtained from the chopped roots of *Moringa pterygosperma*. The roots are extracted with absolute EtOH, the active material adsorbed on activated carbon, eluted with petroleum ether and the eluate evaporated *in vacuo* to give an oily residue.

Rao and his colleagues have determined the following inhibition dilutions ($\times$ 1000) *in vitro*: *Aerobacter aerogenes* (20); *Bacillus subtilis* (75–100); *Eberthella typhi* (40–50); *Escherichia coli* (20); *Mycobacterium phlei* (30); *Salmonella enteriditis* (30–40); *Shigella paradysenteriae* (40–50) and *Staphylococcus aureus* (75–100).

Rao, George, Pandalai, *Nature*, **158**, 745 (1946)

PUBERULIC ACID
$C_8H_6O_6$
M.p. 316–318°C (*dec.*)

This antibiotic is formed, together with puberulonic acid (q.v.) by *Penicillium aurantio-virens*, *P. cyclopium-viridicatum*, *P. johannioli* and *P. puberulum*, the ratio of the two acids obtained depending upon the organism used in the fermentation. The crude puberulic acid, isolated from the culture filtrate is purified by forming the diacetyl derivative with anhydrous sodium acetate at 140–150°C, pouring into H_2O and removing the associated puberulonic acid by crystallization as the acid sodium salt. Acidifying the mother liquor with H_2SO_4 gives crude puberulic acid diacetate which is dissolved in hot EtOH, treated with activated carbon and recrystallized. It is then hydrolyzed with NaOH in a nitrogen stream and on cooling and acidifying the solution, the free acid is precipitated. The pure compound forms a pale cream-coloured microcrystalline powder which sublimed at 220°C in high vacuum. The diacetyl derivative forms colourless crystals with m.p. 212°C.

Puberulic acid is assayed by serial dilution with *Staphylococcus aureus* as test organism. Oxford and his colleagues have determined the following inhibition dilutions ($\times$ 1000) *in vitro*: *Bacillus anthracis* (17–33); *B. coli-commune* ($>6\cdot0$); *B. typhimurium* ($>6\cdot0$); *Staphylococcus aureus* ($>6\cdot0$); *Staph. citreus* (>67); *Streptococcus pyogenes* ($6\cdot0$); *Strep. viridans* ($>6\cdot0$) and *Vibrio comma* ($>6\cdot0$).

Birkinshaw, Raistrick, *Biochem. J.*, **26**, 441 (1932)
Barger, Dorrer, *ibid.*, **28**, II (1934)
Oxford, Raistrick, Smith, *Chem. Ind.*, **61**, 485 (1942)
Kiser, Zellat, *Trans. N.Y. Acad. Sci.*, **7**, 210 (1945)
Heatley, Philpot, *J. Gen. Microbiol*, **1**, 232 (1947)
Structure
McGowan, *Chem. Ind.*, 205 (1947)
Corbett et al., *ibid.*, 626 (1949)
Corbett et al., *J. Chem. Soc.*, **1** (1950)
Corbett, Johnson, Todd, *ibid.*, 6 (1950)
Johns, Johnson, *ibid.*, 198 (1954)
Biosynthesis
Ferretti, Richards, *Proc. Nat. Acad. Sci.*, **46**, 1438 (1960)

PUBERULONIC ACID
$C_9H_4O_7$
M.p. 296–298°C (*dec.*)

Puberulonic acid is isolated, together with the preceding antibiotic, from the same species of *Penicillium*. It is purified by formation of the acid sodium salt which is then dissolved in H_2O, acidified with dilute HCl thereby precipitating the free acid. When purified in this manner, puberulonic acid forms glistening yellow plates or bright yellow prims. No esters or acetyl derivatives are formed by this compound.

Puberulonic acid is assayed in the same manner as puberulic acid (q.v.) and the following typical inhibition dilutions ($\times$ 1000) have been determined *in vitro*: *Bacillus anthracis* (10–17); *B. coli-commune* ($>6\cdot0$); *B. typhimurium* ($>6\cdot0$); *Staphylococcus aureus* ($>6\cdot0$); *Staph. citreus* (17); *Streptococcus pyogenes* ($>6\cdot0$); *Strep. viridans* ($>6\cdot0$) and *Vibrio comma* ($>6\cdot0$).

Birkinshaw, Raistrick, *Biochem. J.*, **26**, 441 (1932)
Barger, Dorrer, *ibid.*, **28**, II (1934)
Oxford, Raistrick, Smith, *Chem. Ind.*, **61**, 485 (1942)
Kiser, Zellat., *Trans. N.Y. Acad. Sci.*, **7**, 210 (1945)
Heatley, Philpot, *J. Gen. Microbiol.*, **1**, 232 (1947)

Structure
McGowan, *Chem. Ind.*, 205 (1947)
Aulin-Erdtman, *Acta Chem. Scand.*, **4**, 1325 (1950)
Johnson et al., *J. Chem. Soc.*, 1139 (1951)
Synthesis
Nozoe et al., *Bull. Chem. Soc., Japan*, **33**, 1071 (1960)
Biosynthesis
Ferritti, Richards, *Proc. Nat. Acad. Sci.*, **46**. 1438 (1960)

PUCHIIN

An antibiotic substance derived from *Eleocharis tuberosa* (Chinese waterchestnut), puchin is stable between pH 3·0 and 8·0, unstable to heat, not adsorbed by activated carbon, nor extracted by organic solvents. It is active against *Aerobacter aerogenes*, *Escherichia coli* and *Staphylococcus aureus* but not against *Bacillus graveolus*. The activity is destroyed by EtOH.

Chen, Cheng, Cheng, *Nature*, **156**, 234 (1945)

PUROMYCIN (*Achromycin*)

$C_{22}H_{29}O_5N_7$
M.p. 175·5–177°C

This non-pigmented basic antibiotic has been obtained from *Streptomyces alboniger*, the original mode of extraction not having been published. Hydrolysis yields dimethylaminopurine, s-amino-D-ribose and O-methyl-L-tyrosine. Puromycin is laevorotatory with a specific rotation of $[\alpha]_D^{25} - 11°$ (CH_3OH) and the ultraviolet spectrum in 0·1 N-NaOH has a single absorption maximum at 275 nm. Puromycin inhibits gram-positive bacteria including *Bacillus subtilis*, *Escherichia coli*, *Klebsiella pneumoniae*, *Micrococcus pyogenes* var. *aureus* and *Sarcina lutea* at a concentration of 2·0–8·0 µg/ml but has a lower activity against *Proteus vulgaris* (about 300 µg/ml) and *Mycobacterium* 607 (40 µg/ml). In mice it is active against *Trypanosoma equiperum*. The LD_{50} in mice is 675 mg/kg (oral), 350 mg/kg (intravenous) and 525 mg/kg (intraperitoneal). It is being investigated for use as an antiprotozoal agent. The antibiotic also completely inhibited Shope fibroma virus DNA synthesis in secondary rabbit kidney cell cultures at a concentration of 2 µg/ml as determined by autoradiography. This inhibition was, however, reversed following removal of the antibiotic from the cultures. The antibiotic has a marked effect on the rat phrenic nerve diaphragm, inhibiting the contractile response both to direct electrical stimulation of the muscle and to indirect stimulation via the phrenic nerve.

Porter et al., *Antibiotics & Chemotherapy*, **2**, 409 (1952)
Waller et al., *J. Amer. Chem. Soc.*, **75**, 2025 (1953)
Baker, Schaub, *ibid.*, **75**, 3864 (1953)
Baker et al., *ibid.*, **76**, 4044 (1954)
Porter et al., *U.S. Patent*, 2,763,642 (1956)
Goodman, *U.S. Patent*, 2,797,187 (1957)
Fryth, Waller, *J. Amer. Chem. Soc.*, **80**, 2736 (1958)
Synthesis
Baker et al., *J. Amer. Chem. Soc.*, **77**, 12 (1955)
Conformation
Jardetsky, *J. Amer. Chem. Soc.*, **85**, 1823 (1963)
See also
Maloney, Minocha, *Can. J. Microbiol*, **16**, 1369 (1970)
Luczak et al., *Acta Virol.* (Prague), **15**, 374 (1971)
Maroli, Scarsella, *Boll. Soc. Ital. Biol. Sper.*, **49**, 449 (1973)
Scarsella, Maroli, *ibid.*, **49**, 452 (1973)
Wulff, *Pharmacol. Biochem. Behav.*, **1**, 177 (1973)
Sturgess, Moscarello, *Proc. Electron Microsc. Soc. Amer.*, **31**, 544 (1973)
Szell et al., *Hung. Teljes.*, 6301 (1973)
Abou-Zeid et al., *J. Appl. Chem. Biotechnol.*, **23**, 837 (1973)

PURPUROMYCIN

$C_{26}H_{18}O_{13}$
Dec. 212°C

A naphthoquinone antibiotic related to the rubromycins (q.v.), this compound was produced by culturing *Actinoplanes ianthinogenes* on a medium containing peptone, meat extract, yeast extract, soybean flour, glucose and inorganic salts at pH 5·0 and 45°C. It is isolated by treatment of the filtrate with light petroleum and CH_3OH followed by purification on a silica gel column. Purpuromycin forms dark red crystals which decompose without melting. It is active in the concentrations given (µg/ml) against gram-positive bacteria (0·005–0·02), gram-negative bacteria (1·0–20) and fungi (0·2–0·5).

Coronelli et al., *J. Antibiotics* (Japan), **27**, 161 (1974)
Bardone et al., *Tetrahedron*, **30**, 2747 (1974)

PUUPEHENONE
$C_{21}H_{28}O_3$

An antibiotic isolated from a marine sponge of unknown genus, this compound has the structure given above which is based upon chemical and spectroscopic evidence. It is effective against gram-positive and gram-negative bacteria both *in vitro* and *in vivo*.

Ravi., *PhD Thesis*, University of Hawaii (1976)
Total synthesis
Trammell, *Tetrahedron Lett*, 1525 (1978)

PYO COMPOUNDS

A number of complex antibiotic substances have been isolated from cultures of *Pseudomonas pyocyanea* and characterized as, more or less, pure compounds. Those which have been described are Pyo Ib, Pyo Ic, Pyo II, Pyo III and Pyo IV. All are active against a wide range of bacteria (mainly gram-positive organisms) and are assayed by serial dilution with *Staphylococcus aureus* as the test organism or by acid-production inhibition with the same organism on lactose. The individual compounds are described below.

Schoental, *Brit. J. Exptl. Path.*, **22**, 137 (1941)

PYO Ib
$C_{31}H_{40}O_2N_2$
M.p. 146·2–147°C

The culture filtrate obtained from *Pseudomonas pyogenes* is centrifuged after acidifying with HCl to pH 3·5 and the precipitate extracted with hot 95 per cent EtOH, diluted to 80 per cent EtOH, extracted with petroleum ether and the petroleum ether extracts discarded. The EtOH layer is then evaporated, the aqueous fraction extracted with Et_2O and the ethereal layer washed with sodium bicarbonate solution, following which it is extracted with dilute sodium carbonate solution. The carbonate solution is then extracted with Et_2O and then with dilute NaOH solution. This procedure removes the Pyo II and leaves Pyo I, III and IV in the sodium carbonate phase. The latter mixture is then fractionated on a 'Permutit' column after dissolving in $CHCl_3$ using increasing amounts of EtOH in $CHCl_3$. Pyo Ib is stable and forms colourless crystals which are soluble in alcohols, C_6H_6, dioxan, Et_2O, $(CH_3)_2CO$ and $CHCl_3$. It is precipitated from Et_2O by flavianic, hydrochloric and oxalic acids and may be catalytically hydrogenated with PtO_2 in AcOH to give the octahydro derivative. The biological properties are similar to those of Pyo Ic (q.v.).

Structure
Wells, *J. Biol. Chem.*, **196**, 331 (1952)

PYO Ic
$C_{34}H_{48}O_2N_2$
M.p. 138·8–139·2°C

This antibiotic forms colourless crystals, soluble in alcohols, $CHCl_3$, dioxan, C_6H_6, $(CH_3)_2CO$ and Et_2O. It is separated from the accompanying components by adsorption on a 'Permutit' column and elution with EtOH—$CHCl_3$. It has a potency of 1280 *Staphylococcus aureus* units/mg. Like the preceding antibiotic, it may be catalytically hydrogenated to give the octahydro derivative. It is also precipitated from Et_2O solution by flavianic, hydrochloric and oxalic acids.

Hays has determined growth inhibition dilutions against a number of bacteria, measured in Pyo II units causing a 50 per cent acid-production inhibition (2 units being equivalent to 1 growth inhibition unit): *Bacillus subtilis* (20); *Corynebacterium xerose* (320); *Escherichia coli* (20); *Staphylococcus aureus* (320); *Staph. aureus*, penicillin-resistant (20) and *Streptococcus hemolyticus* (40).

Hays et al., *J. Biol. Chem.*, **159**, 725 (1945)
Wells, *ibid.*, **196**, 331 (1952)

PYO II
$C_{34}H_{46}O_4N_2$
M.p. 149–149.5°C

This antibiotic is present in the ethereal extract from the treatment of the culture filtrate of *Pseudomonas pyocyanea* and may be purified by dissolving in C_6H_6, passing through an oxalic acid column, washing with C_6H_6, dissolving the column in Et_2O and saturated potassium bicarbonate and extracting the ethereal fraction with dilute sodium carbonate, acidifying the aqueous layer and re-extracting into Et_2O. The solvent is evaporated and the residue crystallized from C_6H_6 to give crude Pyo II. This material is purified further by dissolving the crystals in EtOH, decolourizing with activated carbon, recrystallizing from $(CH_3)_2CO$, from CH_3OH and finally from EtOH.

Pyo II contains 10,000 *Staphylococcus aureus* units/mg and has been tested against a large number of bacteria by Hays, giving the following Pyo II units *in vitro*: *Bacillus anthracis* (8·0); *B. subtilis* (4·0); *Brucella abortus* (64–256); *Br. melitenis* (256); *Br. suis* (128); *Corynebacterium diphtheriae* (4·0); *C. hoffmanni* (1·0); *C. xerose* (256); *Diplococcus pneumoniae* (64); *Eberthella typhi* (256); *Escherichia coli* (256); *Neisseria catarrhalis* (256); *Serratia marcescens* (256); *Staphylococcus aureus* (1·0–4·0); *Streptococcus hemolyticus* (65) and *Strep. viridians* (256).

When tested *in vivo*, Pyo II did not protect mice against *Diplococcus pneumoniae* when administered intraperitoneally, nor guinea pigs against *Mycobacterium tuberculosis* when given subcutaneously. Pyo II is highly toxic to mammals, the LD_{50} in mice being about 0·75 mg/kg given intraperitoneally.

Schoental, *J. Brit. Exptl. Path.*, **22**, 137 (1941)
Hays, *J. Biol. Chem.*, **196**, 331 (1952)

PYO III
$C_{34}H_{44}O_2N_2$
M.p. 152·8–153·5°C

A minor constituent found in the culture filtrate of *Pseudomonas pyocyanea*, this compound forms colourless crystals from EtOH. Catalytic hydrogenation yields the tetrahydro and dodecahydro derivatives. The antibiotic has a potency of 300 *Staphylococcus aureus* units/mg.

Schoental, *J. Brit. Exptl. Path.*, **22**, 137 (1941)
Wells, *J. Biol. Chem.*, **196**, 331 (1952)

PYO IV
$C_{16}H_{22}O_2N$
M.p. 139·5–140°C

This antibiotic from *Pseudomonas pyocyanea* forms colourless needles from EtOH. It has a potency of 120 *Staphylococcus aureus* units/mg. Pyo IV may be characterized as the crystalline dibenzoate and the 2:4-dinitrophenylhydrazone.

Schoental, *J. Brit. Exptl. Path.*, **22**, 137 (1941)

PYOPEN
See Carbenicillin

PYRACRIMYCIN A
$C_7H_{10}ON_2$

Streptomyces eridani elaborates two metabolites, pyracrimycins A and B which have also been obtained from *S. ticinensis* ATCC 21,619 by aerobic fermentation in a medium containing dextrose cultured at 28–30°C. The mixture of metabolites was obtained by filtration of the medium and addition of excess petroleum ether and pyracrimycin A separated by extraction with CH_2Cl_2 and crystallization from CH_3OH. The antibiotic is primarily active against several strains of *Escherichia coli* having a minimum inhibition concentration of 10–20 µg/ml. Reduction of the antibiotic yielded the dihydro derivative, also active against *E. coli* with a minimum inhibition concentration of 50 µg/ml.

Coronelli, Gallo, Beretta, *German Patent*, 2,061,056 (1972)
Coronelli *et al.*, *J. Antibiotics* (Japan), **24**, 491 (1971)

PYRACRIMYCIN B
$C_7H_{10}O_2N_2$
M.p. 222–4°C

This compound is elaborated by *Streptomyces eridani* and *S. ticinensis*. It forms pale yellow crystals from $CHCl_3$ and has no antibiotic activity.

Coronelli *et al.*, *J. Antibiotics* (Japan), **24**, 491 (1971)
Coronelli, Gallo, Beretta, *German Patent*, 2,061,056 (1972)

PYRAZOMYCIN (*Antibiotic A23812*)
$C_9H_{13}O_6N_3$
M.p. 112–115°C

An antibiotic isolated from *Streptomyces candidus* NRRL 3601, pyrazomycin is prepared by fermentation on a medium containing dextrose, dextrin, soybean peptone, Nadrisol Distillers Solubles and H_2O and cultured for 3–6 days at 30°C. Filan purification is carried out by filtration of the medium and chromatography. The antibiotic forms colourless crystals from H_2O and the structure has been determined from chemical and spectroscopic investigations. Pyrazomycin shows antifungal activity, particularly against *Neurospora* and is active *in vivo* against Herpes simplex viruses and vaccinia. Its use has been proposed for the treatment of viral infections, e.g. cold sores and smallpox at a dose of 0·5–250 mg/kg given daily.

Hoehn, Williams, *German Patent*, 2,019,838 (1971)
Farkas, Flegelova, Sorm, *Tetrahedron Lett.*, 2279 (1972)
Williams, Hoehn, *U.S. Patent*, 3,802,999 (1974)

PYRIDINDOLOL
$C_{14}H_{14}N_2O_3$

An unclassified species of *Streptomyces* yields this antibiotic substance which has the structure shown above based upon spectroscopic analysis and X-ray structure determinations. It possesses antibacterial, antifungal and antiviral activity and also inhibits bovine livergalactosidase.

Aoyagi *et al.*, *J. Antibiotics* (Japan), **28**, 555 (1975)
Kumagai *et al.*, *ibid.*, **28**, 876 (1975)

2-PYRROLIDINE-2-ACRYLAMIDE

This antibiotic has been produced by cultivating *Streptomyces eridani* ATCC 21,619 under aerobic conditions in nutrient media containing assimilable sources of carbon and nitrogen together with inorganic salts at 28–37°C for 3 days. 2-Pyrrolidine-2-acrylamide was isolated by extraction of the filtered medium with saline followed by extraction with an organic solvent. The antibiotic is active against a number of gram-positive bacteria.

Coronelli *et al.*, *U.S. Patent*, 3,737,439 (1973)

PYRROLNITRIN
$C_{10}H_6O_2N_2Cl_2$
M.p. 124–125°C

Pyrrolnitrin was first isolated from cultures of *Pseudomonas pyrrocina* and subsequently from *Ps. acidula*, strains B 76, CB 2318 and CB 2681. When purified by recrystallization from hot cyclohexane it forms pale yellow crystals which gradually become red or brown and lose antibiotic activity on exposure to air. The ultraviolet spectrum has a single absorption maximum at 252 nm. Pyrrolnitrin is soluble in AcOH and most organic solvents, slightly soluble in H_2O, cyclohexane and petroleum ether. The structure has been shown to be 3-chloro-4-(2'-nitro-3'-chlorophenyl)pyrrole, this having been confirmed by synthesis. The antibiotic has little activity against bacteria and is primarily active against various fungi including *Epidermophyton*, *Microsporum*, *Penicillium* and *Trichophyton*. The LD_{50} in mice has been given as 680 mg/kg (suspension in 5 per cent carboxymethylcellulose) administered intraperitoneally.

A large number of pyrrolnitrin analogues have been prepared by American and Japanese workers, by fermentation of a nutrient medium containing a substituted tryptophan in the presence of a pyrrolnitrin-producing organic such as *Pseudomonas* species ATCC 15,926. These compounds have been shown to possess an inhibitory action against a broad spectrum of bacteria and fungi.

Arima *et al.*, *Agr. Biol. Chem.*, **28**, 575 (1964)
Arima *et al.*, *J. Antibiotics* (Japan), **18A**, 201 (1965)

Pyrrolnitrin

Structure
    Imanaka *et al.*, *J. Antibiotics* (Japan), **18A**, 207 (1965)
Synthesis
    Nakano, *Tetrahedron Lett.*, 737 (1966)
Modified pyrrolnitrins
    Ajisaka *et al.*, *Progr. Antimicrob. Anticancer Chemother.*, *Proc. Int. Congr. Chemother.*, 6th (1969) p. 77.
    Gorman *et al.*, *U.S. Patent*, 3,590,051 (1971)

Q

QUADRONE
$C_{15}H_{20}O_3$
M.p. 185–186°C

Isolated from cultures of *Aspergillus tereus*, this unique antibiotic has the above structure based upon chemical and spectroscopic evidence. X-ray analysis has shown that the crystals are orthorhombic with space group $P2_12_12_1$ and a = 10·859, b = 12·890 and c = 18·550 Å with Z = 8. Quadrone is an antineoplastic having a marked inhibitory action against human epidermoid carcinoma of the nasopharynx (KB) *in vitro* and against P388 lymphocytic leukemia *in vivo* in mice.

Ranieri, Calton, *Tetrahedron Lett.*, 499 (1978)

QUINACILLIN
$C_{16}H_{16}O_6N_4S$

A semi-synthetic antibiotic of the penicillin class, this compound is a dicarboxylic acid and is normally employed as the crystalline disodium salt. It has been shown to have the advantage of a higher resistance to acid hydrolysis and a higher bacteriostatic activity than most of the semi-synthetic penicillin type compounds; e.g. cloxacillin, nafcillin, methicillin and oxacillin. Tests *in vitro* have shown that when given orally or subcutaneously at a dose of 50 mg/kg twice a day for 2 days to mice that have been experimentally infected with septicemia due to staphylococci, the therapeutic effects are greater with quinicillin than with the above mentioned antibiotics.

Rudzit et al., *Farmakol. Toksikol.* (Moscow), **37**, 219 (1974)

QUINOMYCIN A
$C_{51}H_{78}O_{12}N_{12}S_2$
M.p. Indefinite

This complex macrocyclic antibiotic is formed by the cultivation of *Streptomyces* 731-I in a common nutrient medium. The structure has recently been revised to that given above which is based upon carbon-13 NMR and infrared spectral examination. Quinomycin A is active against gram-positive bacteria and against Ehrlich ascites sarcoma.

Yosida et al., *J. Antibiotics* (Japan), **21**, 465 (1968)
Revised structure
Martin et al., *J. Antibiotics* (Japan), **28**, 332 (1975)

NX-QUINOMYCIN A
M.p. Indefinite

This antibiotic is prepared by cultivating *Streptomyces* strain 731-I in a medium containing quinaldinic acid. In this compound, one of the quinoxaline-2-carboxylic moieties in quinomycin A is replaced by one mole of quinaldinic acid. The antibiotic is active against a range of gram-positive bacteria and inhibits HeLa cells in suspension culture by 87 per cent. When given subcutaneously to mice it is effective against Ehrlich ascites sarcoma at a dose of 0·2 mg/kg daily for 5 days. The LD_{50} in mice is 0·84 mg/kg given intraperitoneally.

Yoshida et al., *J. Antibiotics* (Japan), **21**, 465 (1968)

QN-QUINOMYCIN A
M.p. Indefinite

A further semi-synthetic antibiotic, this compound occurs with the preceding substance in the culture filtrate after incubating *Streptomyces* strain 731-I in a medium to which quinaldinic acid is added. Here, both of the quinoxaline-2-carboxylic acid residues of quinomycin A are substituted by quinaldinic acid moieties. QN-quinomycin A inhibits the growth of gram-positive bacteria and HeLa cells in suspension culture at 0·01 μg/ml by 76 per cent. It also has a similar effect against Ehrlich ascites carcimona at twice the dose given for the preceding antibiotic. The LD_{50} in mice is 1·68 mg/kg given intraperitoneally.

Yoshida et al., *J. Antibiotics* (Japan), **21**, 465 (1968)

QUINOMYCIN C
$C_{55}H_{86}O_{12}N_{12}S_2$
M.p. Indefinite

Streptomyces strain 731–I, incubated on a common nutrient medium, yields this antibiotic which closely resembles quinomycin A in structure. It has a similar antibiotic activity and toxicity.

Martin et al., *J. Antibiotics* (Japan), **28**, 332 (1975)

QUINTOMYCIN D
$C_{23}H_{45}O_{13}N_5$

This antibiotic obtained from a number of *Streptomyces* species has been isolated as the pentahydrochloride which forms colourless crystals with m.p. 203°C (*dec.*). This salt is dextrorotatory with a specific rotation of $[\alpha]_D^{27} + 36°$ (c 1·0, H_2O). It is active against a range of gram-positive bacteria.

Munakata et al., *Japanese Patent*, 7,026,080 (1970)

R

RABELOMYCIN
$C_{19}H_{14}O_6$
M.p. 193°C (dec.)

A quinoid antibiotic obtained from cultures of *Streptomyces olivaceus* ATCC 21,549, rabelomycin is produced using a soybean medium and incubating at 25°C for 3 days. The mycelium is extracted with CH_3OH and extraction of the supernatant liquor with AcOEt yields the antibiotic. Rabelomycin crystallizes as yellow needles from $EtOH-C_6H_6$. It is laevorotatory with a specific rotation of $[\alpha]_D - 102°$ (c 1·0, $CHCl_3$). The ultraviolet spectrum in CH_3OH has absorption maxima at 228, 276 and 433 nm. The structure has been established as 1:2:3:4:7:12-hexahydro-3:6:8-trihydroxy-3-methylbenz a anthracene-1:7:12-trione.

Rabelomycin is assayed by serial dilution using *Staphylococcus aureus* as the test organism. It is active against a number of bacteria, and the following minimum inhibition concentration (μg/ml) have been measured: *Bacillus subtilis* (4·7); *Staphylococcus aureus* (6·3) and *Streptococcus pyogenes* (1·2).

Liu *et al.*, *J. Antibiotics* (Japan), **23**, 437 (1970)
Meyers *et al.*, German Patent, 2,124,711 (1971)

RACEMOMYCIN A
$C_{19}H_{34}O_8N_8$

A streptothricin-type antibiotic obtained from *Streptomyces racemochromogenes*, this compound has the structure given below based upon chemical and spectroscopic data. It is active against both gram-positive and gram-negative bacteria and also against mycobacteria. A number of N-phenyl-alkylidene derivatives have been prepared and examined for antibiotic activity, all being active in the same manner as the base antibiotic but with a tendency of lower delayed toxicity in mice. When acetylated with N-acetoxysuccinide, the N-acetyl derivative is formed, the antimicrobial activity of this compound being 500-fold lower than that of racemomycin A.

Taniyama, Takemura, *J. Pharm. Soc.*, Japan, **77**, 1210, 1217 (1957)
Taniyama, Takemura, *ibid.*, **78**, 742 (1958)
Taniyama, Sawada, Tanaka, *Chem. Pharm. Bull.*, **22**, 337 (1974)
Sawada, Sakamoto, Taniyama, *Yakugaku Zasshi*, **94**, 176 (1974)

RACEMOMYCIN B
$C_{60}H_{128}O_{32}N_{20}$
M.p. Indefinite

This antibiotic metabolite of *Streptomyces racemochromogenes* has a much more complex structure than either of the two accompanying antibiotics. When hydrolysed it yields β-lysine and streptolidine. It may be characterized as the chloride, m.p. 175°C (dec.) which is laevorotatory with a specific rotation of $[\alpha]_D^{19} - 45°$ (c 0·5, H_2O). Racemomycin B has a lower antibiotic activity than either racemomycins A and C.

Taniyama, Takemure, *J. Pharm. Soc., Japan,* **77**, 1210, 1217 (1957)
Taniyama, Takemura, *ibid.*, **78**, 742 (1958)

RACEMOMYCIN C
$C_{25}H_{46}O_9N_{10}$

The structure of this antibiotic closely resembles that of racemomycin A, differing only in the nature of the glysidic side-chain. It is also active against gram-positive and gram-negative bacteria and mycobacteria.

Taniyama, Takemura, *J. Pharm. Soc., Japan*, **77**, 1210, 1217 (1957)
Taniyama, Takemura, *ibid.*, **78**, 742 (1958)
Taniyama, Sawada, Tanaka, *Chem. Pharm. Bull.*, **22**, 337 (1974)

RACTINOMYCIN A
$C_{33}H_{30}O_{14}N_3$
M.p. 157°C (*dec.*)
A complex antibiotic, ractinomycin A is produced by *Streptomyces phaeochromogenes*. It forms orange needles which melt at 157°C with browning, turning black at 208°C. The ultraviolet spectrum in CH_3OH has two absorption maxima at 245 and 440–450 nm. In alkalies, the compound gives purple solutions. It is readily soluble in $(CH_3)_2CO$ and $CHCl_3$, moderately soluble in AcOEt, butyl acetate, CH_3OH, EtOH, CS_2 and C_6H_6, insoluble in H_2O and petroleum ether. Ractinomycin A is unstable in solutions with pH above 6·4–6·6. It is active against a number of gram-positive bacteria and is comparatively toxic, the LD_{50} in mice being 5·0–12·5 mg/kg when given intravenously.

Utahara *et al.*, *J. Antibiotics* (Japan), **8A**, 132 (1955)
Utakara *et al.*, *ibid.*, **10A**, 115 (1957)
Wakiki *et al.*, *Antibiotics & Chemotherapy*, **8**, 228 (1958)

RACTINOMYCIN B
M.p. 172–175°C (*dec.*)
Streptomyces phaeochromogenes also yields this antibiotic which forms orange-red needles from $CHCl_3$. It has a similar antibiotic spectrum to that of ractinomycin A but is somewhat less active.

Utahara *et al.*, *J. Antibiotics* (Japan), **8A**, 132 (1955)
Utakara *et al.*, *ibid.*, **10A**, 115 (1957)
Wakiki *et al.*, *Antibiotics & Chemotherapy*, **8**, 228 (1958)

RANCINAMYCIN Ia
$C_{11}H_{16}O_6$

Streptomyces lincolnensis elaborates a series of relatively simple antibiotics when cultured in a sulphur deficient medium. This antibiotic is isomeric with the following substance and has the structure given above based upon chemical analysis and spectroscopic data. It is active against a range of bacteria but failed to protect mice against lethal doses of *Straphylococcus aureus* when given orally or injected subcutaneously.

Argoudelis *et al.*, *J. Antibiotics* (Japan), **29**, 777 (1976)
Structure
Argoudelis *et al.*, *J. Antibiotics* (Japan), **29**, 787 (1976)

RANCINAMYCIN Ib
$C_{11}H_{16}O_6$

An isomer of the preceding compound, this antibiotic is one of the major constituents of the rancinamycin complex produced by *Streptomyces lincolnensis* when grown on a medium deficient in sulphur. The structure has been shown to be that given above. It has a similar antibiotic activity to that of the preceding compound.

Argoudelis *et al.*, *J. Antibiotics* (Japan), **29**, 777 (1976)
Structure
Argoudelis *et al.*, *J. Antibiotics* (Japan), **29**, 787 (1976)

RANCINAMYCIN IIa
$C_{12}H_{18}O_6$

Rancinamycin II, isolated from sulphur deficient cultures of *Streptomyces lincolnensis* has been shown to consist of three isomers, rancinamycins IIa, IIb, and IIc. These have been separated and purified chromatographically. This component has the structure shown above which has been determined from chemical and spectroscopic analysis.

Argoudelis *et al.*, *J. Antibiotics* (Japan), **29**, 777 (1976)
Structure
Argoudelis *et al.*, *J. Antibiotics* (Japan), **29**, 787 (1977)

RANCINAMYCIN IIb
$C_{12}H_{18}O_6$

An isomer of rancinamycin IIa, this antibiotic also occurs in the fermentation broth of *Streptomyces lincolnensis* when grown under sulphur deficient conditions. The structure has been established from chemical and spectroscopic data.

Argoudelis *et al.*, *J. Antibiotics* (Japan), **29**, 777 (1976)
Structure
Argoudelis *et al.*, *J. Antibiotics* (Japan), **29**, 787 (1976)

RANCINAMYCIN IIc
$C_{12}H_{18}O_6$

A further isomer of rancinamycin IIa, this substance has also been isolated from sulphur deficient cultures of *Streptomyces lincolnensis*. It has been assigned the structure given above.

Argoudelis *et al.*, *J. Antibiotics* (Japan), **29**, 777 (1976)
Structure
Argoudelis *et al.*, *J. Antibiotics* (Japan), **29**, 787 (1976)

RANCINAMYCIN III
$C_7H_{10}O_5$

Streptomyces lincolnensis also elaborates this antibiotic when grown on a medium deficient in sulphur. The structure has been elucidated from chemical and spectroscopic examination. It is one of the minor components of the rancinamycin complex.

Argoudelis *et al.*, *J. Antibiotics* (Japan), **29**, 777 (1976)
Structure
Argoudelis *et al.*, *J. Antibiotics* (Japan), **29**, 787 (1976)

RANCINAMYCIN IV
$C_7H_6O_3$

This antibiotic isolated from sulphur deficient cultures of *Streptomyces lincolnensis* has been shown to be 3,4-dihydroxybenzaldehyde. It is a minor component of the antibiotic complex and has only weak antibiotic properties.

Argoudelis et al., *J. Antibiotics* (Japan), **29**, 777 (1976)
Structure
Argoudelis et al., *J. Antibiotics* (Japan), **29**, 787 (1976)

RAPAMYCIN
$C_{56}H_{89}O_{14}N$
M.p. 183–185°C
A recently discovered antibiotic, rapamycin is produced by aerobic fermentation of the first inoculum of *Streptomyces hygroscopicus* NRRL 5491 in a common medium incubated at pH 7·1–7·3 and 28°C for 5 days. The antibiotic has only a limited activity against bacteria or mycobacteria but is active against fungi, particularly *Candida albicans*. Its use has been proposed for the disinfection of surgical instruments and in pharmaceutical preparations.

Sehgal et al., *German. Patent*, 2,347,682 (1974)
Sehgal, Baker, Vezina, *J. Antibiotics* (Japan), **28**, 727 (1975)

RAPHANIN
$C_{17}H_{26}O_3N_3S_5$?
B.p. 135°C/0·06 mm
Raphanin has been described as an antibiotic substance derived from the seeds of the radish (*Raphanus sativus*). In the seed it is present as a precursor which is antibiotically inactive being converted into the active form by a concomitant enzyme when incubated in aqueous solution. Care must be taken not to over-incubate since raphanin is then converted enzymatically into an inactive product. Following extraction from the seeds, the aqueous solution is extracted with butyl acetate, the solvent removed and the brown residue shaken with phosphate buffer at pH 7·2. The H_2O-soluble fraction is then extracted with $CHCl_3$, washed with phosphate buffer and passed through an alumina column before being distilled *in vacuo*. Raphanin is a yellow liquid which is soluble in EtOH, BuOH, AcOEt, butyl acetate, $CHCl_3$ and H_2O. It is fairly soluble in Et_2O and petroleum ether and is laevorotatory with a specific rotation of $[\alpha]_D^{20} - 141°$ (c 1·0, EtOH).

Raphanin is active against *Bacillus anthracis*, *B. prodigiosus*, *B. subtilis* and *Shigella dysenteriae* and the following inhibition dilutions (× 1000) have been determined *in vitro* by Ivanovics and Horvath: *Escherichia coli* (1–125); *Pseudomonas aeruginosa* (5·0–16); *Salmonella schottmuelleri* (8·0); *S. typhi* (4·0–16) and *Staphylococcus aureus* (1·0–15).

The antibiotic is comparatively toxic, a dose of 7–10 mg being lethal when administered subcutaneously or intravenously to mice. When given to guinea pigs, a dose of 50 mg, given intracardially, was also lethal.

Ivanovics, Horvath, *Nature*, **160**, 297 (1947)
Ivanovics, Horvath, *Proc. Soc. Exptl. Biol. Med.*, **66**, 625 (1947)

RAROMYCIN
M.p. Indefinite
A species of *Streptomyces* produces this antitumour antibiotic which is obtained in the form of a light yellow microcrystalline powder. The antibiotic has no definite melting point but begins to darken at 210°C. It is soluble in H_2O, CH_3OH, EtOH, BuOH and AcOEt, slightly soluble in C_6H_6 and $(CH_3)_2CO$ and insoluble in Et_2O and petroleum ether. Raromycin is active against a number of experimental tumours in mice.

Tanaka et al., *J. Antibiotics* (Japan), **10A**, 189 (1957)
Sumiki, Umezawa, *British Patent*, 822,226 (1959)
Sumiki, Umezawa, *Japanese Patent*, 10,996 (1960)

RECTILAVENDOMYCIN
A strain of *Actinomyces rectilavendulae* yields this antibiotic which has been isolated and studied by Russian workers. It is stated to have a pentaenic structure although the complete structure is not yet known.

Mitshevich et al., *Antibiotiki*, **20**, 202 (1975)

REQUINOMYCIN
$C_{40}H_{54}O_{16}N_2$
M.p. 215°C (*dec.*)
This antibiotic is elaborated by *Streptomyces filamentosus* and forms yellow crystals when recrystallized from EtOH. It is dextrorotatory with a specific rotation of $[\alpha]_D^{28} + 214°$ (c 1·09, $CHCl_3$).

Hori et al., *J. Antibiotics* (Japan), **25**, 393 (1972)

RESISTAPHYLLIN
$C_{24}H_{34}O_7N_2$
M.p. 91–92°C
Streptomyces antibiotics and *Streptomyces* species K-869 yield this antibiotic which has been shown to contain a conjugated triene system. It has a

specific rotation of $[\alpha]_D^{22} + 65°$ (c 1·0, CH_3OH) and forms a crystalline acetate with m.p. 79–80°C. The antibiotic is highly active against gram-positive bacteria. The following minimum growth inhibition concentrations (μg/ml) have been reported by Shirado et al. in vitro: *Bacillus cereus* (0·1); *B. megaterium* (0·1); *B. subtilis* (0·05); *Micrococcus fulvus* (0·025); *Sarcina lutea* (0·05); *Staphylococcus aureus* (0·006); *Staph. aureus*, resistant strains (0·025) and *Staph. epidermidis* (0·006).

Aizawa, Shibuya, Shirato, *J. Antibiotics* (Japan), **24**, 393 (1971)
Shirado et al., *Japanese Patent*, 7.205,000 (1972)

RESISTOFLAVIN
$C_{22}H_{16}O_7$
M.p. 238–240°C (dec.)

A pentacyclic antibiotic isolated from *Streptomyces resistonacificus* JA 3733, resistoflavin may be purified by crystallizing from AcOEt. It is laevorotatory with a specific rotation of $[\alpha]_D^{23} - 96°$ (c 0·5, pyridine). The ultraviolet spectrum in $CHCl_3$ has absorption maxima at 267 and 391 nm and a shoulder at 294 nm. The antibiotic is active against a number of gram-positive bacteria.

Eckardt et al., *Z. Chem.*, **10**, 221 (1970)
Eckardt, Fritzsche, Tresselt, *Tetrahedron*, **26**, 5875 (1970)
Eckardt, Bradler, Scoenfeld, *East German Patent*, 84,898 (1971)

RESISTOMYCIN
$C_{22}H_{16}O_6$
Dec. 315°C

Streptomyces resistomycificus elaborates this antibiotic which forms yellow needles when recrystallized from dioxan. It sublimes at 200–204°C at 0·0001 mm without any significant loss of activity. This substance is a weak acid, moderately soluble in EtOH, $(CH_3)_2CO$, C_6H_6, Et_2O and AcOH, slightly soluble in H_2O. The solutions in pyridine and piperidine vary from red to orange. In solution in H_2SO_4, EtOH, C_6H_6 and $(CH_3)_2CO$ it shows a marked fluorescence. Resistomycin is characterized by a number of derivatives including the monomethyl ether as colourless needles from dioxan, m.p. 277°C; the tetrabenzoyl derivative, colourless needles from C_6H_6-light petroleum, m.p. 264°C; the tetraacetate as an amorphous powder, m.p. 204–206°C and the 5:7:10-trimethyl ether, red prisms from CH_3OH with m.p. 280°C. It is highly active against gram-positive bacteria, inhibiting *Mycobacterium tuberculosis* at a dilution of 1:1,000,000 and both *Bacillus subtilis* and *Staphylococcus aureus* at 1:20,000,000.

Brockmann, Schmidt-Kastner, *Naturwiss*, **38**, 479 (1951)
Brockmann, Schmidt-Kastner, *Chem. Ber.*, **87**, 1460 (1954)
Brockmann, *German Patent*, 888,918 (1953)
Structure
Brockmann, *Angew. Chem.*, **76**, 863 (1964)
Brockmann et al., *Chem. Ber.*, **102**, 1224 (1969)

RETAMYCIN

Streptomyces olindensis produces an antibiotic complex, retamycin, which countercurrent distribution indicates contains at least two components. The mould was grown in submerged culture in a medium containing glucose, soy flower and inorganic salts at 27°C for 2 days. After adjusting the final pH to 6·6–6·8, the mycelium was extracted with $(CH_3)_2CO$, concentrated *in vacuo*, and back extracted with $CHCl_3$. Anhydrous sodium sulphate was then added and the solution concentrated, the antibiotic being precipitated by addition of *n*-hexane or petroleum ether. Retamycin complex is active against gram-positive and some gram-negative bacteria, *Neurospora crassa* and *Streptococcus fecalis* and also inhibits the growth of Walker carcinosarcoma and Yoshida sarcoma.

Goncalves de Lima et al., *Rev. Inst. Antibiot. Univ. Fed. Pernambuco, Recife*, **9**, 27 (1969)

REUMYCIN
$C_6H_5O_2N_5$
M.p. 244–5°C

A strain of *Actinomyces* elaborates this simple antibiotic which has the structure 6-methylpyrimido 5,4-e-*as*-triazine-5:7-(6*H*, 8*H*)-dione. Reumycin forms yellow crystals from EtOH and gives an ultraviolet spectrum in EtOH with absorption maxima at 235, 340 and 400 nm with a shoulder at

265 nm. Reumycin is an antineoplastic and antitumour agent. Experiments *in vitro* have shown that it possesses a significant cytostatic effect on transplantable Hep-12 HeLa cells at 12·5–50 µg/ml and at the higher concentration it strongly suppresses DNA, RNA and protein synthesis in these cells. With human tumours *in vitro*, the antibiotic exhibits a cytotoxic effect on Wilms tumour at 6·0–12·5 µg/ml. When incubated with 5-day-old primary explanations from Crocker sarcoma, Ehrlich carcinoma and lymphosarcoma LIO-1, inhibition of RNA synthesis and destruction of the electron transport system was observed. The drug appears to destroy protoplasm membranes and the lipoprotein complex of mitochondrial membranes. Reumycin produced a significant inhibition of the growth of Harding-Passay melanoma and Ehrlich ascites carcinoma in mice and rats at a dose of 20–30 mg/kg.

Shtegel'man, *Antibiotiki*, **15**, 1021 (1970)
Esipov, Kolosov, Saburova, *J. Antibiotics* (Japan), **26**, 537 (1973)
Navashin *et al.*, *Aktual. Vop. Sovrem. Onkol.*, No. 3, 273 (1973)

RHIZOMYCIN
$C_{19}H_{30}O_5N_4$
M.p. 250–253°C (*dec.*)
Streptomyces novoverticillus elaborates this antibiotic which has been described by Japanese workers. It has been isolated from the culture filtrate by extraction with AcOEt followed by chromatography on Florisil and Sephadex G-10. Rhizomycin is a neutral substance, giving positive Benedict, biuret and Fehling reactions and negative anthrone, Ehrlich, $FeCl_3$ and ninhydrin reactions. It is stable under neutral and alkaline conditions but unstable in acid solutions. Rhizoymcin is active against gram-positive bacteria.

Takashi Tsuoroka *et al.*, *Meiji Seika Kenkyu Nempo.*, **11**, 26 (1970)

RHIZOPCHIN
$C_{34}H_{49}O_{10}N$
M.p. Indefinite
An antifungal antibiotic, rhizopchin is produced by *Rhizopus chinensis* MP-816, freshly isolated from soil and cultivated in common media at 28°C for 50 hours. The culture extract is chromatographed to give the polyene antibiotic. Rhizopchin exhibits no activity against bacteria but is effective against *Penicillium chrysogenum* and *Piricularia oryzae*. It is moderately toxic with LD_{50} in mice of 15 mg/kg when administered intraperitoneally.

Arima, Odahara, *Japanese Patent*, 7,130,793 (1971)

RHODIRUBIN A
$C_{42}H_{55}NO_{16}$

A strain of *Streptomyces* yields a number of antibiotics, the rhodirubins, when grown on a common nutrient medium. The culture broth is extracted with an organic solvent and the various components separated and purified by column and preparative thin layer chromatography. The structure of this antibiotic has been elucidated from a chemical and spectroscopic study of the hydrolysis products. Rhodorubin A is highly active against gram-positive bacteria and also possesses antifungal and antileukemic activity. The LD_{50} in mice has been reported as 7·5–10·0 mg/kg given intraperitoneally.

Kitamura *et al.*, *J. Antibiotics* (Japan), **30**, 616 (1977)

RHODIRUBIN B
$C_{42}H_{55}NO_{15}$

A further major component of the rhodirubin complex produced by an unclassified strain of *Streptomyces*, this antibiotic has a structure very similar to that of rhodirubin A. Acid hydrolysis at 85°C for 30 minutes with $0 \cdot 1N$ HCl furnishes ε-pyrromycinone and various sugars. It is strongly active against a wide range of gram-positive bacteria and also has some antifungal and antileukemic activity.

Kitamura *et al.*, *J. Antibiotics* (Japan), **30**, 616 (1977)

RHODIRUBIN C
An unclassified strain of *Streptomyces* also produces this antibiotic which is a minor constituent of the rhodirubin complex. The structure has not yet been fully elucidated. Hydrolysis with $0 \cdot 1N$ HCl at 85°C for 30 minutes gives ε-pyrromycinone and a number of sugars. It appears to possess a similar antibiotic spectrum to those of the other rhodirubins.

Kitamura *et al.*, *J. Antibiotics* (Japan), **30**, 616 (1977)

RHODIRUBIN D
A further component of the rhodirubin complex produced by an unclassified strain of *Streptomyces*, this antibiotic has been isolated only in small amounts and its structure is not yet known.

Kitamura *et al.*, *J. Antibiotics* (Japan), **30**, 616 (1977)

RHODIRUBIN E
Also present in the rhodirubin complex isolated from the culture broth of an unclassified *Streptomyces* species, this minor component of the mixture has not been fully investigated.

Kitamura *et al.*, *J. Antibiotics* (Japan), **30**, 616 (1977)

RHODIRUBIN G
A minor constituent of the rhodirubin complex, isolated from a species of *Streptomyces*, this antibiotic occurs only in small quantities and the structure has not yet been elucidated.

Kitamura *et al.*, *J. Antibiotics* (Japan), **30**, 616 (1977)

RHODOCIDIN
An antibiotic isolated from a species of *Streptomyces* termed *S. phoenix*, rhodocidin is an amorphous red powder which gives an ultraviolet and visible spectrum showing a broad absorption maximum between 500 and 530 nm. It is soluble in H_2O and a number of common organic solvents and is rapidly deactivated on addition of acids or alkalies. It has also been shown to be deactivated by the mycelium of *S. phoenix* unless excess oxygen is present. The dry powder and solutions in organic solvents are indefinitely stable at 55°C. Rhodocidin is active against gram-positive, gram-negative bacteria and mycobacteria. It is active *in vivo* against *Streptococcus pyogenes* and is found to be appreciably more active when given intraperitoneally than when administered by the intramuscular or intravenous routes. The LD_{50} in mice is 3 mg/kg (intramuscular), $2 \cdot 1$ mg/kg (intraperitoneally) and 2 mg/kg (intravenous). It is doubtful, however, if it will find any use in medicine.

Charney *et al.*, *Antibiotics & Chemotherapy*, **3**, 788 (1953)

RHODOMYCETIN
M.p. Indefinite

Produced by a red mutant strain of *Streptomyces griseus*, rhodomycetin is obtained by precipitation of the broth with acid and extraction of the precipitate with CH_3OH. The compound gives a red colour with acids and a blue colour with alkalies and is unstable under alkaline conditions. It is soluble in Et_2O, $(CH_3)_2CO$, AcOH, the lower alcohols and ethyleneglycol monomethyl ether but insoluble in H_2O. The ultraviolet spectrum shows absorption maxima at 235, 540 and 580 nm. The antibiotic is active against gram-positive bacteria and moderately active against mycobacteria. It has no activity against gram-negative bacteria and none *in vivo* in mice. No data are available concerning its toxicity.

Shockman, Waksman, *Antibiotics & Chemotherapy*, **1**, 68 (1951)

RHODOMYCIN A (*β-Rhodomycin II*)
$C_{36}H_{46}O_{12}N_2$
M.p. 189°C

One of two closely related antibodies isolated from cultures of *Streptomyces purpurascens*, this substance forms red prisims when recrystallized from $CHCl_3$-light petroleum. The ultraviolet and visible spectrum in CH_3OH consists of absorption maxima at 496, 532 and 566 nm. The antibiotic yields a dihydrochloride as red prisims, m.p. 205°C and a perchlorate, reddish needles, m.p. 188°C.

Brockmann, Patt., *Chem. Ber.*, **88**, 1455 (1955)
Structure
Brockmann, Valhneldt, Niemeyer, *Tetrahedron Lett.*, 415 (1969)

RHODOMYCIN B
$C_{28}H_{33}O_{10}N$

This antibiotic is also present in cultures of *Streptomyces purpurascens* and yields red crystals from CH_3OH. It forms a hydrochloride, m.p. 180°C and can be hydrolysed to rhodosamine and β-rhodomycinone.

Brockmann, Patt, *Chem. Ber.*, **88**, 1455 (1955)
Structure
Brockmann, Valhneldt, Niemeyer, *Tetrahedron Lett.*, 415 (1969)

β-RHODOMYCIN II
See Rhodomycin A

RHODOSPORIN
M.p. 210–220°C
This antibiotic from cultures of *Nigrospora oryzae* has been described by Japanese workers. It forms deep red crystals from EtOH. The structure is not yet known with certainty.

Furuya, Shirasaka, *Japanese Patent*, 7,012,637 (1970)

RICKAMYCIN
See Sisomicin

RIFAMAZINE
$C_{76}H_{92}O_{24}N_4$
A dimeric antibiotic of the rifamycin class, this compound is active against viral RNA-dependent DNA polymerase, bacterial DNA-dependent RNA polymerase and DNA-dependent RNA polymerase extracted from

rifampicin-resistant strains of *Escherichia coli*. While the antibiotic blocks initiation there is no interference with enzyme-template interation or with RNA elongation. It has been suggested that the activity of this antibiotic against RNA polymerase from rifampicin-resistant mutants is due to the binding of the dimer to both the rifamycin-specific binding site and a weak second site.

Fietta, Silvestri, *Eur. J. Biochem.*, **52**, 391 (1975)

RIFAMINE (*Rifamycin B diethylamide*)
$C_{43}H_{58}O_{13}N_2$
M.p. 170°C (*dec.*)

A semi-synthetic antibiotic, this substance is prepared from rifamycin B by normal chemical methods. It forms an orange-yellow precipitate which crystallizes from C_6H_6 with one mole of solvent. The crystals soften at 140°C and melt gradually up to 170°C with some decomposition. The antibiotic is laevorotatory with a specific rotation of $[\alpha]_D^{20} - 48 \cdot 7°$ (c 0·4, CH_3OH). The ultraviolet spectrum in a phosphate buffer has absorption maxima at 222, 302 and 421 nm. It has found some use as an antimicrobial.

Sensi *et al.*, *J. Med. Chem.*, **7**, 596 (1964)

RIFAMPICIN (*Rifampin*)
$C_{43}H_{58}O_{12}N_4$

A macrocyclic naphthalene type antibiotic, rifampicin is structurally related to the rifamycins (q.v.), both being produced by *Streptomyces mediterranei*. The structure given above has been established from chemical degradative studies and spectroscopic data. Rifampicin is active against gram-positive bacteria and a number of viruses, e.g. *Escherichia coli*, *Neisseria meningitidis* and *Staphylococcus aureus*. In the case of the meningococci there is often a rapid emergence of resistant cells when treated with this antibiotic. Volk and Dorozhkova have shown that rifampicin has the ability to induce L-forms in *Mycobacterium tuberculosis*, this process being realized mainly through the phase of spheroplast-like formations. Using the same organism, Westfal *et al.* have demonstrated that both continuous and intermittent oral treatment with rifampicin in guinea pigs markedly decreased the bacilli count in the spleen and the combined treatment with rifampicin and isoniazid was even more effective. Rifampicin also has an immunosuppressant effect, the antibiotic probably acting at a very early stage of the immune response, thereby blocking recognition of the antigen.

Rifampicin inhibits H-1 virus infection in hamsters at a dose of 300 mg/kg/day given orally for 9 days.

Engle, Lasinski, Gelzer, *Nature*, **228**, 1190 (1970)
Paunesco, *ibid.*, **228**, 1188 (1970)
Fisher, Hillegas, Nazeeri, *Appl. Microbiol.*, **22**, 13 (1971)
O'Beirne, Robinson, *Amer. J. Med. Sci.*, **262**, 33 (1971)
Zimmermann, Rosselet, Kneusel, *Ann. N.Y. Acad Sci.*, **182**, 329 (1971)
Passent, Kaesberg, *J. Virol.*, **8**, 286 (1971)
Erhlich, Laffler, Gallant, *J. Biol. Chem.*, **246**, 6121 (1971)
White, Lancini, *Biochim. Biophys. Acta*, **240**, 429 (1971)
Acocella et al., *Chemotherapy*, **16**, 356 (1971)
Finkel, Pittillo, Mellett, *ibid.*, **16**, 380 (1971)
Dworsky, Schaechter, *J. Bact.*, **116**, 1364 (1973)
Arioli et al., *Scand. J. Resp., Dis., Suppl.*, **84**, 20 (1973)
Homberg, Pujet, Salmon, *ibid.*, **84**, 36 (1973)
Aoyagi, *ibid.*, **84**, 44 (1973)
Araszkiewicz et al., *C.R. Soc. Biol.*, **167**, 875 (1973)
Volk, Dorozhkova, *Antibiotikii*, **18**, 706 (1973)
Kenwright, Levi, *Lancet*, **2** (7843), 1401 (1973)
Keln et al., *Folia Biol.* (Prague), **19**, 354 (1973)
Westfal et al., *Poznan. Tow. Przyi. Nauk. Pr. Kom. Med. Dosw.*, **45**, 309 (1973)
Lobo, Mandell, *Proc. Soc. Exptl. Biol. Med.*, **142**, 1048 (1973)
Marseillan, Corrado, *Arzneim.-Forsch*, **24**, 793 (1974)
Nessi et al., *ibid.*, **24**, 832 (1974)
Srb et al., *Experientia*, **30**, 484 (1974)
Lipkina et al., *Antibiotiki*, **19**, 6 (1974)
Soska et al., *Folia Microbiol.* (Prague), **19**, 358 (1974)
Scherbel, Arnold, *Deut. Apoth.-Ztg.*, **114**, 787 (1974)
Trnka, Mison, Staflova, *Chemotherapy*, **20**, 82 (1974)
Drabkina, Ginzburg, *Probl. Tuberk.*, **69** (1975)

RIFAMPIN
See Rifampicin

RIFAMYCIN A
One of the group of antibiotics isolated from certain species of *Streptomyces*, cultured in the absence of diethylbarbituric acid which is normally employed to inhibit the formation of this substance, together with rifamycins C, D and E. Rifamycin A has not been studied as extensively as most of the other members of this group.

Sensi et al., *Antibiotics Annual*, 262 (1959–1960)

RIFAMYCIN AG
This antibiotic is a condensation product formed from rifamycin O (q.v.) and aminoguanidine. It possesses good antibacterial activity against a number of gram-negative organims.

Sensi et al., *Antibiotics & Chemotherapy*, **12**, 448 (1962)

RIFAMYCIN B
$C_{39}H_{49}O_{14}N$
M.p. 300°C (*dec.* 160–164°C)

Rifamycin B has been isolated from the cultures of a number of *Streptomyces* species including *S. mediterranei*, *S. tolypophorus* and *Streptomyces* G5/A which is a mutant of *S. albovinaceous*, also *Nocardia asiatica*. In most of these cases, rifamycin O is produced at the same time and the two compounds may be separated chromatographically on alumina. Rifamycin B forms yellow prismatic needles from C_6H_6 which begin to decompose at 160–164°C before melting at 300°C. It is slightly laevorotatory with a specific rotation of $[\alpha]_D^{20} - 11°$ (c 1·0, CH_3OH) and gives an ultraviolet spectrum in phosphate buffer at pH 7·3 with absorption maxima at 223, 304 and 425 nm. It is a very stable dibasic acid and is active against gram-negative bacteria. The antibiotic is comparatively non-toxic, the LD_{50} in mice being 2040 mg/kg given intravenously and > 3000 mg/kg administered orally, subsutaneously or intraperitoneally.

Sensi et al., *Antibiotics & Chemotherapy*, **12**, 448 (1962)
Gallo et al., *Farmaco (Pavia), Ed. Sci.*, **17**, 668 (1962)
Shibata et al., *German Patent*, 2,026,595 (1970)
Takeda Chem. Indust., *French Patent*, 2,043,847 (1971)
Gauze et al., *French Patent*, 2,183,837 (1974)

Structure
  Prelog, *Pure Appl. Chem.*, **7**, 551 (1963)
  Prelog, *Chemotherapia*, **7**, 133 (1963)
  Oppolzer *et al.*, *Experientia*, **20**, 336 (1964)

RIFAMYCIN G
$C_{38}H_{51}NO_{12}$

A rifamycin antibiotic, this substance has been isolated from cultures of *Nocardia mediterranei*. The structure has been elucidated from chemical analysis and a study of the infrared, ultraviolet, NMR and mass spectra. It is active against gram-negative bacteria.

  Lancini, Sartori, *J. Antibiotics* (Japan), **29**, 466 (1976)

RIFAMYCIN L (*Rifamycin SV-4-glycollate*)
$C_{39}H_{49}O_{14}N$
M.p. 152–153°C (*dec.*)

One of the number of antibiotics possessing a similar structure, this compound is obtained from cultures of *Streptomyces mediterranei*. It crystallizes from $(CH_3)_2CO—C_6H_6$ and gives an ultraviolet spectrum having absorption maxima at 297 and 412 nm. The antibiotic activity is similar to that of the other rifamycins.

  Lancini *et al.*, *J. Antibiotics* (Japan), **22A**, 369 (1969)
Configuration
  Oppolzer, Prelog, *Helv. Chim. Acta*, **56**, 2287 (1973)

RIFAMYCIN O
$C_{39}H_{47}O_{14}N$
M.p. 300°C (*dec.* 160°C)

This particular rifamycin antibiotic occurs in cultures of *Streptomyces mediterranei* and *S. tolypophorous*. It forms pale yellow crystals when recrystallized from CH_3OH and is dextrorotatory with $[\alpha]_{589}^{20} + 71·5°$ (c 1·0, dioxan). The ultraviolet spectrum at pH 4·62 in CH_3OH containing 5 per cent acetate buffer solution has absorption maxima at 226, 273 and 370 nm. Rifamycin O is a weak acid, soluble in $(CH_3)_2CO$ and tetrahydrofuran, slight soluble in CH_3OH, EtOH and AcOEt, virtually insoluble in Et_2O, petroleum ether, H_2O and dilute acids. It dissolves slowly in dilute alkalies with the formation of a red-violet colour.

  Sensi *et al.*, *Antibiotics & Chemotherapy*, **12**, 448 (1962)
  Gallo *et al.*, *Farmaco* (Pavia), *Ed. Sci.*, **17**, 668 (1962)
Structure
  Prelog, *Pure Appl. Chem.*, **7**, 551 (1963)
  Prelog, *Chemotherapia*, **7**, 133 (1963)
  Oppolzer *et al.*, *Experientia*, **20**, 336 (1964)

RIFAMYCIN S
$C_{37}H_{45}O_{12}N$
Dec. 179–181°C

This antibiotic is an activation compound isolated from solutions of rifamycins B and O. It forms yellow-orange crystals when crystallized from CH_3OH and is dextrorotatory with a specific rotation of $[\alpha]_D^{20} + 476°$ (c 0·1, CH_3OH). The ultraviolet and visible spectra in phosphate buffer at pH 7·3 have absorption maxima at 317 and 525 nm. The antibiotic is active against gram-negative organisms and is relatively non-toxic to mammals with LD_{50} in mice of 122 mg/kg (intravenous), 258 mg/kg (intraperitoneal) and 3000 mg/kg (oral).

Sensi et al., Experientia, **16**, 412 (1960)

RIFAMYCIN SV (*Rifocin*)
$C_{37}H_{47}O_{12}N$
M.p. 300°C (*dec.* 140°C)

Perhaps the most important of the rifamycin group of antibiotics, this compound is produced by *Micromonospora chalcea* and *Streptomyces mediterranei*. It forms yellow-orange crystals from EtOH and is slightly laevorotatory with a specific rotation of $[\alpha]_D^{20} - 4°$ (c 1·0, CH_3OH). The ultraviolet spectrum in phosphate buffer solution at pH 7·3 has absorption maxima at 223, 314 and 445 nm. It is slightly acidic, freely soluble in CH_3OH, EtOH, AcOEt and $(CH_3)_2CO$, moderately soluble in Et_2O and sodium bicarbonate solution and only slightly soluble in H_2O and petroleum ether.

Rifamycin SV has a high activity against gram-positive organisms *in vitro* but only a slight activity against gram-negative bacteria. It has proved therapeutically effective in the treatment of pneumonococcal, staphylococcal and streptococcal infections. It also inhibits the *in vitro* infected cell culture multiplication of adenovirus, the inhibition being reversed on removal of the antibiotic. Berman has also shown that rifomycin SV-pretreated normal mouse lymphocytes destroyed allogenic tumour target cells accompanied by an increase in the cytotoxicity of the normal lymphocytes.

Sensi et al., Experientia, **16**, 412 (1960)
Sensi et al., Farmaco (Pavia), Ed. Sci., **16**, 165 (1961)
Shorin, Shapovalova, Antibiotiki, **19**, 3 (1974)
Gol'dberg et al., ibid., **19**, 344 (1974)
Wigand, Vujic, Schoener, Acta Virol., **18**, 113 (1974)
Berman, Byull. Eksp. Biol. Med., **77**, 83 (1974)
Ziv, Sulman, Antimicrobial Agents & Chemotherapy, **5**, 139 (1974)
Celmer, Cullen, Routien, U.S. Patent, 3,884,763 (1975)

RIFAMYCIN SV-4 GLYCOLLATE
See Rifamycin L

RIFAMYCIN W
$C_{35}H_{45}O_{11}N$
M.p. Indefinite

A further rifamycin antibiotic isolated from cultures of *Nocardia Mediterranei*, this compound has the structure given above which is based upon chemical and spectroscopic data and comparison with the other rifamycins. It forms yellow crystals from AcOEt which decompose before melting. It is active against a number of gram-positive bacteria but has only a weak activity against gram-negative organisms.

Martinelli *et al.*, *Tetrahedron*, **30**, 3087 (1974)

RIFAMYCIN X
$C_{37}H_{45}O_{11}N_3$
Dec. 135–140°C

This antibiotic occurs in cultures of *Streptomyces mediterranei*. It crystallizes from EtOH as yellow crystals which have no definite melting point. It is unstable to light and is dextrorotatory with a specific rotation of $[\alpha]_D^{20} + 491 \cdot 8°$ (c 0·981, dioxan). The antibiotic is soluble in CH_3OH, EtOH, C_6H_6 and AcOEt but insoluble in H_2O. The ultraviolet spectrum in acetate buffer solution has absorption maxima at 286, 317 and 402 nm. Like the majority of the rifamycin antibiotics, it inhibits the growth of gram-positive bacteria, having only a slight activity against gram-negative organisms.

Sensi, *Res. Progress in Organic-Biological & Medicinal Chemistry*, Vol. 1, 337 Milano, Italy, (1964)

RIFAMYCIN Y
$C_{39}H_{47}O_{15}N$

A further antibiotic obtained from *Streptomyces mediterranei*, rifamycin Y is dextrorotatory with a specific rotation of $[\alpha]_D + 325°$ (c 1·0, CH_3OH). The crystal structure has been established by X-ray analysis. It is also active against gram-positive bacteria.

Leitich, Prelog, Sensi, *Experientia*, **23**, 505 (1967)
Lancini *et al.*, *ibid.*, **23**, 899 (1967)
Crystal structure
Brufani *et al.*, *Experientia*, **23**, 508 (1967)

RIFOCIN
See Rifamycin SV

RIMOCIDIN
$C_{39}H_{61}O_{14}N$
M.p. 151°C (*dec.*)

Rimocidin has been isolated from the mycelium of *Streptomyces rimosus* by extraction with *n*-BuOH. It is amphoteric in nature and has a specific rotation of $[\alpha]_D^{25} + 75 \cdot 2°$. The ultraviolet spectrum in EtOH has absorption maxima at 279, 289, 304 and 318 nm. It is slightly soluble in H_2O and the lower alcohols and begins to decompose when heated above 110°C. The sodium salt is crystalline and the antibiotic forms a sulphate as the crystalline heptahydrate, m.p. 151°C, which is soluble in H_2O.

Rimocidin is active against a large number of pathogenic fungi including *Candida albicans*, *Histoplasma capsulatum* and *Trichophyton gypseum*, the minimum inhibition concentration being 1–5 µg/ml. It is less active, however, against *Candida neoformans*. The antibiotic also inhibits protozoa such as *Endamoeba histolytica*, *Leishmania donovani*, *Leishmania tropica* and *Trypanosoma cruzi*. At a concentration of 30 µg/ml it is hemolytic for human and rabbit erythrocytes. The LD_{50} for mice is 20 mg/kg when given intravenously.

Davisson *et al.*, *Antibiotics & Chemotherapy*, **1**, 289 (1951)
Seneca, Kane, Rockenbach, *ibid.*, **2**, 435 (1952)
Davisson *et al.*, *U.S. Patent*, 2,963,401 (1960)
Partial structure
Cope *et al.*, *J. Amer. Chem. Soc.*, **87**, 5452 (1965)
Structure
Falkowski *et al.*, *J. Antibiotics* (Japan), **29**, 197 (1976)

RINAMYCIN
$C_{20}H_{35}NO_8$

Isolated from the culture mycelium of *Streptomyces venezuelae*, this antibiotic has been obtained as a honey-yellow powder which has an inhibitory action against gram-positive, some gram-negative bacteria, fungi and yeasts. Experiments indicate that the primary site of action of rinamycin in the RNA metabolism of rinomycin-sensitive cells.

Uchida, Zahner, *J. Antibiotics* (Japan), **28**, 185 (1975)

RIOMYCIN
See Fluvomycin

RISTOCETIN A
Nocardia lurida produces two closely related antibiotics, ristocetins A and B which have been differentiated by paper strip chromatography. The structure of this compound is unknown although it has been shown to contain amino and phenolic groups in the molecule together with a number of sugar moieties. The sulphate is crystalline and laevorotatory with a specific rotation varying between $[\alpha]_D^{25} - 120°$ to $- 133°$. It is insoluble in organic solvents, soluble in aqueous solutions at an acidic pH and considerably less soluble at a neutral reaction. It has a maximum stability in acid solution, but is readily inactivated above pH 7·0. Ristocetin is active against gram-positive bacteria and has found some use in medicine as an antimicrobial. The normal dose given is 25–80 mg/kg/day although certain side effects such as rash, transient neutropenia and venous irritation have been observed.

Philipi, Schenk, Hargia, *Antibiotics Annual*, 699 (1956–1957)
Philip, Schenk, Hargie, *U.S. Patent*, 2,990,329 (1961)

RISTOCETIN B
Also produced by *Nocardia lurida*, the structure of this antibiotic appears to be very similar to that of the preceding substance. The crystalline sulphate is laevorotatory with a specific rotation varying from $[\alpha]_D^{25}$ to $- 149°$. The biological activity is similar to that of ristocetin A but this antibiotic is considerably more potent.

Philip, Schenk, Hargie, *Antibiotics Annual*, 699 (1956–1957)
Philip, Schenk, Hargie, *U.S. Patent*. 2,990,329 (1961)

RISTOMYCIN
M.p. Indefinite

A crystalline antibiotic has been obtained from cultures of *Proactinomyces fructifera* var. *ristomycini*. When examined by paper chromatography, it is found that different preparations of this substance show the presence of at least two active components, ristomycins A and B. Chemical evidence shows that these have the same aminoacid composition but differ in the carbohydrate content. Hydrolysis of ristomycin A furnishes ristomycin B, arabinose and mannose. Both component are active *in vitro* against a range of gram-positive and some gram-negative bacteria with the activity of ristomycin B being twice as great as that of ristomycin A.

Brazhnikova *et al.*, *Upr. Biosin*, 252 (1966)
Trenina *et al.*, *Antibiotiki*, **18**, 422 (1973)

ROBIGOCIDIN A
$C_{36}H_{50}O_8N_2$
M.p. 105–107°C (dec.)

Streptomyces platensis robigocidicus elaborates this antibiotic which forms yellow crystals when recrystallized from EtOH. It is dextrorotatory with a specific rotation of $[\alpha]_D^{22} + 42°$ (c 1·0, CH_3OH) and gives an ultraviolet spectrum in EtOH with absorption maxima at 263, 272 and 282 nm. It is active against gram-positive and some gram-negative bacteria.

Misato *et al.*, *Japanese Patent*, 7,017,598 (1970)

ROLITETRACYCLINE
$C_{27}H_{33}O_8N_3$
M.p. 162–165°C

A semi-synthetic antibiotic, this compound is prepared from tetracycline (q.v.) by a Mannich reaction. It crystallizes as slender, pale yellow needles and is amphoteric. It is more soluble than tetracycline, being readily soluble in EtOH, H_2O and dilute acids and alkalies. The antibiotic has been marketed under a variety of trade names including Bristacin, Reverin, Supercilin, Syntetrex, Syntetrin, Synotodecin, Transcycline, Velacicline and Velacycline. The nitrate forms colourless crystals of the sesquihydrate (Bristacin-A, Pyrrocycline-N). Rolitetracycline finds a use in medicine as antimicrobial and may be administered either intravenously or intramuscularly. The normal dose is 275 mg and the side effects are similar to those of terramycin (q.v.).

Siedel et al., *Münich. med. Wochschr.*, **100**, 661 (1958)
Gottstein et al., *J. Amer. Chem. Soc.*, **81**, 1198 (1959)
Cheney et al., *U.S. Patent*, 3,104,240 (1963)

ROMICIL
See Oleandomycin

RORIDIN E
$C_{29}H_{38}O_8$
M.p. 183–184°C; 220–222°C

An antibiotic isolated from cultures of *Myrothecium* spp., roridin E exists two crystal modifications having the melting points given above. It is laevorotatory with $[\alpha]_D^{23} - 16°$ (c 1·0, $CHCl_3$). The macrocyclic structure has been elucidated by means of chemical and spectroscopic techniques.

Böhner et al., *Helv. Chim. Acta*, **48**, 1079 (1965)
Structure
Traxler, Zurcher, Tamm, *Helv. Chim. Acta*, **53**, 2071 (1970)

RORIDIN H (*Verrucarin H*)
$C_{29}H_{36}O_8$
M.p. >325°C

Myrothecium verrucaria produces this antibiotic whose structure closely resembles that of the preceding antibiotic. Roridin H crystallizes as colourless needles and has a specific rotation of $[\alpha]_D^{23} + 31°$ (c 1·16, $CHCl_3$).

Böhner et al., *Helv. Chim. Acta*, **48**, 1079 (1965)
Structure
Traxler, Tamm, *Helv. Chim. Acta*, **53**, 1846 (1970)

ROSAMICIN (*Rosaramicin*)
$C_{31}H_{51}O_9N$
M.p. 119–122°C

A glycosidic antibiotic isolated from *Micromonospora rosaria*, rosamicin crystallizes from $CHCl_3$ and is laevorotatory with a specific rotation of $[\alpha]_D^{26} - 36°$ (c 1·0, EtOH). In CH_3OH solution it gives an ultraviolet spectrum having a single absorption maximum at 240 nm. The structure has been determined from chemical and spectroscopic data. Rosamicin exhibits bacteriostatic activity against many gram-positive bacteria, its activity being comparable to that of erythromycin (q.v.). It is slightly active against gram-negative bacteria, alkali enhancing this activity. The antibiotic shows some activity at physiological pH, this not being the case for erythromycin.

Reimann, Jaret, *J. Chem. Soc., Chem. Commun.*, 1270 (1972)
Wagman et al., *J. Antibiotics* (Japan), **25**, 641 (1972)
Waitz et al., *ibid.*, **25**, 647 (1972)

ROSARAMICIN
See Rosamicin

ROSEOFLAVIN
$C_{18}H_{23}O_6N_5$
M.p. 276–278°C

Roseoflavin has been isolated from cultures of *Streptomyces davawensis*. It forms deep red crystals and yields a characteristic tetraacetate with m.p. 279–280°C.

Miura et al., *J. Chem. Soc., Chem. Commun.*, 703 (1973)
Otani et al, *J. Antibiotics* (Japan), **27**, 88 (1974)

ROSEOFUNGIN
This antibiotic is produced by a proactinomycete variant of *Streptomyces roseoflavus* var. *roseofungini* grown in submerged culture at 27°C. The maximum accumulation of the antibiotic occurs after 72–96 hours fermentation. Roseofungin is active against a number of pathogenic fungi.

Nikitina, Kazakova, *Antibiotiki*, **17**, 114 (1972)

ROSEOMYCIN
This antibiotic is similar in many respects to streptomycin and streptothricin and is obtained by the same methods from cultures of *Streptomyces roseochromogenes*. It is a basic substance and is characterized as the crystalline helianthate, m.p. 211–216°C and the reineckate, m.p. 114°C (*dec.*). Roseomycin is active against both gram-positive and gram-negative bacteria but has little activity against clostridia. It is active *in vitro* against *Vibrio comma*, and *in vivo* against *Eberthella typhosa*. The LD_{50} in mice is about 1000 mg/kg when given either intramuscularly or intravenously.

Ishida, *J. Antibiotics* (Japan), **3**, 839 (1950)
Nagao, *ibid.*, **3C**, 20 (1950)
Nagao, *ibid.*, **4**, 24 (1951)
Ishida, Tohoku, *J. Exptl. Med.*, **58**, 153 (1953)

ROTAVENTIN
M.p. 170–175°C

An antibiotic obtained from *Streptomyces reticuli*, rotaventin is isolated by extraction of the mycelium with CH_3OH, concentration *in vacuo*, followed by precipitation at pH 2·0. The precipitate is then washed with Et_2O, the residue dissolved in CH_3OH and precipitated with H_2O. Further purification is then carried out by countercurrent distribution. When crystallized from CH_3OH, rotaventin forms colourless platelets which turn yellow at about 130°C and also become yellow gradually on exposure to air. When treated with concentrated H_2SO_4, the substance gives a deep red colour. The antibiotic is soluble in CH_3OH, $(CH_3)_2CO$, BuOH and amyl alcohol but insoluble in Et_2O, $CHCl_3$, C_6H_6, AcOEt, amyl acetate, petroleum ether and H_2O. Rotaventin is not precipitated from solution in CH_3OH with either picric acid or phosphotungstic acid.

The antibiotic is active *in vitro* against *Aspergillus niger*, *Penicillium glaucum* and *Saccharomyces sake* at a concentration of 6 µg/ml. It exhibits little activity against *Candida albicans*, *Mucor*, *Rhizopus* or *Trichophyton* and none against bacteria. The LD_{50} in mice is 150 mg/kg (intraperitoneal) and 770 mg/kg (subcutaneous).

Hosoya, Komatsu, Soeda, *J. Antibiotics* (Japan), **5**, 451 (1952)

ROVAMYCIN
See Spiramycin

RUBIDIN
An antibiotic substance obtained from an unclassified *Streptomyces* species, this compound forms a dark red amorphous powder having no definite melting point. Physical evidence suggests that rubidin is a mixture of several compounds and following successive extraction with petroleum ether, Et_2O and $CHCl_3$, an insoluble residue remains which may be dissolved in hot CH_3OH, giving red crystals on cooling. Chemical evidence indicates that this compound is a quinone containing four hydroxyl groups

and two lactone rings in the molecule. NMR studies show the presence of two secondary methyl groups.

Pure rubidin, obtained in the crystalline form, shows activity against *Bacillus subtilis*, *Staphylococcus aureus* and *Streptococcus fecalis*.

Barua et al., *J. Indian Chem. Soc.*, **50**, 223 (1973)

RUBOMYCIN

Actinomyces coeruleorubidis elaborates an antibiotic, rubomycin, which consists of at least three components, rubomycins A, B and C. The fungus is incubated at 28–30°C for 4 days and the mycelium extracted with $(CH_3)_2CO$ at pH 4·0, the antibiotic mixture being isolated by extraction with $CHCl_3$ at pH 8·8–9·0, the extract acidified with HCl to pH 3·5–3·9 and chromatographed on a silica gel column. Elution with $CHCl_3$—C_6H_6—CH_3OH (100:10:5) gives rubomycin A, elution with the same solvent mixture (10:10:15) gives rubomycin B and the remaining component is obtained by elution with CH_3OH. The three compounds exhibit similar biological activities against gram-positive and gram-negative bacteria.

Brazhnikova et al., *Soviet Patent*, 324,770 (1973)

RUFOMYCIN A

M.p. Indefinite

An antibiotic mixture is elaborated by *Streptomyces atratus* nov. species ATCC 14,046 which yields rufomycins A and B. The former is obtained by extraction of the culture filtrate with AcOEt or EtOH at pH 2·0, the organic fraction being further diluted and chromatographed on an alumina column, the mixture forming an orange-yellow band. The concentrated fraction yields crystals of rufomycin B, with rufomycin A being obtained from the mother liquor by rechromatography. Rufomycin A is a broad-spectrum antibiotic, more active against gram-positive bacteria than against gram-negative organisms.

Nakazawa et al., *U.S. Patent*, 3,655,879 (1972)

RUFOMYCIN B

M.p. 165–168°C

This component of rufomycin, isolated from cultures of *Streptomyces atratus* nov. species ATCC 14,046 forms orange-yellow crystals and has an antibiotic spectrum similar to that of the accompanying rufomycin A.

Nakazawa et al., *U.S. Patent*, 3,655,879 (1972)

S

SAGAMICIN (*Antibiotic XK-62-2*)
$C_{20}H_{41}O_7N_5$
M.p. 260°C (*dec.*)

Micromonospora sagamiensis elaborates this antibiotic which forms a colourless, amorphous powder. It is dextrorotatory with a specific rotation of $[\alpha]_D^{20} + 116°$ (c 1·0, H_2O). Sagamicin is active against a number of gram-positive bacteria.

Okachi *et al.*, *J. Antibiotics* (Japan), **27**, 793 (1974)
Structure
Egan *et al.*, *J. Antibiotics* (Japan), **28**, 29 (1975)

SAIHOCIN
Pseudomonas allicola TPR-NI-I produces a mixture of saihocins A and B when aerobically cultured in a medium containing glycerol and peptone at 30°C for 18 hours. After centrifuging the culture, the supernatant liquor is extracted with BuOH, while the cells are extracted with $(CH_3)_2CO$, the extract concentrated under reduced pressure and the residue extracted with BuOH. The two BuOH fractions are combined and sodium sulphate is added which precipitates the crude material. This is washed successively with BuOH, $(CH_3)_2CO$ and Et_2O, the residue dissolved in $(CH_3)_2SO$ and precipitated with BuOH. Saihocins A and B are primarily active against gram-positive bacteria.

Shibata *et al.*, *Japanese Patent*, 7,445,596 (1974)

SALINOMYCIN
$C_{42}H_{70}O_{11}$
M.p. 117–118°C

A polycyclic antibiotic, salinomycin is elaborated by *Streptomyces albus* 80,614 which is cultured in a common nutrient medium with aerobic stirring at 27°C for 84 hours at pH 7·0. The broth is extracted with $(CH_3)_2CO$, $CHCl_3$ or butyl acetate and the extract chromatographed on alumina and Sephadex columns. The structure given above is based upon chemical and spectroscopic evidence. Salinomycin is laevorotatory with a specific rotation of $[\alpha]_D^{20} - 25°$ (c 1·0, CH_3OH), is insoluble in H_2O and unstable under acid conditions. The ultraviolet spectrum in acidified CH_3OH has absorption maxima at 220 and 285 nm. The antibiotic inhibits the growth of gram-positive bacteria but is mainly active against coccidia in poultry, particularly *Eimeria tenella* infections.

Tanaka *et al.*, *German Patent*, 2,253,031 (1973)
Tanaka *et al.*, *German Patent*, 2,353,998 (1975)

SAMBUCININ
$C_{24}H_{42}O_7N_2$
M.p. 86°C
An antibiotic elaborated by a species of *Fusarium*, this compound is

laevorotatory with a specific rotation of $[\alpha]_D^{20} - 83°$ and on hydrolysis it furnishes N-ethyl-L-valine and D(−)-α-hydroxyisovaleric acid. The structure is not yet known with certainty.

Cook et al., Nature, **160**, 31 (1947)
Cook, Cox, Farmer, J. Chem. Soc., 1022 (1949)

SANCYCLINE (*Bonomycin, Norcycline*)
$C_{21}H_{22}O_7N_2$
M.p. Indefinite

A semi-synthetic tetracycline antibiotic, sancycline has the structure given above which is based upon a total synthesis of the compound. It forms a crystalline hydrochloride hemihydrate, m.p. 215–220°C (dec.). The antibiotic has found some use in medicine as an antimicrobial.

Beereboom et al., J. Amer. Chem. Soc., **82**, 1003 (1960)
McCormick et al., ibid., **82**, 3381 (1960)
McCormick, Jensen, U.S. Patent, 3,019,260 (1962)
McCormick, Jensen, British Patent, 901,209 (1962)
Total synthesis
Conover et al., J. Amer. Chem. Soc., **84**, 3222 (1962)

SANGIVAMYCIN
$C_{12}H_{15}O_5N_5$

This antitumour antibiotic has been isolated from cultures of several *Streptomyces* species. When administered intraperitoneally to mice it is incorporated into the nucleic acids of the tissues after phosphorylation. In the kidney and spleen, the antibiotic is found intact whereas in the liver, it is mainly present as the 5′-monophosphate. Sangivamycin is incorporated into DNA and RNA of all tissues with the exception of the brain where labelling occurs only in RNA.

Hardesty et al., Cancer Res., **34**, 1005 (1974)

SARAMYCETIN

A recently discovered antibiotic, saramycetin is a polypeptide produced by incubating *Streptomyces saraceticus* NRRL 2831 aerobically on a medium containing corn steep liquor, brown sugar, lard oil and potassium dihydrogen phosphate at 28°C for 4 days. The medium is adjusted to pH 3·5 with dilute H_2SO_4, filtered, the filter cake extracted with CH_3OH and the CH_3OH removed at pH 7·0. The aqueous concentrate is then concentrated further at pH 7·0–7·5, extracted with BuOH and hexane added which precipitates crude saramycetin. Further purification is carried out by chromatography on a partially deactivated alumina column. So far, a product of approximately 85 per cent purity has been obtained. The antibiotic possesses both antibacterial and fungicidal properties.

Aszalos et al., German Patent, 2,224,145 (1973)

SARCIDIN
M.p. 274–275°C

Sarcidin is obtained from *Streptomyces achromogenes* by adsorption on activated carbon at pH 7·0 followed by elution with acidified EtOH, concentration *in vacuo*, crystallization at low temperatures between 0°C and 5°C and recrystallization from 80 per cent aqueous EtOH. Nitrogen is present in the molecule and possibly sulphur and halogen. It has a maximum stability at pH 2·0.

Sarcidin is active against *Sarcina lutea* at low concentrations of between 1·0 and 1·5 μg/ml but shows no activity against most of the bacteria and fungi that have been tested with this antibiotic. The LD_{50} in mice is greater than 600 mg/kg when given intraperitoneally.

Takeuchi, Nitta, Umezawa, J. Antibiotics (Japan), **6A**, 31 (1953)

SARCOMYCIN A
See Sarkomycin A

SARKOMYCIN A (*Sarcomycin A*)
$C_7H_8O_3$
Streptomyces erythrochromogenes strain W-115-C, isolated from soil found

at Kamakura, Japan, elaborates an antibiotic substance named sarkomycin. The active constituent is sarkomycin A, the structure of which is 2-methylene-3-oxocyclopentane carboxylic acid. The antibiotic is an oily liquid having no definite boiling point. It is laevorotatory with a specific rotation of $[\alpha]_D^{15} - 32\cdot 5°$ (c 1·0, CH_3OH) and gives an ultraviolet spectrum in H_2O consisting of a single absorption maximum at 230 nm. It is soluble in H_2O, CH_3OH, EtOH, BuOH and AcOEt, sparingly so in petroleum ether. The antibiotic reacts with H_2S to give sarkomycins S_1, S_2 and S_3. The sodium salt decomposes to give sarkomycin B and both decompose to yield sarkomycin E in the presence of formic acid. Sarkomycin A has both antibacterial and antitumour properties.

Umezawa et al., *J. Antibiotics* (Japan), **6A**, 101, 147, 153 (1953)
Umezawa et al., *Antibiotics & Chemotherapy*, **4**, 514 (1954)
Hooper et al., *ibid.*, **5**, 585 (1955)
Tatsuoka et al., *J. Antibiotics* (Japan), **9B**, 107, 110 (1956)
Maeda, Kondo, *ibid*, **11A**, 37 (1958)
Synthesis
Toki, *J. Antibiotics* (Japan), **10A**, 35, 226 (1957)
Toki, *Bull. Chem. Soc., Japan*, **30**, 450 (1957)
Absolute configuration
Sato et al., *Chem. Pharm. Bull.*, **11**, 829 (1963)

SCHLEROTHRICIN
$C_{16}H_{30}O_8N_6$
M.p. Indefinite
An amorphous antibiotic, schlerothricin has been isolated from cultures of *Streptomyces schlerogranulatus* Shimazu et Yonehara. The substance is laevorotatory with a specific rotation of $[\alpha]_D^{23} - 74°$ (c 1·1, H_2O) and may be characterized as the hydrochloride, an amorphous powder, m.p. 214°C (*dec.*). The antibiotic is active against a variety of gram-positive bacteria.

Kono et al., *J. Antibiotics* (Japan), **22A**, 583 (1969)

SCOPAFUNGIN
M.p. 119·3°C
Streptomyces hygroscopicus var. *enhygrus* var. nova elaborates this nonpolyenic antimicrobial antibiotic which forms colourless crystals from aqueous $(CH_3)_2CO$. It has a specific rotation of $[\alpha]_D^{25} + 20°$ (dimethylformamide) and inhibits *in vitro* a wide variety of gram-positive bacteria, yeasts and pathogenic fungi.

Johnson, Dietz, *Appl. Microbiol*, **22**, 303 (1971)
Bergy, Hoeksema, *J. Antibiotics* (Japan), **25**, 39 (1972)

SELDOMYCIN FACTOR I (*Antibiotic XK-88-1*)
$C_{17}H_{34}N_4O_{10}$

Cultures of *Streptomyces hofunensis* sp. nov. yield an antibiotic complex from which four antibiotics have been isolated, seldomycin factors 1, 2, 3 and 5. This component has the structure given above which is based upon chemical and spectroscopic evidence. It is active against gram positive bacteria.

Saito et al., *J. Antibiotics* (Japan), **30**, 25 (1977)
Structure
Egan et al., *J. Antibiotics* (Japan), **30**, 31 (1977)

SELDOMYCIN FACTOR 2
$C_{12}H_{26}N_4O_5$

A second constituent of the seldomycin complex obtained from cultures of *Streptomyces hofunensis* sp. nov., this antibiotic has been assigned the above structure from chemical and spectroscopic data. It is effective against a number of gram-positive organisms.

Saito *et al.*, *J. Antibiotics* (Japan), **30**, 25 (1977)
Structure
Egan *et al.*, *J. Antibiotics* (Japan), **30**, 31 (1977)

SELDOMYCIN FACTOR 3
$C_{17}H_{35}N_5O_9$

Streptomyces hofunensis sp. nov. also elaborates this antibiotic, the structure of which is most probably that given above based upon chemical analysis and the infrared, NMR and mass spectra.

Saito *et al.*, *J. Antibiotics* (Japan), **30**, 25 (1977)
Structure
Egan *et al.*, *J. Antibiotics* (Japan), **30**, 31 (1977)

SELDOMYCIN FACTOR 5
$C_{18}H_{38}N_6O_7$

This aminoglycosidic antibiotic is a constituent of the culture broth of *Streptomyces hofunensis* sp. nov. It has been separated from the accompanying substances and purified by chromatographic methods. It has a similar antibiotic spectrum to the other seldomycin factors.

Saito *et al.*, *J. Antibiotics* (Japan), **30**, 25 (1977)
Structure
McAlpine *et al.*, *J. Antibiotics* (Japan), **30**, 39 (1977)

SELECTOMYCIN
See Spiramycin

SELENOMYCIN
M.p. 135–138°C

This antibiotic has been obtained by culturing *Streptosporangium brasiliense*, ATCC 21,393 on an agar-oatmeal medium and fermenting for 10 days at 32°C. The medium was then used to inoculate a medium containing peptone, glucose, meat extract, yeast and sodium chloride and cultured with shaking at pH 7·2 and 28°C for 3 days, when this medium was used for the final inoculation of a medium consisting of glucose, peptone, yeast, meat extract, soybean flour and inorganic salts. After fermenting for 3 days the pH was adjusted to 5·5 with dilute HCl and sodium chloride added. Extraction of the medium with $CHCl_3$ was followed by precipitation with petroleum ether. Selenomycin is a broad-spectrum antibiotic, primarily active against gram-positive bacteria.

Coronelli, Thiemann, *German Patent*, 2,028,986 (1971)

SEPTAMYCIN
$C_{48}H_{82}O_{16}$
M.p. Indefinite

A polycyclic antibiotic, septamycin has been isolated from cultures of *Streptomyces hygroscopicus*. The crystal structure has been determined by X-ray analysis. Septamycin is an organic acid and has proved effective against experimental infections in mice due to gram-positive organisms.

Petcher, Weber, *J. Chem. Soc., Chem. Commun.*, 697 (1974)
Keller-Juslen *et al.*, *J. Antibiotics* (Japan), **28**, 854 (1975)

SEQUAMYCIN
See Spiramycin

SERINOMYCIN

This antibiotic from *Streptomyces* species RK-9755 has been obtained by Japanese workers by culturing the fungus at pH 7·0 on a medium containing glucose, starch, meat extract, soybean flour, yeast and inorganic salts at 27°C for 24 hours. After heating the culture broth to 80°C for 10 minutes at pH 3·0, the filtrate is extracted with AcOEt and the residue then extracted with 90 per cent aqueous $(CH_3)_2CO$, concentrated and the antibiotic isolated as the sulphate. The hydrochloride has also been prepared as white needles from H_2O with m.p. 158–161°C (*dec.*). Serinomycin is active against a number of gram-positive bacteria. The LD_{50} of the sulphate in mice is 100 mg/kg when administered intraperitoneally.

Suzuki *et al.*, *Japanese Patent*, 7,425,197 (1974)
Kasakabe *et al.*, *J. Antibiotics* (Japan), **25**, 541 (1972)

SESQUICILLIN
$C_{29}H_{42}O_5$

A substituted decalin, sesquicillin is obtained by aerobic fermentation of *Sesquicillium globulisporum* NRRL 5433 in a common nutrient medium containing sucrose, glycine and inorganic salts. The structure has been established by chemical and spectroscopic methods. Sesquicillin has proved useful in medicine as an inflammation inhibitor and bronchospasmolytic agent.

Thiele, Tscherter, *German Patent*, 2,316,429 (1973)

SHINCOMYCIN A
M.p. 134–136°C

One of two macrolide antibiotics elaborated by *Streptomyces phaeochromogenes* ATCC 19,081 when cultured aerobically on a nutrient medium at pH 5·0–8·0 and 28–30°C. The mixture of components is adsorbed from the culture filtrate on activated carbon, extracted with $(CH_3)_2CO$ and chromatographed on an activated alumina column. The antibiotic is purified by repeated crystallization from Et_2O. This antibiotic is laevorotatory with a specific rotation of $[\alpha]_D - 61·2°$ and gives an ultraviolet spectrum with a single absorption maximum at 240 nm. It gives a positive test with Fehling's solution. Shincomycin A is stable at 100°C for 2 hours but is rapidly inactivated in alkaline solution.

The antibiotic is assayed by serial dilution with *Bacillus subtilis* as the test organism. It is active against gram-positive bacteria and has a minimum inhibitory concentration of 3·2 µg/ml against *Staphylococcus aureus*.

Ishida, Kumagai, Nishimura, *French Patent*, 1,486,376 (1967)
Ishida, Kumagai, Nishimura, *British Patent*, 1,101,361 (1968)
Ishida, Kumagai, Nishimura, *U.S. Patent*, 2,534,138 (1970)

SHINCOMYCIN B
M.p. 128–129°C

The second antibiotic obtained from cultures of *Streptomyces phaeochromogenes* ATCC 19,081, this compound has a specific rotation of $[\alpha]_D 0°$ and gives an ultraviolet spectrum identical to that of shincomycin A with an absorption maximum at 240 nm. Unlike the preceding antibiotic it gives a negative test with Fehling's solution. It is also stable for 2 hours at 100°C and inactivated by alkalies. The antibiotic activity is identical to that of shincomycin A.

Ishida, Kumagai, Nishimura, *French Patent*, 1,486,376 (1967)
Ishida, Kumagai, Nishimura, *British Patent*, 1,101,361 (1968)
Ishida, Kumagai, Nishimura, *U.S. Patent*, 2,534,138 (1970)

SHOWDOMYCIN

$C_9H_{11}O_6N$
M.p. 160–161°C

Streptomyces showdoensis produces this simple maleimide antibiotic which has the structure 3-(β-D-ribofuranosyl)-maleimide. It forms colourless crystals from $(CH_3)_2CO$ and is dextrorotatory with a specific rotation of $[\alpha]_D^{22.4}$ + 149.9° (c 1.0, H_2O). The ultraviolet spectrum in EtOH consists of a single absorption maximum at 222 nm. The antibiotic forms a crystalline triacetate, m.p. 115–116°C and the 2′:3′-isopropylidene derivative, m.p. 140.5–141°C. Showdomycin is active against a number of gram-positive bacteria.

Nishimura *et al.*, *J. Antibiotics* (Japan), **17A**, 148 (1964)
Darmall, Townsend, Robins, *Proc. Nat. Acad. Sci., U.S.*, **57**, 548 (1967)
Nakagawa *et al.*, *Tetrahedron Lett.*, 4105 (1967)
Crystal structure
 Tsukuda *et al.*, *Chem. Commun.*, 975 (1967)
 Tsukuda *et al.*, *J. Chem. Soc., B*, 843 (1969)
Mass spectrum
 Townsend, Robins, *J. Heterocyclic Chem.*, **6**, 459 (1969)
Biosynthesis
 Elstner, Suhadolnik, *Biochemistry*, **10**, 3608 (1971)

SIBIROMCIN

$C_{24}H_{31}O_7N_3$
M.p. Indefinite

An antibiotic obtained from cultures of *Streptosporangium sibiricum*, sibiromycin decomposes above 120°C with no definite melting point and has a specific rotation of $[\alpha]_D$ + 525° (dimethylformamide). The ultraviolet spectrum consists of two absorption maxima at 230 and 310 nm. The antibiotic brings about significant changes in the CD spectra of the double-stranded DNA obtained from *Escherichia coli*, *Sarcina maxima* and *Streptomyces chrysomallus* when added to the DNA solutions at molar ratios of 1:7.5 to 1:30. The effects were greater the higher the G-C pairs in DNA. When administered intravenously to dogs at doses from 0.75–1.5 µg/kg daily, the antibiotic caused lymphopenia and thrombocytopenia and at higher doses up to 20 µg/kg caused leukocytosis and lymphopenia and, to a somewhat lesser extent, thrombocytopenia. Given intravenously to rabbits in single doses of 300 or 500 µg/kg, the antibiotic was detected in the blood within 15–30 minutes and although small amounts penetrated to all of the body organs, between 35–40 per cent of the administered dose was excreted through the urine within 6 hours.

Vertogradova, Kunrat, *Antibiotiki*, **16**, 316 (1971)
Pokras *et al.*, *ibid.*, **17**, 697 (1972)
Brazhnikova, Konstantinova, Mesentsev, *J. Antibiotics* (Japan), **25**, 668 (1972)
Dudnik, Zimmer, Luck, *Antibiotiki*, **18**, 895 (1973)
Structure
 Mesentsev, Kuljaeva, Rubasheva, *J. Antibiotics* (Japan), **27**, 866 (1974)

SICCANIN

$C_{22}H_{30}O_3$
M.p. 138°C

Siccanin is produced by *Helminthosporium siccans*, a parasitic organism of rye-grass, which is cultured on a common nutrient medium with the final pH kept at 2·5–3·0, thereby reducing the production of side products. Siccanin forms colourless crystals and is laevorotatory with a specific rotation of $[\alpha]_D^{18} - 150°$ (c 7·75, CHCl$_3$). The ultraviolet spectrum in EtOH has an absorption maximum at 285 nm and a shoulder at 278 nm. The antibiotic may be characterized as the p-bromobenzenesulphonate, m.p. 156°C.

The antibiotic is not active against bacteria, but is highly effective against fungi, particularly *Trichophyton interdigitale* and *T. mentagrophytes*, the growth of the germinating conidia being markedly inhibited and viability decreased.

Ishibashi, *J. Antibiotics* (Japan), **15A**, 161 (1962)
Endo, *Sankyo Kenkyusho Nempo*, **22**, 25 (1970)
Shimagata *et al.*, *Japanese Patent*, 7,200,676 (1972)
Configuration
Hirai *et al.*, *Tetrahedron Lett.*, 2177 (1967)
Biosynthesis
Suzuki, Nozoe, *Biiorg. Chem.*, **3**, 72 (1974)

SIMPLEXIN
M.p. Indefinite

Derived from *Bacillus simplex*, this antibiotic substance is obtained by growth on a medium containing corn steep liquor. The material is isolated by adsorbing the activity of the culture filtrate on activated carbon, eluting with CH$_3$OH, evaporating the eluate to dryness *in vacuo* and taking up the residue in H$_2$O. Simplexin is stable in acid solution, unstable towards alkalies. It is soluble in H$_2$O, CH$_3$OH and 95 per cent EtOH, insoluble in Et$_2$O, CHCl$_3$, AcOEt, BuOH and C$_6$H$_6$.

The antibiotic is active *in vitro*, inhibiting *Rhizoctonia solani*. It has no activity *in vivo*, giving no protection to mice which have been experimentally infected with *Diplococcus pneumoniae* or *Staphylococcus aureus*. When tested in mice, 20 mg was the highest tolerated dose given intraperitoneally.

Cordon, Haenseler, *Soil Science*, **47**, 207 (1939)
Katznelson, *J. Bact.*, **39**, 101 (1940)
Katznelson, *Can. J. Res.*, **20**, 169 (1942)
Foster, Woodruff, *J. Bact.*, **51**, 363 (1946)

SIOMYCIN A
C$_{74}$H$_{92}$O$_{19}$N$_{19}$S$_5$
M.p. 255–260°C

One of the three closely related antibiotics containing sulphur that have been isolated by Japanese workers from *Streptomyces sioyaensis*. This substance crystallizes well from a mixture of CH$_3$OH and ligroin and has a specific rotation of $[\alpha]_D^{23} - 90·0°$ (c 1·0, dioxan). The structure is not yet known.

Nishimura *et al.*, *J. Antibiotics* (Japan), **14A**, 255 (1961)
Ebata, Miyazaki, Otsuka, *ibid.*, **22A**, 364, 423, 434 (1969)

SIOMYCIN B
C$_{63}$H$_{80}$O$_{32}$N$_{16}$S$_5$
M.p. 255–260°C (*dec.*)

A second highly complex antibiotic obtained from cultures of *Streptomyces sioyaensis*. This compound is also laevorotatory with a specific rotation of $[\alpha]_D^{23} - 102·9°$ (c 0·5, dioxan).

Ebata, Miyazaki, Otsuka, *J. Antibiotics* (Japan), **22A**, 364 (1969)
Nishimura, Otsuka, Ebata, *Japanese Patent*, 7,005,034 (1970)

SIOMYCIN C
C$_{69}$H$_{87}$O$_{31}$N$_{14}$S$_{4-5}$
M.p. 255–260°C

Streptomyces sioyaensis also elaborates this antibiotic substance which crystallizes from CH$_3$OH-CHCl$_3$. It has a specific rotation of $[\alpha]_D^{23} - 84·5°$ (c 0·5, dioxan).

Ebata, Miyazaki, Otsuka, *J. Antibiotics* (Japan), **22A**, 364 (1969)
Nishimura, Otsuka, Ebata, *Japanese Patent*, 7,005,034 (1970)

SIRODESMIN A
C$_{20}$H$_{26}$N$_2$O$_8$S$_2$

Sirodesmum diversum elaborates an antibiotic complex which has, so far, been separated into four components by chromatographic methods. This antibiotic forms an amorphous white powder having no definite melting point. It has been characterized as the deacetyl derivative, m.p. 193–195°C;

monoacetate which is amorphous with an indefinite melting point, and the diacetate, colourless needles with m.p. 186–189°C. The antibiotic has little, or no, activity against bacteria but is effective against a number of viruses.

Curtis et al., J. Chem. Soc., Perkin I, 180 (1977)

SIRODESMIN B
$C_{20}H_{26}N_2O_8S_4$

A constituent of the sirodesmin complex obtained from cultures of *Sirodesmum diversum*, this substance has a structure similar to that of the preceding antibiotic, having four sulphur atoms in the intramolecular bridge. It possesses antiviral activity.

Curtis et al., J. Chem. Soc., Perkin I, 180 (1977)

SIRODESMIN C
$C_{20}H_{26}N_2O_8S_3$

A further constituent of the sirodesmin complex, this antibiotic differs in structure from the two preceding compounds only in having three sulphur atoms in the bridge. It has antiviral activity similar to that of the other sirodesmins.

Curtis et al., J. Chem. Soc., Perkin I, 180 (1977)

SIRODESMIN G
$C_{20}H_{26}N_2O_8S_2$

Sirodesmin G has been isolated from the culture broth of *Sirodesmum diversum* and purified by column and thin layer chromatography. It is a stereoisomer of sirodesmin A having the structure given above derived from chemical and spectroscopic data. It is active against a range of viruses.

Curtis et al., J. Chem. Soc., Perkin I, 180 (1977)

SISOMICIN *(Antibiotic 6640, Rickamycin Sissomicin)*
$C_{19}H_{37}O_7N_5$
M.p. 198–201°C

Cultures of *Micromonospora inyoensis* yield this antibiotic which crystallizes from EtOH as the hemihydrate. It is dextrorotatory with a specific rotation of $[\alpha]_D^{26} + 189°$ (c 0·3, H_2O). The compound may be characterized as the pentaacetate which is an amorphous powder with m.p. 185–190°C. The structure has been shown to be that given above, which is a dehydro derivative of gentamicin 1a (q.v.). Sisomycin has an antibiotic spectrum both *in vitro* and *in vivo* which is very similar to that of gentamycin. It has a marked activity against penicillin-sensitive and pencillin-resistant strains of *Escherichia*, *Klebsiella*, *Proteus*, *Pseudomonas*, *Salmonella* and *Staphylococcus*. It is, however, inactive against cellular and filamentous fungi. Although sisomycin is effective against most strains of *Pseudomonas aeruginosa*, certain resistant strains have been encountered, sisomycin being inactivated by cell-free extracts from these isolates. This inactivation has been shown to be due to enzymic acetylation of the antibiotic.

Weinstein et al., *J. Antibiotics* (Japan), **23**, 551 (1970)
Wagman, Testa, Marquez, *ibid.*, **23**, 555 (1970)
Cooper, Jaret, Reimann, *Chem. Commun.*, 285 (1971)
Reimann, Jaret, Cooper, *ibid.*, 924 (1971)
O'Hara, Kono, *Antimicrobial Agents & Chemotherapy*, **5**, 558 (1974)
Reimann et al., *J. Org. Chem.*, **39**, 1451 (1974)

SOFRAMYCIN
See Neomycin B

SORBISTIN A$_1$
$C_{15}H_{31}N_3O_9$

A new strain *Pseudomonas sorbicinii* elaborates an aminoacid complex which has been separated by ion-exchange chromatography into sorbistins A$_1$, A$_2$ and B which are antibiotics and sorbistins C and D which are bio-active. Sorbistin A$_1$ is moderately active against a wide range of gram-positive and gram-negative bacteria, inhibiting most aminoglycoside-resistant organisms. This component of the complex shows the highest antibiotic activity and also possesses a low acute toxicity in mice.

Tsukiura et al., *J. Antibiotics* (Japan), **29**, 1137 (1976)
Structure
Konishi et al., *J. Antibiotics* (Japan), **29**, 1152 (1976)
See also
Kirby et al., *J. Antibiotics* (Japan), **30**, 344 (1977)

SORBISTIN A$_2$
$C_{16}H_{33}N_3O_9$

A homologue of sorbistin A$_1$, this antibiotic has been obtained by ion-exchange chromatography of the complex isolated from cultures of *Pseudomonas sorbicinii*. It is active against gram-positive and gram-negative bacteria and, like the preceding antibiotic, inhibits most aminoglycoside-resistant bacteria.

Tsukiura et al., *J. Antibiotics* (Japan), **29**, 1137 (1976)
Structure
Konish et al., *J. Antibiotics* (Japan), **29**, 1152 (1976)

SORBISTIN B
$C_{14}H_{29}N_3O_9$

The lowest of the homologous series of antibiotics obtained from cultures of *Pseudomonas sorbicinii*, this substance has the structure given above derived from chemical analysis and correlations and spectroscopic evidence. It has a lower antibiotic activity than sorbistin A$_1$.

Tsukiura et al., *J. Antibiotics* (Japan), **29**, 1137 (1976)
Structure
Konishi et al., *J. Antibiotics* (Japan), **29**, 1152 (1976)

SORDARIN
$C_{27}H_{40}O_8$

Sordaria araneosa elaborates this antifungal metabolite which is a colourless oil. It is laevorotatory with a specific rotation of $[\alpha]_D^{20} - 45 \cdot 2°$ (c 0·57, CH_3OH). Hydrolysis yields 6-deoxy-4-O-methyl-D-altrose and an aglycone, sordaricin, $C_{20}H_{28}O_4$, m.p. 188–109°C (*dec.*); $[\alpha]_D^{20} - 62°$ (c 0·33, CH_3OH). The antibiotic forms a crystalline sodium salt, m.p. 253–255°C and a methyl ester as an amorphous white powder with $[\alpha]_D^{20} - 53°$. The antibiotic is active against a range of gram-positive bacteria.

Hauser, Sigg, *Helv. Chem. Acta*, **54**, 1178 (1971)

SOVIET GRAMICIDIN
See Gramicidin S

SPARSOMYCIN
M.p. Indefinite

Streptomyces cuspidosporus yields two antibiotics when cultivated on a common nutrient medium for 90 hours at 28°C, one being this antibiotic and the other tubercidin (q.v.). The culture filtrate is stirred with activated carbon at pH 4·0–5·0, the cake extracted with CH_3OH-NH_4OH and the extracted treated with Dowex 1-X2. Sparsomycin has anti-tubercular properties similar to those of tubercidin.

Higashide *et al.*, *Japanese Patent*, 7,134,196 (1971)

SPECTINOMYCIN
See Actinospectacin

SPHAEROPSIDIN
$C_7H_8O_4$
M.p. Indefinite

A simple antibiotic substance isolated from cultures of *Phoma* species NRRL 3188 under aerobic conditions, the structure of sphaeropsidin has been shown to be 5,6-epoxy-4-hydroxy-2-hydroxymethylcyclohex-2-enone. The antibiotic is dextrorotatory with a specific rotation of $[\alpha]_D^{25} + 80°$ (c 1·0, H_2O) and the ultraviolet spectrum in H_2O consists of a single absorption maximum at 238 nm. Sphaeropsidin is active against gram-positive and gram-negative bacteria and also a range of pathogenic fungi. It also exhibits an inhibitory action against Eagle's KB epidermoid carcinoma cells grown on a modified Miyamura agar and incubated at 37°C for 16 hours.

Upjohn Co., *British Patent*, 1,159,502 (1969)

SPINAMYCIN
$C_{16}H_{16}O_2N_2$
M.p. 143°C

This antibiotic is produced by a new species of *Streptomyces*, *S. albospinus* which is allied to *S. albus*. The organism is cultured with shaking on a medium containing glucose, soybean flour, starch, yeast extract and inorganic salts at 27–29°C and pH 7·4 for 5 days. Spinamycin is isolated by stirring the broth with CH_3OH, centrifuging, leaving overnight at 5°C, clarifying, evaporating under reduced pressure, extracting with AcOEt, the extract concentrated and kept overnight with added petroleum ether. The precipitate which forms is then dissolved in AcOEt and chromatographed twice on silica gel, eluting with AcOEt-$CHCl_3$. Spinamycin gives positive tests with $FeCl_3$, Kostanecki and Erhlich reagents.

The antibiotic has little activity against bacteria but inhibits the growth of fungi including *Candida albicans, Histoplasma capsulatum, Piricularia oryzae* and *Trichophyton mentagrophytes*, the respective minimum inhibition concentrations (μg/ml) being 25–50, 0·78, 3·12–6·25 and 3·12–6·25. Spinamycin also gives a 50 per cent inhibition of Yoshida sarcoma cells at a concentration of 1·5 μg/ml.

Umezawa, Wang, *Japanese Patent*, 5719 (1968)

SPINULOSIN
$C_8H_8O_5$
M.p. 201–203·5°C

A simple quinoid antibiotic, spinulosin is elaborated by *Aspergillus fumigatus, Penicillium cinarescens* and *P. spinulosum* and is also obtained by synthesis. The two species of *Penicillium* are grown on a Czapek-Dox medium, iron being added in the case of *P. spinulosum*. *Aspergillus fumigatus* is fermented on a medium containing glucose, tartaric acid, ammonium tartrate and inorganic salts including ferrous sulphate heptahydrate. Various methods of isolation have been employed and purification is carried out by sublimation *in vacuo* followed by recrystallization from toluene. The structure of the antibiotic is 3:6-dihydroxy-4-methoxy-2:5-toluquinone. It forms black crystals with a metallic lustre, moderately soluble in hot H_2O, only slightly so in the cold. Unsaturation is shown by the decolourization of acidified potassium permanganate solution.

Spinulosin is assayed by cylinder plate with *Staphylococcus aureus* as the test organism. Both Kavanagh and Oxford and Raistrick have determined typical inhibition concentrations (μg/ml) *in vitro*, these being as follows: *Bacillus anthracis* (170); *B. mycoides* (125); *B. subtilis* (125); *Escherichia coli* (100–250); *Klebsiella pneumoniae* (250); *Mycobacterium phlei* (250); *Myco. smegmatis* (500); *Photobacterium fischeri* (16); *Pseudomonas aeruginosa* (500); *Salmonella typhimurium* (170); *Staphylococcus albus* (170); *Staph. aureus* (63–170) and *Vibrio comma* (170).

Birkinshaw, Raistrick, *Roy. Soc. London, Phil Trans*, **220B**, 245 (1931)
Anslow, Raistrick, *Biochem. J.*, **32**, 687 (1938)
Anslow, Raistrick, *ibid.*, **32**, 803 (1938)
Anslow, Raistrick, *ibid.*, **32**, 2288 (1938)
Anslow, Raistrick, *J. Chem. Soc.*, 1446 (1939)
Oxford, Raistrick, *Chem. Ind.*, **61**, 128 (1942)
Page, Robinson, *J. Chem. Soc.*, 1446 (1943)
Waksman, Geiger, *J. Bact.*, **47**, 391 (1944)
Kavanagh, *ibid.*, **54**, 761 (1947)
Bracken, Raistrick, *Biochem. J.*, **41**, 569 (1947)

SPIRAMYCIN (*Foromacidin, Rovamycin, Selectomycin, Sequamycin*)

This antibiotic substance has been isolated from cultures of *Streptomyces ambofaciens* found in soil from northern France. Recent work has shown that it consists of three closely related macrocyclic antibiotics, details of which are given below.

Cosar *et al.*, *Compt. rend. soc. biol.*, **234**, 1498 (1952)
Cosar *et al.*, *Antibiotics Annual*, 724 (1954–1955)
Cosar *et al.*, *U.S. Patent*, 2,943,023 (1960)

SPIRAMYCIN I
$C_{43}H_{74}O_{14}N_2$
M.p. 134–137°C

Chromatography of the spiramycin complex from *Streptomyces ambofaciens* yields three crystalline components of which this antibiotic predominates. Most of the antibiotic studies have been carried out with spiramycin I. The antibiotic forms colourless crystals and is laevorotatory with a specific rotation of $[\alpha]_D^{20} - 96°$. It forms a crystalline triacetate, m.p. 140–142°C; $[\alpha]_D^{20} - 92.5°$. Catalytic hydrogenation with Pd/C gives the dihydro derivative, with $NaBH_4$ the tetrahydro compound and with PtO_2 the hexahydro derivative. Spiramycin I is active against gram-positive bacteria, particularly *Bacillus subtilis*. When administered to guinea pigs in a single 50 mg/kg oral dose, only low levels of the antibiotic are found in the blood, but high levels are reached in the heart, kidney and liver, and particularly in the lungs and spleen. Evidently this antibiotic permeates the tissues of the major organs where it is bound for a considerable period. These observations show quite clearly that it is not always wise to judge the efficacy of an antibiotic solely upon the blood levels which are attained.

Preud'homme, Charpentier, *U.S. Patent*, 2,978,380 (1961)
Preud'homme, Charpentier, *U.S. Patent*, 3,011,947 (1961)
Takahira, *J. Antibiotics* (Japan), **23**, 424 (1970)
Curci, D'Alessio, Malagoli, *G. Ital. Chemoter.*, **18**, 1 (1971)
Structure
Kuehne, Benson, *J. Amer. Chem. Soc.*, **87**, 4660 (1965)

SPIRAMYCIN II
$C_{45}H_{76}O_{15}N_2$
M.p. 130–133°C

A second constituent of the spiramycin complex elaborated by *Streptomyces ambofaciens*, the structure of this compound is very similar to that of the preceding antibiotic. It is also laevorotatory with a specific rotation of $[\alpha]_D^{20} - 86°$ and yields a crystalline diacetate, m.p. 156–160°C and

$[\alpha]_D^{20} - 98.4°$. The antibiotic activity of this antibiotic is similar to that of spiramycin A, being effective against gram-positive bacteria.

Preud'homme, Charpentier, *U.S. Patent*, 2,978,380 (1961)
Preud'homme, Charpentier, *U.S. Patent*, 3,011,947 (1961)
Structure
Kuehne, Benson, *J. Amer. Chem. Soc.*, **87**, 4660 (1965)

SPIRAMYCIN III

$C_{46}H_{78}O_{15}N_2$
M.p. 128–131°C

This antibiotic is the homologue of spiramycin II and forms colourless crystals which are laevorotatory with $[\alpha]_D^{20} - 83°$. It yields a crystalline diacetate, m.p. 140–142°C and a specific rotation of $[\alpha]_D^{20} - 90.4°$. It is also active against gram-positive bacteria.

Preud'homme, Charpentier, *U.S. Patent*, 2,978,380 (1961)
Preud'homme, Charpentier, *U.S. Patent*, 3,011,947 (1961)
Structure
Kuehne, Benson, *J. Amer. Chem. Soc.*, **87**, 4660 (1965)

SPORACURACIN

Streptosporangium vulgare var. *eborea* strain A-11166 elaborates an antibiotic substance when fermented aerobically at 30°C for 48 hours on a medium consisting of glucose, starch, peptone, meat extract, defatted soybean flour, soybean oil and inorganic salts. The cells are extracted with AcOEt after centrifuging and the extract treated with an ion-exchange resin when the compound may be separated into two components, sporacuracins A and B. The antibiotic mixture is active against gram-positive bacteria.

Tamura, Furuta, Kotani, *Japanese Patent*, 75 125,094 (1975)

SPORAVIRIDIN

$C_{34-6}H_{63-7}O_{16}N$
M.p. Indefinite

Japanese workers have isolated this antibiotic from cultures of *Streptosporangium viridogriseum* by culturing the organism at 27°C for 3 days in a medium at pH 7·0 containing glucose, glycerol, soybean flour, starch and inorganic salts. Following extraction from the culture filtrate by conventional methods, the antibiotic is purified by precipitation from EtOH with $(CH_3)_2CO$. It forms an amorphous white powder with no definite melting point. It has a specific rotation of $[\alpha]_D^{29} - 12°$ (c 1·0, CH_3OH) and gives an ultraviolet spectrum having a single absorption maximum at 238 nm in both H_2O and 0·1 N-NaOH. Sporaviridin is a broad spectrum antibiotic, active against bacteria, yeasts and fungi, e.g. *Staphylococcus aureus* strains resistant to other antibiotics, *Torulopsis utilis* and *Trichophyton mentagyrophytes*. Mice tolerate a dose of 1·5 mg/kg administered intraperitoneally.

Okuda *et al.*, *Japanese Patent*, 6,806,995 (1968)

STABICILLIN

See Penicillin V

STAPHOCILLIN
See Methicillin

STAPHYLOCOCCIN
M.p. Indefinite

A number of apathogenic staphylococci produces this complex of antibiotics. e.g. *Staphylococcus epidermidis* grown on a protein hydrolysate alanine, cystine, tryptophan and vitamin B complex. The mixture of staphylococcins is isolated from the culture filtrate by the addition of ammonium sulphate followed by purification by chromatography on a Sephadex column. Staphylococcin forms an amorphous white powder and is inactivated by sulphosalicyclic acid, trichloroacetic acid or trypsin. The antibiotic is active against gram-positive bacteria, inhibiting *Corynebacterium diphtheriae*, *Diplococcus pneumoniae*, *Staphylococcus aureus* and *Streptococcus hemolyticus* at a minimum inhibition concentration of 30 µg/ml.

Bukharin, Suleimanov, Frolov, *Antibiotiki*, **15**, 1068 (1970)
Hale, Hinsdill, *Antimicrobial Agents & Chemotherapy*, **4**, 634 (1973)
Hoehne, Fink, Ortel, *East German Patent*, 99,601 (1973)

STAPHYLOMYCIN (*Virginiamycin, Virgimycim*)

A *Streptomyces* species related to *S. virginiae* produces an antibiotic complex, staphylomycin, which has been separated by Gosselinck and Parmentier into six components of which only two are of importance, namely staphylomycins M_1 and S. The mixture of antibiotics is a white, amorphous powder with a neutral reaction which decomposes at 138–140°C and is laevorotatory with a specific rotation of $[\alpha]_D^{20} - 124°$ (c 0·5, CH_3OH). It is active *in vivo*, protecting mice against experimental infections due to gram-positive bacteria. The LD_{50} in mice is 450 mg/kg given intraperitoneally.

Somer, Van Dijck., *Antibiotics & Chemotherapy*, **5**, 632 (1955)

STAPHYLOMYCIN M
See Ostreogrycin A

STAPHYLOMYCIN M_1
$C_{28}H_{36}O_8N_3$
Dec. 165–167°C

This component of the staphylomycin complex forms a tan-coloured, amorphous powder from $(CH_3)_2CO$-petroleum ether. It has a specific rotation of $[\alpha]_D - 191°$ (c 0·5, EtOH) and gives an ultraviolet spectrum in CH_3OH with a single absorption maximum at 216 nm. It is freely soluble in $CHCl_3$ and dimethylformamide, practically insoluble in H_2O and petroleum ether. The antibiotic is active against gram-positive bacteria, particularly *Micrococcus* spp. The commerical product contains approximately 75 per cent of this antibiotic and 5 per cent of staphlomycin S.

Vanderhaeghe et al., *Antibiotics & Chemotherapy*, **7**, 606 (1957)

STAPHYLOMYCIN S
$C_{28}H_{36}O_8N_3$
M.p. 240–242°C

A macrocyclic antibiotic, staphylomycin S has a structure very similar to that of mikamycin (q.v.). It forms colourless crystals from CH_3OH and is laevorotatory with a specific rotation of $[\alpha]_D^{20} - 28°$ (c 1·0, EtOH). The ultraviolet spectrum in EtOH has one absorption maximum at 305 nm. Staphylomycin S is readily soluble in $CHCl_3$ and dimethylformamide, slightly soluble in C_6H_6, $(CH_3)_2CO$ and AcOEt and insoluble in H_2O and petroleum ether. It has found some use in medicine as an antimicrobial and in veterinary use as a treatment for gram-positive bacterial infections of the eye and ear.

Gosselinckx, Parmentier, *Chromatog. Sym., 2nd Brussels*, 181 (1962)
Structure
Vanderhaeghe, Parmentier, *J. Amer. Chem. Soc.*, **82**, 4414 (1960)
Compernolie, Vanderheighe, Janssen, *Org. Mass Spectrom.*, **6**, 151 (1972)

STEFFIMYCIN
Streptomyces elgreteus NRRL 5634 produces this antibiotic when cultivated in a nutrient medium containing an assimilable carbohydrate and a source

of nitrogen under submerged aerobic conditions at 18–40°C for 2–10 days. The antibiotic is isolated by extraction of the broth with BuOH and purified by crystallization from EtOH. The structure is not yet known. Steffimycin is active in inhibiting the growth of a range of gram-positive bacteria.

Broadasky, Reusser, *U.S. Patent*, 3,794,721 (1974)

STEFFIMYCIN B
$C_{29}H_{32}O_{13}$

This antibiotic has been isolated from cultures of *Streptomyces elgretens* by extraction with organic solvents and purification on a silica gel column. The structure has been established from chemical and spectroscopic examination. Steffimycin B shows little, if any, activity against bacteria in experimentally infected laboratory animals. It has, however, shown some potential antitumour activity in an *in vitro* screening programme.

Brodasky, Ruesser, *J. Antibiotics* (Japan), **27**, 809 (1974)

STILBELLIN
M.p. 228–230°C

A neutral polypeptide antibiotic, this compound is elaborated by a species of *Stilbella*. The structure of the antibiotic is not known but hydrolysis experiments show that it contains the aminoacids, glutamic acid, glycine, hydroxyproline, leucine, phenylalanine, proline and an unknown aminoacid in the ratio of 1:2:3:2:2:2:2. The molecular weight has been determined as 1470–1500. Stilbellin has weak antibacterial activity and does not inhibit the growth of HeLa cells. The LD_{50} in mice is 47·5 mg/kg, given intraperitoneally.

Sasaki *et al.*, *J. Antibiotics* (Japan), **24**, 67 (1971)

STREPTIN
An antibiotic isolated from a *Streptomyces* species resembling *S. lavendulae* and *S. reticulus-ruber*, this basic substance is soluble in H_2O and active gram-positive, gram-negative bacteria and mycobacteria. It has a greater activity against staphylococci and micrococci than either streptomycin or streptothricin. No information is available regarding its toxicity.

Woodruff, Foster, *J. Bact.*, **52**, 502 (1946)

STREPTOCIN
Streptomyces griseus elaborates this antibiotic which is obtained by Et_2O extraction of the mycelium, concentration *in vacuo*, extraction of the residue with EtOH, further concentration *in vacuo* and extraction with petroleum ether. The substance is then purified by chromatography on an alumina column and elution with 1 per cent AcOH in CH_3OH. Streptocin forms colourless needles which sublime readily and are soluble in H_2O, CH_3OH, EtOH but not in $CHCl_3$. It is active against trichonomads although it has only a slight activity against gram-positive bacteria and mycobacteria.

Streptocin is normally assayed by serial dilution with *Trichomonas vaginalis* using penicillin and streptomycin in the test to prevent contamination. Waksman and his colleagues have measured the following inhibition concentrations (units/mg) *in vitro*: *Bacillus mycoides* (3·0); *B. subtilis* (5·0); *Escherichia coli* (>3·0); *Mycobacterium avium* (8·0); *Myco. ranae* (>8·0) and *Staphylococcus aureus* (3·0). The antibiotic inhibits *Trichomonas vaginalis* but there is only partial inhibition of *T. foetus* Br. at a concentration of 50 μg/ml and no inhibition of *T. gallinae* at the same concentration.

Schatz, Waksman, *Proc. Soc. Exptl. Biol. Med.*, **57**, 244 (1944)
Waksman, Schatz, Reilly, *J. Bact.*, **51**, 753 (1946)
Waksman *et al.*, *Proc. Soc. Exptl. Biol. Med.*, **70**, 308 (1949)
Kupferberg *et al.*, *J. Bact.*, **59**, 523 (1950)

STREPTOGRAMIN
M.p. *ca.* 155°C

Streptomyces graminofaciens, isolated from Texas soil, produces this antibiotic substance. The purest product obtained so far consists of solid spherules which melt at about 155°C. The substance is laevorotatory with a specific rotation of $[\alpha]_D - 134°$. It is readily soluble in CH_3OH, EtOH, AcOEt, $(CH_3)_2CO$, sparingly soluble in H_2O and dilute acids, insoluble in petroleum ether. Streptogramin has been shown to consist of an antibiotic factor which is able to inhibit the synthesis of protein and a synergizing factor, the latter being a macrocyclic polypeptide having a lactone structure. The antibiotic is active against a number of gram-positive bacteria.

Charney et al., Antibiotics & Chemotherapy, **3**, 1283 (1953)
Charney et al., British Patent, 776,035 (1957)

STREPTOLIN
$C_{25}H_{48}O_9N_{10}$

This antibiotic, isolated from *Streptomyces* species, is normally obtained as the crystalline helianthate, m.p. 207–211°C (*dec.*). It is prepared by submerged culture in various media and purified by precipitation of the helianthate and conversion to the hydrochloride.

The antibiotic is assayed by a turbidimetric method using *Escherichia coli* as the test organism. The helianthate normally has between 15,200 and 15,400 units/mg and the hydrochloride 33,000–34,000 units/mg. Inhibition concentrations (given in units/ml) have been determined *in vitro* as follows: *Aerobacter aerogenes* (3·3); *Aero. polymyxa* (1·0); *Bacillus cereus* (3·3); *B. fusiformis* (0·1); *B. megatherium* (0·3); *B. mycoides* (10); *Escherichia coli* (1·0); *Proteus vulgaris* (3·3); *Pseudomonas aeruginosa* (10) and *Ps. fluorescens* (33). When tested in mice, 8–10 mg/kg proved lethal when administered intravenously.

Rivers, Peterson, *J. Amer. Chem. Soc.*, **69**, 3006 (1947)
Smissman et al., *ibid.*, **75**, 2020 (1953)
Larson, Sternberg, Peterson, *ibid.*, **75**, 2035 (1953)
van Tamelen et al., *ibid.*, **83**, 4295 (1961)

STREPTOLYDIGIN (*Portamycin*)
$C_{32}H_{44}O_9N_2$
M.p. 147–148°C

Streptomyces lydicus elaborates this antibiotic which has been shown to possess the above structure based upon chemical and spectroscopic evidence.

Streptolydigin crystallizes from aqueous $(CH_3)_2CO$ and is laevorotatory with a specific rotation of $[\alpha]_D^{25} - 93°$ (c 1·6, $CHCl_3$). The ultraviolet spectrum in ethanolic H_2SO_4 has absorption maxima at 234, 357·5 and 370 nm, shifted to 261, 291 and 336 nm in ethanolic KOH. The antibiotic is soluble in $CHCl_3$, AcOEt, Et_2O and EtOH, insoluble in H_2O and hydrocarbons. A crystalline sodium salt, m.p. 225°C and $[\alpha]_D^{25} + 153°$ (c 1·35, $CHCl_3$) has been prepared. Streptolydigin is active against gram-positive bacteria except micrococci.

Eble et al., *Antibiotics Annual*, 893 (1955–1956)
Eble et al., *British Patent*, 779,570 (1957)

STREPTOMYCIN A
$C_{21}H_{39}O_{12}N_7$
M.p. Indefinite

One of two aminoglycosidic antibiotics isolated from cultures of *Streptomyces griseus* (Krainsky) Waksman et Henrici, the structure of this compound in N-methyl-L-glucosamindostreptosido-streptidine. The antibiotic is normally used as the trihydrochloride, m.p. indefinite; $[\alpha]_D^{25} - 84°$ (c 1·0, H_2O); the trihydrochloride double salt with calcium chloride, dec. 200°C; $[\alpha]_D^{25} - 76°$ (c 1·0, H_2O) or the sesquisulphate. Almost all of the salts are highly deliquescent but are not affected by light or air, freely soluble in H_2O, insoluble in EtOH, Et_2O and $CHCl_3$. The antibiotic is active against a range of gram-positive, gram-negative bacteria and mycobacteria, particularly against *Mycobacterium tuberculosis*. The normal medicinal dose is 0·5–1·0 g and side effects include rash, fever and possibly disturbances of the eigth nerve. It also finds a use in veterinary medicine in the treatment of leptospira, chronic respiratory disease, infectious sinusitis of turkeys and infectious synovitis of chickens. Priezzheva has also reported that when injected intramuscularly into rats at a dose of 20,000 units/kg/day for 5–60 days, the antibiotic inhibited oxidative phosphorylation in the brain cerebrum and cerebellum. In the former the oxygen uptake was increased while in the latter it was decreased. Submicroscopic alteration of the Reissner membrane has been reported by Novak when streptomycin was given to healthy guinea pigs at a dose of 250 mg/kg.

Schatz, Bugie, Waksman, *Proc. Soc. Exptl. Biol. Med.*, **55**, 66 (1944)
Weiss *et al.*, *Antibiotics & Chemotherapy*, **7**, 374 (1957)
Tishler, *Streptomycin*, Ed. Waksman, Baltimore (1949)
Bartels *et al.*, *Chem. Eng. Progress*, **54**, No. 8, 49 (Aug. 1958)
Structure
Brink, Folkers, *J. Amer. Chem. Soc.*, **69**, 1234 (1947)
See also
Heding, Fredericks, Lutzen, *Acta Chem. Scand.*, **26**, 3251 (1972)
Parfenov, *Veterinariya* (Moscow), **100** (1973)
Priezzheva, *Farmakol. Toksikol.*, **36**, 414 (1973)
Wallace *et al.*, *Proc. Nat. Acad. Sci., U.S.*, **70**, 1234 (1973)
Novak, *Tsitologiya*, **17**, 495 (1975)

STREPTOMYCIN B

$C_{27}H_{49}O_{17}N_7$
M.p. Indefinite

This antibiotic occurs in the concentrates from the isolation of streptomycin A. It is usually obtained as the trihydrochloride monohydrate which forms an amorphous white powder, m.p. 190–200°C after drying *in vacuo* at 100°C. This salt is laevorotatory with a specific rotation of $[\alpha]_D^{25} - 47°$ (c 1·35, H_2O). The reineckate is also amorphous with m.p. 178–179°C (*dec.*). The antibiotic activity of the trihydrochloride is about a quarter of that of streptomycin A trihydrochloride.

Fried, Titus, *J. Biol. Chem.*, **168**, 391 (1947)
Fried, Staveley, *J. Amer. Chem. Soc.*, **69**, 1549 (1947)
Fried, Staveley, *ibid.*, **70**, 3615 (1948)
Fried, Staveley, *J. Biol. Chem.*, **174**, 57 (1948)
O'Keefe *et al.*, *J. Amer. Chem. Soc.*, **71**, 2452 (1949)
Structure
Peck *et al.*, *J. Amer. Chem. Soc.*, **70**, 3968 (1948)
Staveley, Fried, *ibid.*, **71**, 135 (1949)
Staveley, Fried, *ibid.*, **74**, 5461 (1952)

STREPTONIGRIN

$C_{25}H_{22}O_8N_4$
Dec. 275°C

Streptonigrin is an antitumour antibiotic isolated from cultures of *Streptomyces flocculus*. When recrystallized from $(CH_3)_2CO$ or dioxan, it forms black rectangular plates which decompose without melting. The substance is weakly acidic, soluble in dimethylformamide, pyridine, dioxan and aqueous sodium bicarbonate with some decomposition. It is only slightly soluble in H_2O, $CHCl_3$, AcOEt and the lower alcohols. The antibiotic has an inhibitory effect upon a murine sarcoma virus-induced tumour cell line, being RNA-dependent DNA polymerase inhibitor. Price and his colleagues have shown that streptonigrin, given in a non-toxic dose (0·16 µg/ml) protected cultured Fischer rat embryo from *in vitro* transformation by 3-methylcholanthrene, a potent carcinogen. The LD_{50} in dogs is 4·0–5·0 µg/kg/day for 10 days. In man the tolerated dose lies in the range 1·75–2·25 mg for a given course of treatment. It is highly toxic to mammals and can cause severe and prolonged bone marrow depression.

Rao, Cullen, *Antibiotics Annual*, 950 (1959–1960)
Woods *et al.*, *In Vitro*, **9**, 24 (1973)
Chirigos *et al.*, *Cancer Chemother. Rep. Part I*, **57**, 305 (1973)
Pittillo, Woolley, *Antimicrobial Agents & Chemotherapy*, **5**, 82 (1974)
Price *et al.*, *Proc. Soc. Exptl. Biol. Med.*, **145**, 1197 (1974)

STREPTOTHRICIN
$C_{19}H_{34}O_8N_8$

This antibiotic, isolated from *Streptomyces lavendulae*, should not be confused with that obtained from *S. fradiae* and now named neomycin A or neamine (q.v.). Streptothricin may be produced by both surface and submerged growth on various media. It is not normally purified as the free base but as a salt or derivative, e.g. the hydrochloride which is an amorphous white powder, soluble in H_2O and dilute mineral acids, insoluble in organic solvents; the sulphate which is a hygroscopic microcrystalline powder, the helianthate, colourless crystals with m.p. 225–230°C (*dec.*), insoluble in H_2O or CH_3OH, or the reineckate, clusters of colourless small plates, decomposing at 192–194°C. The free base is thermostable when purified, but unstable to heat in the culture filtrate and is destroyed by concentrated mineral acids. It is not digested by proteolytic enzymes. It gives positive ninhydrin and biuret reactions, negative Molisch, Sakaguchi and Schiff reactions and decolourizes neutral potassium permanganate solution. It forms sparingly soluble salts with flavianic, rhodanilic and nitranilic acids and a crystalline *p*-(*w*-hydroxy-1-naphthylazo)-benzenesulphonate.

Several methods of assay have been employed, e.g. serial dilution with *Escherichia coli* in the presence of streptomycin, agar plate dilution with *Bacillus subtilis* or *Escherichia coli* and cylinder plate with *Bacillus subtilis*. Typical inhibition concentrations (units activity × 1000) with the purified material *in vitro* have been determined by Waksman as follows: *Aerobacter aerogenes* (30); *Bacillus cereus* (>10); *B. mycoides* (>10); *B. subtilis* (750); *Escherichia coli* (100); *Pseudomonas fluorescens* (>10); *Shigella dysenteriae* (30–100); *Shig. gallinarum* (300); *Shig. paradysenteriae* (50); *Sarcina lutea* (100) and *Staphylococcus aureus* (200).

Robinson *et al.* have also determined the following inhibition concentrations (*E. coli* units/ml) against a number of fungi: *Aspergillus niger* (250); *Cryptococcus neoformans* (250); *Epidermophyton inguineae* (1000); *Microsporum canis* (1000); *Penicillium chrysogenum* (250); *Sabouraudites schenki* (250); *Trichophyton gypseum* (500); and *Trich. interdigitale* (1000).

The antibiotic exerts both a bacteriostatic and bactericidal effect and the only factors which appear to affect the activity are the pH and the presence of inorganic salts.

Streptothricin is active *in vivo*. A dose of 1600 units protects mice infected with *Streptococcus hemolyticus* and 100 units gives 50 per cent protection against *Eberthella typhi*, *Escherichia coli* and *Salmonella aertrycke*. Complete survival is also provided against *Salmonella schottmuelleri* by 50 units per day for 3 days given intravenously and a single dose of 200 units given subcutaneously. No protection is given, however, against *Diplococcus pneumoniae*, nor against *Serratia marcescens* and *Proteus vulgaris*. The antibiotic is active against *Brucella abortus* in chick embryos and guinea pigs but not against *Trepanoma equipertum*, the viruses of feline pneumonitis, influenza and lymphogranuloma venereum, the toxins of *Clostridium tetani* and *Cl. welchii*.

The LD_{50} in mice, using a preparation of 5–300 *E. coli* units/mg is 750,000 mg/kg (oral), 500,000–750,000 mg/kg (intravenous) and 250,000–750,000 mg/kg (subcutaneous). The acute toxicity in mice when given intravenously depends upon the purity of the streptothricin, decreasing as the purity increases. Side effects in mice include gangrene of the small intestine and lesions, acute arteritis and myocarditis when given intravenously and toxic symptoms, convulsions and anorexia when administered orally by stomach tube.

Waksman, Woodruff, *J. Bact.*, **42**, 816 (1941)
Waksman *et al.*, *Soil Science*, **54**, 281 (1942)

Woodruff, Foster, *Arch. Biochem.*, **2**, 301 (1942)
Waksman, Woodruff, *Proc. Soc. Exptl. Biol. Med.*, **49**, 207 (1942)
Foster, Woodruff, *J. Bact.*, **45**, 408 (1942)
Foster, Woodruff, *Arch. Biochem.*, **3**, 241 (1943)
Woodruff, Foster, *J. Bact.*, **45**, 30 (1943)
Waksmann, *ibid.*, **46**, 299 (1943)
Schatz, Bugie, Waksman, *Proc. Soc. Exptl. Biol. Med.*, **55**, 66 (1944)
Robinson, Smith, *J. Pharmacol. Exper. Therapy*, **81**, 390 (1944)
Waksman, Bugie, Schatz, *Proc. Staff Meet. Mayo Clin.*, **19**, 537 (1944)
Fried, Wintersteiner, *Science*, **101**, 613 (1945)
Waksman, Schatz, *Proc. Nat. Acad. Sci.*, **31**, 208 (1945)
Donovick *et al.*, *J. Bact.*, **50**, 623 (1945)
Peck *et al.*, *J. Amer. Chem. Soc.*, **68**, 772 (1946)
Smith, *Proc. Soc. Exptl. Biol. Med.*, **61**, 214 (1946)
Kocholaty, Junowicz-Kocholaty, *Arch. Biochem.*, **15**, 55 (1947)
Trussel, Fulton, Grant, *J. Bact.*, **53**, 769 (1947)
Foster, Woodruff, *Brit. Patent*, 584,955 (1947)
Peterson *et al.*, *J. Amer. Chem. Soc.*, **69**, 3145 (1947)
Carter *et al.*, *ibid.*, **76**, 566 (1954)
van Tamelen., *ibid.*, **78**, 4817 (1956)
van Tamelen *et al.*, *ibid.*, **83**, 4295 (1961)
Chemotherapeutic properties
Kocholaty, *J. Bact.*, **44**, 143 (1942)
Waksman, Woodruff, *ibid.*, **44**, 373 (1942)
Welsch, *ibid.*, **44**, 571 (1942)
Metzger, Waksman, Pugh, *Proc. Soc. Exptl. Biol. Med.*, **51**, 251 (1942)
Perlman, *J. Bact.*, **48**, 116 (1944)
Woodruff, Foster, *Proc. Soc. Exptl. Biol. Med.*, **57**, 88 (1944)
Robinson, Smith, Graessle, *ibid.*, **57**, 226 (1944)
Schatz, Waksman, *ibid.*, **57**, 244 (1944)
Denkelwater, Cook, Tishler, *Science*, **102**, 12 (1945)
Perlman, McCoy, *J. Bact.*, **49**, 271 (1945)
Reilley, Schatz, Waksman, *ibid.*, **49**, 585 (1945)
Feldman, Hinshaw, *Amer. Rev. Tuberculosis*, **52**, 191, 299 (1945)
Neter, *Proc. Soc. Exptl. Biol. Med.*, **58**, 126 (1945)
Roessler *et al.*, *J. Inf. Diseases*, **79**, 23 (1946)
Meyer, Ordal, *ibid.*, **79**, 199 (1946)
Tonkin, *Brit. J. Pharm. Chemotherapy*, **1**, 163 (1946)
Hamre, Rake, *J. Inf. Diseases*, **81**, 175 (1947)
Toxicity
Rake *et al.*, *Amer. J. Med. Sci.*, **210**, 61 (1945)
Stanley, *J. Bact.*, **52**, 399 (1946)
Johnson, Walker, Kollros, *Arch. Neur. Psych.*, **56**, 184 (1946)
Pharmacology
Robinson *et al.*, *J. Pharm. Exper. Therapy*, **86**, 22 (1946)
Molitor, *Ann. N.Y. Acad. Sci.*, **48**, 101 (1946)

STREPTOTHRICIN A
$C_{49}H_{94}O_{13}N_{18}$
M.p. Indefinite.

Streptothricin has recently been separated into a number of components which differ only in the length of the peptide chain. In every case it has been shown that these are unbranched and the lysine residues are joined at the terminal amino groups.

Khokhlov, Shutova, *J. Antibiotics* (Japan), **25**, 501 (1972)
Shutova, Khokhlov, *Dokl. Akad. Nauk SSSR*, **205**, 1119 (1972)

STREPTOTHRICIN B
$C_{43}H_{82}O_{12}N_{16}$
M.p. Indefinite

A further component of the streptothricin complex, the structure of this compound has been elucidated from the products of partial hydrolysis.

Khokhlov, Shutova, *J. Antibiotics* (Japan), **25**, 501 (1972)
Shutova, Khokhlov, *Dokl. Akad. Nauk. SSSR*, **205**, 1119 (1972)

STREPTOTHRICIN BI
See Neomycin C

STREPTOTHRICIN BII
See Neomycin B

STREPTOTHRICIN C
$C_{37}H_{70}O_{11}N_{14}$
M.p. Indefinite

Also isolated from the streptothricin complex, the above structure for this antibiotic has been deduced from quantitative determination of L-lysine, streptolidine and 2-amino-2-deoxygulose in the hydrolysate.

Khokhlov, Shutova, *J. Antibiotics* (Japan), **25**, 501 (1972)
Shutova, Khokhlov, *Dokl. Akad. Nauk SSSR*, **205**, 1119 (1972)

STREPTOTHRICIN D
$C_{31}H_{58}O_{10}N_{12}$
M.p. Indefinite
The aminoacid side chain in this antibiotic has been shown to consist of three L-lysine moieties from an examination of the products of partial hydrolysis.

Khokhlov, Shutova, *J. Antibiotics* (Japan), **25**, 501 (1972)
Shutova, Khokhlov, *Dokl. Akad. Nauk SSSR*, **205**, 1119 (1972)

STREPTOTHRICIN E
$C_{25}H_{46}O_9M_{10}$
M.p. Indefinite

A further component of the streptothricin complex elaborated by *Streptomyces lavendulae*, this compound has the structure given above which is based upon a quantitative determination of the hydrolysis products.

Khokhlov, Shutova, *J. Antibiotics* (Japan), **25**, 501 (1972)
Shutova, Khokhlov, *Dokl. Akad. Nauk SSSR*, **205**, 1119 (1972)

STREPTOTHRICIN F
This antibiotic is identical with streptothricin (q.v.).

STREPTOTHRICIN X
$C_{55}H_{110}O_{14}N_{20}$
M.p. Indefinite
The most complex of the streptothricins, this antibiotic has an aminoacid

side chain consisting of seven L-lysine groups as determined from the quantitative estimation of L-lysine, streptolidine and 2-amino-2-deoxy-gulose present in the hydrolysate.

Khokhlov, Shutova, *J. Antibiotics* (Japan), **25**, 501 (1972)
Shutova, Khokhlov, *Dokl. Akad. Nauk SSSR*, **205**, 1119 (1972)

STREPTOVARICIN

This substance is actually a complex mixture of several closely related antibiotics. It is obtained from cultures of *Streptomyces spectabilis* and so far the following pure compounds have been isolated and characterized.

STREPTOVARICIN A

$C_{41}H_{53}O_{16}N$
M.p. 182–184°C

This component of the streptovaricin complex forms yellow crystals from CH_3OH or EtOH. It is strongly dextrorotatory with a specific rotation of $[\alpha]_D^{24} + 454°$ (c 1·0, $CHCl_3$). The structure has recently been revised to that given above. It inhibits the incorporation of nucleosides into HeLa cells, but less so than streptovaricin D (q.v.).

Siminoff et al., *Amer. Rev. Tuberc. Pulmonary Diseases*, **75**, 576 (1957)
Whitfield et al., *ibid.*, **75**, 584 (1957)
Upjohn Ltd., *British Patent*, 811,757 (1959)
Dietz et al., *U.S. Patent*, 3,116,202 (1963)
Revised structure
Rinehart et al., *J. Amer. Chem. Soc.*, **93**, 6273 (1971)

STREPTOVARICIN B

$C_{41}H_{53}O_{15}N$
M.p. 195–200°C

A second constituent of streptovaricin isolated from *Streptomyces spectabilis*, this antibiotic forms yellow crystals from EtOH and has a specific rotation of $[\alpha]_D^{24} + 168°$ (c 1·0, $CHCl_3$). It is less inhibitory than streptovaricin D against the incorporation of nucleosides into HeLa cells.

Siminoff et al., *Amer. Rev. Tuberc. Pulmonary Diseases*, **75**, 576 (1957)
Whitfield et al., *ibid.*, **75**, 584 (1957)
Upjohn Ltd., *British Patent*, 811,757 (1959)
Dietz et al., *U.S. Patent*, 3,116,202 (1963)
Structure
Rinehart et al., *J. Amer. Chem. Soc.*, **93**, 6273 (1971)

STREPTOVARICIN C

$C_{39}H_{51}O_{14}N$
M.p. 168–171°C

This antibiotic, which has been separated from streptovaricin complex, forms yellow crystals from EtOH and is also dextrorotatory with a specific rotation of $[\alpha]_D^{24} + 317°$ (c 1·0, $CHCl_3$).

Simonoff et al., *Amer. Rev. Tuberc. Pulmonary Diseases*, **75**, 576 (1957)
Whitfield et al., *ibid.*, **75**, 584 (1957)
Revised structure
Rinehart et al., *J. Amer. Chem. Soc.*, **93**, 6273 (1971)

STREPTOVARICIN D
$C_{40}H_{51}O_{13}N$
M.p. 115–118°C

A further component of streptovaricin, this antibiotic yields light yellow crystals from EtOH and has a specific rotation of $[\alpha]_D^{24} + 102°$ (c 1·0, CHCl$_3$). The structure has recently been revised to that given above. It selectively inhibits the incorporation of nucleosides into HeLa cells. This incorporation occurs rapidly and it appears likely that it reflects an inhibition of transport of nucleosides into the cells. The antibiotic is the most active in this respect of all the streptovaricins.

Siminoff et al., Amer. Rev. Tuberc. Pulmonary Diseases, **75**, 576 (1957)
Whitfield et al., ibid., **75**, 584 (1957)
Tan, McAuslan, Biochem. Biophys. Res. Commun., **42**, 230 (1971)
Revised structure
Rinehart et al., J. Amer. Chem. Soc., **93**, 6273 (1971)

STREPTOVARICIN E
$C_{40}H_{49}O_{14}N$
M.p. 102–105°C
Also separated from streptovaricin, this compound crystallizes as yellow needles from EtOH. It is slightly dextrorotatory having $[\alpha]_D^{24} + 6·13°$ (c 1·0, CHCl$_3$). The structure of this antibiotic has also been revised.

Siminoff et al., Rev. Amer. Tuberc. Pulmonary Diseases, **75**, 576 (1957)
Whitfield et al., ibid., **75**, 584 (1957)
Revised structure
Rinehart et al., J. Amer. Chem. Soc., **93**, 6273 (1971)

STREPTOVARICIN F
$C_{39}H_{47}O_{14}N$

This antibiotic has recently been isolated from cultures of *Streptomyces spectabilis* and assigned the structure given above. It has a slight effect upon the inhibition of nucleosides into HeLa cells.

Rinehart et al., J. Amer. Chem. Soc., **93**, 6273 (1971)

STREPTOVARICIN G
$C_{40}H_{51}O_{15}N$
A further antibiotic obtained from cultures of *Streptomyces spectabilis*, the structure of this compound has recently been shown to be the secondary alcohol corresponding to streptovaricin E as the ketone.

Rinehart et al., J. Amer. Chem. Soc., **93**, 6273 (1971)

STREPTOVIRUDIN

Streptomyces griseoflavus var. *thuringiensis* elaborates a complex of antibiotics when grown aerobically upon a nutrient medium at 27–30°C. Extraction of the culture filtrate with EtOH yields streptovirudin complex KF while the mycelium furnishes a different complex, streptovirudin M. Chromatography of the two complexes has so far yielded eight components designated streptovirudins A_1, A_2, B_1, B_2, C_1, C_2, D_1 and D_2. The individual components, as well as the complex itself, are active against gram-positive bacteria and a number of DNA and RNA viruses.

Eckardt *et al.*, *East German Patent*, 102,162 (1973)

STREPTOVIRUDINS

A strain of *Streptomyces* yields an antibiotic complex when fermented on a common nutrient medium. Eight components have so far been isolated and purified by column and thin layer chromatography; streptovirudins A_1, A_2, B_1, B_2, C_1, C_2, D_1 and D_2. The antibiotics are active against gram-positive bacteria, mycobacteria and a number of DNA- and RNA-viruses.

Eckardt *et al.*, *J. Antibiotics* (Japan), **28**, 274 (1975)

STREPTOVITACIN A
$C_{15}H_{23}O_5N$
M.p. 156–159°C

STREPTOVITACIN C_2

One of a number of isomeric antibiotics obtained from *Streptomyces griseus*, this substance crystallizes from EtOH as colourless, irregular crystals. The structure has been determined from chemical and spectroscopic evidence. The addition of 10 µg/ml of the antibiotic to a medium containing the BS-C-1 line of *Cercopithecus* monkey kidney cells 1 hour before the end of the eclipse phase completely inhibited the synthesis of RNA poliovirus type 1 and the cytopathogenic effect.

Eble *et al.*, *Antibiotics Annual*, 555 (1958–1959)
Giulio Tarro, *Proc. Soc. Exptl. Biol. Med.*, **126**, 535 (1967)

STREPTOVITACIN B
$C_{15}H_{23}O_5N$
M.p. 124–128°C

This antibiotic from *Streptomyces griseus* is a positional isomer of the preceding substance. It forms colourless crystals from EtOH.

Eble *et al.*, *Antibiotics Annual*, 555 (1958–1959)
Herr, *J. Amer. Chem. Soc.*, **81**, 1595 (1959)

STREPTOVITACIN C_2
$C_{15}H_{23}O_5N$
M.p. 124–128°C

A further positional isomer, this antibiotic from *Streptomyces griseus* has the above structure which is based upon chemical and spectroscopic determinations. It forms colourless crystals from EtOH.

Herr, *J. Amer. Chem. Soc.*, **81**, 2595 (1959)

STREPTOVITACIN D
$C_{15}H_{23}O_5N$
M.p. 67–69°C
A fourth antibiotic isolated from *Streptomyces griseus*, this substance forms colourless crystals from EtOH. It is isomeric with the three preceding compounds but the structure has not yet been established.

Herr, *J. Amer. Chem. Soc.*, **81**, 2595 (1959)

STREPTOZOTOCIN
$C_8H_{15}O_7N_2$
Dec. 115°C

Streptozoticin is derived from *Streptomyces achromogenes* and forms colourless crystals from 95 per cent aqueous EtOH which decompose without melting. The ultraviolet spectrum in CH_3OH consists of a single absorption maximum at 228 nm. It is soluble in H_2O and the lower alcohols, insoluble in less polar organic solvents. Streptozoticin is active against gram-positive bacteria and Reusser has shown that in the case of *Bacillus subtilis*, the antibiotic rapidly degrades DNA in either resting or actively dividing cells, probably due to an interaction with the cytosine residues in DNA.

Herr et al., *Antibiotics Annual*, 236 (1959–1960)
Reusser, *J. Bact.*, **105**, 580 (1971)
Bhuyan et al., *Cancer Chemother. Rep. Part I*, **58**, 157 (1974)

STRIATIN A
$C_{27}H_{36}O_7$
Extraction of the mycelia of the Basidiomycete *Cyathus striatus* strain No. 12 yields three closely related antibiotics, striatins A, B and C which have been separated and purified chromatographically. This component exhibits a high activity against a range of gram-positive bacteria, some gram-negative organisms and fungi imperfecti.

Anke et al., *J. Antibiotics* (Japan), **30**, 221 (1977)

STRIATIN B
$C_{27}H_{36}O_8$
A further constituent of the antibiotic complex obtained from cultures of *Cyathus striatus* No. 12, this substance has an antibiotic spectrum similar to that of the preceding antibiotic.

Anke et al., *J. Antibiotics* (Japan), **30**, 221 (1977)

STRIATIN C
$C_{25}H_{34}O_7$
Also present in the antibiotic complex isolated from cultures of *Cyathus striatus* No. 12, this antibiotic is active against fungi imperfecti, gram-positive and gram-negative bacteria.

Anke et al., *J. Antibiotics* (Japan), **30**, 221 (1977)

STROBILURIN A
An antibiotic isolated from cultures of *Strobilurus tenacellus*, this substance has been shown to inhibit the growth of yeasts and a number of filamentous fungi. It also inhibits the synthesis of macromolecules by Ehrlich ascites tumour cells but has no activity against bacteria.

Anke et al., *J. Antibiotics* (Japan), **30**, 806 (1977)

STROBILURIN B
A further antibiotic obtained from the fermentation broth of *Strobilurus tenacellus*, this substance has a similar antibiotic spectrum to strobilurin A.

Anke et al., *J. Antibiotics* (Japan), **30**, 806 (1977)

STYSADIN
M.p. 290–295°C (*dec.*)
Stysanus medius produces this antibiotic when a preculture of the organism is inoculated into a medium consisting of glucose, glycerol and inorganic salts and incubated with aeration for 69 hours at 27°C. The mycelium is extracted with $(CH_3)_2CO$, the extract concentrated and the residue re-extracted with AcOEt. The residue is then washed with Et_2O, dissolved in $CHCl_3$ and treated with petroleum ether to give, on cooling, a precipitate which is chromatographed on a silica column, eluting with CH_3OH. Addition of H_2O to the eluate yields crystals of the antibiotic. Stysadin is dextrorotatory with a specific rotation of $[\alpha]_D^{28} + 110°$ (c 1·0, CH_3OH) and gives positive Tollens and Molisch reactions. It is effective against plant

pathogenic fungi, inhibiting the growth of *Aspergillus niger*, *Hypochnus sasakii* and *Penicillium digitatum* at a concentration of 0·1–0·4 ppm.

Ishibashi, Takiguchi, *Japanese Patent*, 27,317 (1967)

SUBSPORIN A
$C_{88}H_{148}O_{26}N_{20}$
M.p. Indefinite
When *Bacillus subtilis* is cultivated in a citrate-containing medium at 25–35°C, it yields three polypeptide antibiotics, subsporins A, B and C. This particular antibiotic is an acid and forms the major portion of the complex. Hydrolysis experiments have shown that it contains fourteen aminoacids in the molecule. Subsporin A is active against *Piricularia oryzae* and *Trichophyton mentagrophytes*.

Ebata, *Japanese Patent*, 7,140,195 (1971)

SUBSPORIN B
$C_{88}H_{148}O_{24}N_{20}$
M.p. Indefinite
A further polypeptide antibiotic produced by *Bacillus subtilis* when grown on a medium containing citrate, this minor component is neutral in reaction. It possesses a similar activity to subsporin A against *Piricularia oryzae* and *Trichophyton mentagrophytes*.

Ebata, *Japanese Patent*, 7,140,195 (1971)

SUBSPORIN C
$C_{90}H_{147}O_{26}N_{21}$
M.p. Indefinite
A further minor component of the subsporin complex produced by *Bacillus subtilis* fermented in a citrate-containing medium, this substance is also neutral and is equally effective against *Piricularia oryzae* and *Trichophyton mentagrophytes*.

Ebata, *Japanese Patent*, 7,140,195 (1971)

SUBTENOLIN
M.p. Indefinite
Hirschhorn, Bucca and Thayer first obtained this antibiotic from a culture of *Bacillus subtilis* grown on a medium containing DL-alanine, magnesium citrate, potassium dihydrogen phosphate and inorganic salts, the medium being inoculated with the spore suspension and incubated at 36°C for 3–4 days. The final product had a potency of 1000–1600 *Staphylococcus aureus* units/mg. Subtenolin is a yellow powder with no definite melting point and is slightly hygroscopic. It gives an ultraviolet spectrum with an absorption maximum at 270 nm. The antibiotic is soluble in H_2O and most organic solvents which contain a trace of H_2O. It is, however, insoluble in butanone, $(CH_3)_2CO$, Et_2O and 95 per cent EtOH. Subtenolin is thermostable in aqueous solution and has a maximum stability at pH 2·0. It gives positive Molisch, ninhydrin and enol tests but a negative Millon test. It is not precipitated by either acids or alkalies. The 2:4-dinitrophenylhydrazone crystallizes from EtOH and with picric acid it forms rosettes of minute crystals which are biologically inactive.

The antibiotic is assayed by serial dilution with *Staphylococcus aureus* as the test organism. The spectrum *in vitro* has been examined by Hirschhorn and his colleagues who gives the following inhibition concentrations (units/ml): *Clostridium fallax* (500); *C. histolyticum* (600); *C. novyi* (300); *C. perfringens* (300); *C. tertium* (500); *Eberthella typhi* (165); *Escherichia coli* (370–1500); *Mycobacterium tuberculosis* (>2000); *Neisseria gonorrheae* (600); *Pasteurella pestis* (16·5); *Salmonella schottmuelleri* (600); *Staphylococcus albus* (140); *Staph. aureus* (140–200) and *Streptococcus pyogenes* (1500). It exhibits no activity against *Aerobacter aerogenes*, *Bacillus* spp., *Brucella* spp., *Klebsiella pneumoniae*, *Micrococcus* spp., *Pseudomonas aeruginosa*, *Salmonella enteriditis*, *S. paratyphi*, *S. typhimurium* or *Serratia marcescens*.

The LD_{50} for mice is between 30 and 60 mg (1000 units/ml) given intraperitoneally. At least 50 per cent of the administered dose is detected in the urine after injection.

Hirschhorn, Bucca, Thayer, *Proc. Soc. Exptl. Biol. Med.*, **67**, 429 (1948)
Howell, Tauber, *ibid.*, **67**, 432 (1948)

SUBTILIN (*Subtilin C*)
M.p. Indefinite
A further antibiotic isolated from cultures of *Bacillus subtilis*, subtilin may be produced by both surface and submerged growth on various media. The associated antibiotic subtilin C described by Hassell in 1948 appears to be identical with subtilin in all respects except that it gives no colour reaction with $FeCl_3$ solution. Both materials are purified by washing with 95 per cent EtOH, extracting with 85 per cent EtOH containing AcOH and sodium chloride, discarding the supernatant liquor and extracting the residue with an acetate buffer at pH 4·5. The buffer extract is then deionized with an ion-exchange resin, concentrated and freeze-dried. Subtilin forms an

amorphous white powder with no definite melting point. It is soluble in H$_2$O and the lower aliphatic alcohols provided they are saturated with H$_2$O. In acid solution it is quite stable, is inactivated by light, formaldehyde, CH$_3$OH, pepsin, trypsin and alkali. It gives a blue colour with FeCl$_3$ solution (cf. subtilin C).

Subtilin is assayed by several methods, e.g. paper disc-plate with *Bacillus cereus*, serial dilution with *Lactobacillus casei*, *Micrococcus conglomeratus* and *Staphylococcus aureus* and turbidimetric with the latter organisms. When tested *in vitro* the antibiotic inhibits *Micrococcus conglomeratus* at a concentration of 0·6–1·0 µg/ml, *Streptococcus pyogenes* at 0·034 µg/ml and *Trepanoma pallidum* at 2·0–3·5 µg/ml. It is active against gram-positive bacteria, *Neisseria catarrhalis*, *N. gonorrheae* and certain pathogenic fungi. With *Mycobacterium phlei* and *Staphylococcus aureus*, resistant strains are encountered by serial transfer on a medium containing subtilin.

In both mice and guinea pigs, subtilin afforded protection against experimental infections due to *Bacillus anthracis*, pneumococcus III, *Staphylococcus aureus* and *Streptococcus pyogenes*.

The toxicity in mice was LD$_{50}$ of 60 mg/kg (intravenous) and 2500–3000 mg/kg (subcutaneous). A dose of 5 g/kg given intragastrically proved lethal.

Humfield, Feustel, *Proc. Soc. Exptl. Biol. Med.*, **54**, 232 (1943)
Jansen, Hirschman, *Arch. Biochem.*, **4**, 297 (1944)
Lewis *et al.*, *ibid.*, **14**, 415 (1947)
Stubbs *et al.*, *ibid.*, **14**, 427 (1947)
Dimick *et al.*, *ibid.*, **15**, 1 (1947)
Feeney, Lightbody, Garibaldi, *ibid.*, **15**, 13 (1947)
Dimick *et al.*, *Fed. Proc.*, **6**, 247 (1947)
Feeney *et al.*, *ibid.*, **6**, 250 (1947)
Feeney, Garibaldi, Humphreys, *Arch. Biochem.*, **17**, 435 (1948)
Feeney, Garibaldi, *ibid.*, **17**, 447 (1948)
Fevold, Dimick, Klose, *ibid.*, **18**, 27 (1948)
Garibaldi, Feeney, *Ind. Eng. Chem.*, **41**, 432 (1949)
Chemotherapy
Salle, Jann, *Proc. Soc. Exptl. Biol. Med.*, **60**, 60 (1945)
Salle, Jann, *ibid.*, **61**, 23 (1946)
Salle, Jann, *ibid.*, **62**, 40 (1946)
Salle, Jann, *ibid.*, **63**, 41, 519 (1946)
Salle, Jann, *J. Bact.*, **51**, 592 (1946)
Anderson, Wong, *Tuberculogy*, **8**, 77 (1946)
Anderson *et al.*, *Science*, **103**, 418 (1946)
Goodman, Henry, *ibid.*, **105**, 320 (1947)
Anderson, Chin, *ibid.*, **106**, 643 (1947)
Anderson, *J. Invest. Dermatol.*, **8**, 25 (1947)
Salle, Jann, *J. Bact.* **54**, 269 (1947)
Wong, Hambly, Anderson, *J. Lab. Clin. Med.*, **32**, 837 (1947)
Farber *et al.*, *ibid.*, **33**, 799 (1948)
Knight, Thomsett, *J. Clin. Invest.*, **27**, 544 (1948)
Chin, *Fed. Proc.*, **7**, 211 (1948)
Eagle, Musselman, Fleischman, *J. Bact.*, **55**, 347 (1948)
Salle, Jann, *ibid.*, **55**, 463 (1948)
Housewright, Henry, Birkman, *ibid.*, **55**, 545 (1948)
Steenken, Wolinsky, *ibid.*, **57**, 453 (1949)
Salle, Jann, *J. Clin. Invest*, **28**, 1036 (1949)
Subtilin C
Hassell, *Nature*, **161**, 317 (1948)

SUBTILIN C
See Subtilin

SUBTILYSIN
Also isolated from cultures of *Bacillus subtilis*, this antibiotic is produced by incubating the bacterium on a nutrient broth containing glucose for 20 days. The compound is stated to be unstable to heat and to be active *in vitro* against *Clostridium edematiens*, *Escherichia coli*, *Pasturella* spp., *Salmonella gardneri* and *Vibrio comma*.

Valle, *Compt. rend. soc. biol.*, **139**, 148 (1945)

SULFACTIN
C$_{38}$H$_{55}$O$_7$N$_{11}$S$_4$
M.p. 245–275°C (*dec.*)

Streptomyces roseus elaborates this antibiotic which is obtained by acidification of the culture filtrate to pH 3·0, extraction with BuOH, concentration *in vacuo* and washing the residue with boiling Et$_2$O followed by further extraction with CHCl$_3$. The compound is then recrystallized from boiling EtOH. Sulfactin forms white crystals which are soluble in CHCl$_3$, EtOH, AcOEt, BuOH and dioxan. Sulfactin is virtually insoluble in Et$_2$O, H$_2$O, C$_6$H$_6$ and petroleum ether. It diffuses through a cellophane membrane but with some loss in activity.

Sulfactin is assayed by serial dilution with *Staphylococcus aureus* (one unit being equivalent to 0·0048 µg of crystalline antibiotic) or by agar streak dilution with the same organism (0·0254–0·0270 µg being equal to one unit). Morton has given the following inhibition concentrations (units/ml): *Bacillus anthracis* (8–16); *B. cereus* (16); *B. circulans* (2·0); *B. megatherium* (2·0); *B. mesentericus* (0·5); *B. mycoides* (0·5); *B. subtilis* (0·5); *Corynebacterium diphtheriae* (0·03); *Coryne. xerosis* (0·06); *Diplococcus pneumoniae* I (1·0); *Diplo. pneumoniae* III (0·5); *Gaffkya tetragena* (0·5); *Micrococcus aurantiacus* (0·25); *Micro. lysodeikticus* (0·25); *Micro. roseus* (0·125); *Neisseria sicca* (0·5); *Staphylococcus aureus* (1·0) and *Streptococcus pyogenes* (4·0). All of the other bacteria examined has inhibition concentrations in excess of 32 units/ml.

In mice, sulfactin is active against *Diplococcus pneumoniae* I at a dose of 1–10 µg given intraperitoneally. The LD_{50} in mice is 135 mg/kg when administered intraperitoneally.

Junowicz-Kocholaty, Kocholaty, Kelner, *J. Biol. Chem.*, **168**, 765 (1947)
Morton, *Proc. Soc. Exptl. Biol. Med.*, **66**, 345 (1947)

SULFOCILLIN
$C_{16}H_{18}O_7N_2S_2$

A semi-synthetic antibiotic of the penicillin type, this compound is largely used in medicine as the disodium salt. It is a broad-spectrum antibiotic, mainly active against gram-positive bacteria and is effective *in vivo* against *Clostridium* and *Staphylococcus* species. Sulfocillin has no central nervous system activity in mice and cats and in the latter there is no evidence for any influence on the blood pressure level, heart rate, respiration or electrocardiographic pattern. When administered to rabbits in physiological saline solution it has a local irritant and pain-producing action, the latter being decreased by dissolving in 1 per cent calcium gluconate. Large doses of the drug given to mice, rats and dogs showed a marked decrease in erythrocyte counts, hematocrit values and hemoglobin content.

Kanno *et al.*, *Takeda Kenkyusho Ho*, **30**, 248 (1971)
Murato *et al.*, *ibid.*, **30**, 262 (1971)
Mizutani *et al.*, *ibid.*, **30**, 322 (1971)

SUNCILLIN
$C_{16}H_{19}O_7N_3S_2$

A semi-synthetic penicillin type antibiotic, this compound is used as the disodium salt and is active against gram-positive and some gram-negative bacteria. The minimum inhibition concentrations found against 27 strains of *Pseudomonas aeruginosa* isolated from clinical patients was 8–512 µg/ml. Only in 2 cases, however, was this antibiotic more active than carbenicillin (q.v.).

Chaloupecky, Vymola, *J. Hyg. Epidemiol. Microbiol. Immunol.*, **18**, 123 (1974)

SURGUMYCIN
Actinomyces surgutus strain LIA-0166, a new member of the nonchromogenic actinomycetes, isolated from podzol soils of Western Siberia near Surgut, elaborates this antibiotic which appears to belong to the α-hydroxyoxopentaene group. The antibiotic inhibits the growth of gram-positive bacteria and certain fungi and yeasts.

Konev, Severinets, *Antibiotiki*, **19**, 10 (1974)

SUZUKACILLIN A
A polypeptide antibiotic, suzukacillin A has been obtained by growing *Trichoderma viride* 63C1 on a medium to which asparagine, serine, glycine and arginine are added, all of which stimulate the formation of the antibiotic by the organism. Following extraction of the antibiotic from the culture medium it may be separated chromatographically into this compound and a small amount of suzukacillin B.

Suzukacillin A forms colourless crystals and on hydrolysis yields alanine, 2-amino-2-methylpropanoic acid, leucine, glutamic acid, glycine, proline and valine.

Ooka, Takeda, *Agr. Biol. Chem.*, **36**, 112 (1972)

SUZUKACILLIN B
This polypeptide antibiotic has been isolated from the culture of *Trichoderma viride* 63C1 in small amounts. Very little is known of its constitution and antibiotic properties.

Ooka, Takeda, *Agr. Biol. Chem.*, **36**, 112 (1972)

SYNNEMATIN B
See Penicillin N

TALAMPICILLIN
$C_{24}H_{23}N_3O_6S$

A semi-synthetic antibiotic, this substance is normally prepared as the hydrochloride which is a white powder having m.p. 154–157°C (dec.). It has the same antibiotic activity as ampicillin (q.v.) but has no intrinsic activity, having to be hydrolysed to ampicillin to be effective.

Murakami et al., U.S. Patent, 3,951,954 (1976)
Murakami et al., German Patent, 2,225,149 (1972)
Ferres, Clayton, ibid., 2,228,012 and 2,228,255 (1972)
Clayton et al., Antimicrobial Agents & Chemotherapy, **5**, 670 (1974)

TALARON
Dec. 123–130°C

This new antifungal antibiotic has been obtained from *Talaromyces vermiculatus* which is deep-cultured, with shaking, in a common nutrient medium at pH 7·0 and 23–30°C for 2–3 days. The culture filtrate is adsorbed on diatomaceous earth after adjusting the pH to 3·6 and extracted with buffer solution at pH 7·0. The eluate is then chromatographed on a DEAE-Sephadex A-25 column, the active fraction collected and freeze-dried. Talaron is a pale yellow, amorphous powder which darkens at 123–130°C and has no definite melting point. It is laevorotatory with a specific rotation of $[\alpha]_D^{22} - 324°$ (c 0·5, H_2O). The antibiotic has a polysaccharide structure, contains both nitrogen and phosphorus, has a molecular weight of 7000–8000 and is soluble in H_2O. It exhibits a powerful fungicidal activity against filamentous dermatophytes.

Ando et al., Japanese Patent, 7,243,393 (1972)
Mizuno et al., J. Antibiotics (Japan), **27**, 560 (1974)

TARDIN
$C_{11}H_{15}O_3$

Tardin has been isolated from cultures of *Penicillium tardum* grown by surface culture on a medium consisting of malt extract in tap water incubated at 24°C. The material is isolated by neutralizing the culture medium after filtering, extracting with amyl acetate, distilling the organic extract *in vacuo*, dissolving the brownish residue in C_6H_6 and removing the insoluble material by centrifuging. Tardin is purified further by chromatography on an alumina column previously washed with HCl. It forms a pale yellow oil which is readily soluble in EtOH, Et_2O, $(CH_3)_2CO$, C_6H_6 and amyl acetate, slightly soluble in H_2O and *n*-hexane. It is laevorotatory with a specific rotation of $[\alpha]_D^{20} - 11·4°$.

Tardin is assayed by cylinder plate with *Staphylococcus aureus* as the test organism. It is active against both bacteria and fungi, the following inhibition dilutions ($\times 1000$) having been determined by Borodin and his colleagues *in vitro*: *Clostridium diphtheriae gravis* (8·0); *Cl. xerosis* (64); *Endomycopsis albicans* ($>5·0$); *Escherichia coli* ($>1·0$); *Pseudomonas aeruginosa* ($>1·0$); *Sabouraudites audouini* (5·0); *Sab. lanosus* (5·0); *Salmonella enteriditis* (1·0); *Staphylococcus aureus* (129); *Streptococcus viridans* (8·0); *Trichophyton equinus* (5·0); *Trich. lacticolor* ($>5·0$); *Trich. sabouraudii* (5·0) and *Trich. tonsurans* ($>5·0$).

When administered to mice, 1·8 mg given subcutaneously and 0·8 mg administered intravenously were tolerated although both edema and sloughing occurred at the injection site some hours after administration.

Wilkins, Harris, Brit. J. Exptl. Path., **24**, 141 (1943)
Borodin, Philpot, Florey, ibid., **28**, 31 (1947)

TBILIMYCIN
M.p. Indefinite

An antibiotic isolated from *Streptomyces chartreusis* var. *tsibisus*, this compound has a heptaenic structure although the complete structure is not yet known. It is soluble in EtOH and dimethylformamide and gives an ultraviolet spectrum with absorption maxima at 369, 380, 404 and 450 nm. Tbilimycin is fungistatic towards most common fungi and yeasts at a concentration of 0·32–0·64 µg/ml.

Shenin et al., *Antibiotiki*, **15**, 9 (1970)

TEICHOMYCIN A$_1$
A new species of *Actinoplanes*, *A. trichomyceticus* ATCC 31,121 elaborates a complex of antibiotics from which three components have been isolated by chromatographic methods. This substance is primarily active against gram-positive bacteria.

Coronelli et al., *German Patent*, 2,608,216 (1976)

TEICHOMYCIN A$_2$
A second antibiotic obtained from cultures of *Actinoplanes teichomyceticus* ATCC 31,121, the substance has been obtained from the filtered culture medium by extraction with BuOH followed by paper and thin layer chromatography. Like the accompanying teichomycins it is active against gram-positive bacteria.

Coronelli et al., *German Patent*, 2,608,216 (1976)

TEICHOMYCIN A$_3$
This antibiotic also occurs in the culture filtrate of *Actinoplanes teichomyceticus* ATCC 31,121 and is effective against gram-positive bacteria. The structure, like those of the other teichomycins is not completely known.

Coronelli et al., *German Patent*, 2,608,216 (1976)

TELOMYCIN
$C_{59}H_{79}O_{19}N_{13}$
M.p. Indefinite

```
    COOH
    |
    CHCH₂CO—Ser—Thr—allo-Thr—Ala—Gly—trans-3HO Pro
    |                   |
    NH₂                 O
                        |
                        C—cis-3HOPro—Δ-Try—CH₃Try—HO-Leu
                        ||
                        O
```

A macrocyclic polypeptide antibiotic produced by a *Streptomyces* species isolated from Florida soil, telemycin is laevorotatory with a specific rotation of $[\alpha]_D^{28} - 133°$ (c 1·0, CH$_3$OH aq.). The structure given is based upon chemical and spectroscopic examinations of the hydrolysis products. Telomycin forms an amorphous grey solid with no definite melting point. The ultraviolet spectrum in CH$_3$OH has a single absorption maximum at 339 nm. The antibiotic is soluble in H$_2$O, dilute alkalies, moderately soluble in CH$_3$OH and EtOH, slightly soluble in (CH$_3$)$_2$CO, AcOEt. Telomycin is active against gram-positive bacteria *in vitro* and effective against *Micrococcus pyogenes* var. *aureus in vivo* in mice. The LD$_{50}$ (all routes) in mice is greater than 1000 mg/kg.

Misiek et al., *Antibiotics Annual*, 852 (1957–58)
Bagby et al., *J. Org. Chem.*, **26**, 1261 (1961)
Sheehan et al., *J. Amer. Chem. Soc.*, **85**, 2867 (1963)

TENEBRIMYCIN
Streptomyces tenebrarius ATCC 17,920 elaborates this antibiotic complex which consists of a number of components that have not yet been completely separated and characterized. The complex has been obtained by preparing two successive precultures of the organism and inoculating a medium of glucose, soybean powder, soybean oil and inorganic salts and fermenting at 37°C for 5 days. The filtrate then contains 680 tenebrimycin units/ml.

Thompson, Stark, Higgins, *Japanese Patent*, 76 32,719 (1976)

TENNECETIN
See Pimaricin

TENUAZONIC ACID
$C_9H_{15}O_3N$

A simple antibiotic, tenuazonic acid is produced by *Alternaria tenuis* and is extracted from the culture filtrate with organic solvents and purified by chromatography. It inhibits the growth of a number of human and rodent tumours, the specific locus of action in mammalian cells being related to the suppression of protein synthesis, particularly the inhibition of the release of nascent proteins from microsomes in the cell sap. Tenuazonic acid has no activity against bacteria or yeasts.

Shigeura, *Antibiotics*, **1**, 360 (1967)

TERRAMYCIN (*Oxytetracycline*)
$C_{22}H_{24}O_9N_2$
M.p. 184·5–185·5°C (*dec.*)

This broad-spectrum antibiotic has been isolated from cultures of *Streptomyces rimosus*. It is obtained by extracting the culture filtrate with BuOH and then extracting the organic phase with dilute mineral acid giving an aqueous extract. Purification is carried out by chromatography on an alumina column followed by repetitive solvent and dilute acid extractions, final purification being done by dissolving in dilute acid and then neutralizing to give crystals of the dihydrate. A number of crystalline forms of the antibiotic are known. The free antibiotic, sodium salt and hydrochloride are all soluble in polar organic solvents. The dihydrate is laevorotatory with specific rotations of $[\alpha]_D^{25} - 196·6°$ (c 0·9, 0·1 N-HCl) and $[\alpha]_D^{25} - 2·1°$ (c 0·9, 0·1 N-NaOH). Among the crystalline salts and derivatives that have been prepared are the hydrochloride which forms colourless needles from CH_3OH; the diacetate, colourless crystals from CH_3OH, m.p. 208–213°C; $[\alpha]_D^{25} + 214°$ (CH_3OH) and the sodium salt as lemon-yellow crystals from CH_3OH. The latter decomposes in aqueous solution at room temperature and the acid salts all hydrolyse slowly in solution above pH 1·0 to yield crystals of terramycin.

Terramycin is assayed by cylinder plate or serial dilution with *Bacillus cereus* as the test organism. Finlay has determined the following inhibition concentrations (μg/ml) *in vitro*: *Aerobacter aerogenes* (1·0); *Bacillus subtilis* (3·0); *Brucella bronchiseptica* (3·0); *Escherichia coli* (5·0); *Klebsiella pneumoniae* (3·0); *Proteus* spp. (1000); *Pseudomonas aeruginosa* (100); *Salmonella paratyphi* (1·0); *S. pullorum* (10); *S. schottmuelleri* (1·0); *S. typhi* (3·0); *Staphylococcus albus* (1·0) and *Staph. aureus* (1·0). The antibiotic is also active against several strains of *Hemophilus pertussis*, pneumococci, *Endemeba histolytica* and associated bacterial flora. Resistance to terramycin is induced in coliforms, enterococcus and *Staphylococcus aureus* by serial transfer on a terramycin-containing medium. This is not, however, the case with pneumococci or group A streptococci.

Terramycin produces favourable reactions *in vivo*. It has proved effective in mice against *Hemphilus influenzae*, *Klebsiella pneumoniae*, pneumococcus I and hemolytic streptococcus A. Against brucellosis it is particularly effective when used with streptomycin and it also has a favourable effect against *Pasteurella tularensis*. It acts both as a prophylactic and therapeutic against the spores of *Clostridium septicum* and *Cl. tetani*. When tested in mice and chick embryos it proves effective against a large number of rickettsia, scrub typhus and Rocky Mountain spotted fever.

Numerous clinical tests have been carried out with this antibiotic, favourable results being obtained with pneumonias although in certain cases the bacterial flora of the sputum is replaced by *Staphylococcus* when terramycin is given orally. With a daily dose of 2–6 g given orally, good responses have been obtained in cases of infections of the urinary tract from *Aerobacter aerogenes*, *Escherichia coli*, non-hemolytic streptococci, *Streptococcus fecalis* and a number of other sensitive organisms. Continued therapy also produces favourable results in cases of brucellosis, subacute bacterial endocarditis, septicemia by *Bacteroides* and *Escherichia coli*, follicular tonsillitis, septic sore throat, pneumococcal meningitis, scrub typhus, rickettsial pox and *Hemophilus pertussis*. It is inaffective against *Proteus*, *Pseudomonas*, *Salmonella* and *Staphylococcus* infections, the numbers of *Proteus* tending to show an increase as other bacterial flora declined.

Terramycin is relatively non-toxic. The LD_{50} in mice has been given as 892 mg/kg (subcutaneous); 7200 mg/kg (oral) and 150–200 mg/kg (intravenous) when the hydrochloride is used. When employed in clinical trials, a dose of between 2 and 4 g daily, given orally, showed no hepatic, renal or central nervous system damage. Side effects include vomiting and diarrhoea. The antibiotic is readily absorbed, particularly following oral administration, diffusion occurring into the organs and bodily tissues but not into the intact central nervous system.

Finlay, *Science*, **111**, 85 (1950)
Pasternack *et al.*, *J. Amer. Chem. Soc.*, **73**, 2400 (1951)
Regna *et al.*, *ibid.*, **73**, 4211 (1951)
Hochstein, Pasternack, *ibid.*, **73**, 5008 (1951)
Hochstein *et al.*, *ibid.*, **74**, 3708 (1952)
Hochstein *et al.*, *ibid.*, **75**, 5455 (1953)

TERRAMYCIN X
See 2-Acetyl-2-decarboxamido-oxytetracycline

TETRACYCLINE
$C_{22}H_{24}O_8N_2$
M.p. 170–175°C (*dec.*)

Tetracycline

Tetracycline is an antibiotic produced by several species of *Streptomyces*. It may be purified by recrystallization from toluene when it forms colourless crystals. It is laevorotatory having a specific rotation of $[\alpha]_D^{25} - 239°$ (CH_3OH) and has pK_a 8·3 and 10·2. The structure has been established as 4-dimethylamino-1:4:4a:5:5a:6:11:12a-octahydro-3:6:10:12:12a-pentahydroxy-6-methyl-1:11-dioxanaphthacene-2-carboxyamide. The ultraviolet spectrum in 0·1 N-HCl has absorption maxima at 220, 268 and 355 nm. Tetracycline is quite stable in neutral and alkaline solution in contrast to chlortetracycline (q.v.). The hydrochloride forms colourless crystals from acidified BuOH, decomposing at 214°C and laevorotatory with $[\alpha]_D^{25} - 257·9°$ (c 0·5, 0·1 N-HCl). This salt has been marketed under a variety of trade names including Achromycin V, Ambracyn, Artomycin, Cefracycline, Diacycline, Dumocyclin, Fermentmycin, Quadracycline, Ricycline, Stilciclina, Subamycin, Totomycin and Unimycin. It is readily soluble in H_2O, moderately so in CH_3OH and EtOH and insoluble in Et_2O and hydrocarbons.

A tetracycline phosphate complex has been prepared under the tradenames of Sumycin, Tetrex, Panmycin phosphate and Tetradecin Novum. This is stated to be more rapidly absorbed than either the free base or the salts when ingested. It is prepared by the addition of sodium metaphosphate to a solution of tetracycline or the hydrochloride and although comparatively insoluble, gives higher blood levels following oral administration. The antibiotic is effective *in vivo* against many bacterial infections, both primary pathogens and secondary invaders. The oral dose in humans is 0·25–0·5 g given orally or intravenously and 0·1–0·25 g given intramuscularly. It is also used in the preparation of topical ointments. A number of side effects have been observed including glossitis, diarrhoea, idiosyncrasy and photodynamic reactions. When administered orally to rabbits at a dose of 10–100 mg/kg/day for 20 days there were persistent disturbances in the regeneration of blood cells and also in the proliferation and maturation of bone marrow elements, together with atrophy of the gastric and intestinal mucosa and dystrophic changes in the kidneys, liver and myocardium.

Boothe *et al.*, *J. Amer. Chem. Soc.*, **75**, 4621 (1953)
Stephens *et al.*, *ibid.*, **74**, 4976 (1952)
Stephens *et al.*, *ibid.*, **76**, 3568 (1954)
Conover, *U.S. Patent*, 2,699,054 (1955)
Heinemann *et al.*, *U.S. Patent*, 2,886,595 (1959)
Miller, *U.S. Patent*, 3,005,023 (1961)
Arishima, Sekizawa, *U.S. Patent*, 3,019,173 (1962)
Total synthesis
   Boothe *et al.*, *J. Amer. Chem. Soc.*, **81**, 1006 (1959)
   Conover *et al.*, *ibid.*, **84**, 3222 (1962)
Absolute configuration
   Dobrynin *et al.*, *Tetrahedron Lett.*, 901 (1962)
Biological action
   Paticka, Spratkova, Sestakova, *Advan. Antimicrob. Antineoplastic Chemother.*, *Proc. Int. Congr.* 7th, **1**, 193 (1971)
   Mikaelyan, *Antibiotiki*, **18**, 738 (1973)
   Mikaelyan *et al. ibid.*, **18**, 906 (1973)
   Strippoli, Simonetti, *Mycopathol. Mycol. Appl.*, **51**, 65 (1973)
   Belousova, Zagorodnaya, *Vrach. Delo*, 144 (1973)
   Ma, Jun, Luzzi, *J. Pharm. Sci.*, **62**, 1261 (1973)
   Lanman *et al.*, *Amer. J. Physiol.*, **225**, 1240 (1973)
   Heinrich, Oppitz, *Naturwiss.*, **60**, 524 (1973)
   Martin *et al.*, *J. Infect. Diseases*, **129**, 110 (1974)
   Demidov, Artamonova, *Veterinariya* (Moscow), **65** (1974)
   Madison, Fain, *Arch. Int. Pharmacodyn. Ther.*, **214**, 224 (1975)

5,10,11,11-TETRAHYDRO-9,11-DIHYDROXY-8-METHYL-5-OXO-1H-PYRROLO-[e,2,1][1,4]-BENZODIAZEPIN-2-ACRYLAMIDE
$C_{16}H_{14}N_4O_4$

Streptomyces spadicogriseus ATCC 31,179 yields this antibiotic when grown in a medium of glucose, peptone, meat extract and NaCl with agitation and aeration for 48 hours at 32–34°C. It has been obtained by adsorption of the filtrate on activated carbon, elution with Me_2CO, concentration *in vacuo*, extraction with BuOH, MeOH-$CHCl_3$ added and the resultant mixture chromatographed on a silica gel column. Concentration of the active fractions gives a crude product, purified by addition of Me_2CO-AcOEt. The antibiotic has been shown to prevent the retention of ascites sarcoma 37 in mice two weeks after injection into the abdominal cavity. The dose given was 30 g/kg/day.

Komatsu, *U.S. Patent*, 4,011,140 (1977)

TETRAMYCIN
$C_{34}H_{53}O_{14}N$
M.p. *ca.* 260°C (*dec.*)

Streptomyces noursei var. *jenensis* JA 3789 elaborates this antibiotic which is produced by cultivating the organism in a medium of glucose, soybean flour and inorganic salts at pH 7·0 and 27–29°C for 3–4 days. Tetramycin has an indefinite melting point, is amphoteric, readily soluble in AcOH, dimethylformamide and pyridine, moderately so in aqueous organic solvents but insoluble in H_2O, C_6H_6 and $CHCl_3$. It has a specific rotation of $[\alpha]_D + 89°$ (c 0·5, dimethylformamide) and $[\alpha]_D + 9·5°$ (pyridine). The antibiotic is active against a range of fungi and yeasts but has no activity against bacteria.

Thrum *et al.*, *East German Patent*, 70,706 (1970)
Dornberger *et al.*, *J. Antibiotics* (Japan), **24**, 172 (1971)

TETRAMYCOIN A
A tetraene antibiotic isolated from cultures of *Chainia* species HA234 and HA235, grown by submerged fermentation in a medium containing sorghum meal and inorganic salts at 28°C and pH 6·8–7·0 for 100–120 hours. Both mycelium and filtrate are extracted with BuOH, the extracts combined and concentrated under reduced pressure. Petroleum ether is then added to precipitate the crude antibiotic which is purified by crystallization from hot CH_3OH—$(CH_3)_2CO$. The antibiotic is active against a range of gram-positive and gram-negative bacteria.

Rahalkar, Rahalkar, Thirumalachar, *Hindustan Antibiot. Bull.*, **15**, 1 (1972)

TETRAMYCOIN B
A further tetraene antibiotic produced by *Chainia* species HA234 and HS235, this compound is separated from the preceding substance by chromatography and crystallization from CH_3OH—$(CH_3)_2CO$. It is also active against a variety of gram-positive and gram-negative bacteria.

Rahalkar, Rahalkar, Thirumalachar, *Hindustan Antibiot. Bull.*, **15**, 1 (1972)

TETRANACTIN
$C_{44}H_{72}O_{12}$
M.p. 105–106°C

A macrocyclic antibiotic, tetranactin has been isolated from cultures of *Streptomyces aureus* strain S-3466, being obtained from the filter cake by extraction with $(CH_3)_2CO$. The antibiotic forms colourless, rhombic prisms when crystallized from $(CH_3)_2CO$ and is optically inactive in $CHCl_3$. The symmetrical structure shown above is based upon chemical and spectroscopic evidence. Tetranactin is active against gram-positive bacteria *in vitro* and is also pesticidal against the Azuki-bean weevil. The acute toxicity is very low, mice tolerating 300 mg/kg given intraperitoneally or 15,000 mg/kg administered orally.

Ando *et al.*, *J. Antibiotics* (Japan), **24**, 347, 418 (1971)
Suzuki *et al.*, *ibid.*, **24**, 675 (1971)

THERMOMYCIN
An antibiotic isolated from *Streptomyces thermophilus*, thermomycin is prepared by salting out the broth with ammonium sulphate or by extraction with Et_2O and removal of the solvent *in vacuo*. The antibiotic is thermolabile. Heating at 75°C destroys approximately a quarter of the activity and keeping it at 100°C for 15 minutes destroys the substance completely. Thermomycin is primarily active against *Corynebacterium diphtheriae*. No data are available concerning its toxicity or use in medicine.

Schone, *Antibiotics & Chemotherapy*, **1**, 176 (1951)

THERMORUBIN
See Thermorubin A

THERMORUBIN A (*Antibiotic BT-3-3, Thermorubin*)
$C_{32}H_{24}O_{10}$
M.p. >200°C (*dec.*)

This antibiotic, elaborated by *Thermoactinomyces antibioticus*, forms orange-red needles or rosettes of the dihydrate from $CHCl_3$ or AcOEt. It darkens at 190°C and melt above 200°C with extensive decomposition. The ultraviolet spectrum in EtOH has absorption maxima at 250, 300, 328 and 435 nm with a shoulder at 415 nm. It is soluble in dimethylformamide, pyridine, tetrahydrofuran, AcOH and concentrated acids and alkalies, slightly soluble in CH_3OH, EtOH, BuOH, AcOEt, $CHCl_3$, $(CH_3)_2CO$, C_6H_6, cyclohexane and insoluble in H_2O, hexane, Et_2O and petroleum ether. Thermorubin A is highly active against both gram-positive and gram-negative bacteria. The LD_{50} in mice has been given as 300 mg/kg administered intraperitoneally.

Craveri et al., *Clinical Medicine*, **71**, 511 (1964)
Terao, Furuya, Enokita, *Sankyo Kenkyusho Nempo*, **17**, 110 (1965)
Structure
Moppett et al., *J. Amer. Chem. Soc.*, **94**, 3269 (1972)

THERMOTHIOCIN
$C_{60}H_{110}O_{25}N_{10}S_3$
M.p. 300°C

A complex polypeptide antibiotic, thermothiocin is produced by the submerged culture of *Thermoactinopolyspora coremialis* ATCC 15,974 in a nutrient medium at 48°C and pH 5·0–10·5 for 3 days. The antibiotic is extracted from the broth by adjusting to pH 3·0 and with BuOH. The antibiotic is dextrorotatory with a specific rotation of $[\alpha]_D^{25} + 29\cdot4°$ (c 0·5, dimethylformamide). It forms an amorphous yellow powder which is comparatively stable in alkaline solution. It is active *in vitro* against a range of gram-positive and gram-negative bacteria and *in vivo* protects mice infected with *Streptococcus hemolyticus* and *Staphylococcus aureus*.

Coronelli, Craveri, *British Patent*, 1,106,148 (1968)

THERMOZYMOCIDIN
$C_{21}H_{39}O_6N$
M.p. 170–172°C

Italian workers have described this antibiotic which has been isolated from cultures of a thermophilic Eumycete, *Albomyces* ATCC 20,349 incubated on a medium containing corn flour at 40–43°C, under submerged aerobic conditions. The culture medium is extracted with $(CH_3)_2CO$, filtered and the activity adsorbed on a weak acid exchange resin followed by elution with NH_4OH—CH_3OH, extraction with BuOH and precipitation. A yellow-white powder is obtained which is further purified by chromatography on a silica gel column. The structure has been shown to be 2-amino-3:4-dihydroxy-2-hydroxymethyl-14-oxoeicos-6-enoic acid having the trans configuration about the double bond. It is active against a number of pathogenic fungi but not against bacteria.

Craveri, Manachini, Aragozzini, *Experientia*, **28**, 867 (1972)
Aragozzini et al., *ibid.*, **28**, 881 (1972)
Aragozzini et al., *Tetrahedron*, **28**, 5493 (1972)
Craveri, Manachini, Aragozzini, *U.S. Patent*, 3,758,529 (1973)

THIACTIN
See Thiostrepton

THIAMPHENICOL (*Propacin, Thiocymetin, Urfamycin, Vicemycetin*)
$C_{12}H_{15}O_5NSCl_2$
M.p. 164·3–166·3°C

A synthetic antibiotic, this compound forms colourless crystals from CH_3OH and is dextrorotatory with a specific rotation of $[\alpha]_D^{25} + 12\cdot9°$ (c 1·0, EtOH). The ultraviolet spectrum in 95 per cent EtOH has absorption maxima at 224, 266 and 274 nm. It is soluble in H_2O, CH_3OH and EtOH. Thiamphenicol is active against a wide range of gram-positive and gram-negative bacteria and mycobacteria. Its use has been proposed in the treatment of oriental plague. However, it possesses an *in vivo* immunosuppressant activity in actively immunized mice and rabbits, lowering the production of antibodies, partly by an inhibitory action on antigen-stimulated precursors of the antibody-forming cells. The effect is reversed following withdrawal of the drug. In man, serious suppression of normal and stimulated erythropoiesis has been observed.

Cutler et al., *J. Amer. Chem. Soc.*, **74**, 5475 (1952)
Suter et al., *ibid.*, **75**, 4330 (1953)
Suter et al., *U.S. Patents*, 2,759,927, 2,759,970, 2,759,971, 2,759,972, (1956)

Suter et al., *British Patent*, 770,277 (1957)
Petrescu, *Postgrad. Med. J. Suppl.*, **50**, 97 (1974)
Kaltwasser et al., *ibid.*, **50**, 118 (1974)

THIANOSINE
M.p. Indefinite

A polymyxin type antibiotic isolated from cultures of *Bacillus thiaminolyticus*, this compound is obtained as a white, amorphous powder with no definite melting point. Hydrolysis yields α,γ-diaminobutyric acid, leucine and threonine. It is active against gram-negative bacteria and has LD_{50} in mice of 68 mg/kg given intravenously.

Arima, Beppu, Matsushima, *J. Vitaminol.*, **17**, 163 (1971)

THIOAURIN
$C_{14}H_{12}O_4N_4S_4$
M.p. 179–181°C (*dec.*)

An unclassified *Streptomyces* species produces this antibiotic which forms golden-yellow crystals from $(CH_3)_2CO$. It is only slightly soluble in H_2O and the common organic solvents. The ultraviolet spectrum in CH_3OH shows absorption maxima at 232 and 370 nm. Thioaurin is active against gram-positive and gram-negative bacteria but only slightly so against fungi. The LD_{50} in mice is 16 mg/kg when given intravenously. So far, it shows little promise of use in medicine owing to its relatively high toxicity.

Bolhofer, Machlowitz, Charney, *Antibiotics & Chemotherapy*, **3**, 385 (1953)

THIOCILLIN
Three closely related antibiotics have been isolated from cultures of *Bacillus* species, thiocillins I, II and III. Thiocillins I and II are produced by *B. cereus* strain G-15 and thiocillins II and III by *B. badius* strain AR-91. All of these antibiotics contain a high percentage of sulphur in the molecule and give virtually identical ultraviolet spectrum with absorption maxima about 275 and 348 nm. They are related to micrococcin P and are active against a range of gram-positive bacteria.

Shoji et al., *J. Antibiotics* (Japan), **29**, 366 (1976)

THIOLUTIN (*Aureothricin, Farcinicin*)
$C_8H_8ON_2S_2$
Dec. 270°C

This antibiotic is elaborated by *Streptomyces albus* and *S. celloflavus*. It forms yellow crystals when recrystallized from AcOEt, decomposing at 270°C although a lower decomposition point of 256–257°C has been recorded. Thiolutin is neutral and optically inactive, slightly soluble in H_2O, Et_2O and C_6H_6, readily soluble in CH_3OH, EtOH, $(CH_3)_2CO$, $CHCl_3$, glacial AcOH and methyl *iso*butyl ketone. It gives an ultraviolet spectrum in CH_3OH with absorption maxima at 245, 315 and 365 nm. It is stable in neutral and acid solutions but decomposes under alkaline conditions.

Thiolutin is active against gram-positive and gram-negative bacteria in concentrations of 1–15 µg/ml but both *Brucella* and *Pseudomonas* are resistant to the antibiotic. Pathogenic fungi are inhibited at concentrations of only 1–3 µg/ml but *Candida albicans* is resistant. It possesses a mild but definite microbicidal action against bacteria, fungi and protozoa. The LD_{50} in mice is 25 mg/kg when given orally or subcutaneously. In medicine, it has been recommended as a topical agent against fungus infections.

Umezawa, Maeda, Kosaka, *Jap. Med. J.*, 512 (1948)
Seneca, Kane, Rockenbach, *J. Antibiotics* (Japan), **2**, 357 (1952)
Celmer et al., *J. Amer. Chem. Soc.*, **74**, 6304 (1952)

THIOMYCETIN
See Thiamphenicol

THIOMYCIN
M.p. 176–178°C

A sulphur-containing antibiotic, this compound is produced by an unclassified actinomycete closely resembling *Streptomyces phaeochromogenes* var. *chloromyceticus*. When crystallized from AcOEt it forms golden-yellow needles, soluble in CH_3OH, EtOH, BuOH, $(CH_3)_2CO$, AcOEt, C_6H_6, $CHCl_3$ and amyl acetate, slightly soluble in H_2O, Et_2O and petroleum ether. It gives an ultraviolet spectrum in 0·5 *N*-HCl with a single absorption maximum at 370 nm. The antibiotic is stable at acid pH but unstable under alkaline conditions. It is active against gram-positive bacteria but is highly toxic with LD_{50} in mice of 10 mg/kg given subcutaneously.

Hinuma et al., *J. Antibiotics* (Japan), **8A**, 118 (1955)

THIOPEPTIN A$_1$

Streptomyces tateyamensis elaborates a number of peptide antibiotics, thiopeptins A$_1$, A$_2$, A$_3$ and B. This substance is prepared by preculturing the organism for 2 days at 30°C with stirring in a medium containing starch, corn steep liquor, cottonseed cake and inorganic salts, an inoculum of the liquor then being used with a further batch of the same medium. Thiopeptin A$_1$ is active against gram-positive bacteria.

Miyairi *et al.*, *Japanese Patent*, 7,213,720 (1972)

THIOPEPTIN A$_2$

A further peptide antibiotic isolated from cultures of *Streptomyces tateyamensis*, this substance also possesses activity against gram-positive bacteria, particularly *Staphylococcus aureus*.

Miyairi *et al.*, *Japanese Patent*, 7,213,117 (1972)

THIOPEPTIN A$_3$

This peptide antibiotic is obtained by culturing *Streptomyces tateyamensis* in a nutrient medium at 30°C for 2 days followed by extraction of the culture filtrate with AcOEt, the crude antibiotic being purified by chromatography on an alumina column. Thiopeptin A$_3$ is amphoteric and laevorotatory with a specific rotation of $[\alpha]_D^{23} - 10.8°$ (c 1.0, CHCl$_3$). The minimum inhibition concentration against *Staphylococcus aureus* is 0.25 μg/ml. When hydrolysed with dilute acids it furnishes alanine, cysteine, threonine and valine.

Miyairi *et al.*, *Japanese Patent*, 7,213,117 (1972)

THIOPEPTIN B

$C_{72}H_{90}O_{22}N_{18}S_6$
M.p. 219–222°C

Streptomyces tateyamensis produces this sulphur-containing antibiotic which is separated from the preceding compounds by chromatography on alumina. It is laevorotatory with a specific rotation of $[\alpha]_D^{23} - 80°$ (c 1.0, CHCl$_3$). The ultraviolet spectrum in CH$_3$OH has shoulders at 230–250, 295 and 305 nm. It is active against gram-positive bacteria.

Miyairi *et al.*, *J. Antibiotic* (Japan), **23**, 113 (1970)

THIOSTREPTON (*Thiactin*)

Dec. 246–256°C
A sulphur-containing polypeptide, this antibiotic is elaborated by a species of *Streptomyces* isolated from New Mexican soil. It forms colourless crystals from CHCl$_3$—CH$_3$OH which decompose without melting. It is laevorotatory with the following specific rotations: $[\alpha]_D^{23} - 20°$ (pyridine), $[\alpha]_D^{23} - 61°$ (c 1.0, dioxan) and $[\alpha]_D^{23} - 98.5°$ (c 1.0, AcOH). Thiostrepton is soluble in CHCl$_3$, dioxan, dimethylformamide, pyridine and AcOH, virtually insoluble in H$_2$O, the lower alcohols, hexane and C$_6$H$_6$. The hemisuccinate, m.p. 200–220°C for a potassium salt which is H$_2$O-soluble. Thiostrepton is highly active *in vitro* against gram-positive bacteria but not so active against gram-negative organisms although in veterinary medicine it has been used in the treatment of mastitis caused by a gram-negative bacterium. It is stable in the presence of urine and gastric acid and intestinal juices.

Papano *et al.*, *Antibiotics Annual*, 554 (1955–56)
Vandeputte, Dutcher, *ibid.*, 560 (1955–56)
Donovick *et al.*, *U.S. Patent*, 2,982,689 (1961)
Platt, *U.S. Patent*, 2,982,698 (1961)
Structure
Drey *et al.*, *J. Amer. Chem. Soc.*, **83**, 3906 (1961)
Bodansky *et al.*, *ibid.*, **84**, 2003 (1962)
Cross *et al.*, *J. Chem. Soc.*, 2143 (1963)
Bodansky *et al.*, *J. Amer. Chem. Soc.*, **86**, 2478 (1964)
Identity with Thiactin
Bodansky *et al.*, *J. Antibiotics* (Japan), **16A** 76 (1963)

THRAUSTOMYCIN

$C_{22}H_{28}N_6O_9$

A recently discovered antibiotic, thraustomycin is produced by culturing *Streptomyces exfoliatus* in a medium containing glucose and soybean flour at 27°C for 3–4 days. The antibiotic is extracted from the culture filtrate by adsorbing the activity on activated carbon. eluting with an organic solvent, followed by evaporation of the solvent under reduced pressure.

Thraustomycin is composed of adenine, leucine and a tetrahydroxy-monocarboxylic acid in equal amounts. It is active in inhibiting the growth of a large number of pathogenic fungi.

Kneifel et al., *J. Antibiotics* (Japan), **27**, 20 (1974)

THREOMYCIN
Streptomyces threomyceticus ATCC 15,795 produces this antibiotic when cultivated under submerged aerobic conditions at pH 7·0 and 27°C for 4 days. The crude material is purified by chromatography on silica gel, eluting with $PrOH-H_2O$ (70:30). Threomycin is a wide-spectrum antibiotic.

Katagiri, *U.S. Patent*, 3,642,985 (1972)

TICARCILLIN
$C_{15}H_{16}O_6N_2S_2$

A semi-synthetic antibiotic of the penicillin type, this compound is a wide-spectrum antibiotic which is more active against *Pseudomonas* species than carbenicillin (q.v.). Protein binding in 100 per cent human serum is 65 per cent for ticarcillin compared with 50 per cent for carbenicillin. When administered at a dose of 100–300 mg/kg/day for 3–10 days in healthy volunteers, the antibiotic resulted in defective platelet function in the blood, the effect being dose-related. There was a prolongation of bleeding time, accompanied by decreased prothrombin consumption and abnormal platelet aggregation.

Libke et al., *Clin. Pharmacol. Ther.*, **17**, 441 (1975)
Brown et al., *Antimicrobial Agents & Chemotherapy*, **7**, 652 (1975)

TIRANDAMYCIN
$C_{22}H_{27}O_7N$

An acidic antibiotic, tirandamycin is derived from *Streptomyces tirandis* var. *tirandis* NRRL 3689 cultured in an aqueous nutrient medium. The antibiotic appears to be related structurally to streptolydigin. It is normally isolated as the crystalline sodium salt. Tirandamycin is active against gram-positive bacteria including *Bacillus subtilis*, *Diplococcus pneumoniae*, *Staphylococcus aureus*, *Streptococcus fecalis* and *Strep. hemolyticus*.

Meyer, *J. Antibiotics* (Japan), **24**, 558 (1971)
Sebek, Meyer, *U.S. Patent*, 3,671,628 (1972)

TOBRAMYCIN
$C_{18}H_{37}O_9N_5$
M.p. Indefinite

A broad-spectrum antibiotic, tobramycin is produced by a number of *Streptomyces* species when grown on common nutrient media. It is more active than gentamycin (q.v.) against *Pseudomonas aeruginosa* but less so against other gram-negative bacilli. Both the nephrotoxicity and ototoxicity in guinea pigs are less than those of gentamycin but generally greater than for kanamycin (q.v.). A marked feature of this antibiotic is its high degree of activity against strains of *Pseudomonas* which are resistant to gentamycin. It has also been shown to be active *in vitro* against *Enterobacter*, *Escherichia coli*, *Klebsiella*, *Proteus mirabilis*, indole-positive *Proteus* strains and *Staphylococcus aureus*. Studies with the electron-microscope have shown that short exposures of bacteria to the antibiotic produce morphological changes in the appearance of the bacterial cell.

Smolin et al., *Amer. J. Ophthalmol.*, **76**, 555 (1973)
Burch et al., *Henry Ford Hosp. Med. J.*, **21**, 135 (1973)
Simon, *Med. Welt.*, **24**, 1852 (1973)
Periti, Serra, *G. Ital. Chemioter.*, **20**, 15 (1973)
Geddes et al., *Chemotherapy*, **20**, 245 (1974)

Jedlickova, Rye, *ibid.*, **20**, 303 (1974)
Logan *et al.*, *Arch. Otolaryngol.*, **99**, 190 (1974)
Gevaudan, Gevaudan, *Marseille Med.*, **111**, 77 (1974)
Stratford, Dixson, Cobcroft, *Lancet*, **1** (7854), 378 (1974)
Yamasaku *et al.*, *Chemotherapy* (Tokyo), **23**, 934 (1975)
Takeda *et al.*, *ibid.*, **23**, 1440 (1975)
Yamamoto *et al.*, *ibid.*, **23**, 1460 (1975)
Kuramoto *et al.*, *ibid.*, **23**, 1470 (1975)
Harada *et al.*, *ibid.*, **23**, 1494 (1975)
Akiyoski *et al.*, *ibid.*, **23**, 1522 (1975)
Yoshida *et al.*, *ibid.*, **23**, 1544 (1975)

TOLYPOMYCIN Y
$C_{43}H_{54}O_{14}N_2$
M.p. 300°C

A macrocyclic antibiotic obtained as a metabolite of *Streptomyces tolypophorus*, tolypomycin Y forms clusters of yellow needles from AcOEt which melt above 300°C. It is dextrorotatory with a specific rotation of $[\alpha]_D^{21}$ + 326° (c 1·0, EtOH) and gives an ultraviolet spectrum in EtOH with absorption maxima at 230, 290 and 337 nm. The production of this antibiotic is increased by the addition of iron salts to the culture medium.

Tolypomycin Y is assayed against *Streptococcus alcalophilus* IFO 3531 which is inhibited by this antibiotic but not by other antibiotic components simultaneously produced by this organism. The best method of assay has been shown to be the paper disc. Tolypomycin Y is active against a range of gram-positive bacteria.

Kishi *et al.*, *Tetrahedron Lett.*, **91**, 97 (1969)

Hasegawa, Higashide, Shibata, *J. Antibiotics* (Japan), **24**, 817 (1971)
Kishi *et al.*, *ibid.*, **25**, 11 (1972)
Hasegawa, *ibid.*, **25**, 25 (1972)

TOMAYMYCIN
$C_{16}H_{20}O_4N_2$
M.p. 145–146°C

An antitumour antibiotic isolated from *Streptomyces achromogenes*, this compound crystallizes from CH_3OH with one mole of solvent. It has a specific rotation of $[\alpha]_D^{20}$ + 423° (c 0·5, pyridine) and an ultraviolet spectrum in CH_3OH with absorption maxima at 224, 237, 260 and 320 nm. The antibiotic inhibits nucleic acid biosynthesis in *Bacillus subtilis* although it apparently has little effect upon protein synthesis. It apparently behaves as an inhibitor by forming a complex with DNA and this, in turn, prevents the DNA from taking part as a template in nucleic acid biosynthesis.

Kariyone, Yazawa, Kohsaka, *Chem. Pharm. Bull.*, **19**, 2289 (1971)
Arima *et al.*, *J. Antibiotics* (Japan), **25**, 437 (1972)
Nishioka *et al.*, *ibid.*, **25**, 660 (1972)

TOXOFLAVIN (*Xanthothricin*)
$C_7H_7O_2N_5$
M.p. 172–173°C (*dec.*)

Isolated from cultures of *Pseudomonas cocovenenans* and also from a *Streptomyces* species closely allied to *S. albus*, toxoflavin forms bright yellow plates when crystallized from PrOH. The ultraviolet spectrum in CH_3OH has absorption maxima at 257·5 and 394 nm. The compound is a colour indicator, becoming colourless at pH 10·5 but with complete loss of activity. It is soluble in H_2O, AcOEt, $CHCl_3$ and EtOH. Toxoflavin in active *in vitro* against a number of bacteria including *Bacillus subtilis*, *Eberthella typhosa*, *Escherichia coli*, *Mycobacterium tuberculosis*, *Proteus vulgaris* and

Staphylococcus aureus. It is highly toxic, the LD_{50} in mice being 8·4 mg/kg given orally and only 1·7 mg/kg administered intravenously.

Mertens, Van Veen, *Rec. trav. chim.*, **53**, 257 (1934)
Machlowicz et al., *Antibiotics & Chemotherapy*, **4**, 259 (1954)
Van Damm et al., *Rec. trav. chim.*, **79**, 255 (1960)
Synthesis
Daves et al., *J. Amer. Chem. Soc.*, **83**, 3904 (1961)
Daves et al., *ibid.*, **84**, 1724 (1962)

TOYOCAMYCIN
$C_{12}H_{13}O_4N_5$
M.p. 243°C

Streptomyces toyocaensis produces this antibiotic which is isolated from both the culture filtrate and the mycelium by extraction with organic solvents. It forms fine colourless needles when crystallized from CH_3OH or $(CH_3)_2CO$. When crystallized from H_2O it forms the monohydrate, m.p. 239–243°C with a specific rotation of $[\alpha]_D^{16} - 45·7°$ (c 1·05, 0·1N-HCl). The ultraviolet spectrum in H_2O has absorption maxima at 230 and 277 nm. Toyocamycin is soluble in dilute acids and AcOH, moderately soluble in CH_3OH, EtOH, PrOH, BuOH, $(CH_3)_2CO$, Et_2O and H_2O, virtually insoluble in AcOEt, $CHCl_3$ and petroleum ether. It is active against a range of gram-positive bacteria.

Nishimura et al., *J. Antibiotics* (Japan), **9A**, 60 (1956)
Structure
Ohkuma, *J. Antibiotics* (Japan), **14A**, 343 (1961)
Total synthesis
Tolman, Robins, Townsend, *J. Amer. Chem. Soc.*, **91**, 2102 (1969)

TOYOMYCIN
See Chromomycin A_3

TRICHODERMIN
$C_{17}H_{24}O_4$
M.p. 46°C; B.p. 110–112°C/0·05 mm

An antibiotic related to trichothecin (q.v.), trichodermin has been obtained from cultures of *Trichoderma viride* species ND8. The antibiotic forms colourless crystals from *n*-pentane on cooling to $-70°C$. It is laevorotatory with a specific rotation of $[\alpha]_D^{20} - 11°$ (c 1·0, $CHCl_3$) and gives an ultraviolet spectrum in EtOH having a single absorption maximum at 205 nm. Trichodermin is active against a number of pathogenic fungi *in vitro* and has proved effective in the treatment of infections caused by *Candida albicans* in man. The LD_{50} in mice is 500–1000 mg/kg administered subcutaneously and >1000 mg/kg given orally.

Loevens Kemiske Fabrik Prod., *Netherlands Patent*, 302,527 (1964)
Structure
Godtfredson, Vangedal, *Proc. Chem. Soc.*, 188 (1964)
Gutzwiller et al., *Helv. Chim. Acta*, **47**, 2234 (1964)

TRICHOMYCIN

An antibiotic first isolated from *Streptomyces hachijoensis* Yamaguchi 1954, trichomycin is also produced by the natural mutants of this organism, strains 0680 and 0755 and may be separated into trichomycins A and B, the ratio of these compounds produced being dependent upon the organism used and the medium employed. The antibiotic is obtained by extraction of the mycelium with CH_3OH or $(CH_3)_2CO$, the extract concentrated under reduced pressure and the pH adjusted to 5·4 when a yellow precipitate forms. Trichomycin forms yellow crystals and is very soluble in H_2O at an alkaline reaction, soluble in EtOH, $(CH_3)_2CO$ and BuOH but insoluble in AcOEt, Et_2O and petroleum ether. The ultraviolet spectrum has absorption maxima at 235 and 335 nm. In dilute alkalies the antibiotic is stable, but it is unstable under acid conditions. When treated with concentrated mineral acids it gives a blue colour. Trichomycin has no activity against bacteria, is only weakly active against filamentous fungi but is active against yeasts including *Candida albicans*, *Treponema pallidum*, *Trichomonas vaginalis* and *Trichophyton* species. The LD_{50} in mice is

0·05 mg given intraperitoneally. It has found some use in medicine as an antifungal and trichomonacidal agent. Recent evidence has shown it to be identical with hachimycin (q.v.).

Hosoya et al., *J. Antibiotics* (Japan), **5**, 564 (1952)
Yamaguchi, *ibid.*, **7A**, 10 (1954)

TRICHORIN A
$C_{20}H_{20}N_2O_8S_2$
M.p. 234–236°C

An antibiotic isolated from the culture filtrate of an unclassified *Trichoderma* species, this substance forms colourless crystals when crystallized from $CHCl_3$-EtOH. It is active against gram-positive bacteria.

Katayama et al., *J. Antibiotics* (Japan), **30**, 430 (1977)

TRICHOSTATIN
$C_{17}H_{22}N_2O_3$

One of several antibiotics elaborated by *Streptomyces hygroscopicus*, this substance has the structure given above which has been established from chemical analysis and a study of the infrared, NMR and mass spectra. It is effective against trichophytons and a number of fungi.

Tsuji et al., *J. Antibiotics* (Japan), **29**, 1 (1976)

TRICHOTHECIN
$C_{15}H_{20}O_4$
M.p. 118°C

An antifungal antibiotic, trichothecin is produced by *Trichotherium roseum* Link. It is obtained by surface growth on a medium containing corn steep liquor, glucose, ammonium tartrate and inorganic salts with the pH adjusted to 5·0 and incubated for 12–28 days at 25°C. When purified by chromatography and crystallization from petroleum ether, it forms colourless needles which are soluble in EtOH, $(CH_3)_2CO$, C_6H_6, $CHCl_3$, H_2O, slightly soluble in petroleum ether. Trichothecin is dextrorotatory with a specific rotation of $[\alpha]_D^{18} + 44°$ (c 1·0, $CHCl_3$), the ultraviolet spectrum in hexane or $CHCl_3$ having absorption maxima at 220 and 334 nm. The antibiotic is a neutral substance, thermostable at pH 7·0 and unstable in alkalies. The presence of unsaturation in the molecule is indicated by the decolourization of cold potassium permanganate solution and its ready hydrogenation with a palladium or PtO_2 catalyst.

Trichothecin is assayed by the cylinder plate method. It completely inhibits the germination of the conidia of *Penicillium digitatum* at a concentration of 1·25 µg/ml. Freeman and Morrison have determined the following growth inhibition concentrations *in vitro*: *Aspergillus fumigatus* (80); *A. niger* (16); *Cephalosporium longisporum* (80); *Chaetomium convolutum* (16); *Cladosporium herbarum* (16); *Fusarium graminearum* (16); *Helminthosporium sacchari* (80); *Mucor erectus* (80); *Neurospora crassa* (3·2); *Paecilomyces varioti* (80); *Penicillium citrinum* (80); *P. digitatum* (0·04); *P. expansum* (80); *P. lilacinum* (80); *P. meleagrinus* (16); *P. notatum* (>80); *P. roqueforti* (80); *P. spinulosum* (16); *Saccharomyces carlsbergensis* (16); *Stachybotrys atra* (>80); *Syncephalastrum racemosum* (80); *Thamnidium elegans* (16); *Trichoderma viride* (>80) and *Trichothecium roseum* (>80). The antibiotic has no activity against bacteria.

Brian, Hemming, *J. Gen. Microbiol.*, **1**, 158 (1947)
Freeman, Morrison, *Nature*, **162**, 30 (1948)
Freeman, Morrison, *J. Gen. Microbiol.*, **3**, 60 (1948)
Freeman, Morrison, *Biochem. J.*, **44**, 1 (1949)
Maksimova, Sagdieva, *Antibiotiki*, **16**, 274 (1971)
Sorenson, Sneller, Larsh, *Appl. Microbiol.*, **29**, 653 (1975)

TRICHOVIRIDIN
$C_8H_9O_4N$
M.p. 95–96°C (*dec.*)

A simple antibiotic isolated from cultures of *Trichoderma viride*, trichoviridin forms colourless crystals from $CHCl_3$ and is laevorotatory with a specific rotation of $[\alpha]_D^{24} - 41.2°$ (c 0·5, CH_3OH). It has an inhibitory activity against certain yeasts.

Tamano et al., *Japanese Patent*, 7,015,435 (1970)

TRIEN
M.p. Indefinite
This polyene antibiotic has recently been obtained from cultures of an actinomycete strain 141-18 of the brown group. Hydrolysis furnishes alanine. Trien is active against yeasts and mycelial fungi at a concentration of 0·5–10 µg/ml.

Poltorak et al., *Antibiotiki*, **17**, 738 (1972)

TRIENINE
M.p. Indefinite
An antitumour antibiotic, trienine has been isolated from the fermentation broth of Streptomyces SC3725. Trienine has a molecular weight of approximately 1400 and contains three conjugated double bonds in the molecule. It is active against gram-positive bacteria, some yeasts and fungi and has a minimum inhibition concentration against *Staphylococcus aureus* of 0·37–0·44 µg/ml. It has also been found to inhibit the growth of 5 WM tumour.

Aszalos et al., *J. Antibiotics* (Japan), **21**, 611 (1968)

N-TRIFLUOROACETYLADRIAMYCIN-14-VALERATE
$C_{34}H_{36}O_{13}NF_3$

A semi-synthetic antibiotic, this derivative of adriamycin (q.v.) has been shown to possess a greater antitumour activity than adriamycin or daunorubicin hydrochlorides. It has a reduced toxicity compared with these antibiotics, the normal dose being significantly greater than the lethal dose of adriamycin in mice. It is less effective, however, than adriamycin in inhibiting the growth of human lymphoblastic leukemic cells *in vitro*.

Israel, Modest, Frei, *Cancer Res.*, **35**, 1365 (1975)

3′-5,7-TRIHYDROXY-4′,6-DIMETHOXYISOFLAVONE
$C_{17}H_{14}O_7$

One of two isomeric isoflavone antibiotics isolated from cultures of an unclassified *Streptomyces* species, this compound has the above structure based upon chemical correlations and spectroscopic evidence. It is active against a number of gram-positive bacteria and inhibits catechol-O-methyltransferase and dopa decarboxylase. It also exerts a hypotensive action.

Chimura et al., *J. Antibiotics* (Japan), **28**, 619 (1975)

3′,5,7-TRIHYDOXY-4′,8-DIMETHOXYISOFLAVONE
$C_{17}H_{14}O_7$

An isomer of the preceding compound, this antibiotic also occurs in the cultures of the same unclassified species of *Streptomyces*. It has a very similar antibiotic spectrum and also shows an inhibitory action against catechol-O-methyltransferase and dopa decarboxylase.

Chimura et al., *J. Antibiotics* (Japan), **28**, 619 (1975)

TRIOSTIN C
$C_{54}H_{70}O_{12}N_{12}S_2$
M.p. Indefinite
Streptomyces triostinicus ATCC 21,043, closely allied to *S. aureus*, elaborates a complex of three antibiotics, triostins A, B and C, of which this compound is the most extensively investigated. The complex is obtained by cultivation of the fungus in an aqueous nutrient medium at 27–29°C and pH 7·0 for 3–7 days. Both the culture filtrate and the mycelium are extracted with

organic solvents, the extracts dried with anhydrous sodium sulphate and evaporated under reduced pressure. The components may be separated by chromatography on a silica gel column eluted with $CHCl_3$—CH_3OH. Triostin C forms colourless needles when crystallized from $CHCl_3$—CH_3OH, gradually decomposing above 260°C. It is laevorotatory with a specific rotation of $[\alpha]_D^{24} - 143\cdot9°$ (c 1·2, $CHCl_3$) and gives an ultraviolet spectrum in CH_3OH with absorption maxima at 243 and 315–326 nm. It is active against a number of gram-positive and gram-negative bacteria, including some mycobacteria.

Shoji, Katagiri, *J. Antibiotics* (Japan), **14A**, 335 (1961)
Structure
Otsuka, Shoji, *Tetrahedron*, **21**, 2931 (1965)
Production
Katagiri, *U.S. Patent*, 3,647,631 (1972)

TRYPANOMYCIN
M.p. Indefinite
This anthracycline antibiotic is elaborated by *Streptomyces diastatochromogenes*. It forms reddish crystals and has indicator properties. When tested *in vitro* and *in vivo* it exhibits a marked trypanocidal activity.

Strauss *et al.*, *Advan. Antimicrob. Antineoplast. Chemother., Proc. Int. Congr. Chemother. 7th*, **1**, 413 (1971)

TRYPTANTHRIN
$C_{15}H_8O_2N_2$
M.p. 266–267°C

This antibiotic is produced by *Candida lipolytica* grown in the presence of L-tryptophan. It forms yellow crystals and has the structure given above which is based upon chemical and spectroscopic evidence.

Brufani *et al.*, *Experientia*, **27**, 1249 (1971)

TSUSHUMYCIN
$C_{59}H_{93}O_{20}N_{13}$
M.p. 230–240°C (*dec.*)
A strain of *Streptomyces* Z-237 elaborates this antibiotic which is obtained as an amorphous powder. It is dextrorotatory with a specific rotation of $[\alpha]_D^{23} + 11\cdot9°$ (c 0·99, CH_3OH). It is active against gram-positive bacteria.

Shoji *et al.*, *J. Antibiotics* (Japan), **21**, 439 (1968)
Shoji, Otsuka, *ibid.*, **22**, 473 (1969)

TUBERACTIN
See Tuberactinomycin A

TUBERACTINOMYCIN A (*Tuberactin*)
$C_{25}H_{43}O_{11}N_{13}$

One of a number of structurally similar antibiotics isolated from cultures of *Streptomyces griseoverticillatus* var. *tuberacticus*. This particular compound has been isolated as the hydrochloride which forms colourless crystals with m.p. 244–264°C (*dec.*); $[\alpha]_D^{25} - 31\cdot5°$ (c 1·0, H_2O). The salt gives an ultraviolet spectrum in H_2O with a single absorption maximum at 268 nm. The antibiotic has antifungal and antituberculous properties.

Nagata *et al.*, *J. Antibiotics* (Japan), **21**, 681 (1968)
Wakamiya *et al.*, *Tetrahedron Lett.*, 3497 (1970)
Yoshioka *et al.*, *ibid.*, 2043 (1971)

TUBERACTINOMYCIN B
See Viomycin

TUBERACTINOMYCIN N
$C_{25}H_{43}O_{10}N_{13}$

A further antibiotic produced by *Streptomyces griseoverticillatus* var. *tuberacticus*. The structure has been established from chemical and spectroscopic evidence and comparison with the other antibiotics isolated from the same source. It has a similar antibiotic activity to the other tuberactinomycins.

Yoshioka *et al.*, *Tetrahedron Lett.*, 2043 (1971)

TUBERACTINOMYCIN O
$C_{25}H_{43}O_9N_{13}$

Also present in the culture of *Streptomyces griseoverticillatus* var. *tuberacticus*, the structure of this polypeptide compound differs only slightly from those of the preceding antibiotics.

Yoshioka *et al.*, *Tetrahedron Lett.*, 2043 (1971)

TUBERCIDIN
$C_{11}H_{14}O_4N_4$
M.p. 247–248°C

Streptomyces tubericidus yields this antibiotic which is extracted from the culture filtrate with organic solvents followed by evaporation under reduced pressure and purification by chromatography. The antibiotic forms colourless needles from H_2O and is laevorotatory with a specific rotation of $[\alpha]_D^{17} - 67°$ (c 1·0, 50 per cent AcOH). The ultraviolet spectrum in $0·01N$-NaOH has an absorption maximum at 270 nm. Tubercidin is soluble in dilute acids and alkalies but insoluble in most organic solvents. It is active against gram-positive and mycobacteria and a number of pathogenic fungi and also possesses antineoplastic properties. The LD_{50} in mice is 45 mg/kg administered intravenously.

Anzai *et al.*, *J. Antibiotics* (Japan), **10A**, 201 (1957)
Structure
Suzuki, Marumo, *J. Antibiotics* (Japan), **14A**, 34 (1961)
Production
Shirato, Miyazaki, Suzuki, *Hakko Kogaku Zasshi*, **45**, 60 (1967)

TUMIMYCIN

An antifungal antibiotic, tumimycin is produced by aerobic cultivation of *Streptomyces* strain ATCC 21,501 in a neutral medium containing soybean, soybean flour and corn steep liquor at 25°C for 6 days followed by filtration extraction with C_6H_6 and chromatography on silica gel. The antibiotic is active against bacteria and fungi with minimum inhibition concentrations against *Candida albicans* and *Streptococcus aureus* of 1·2 and 0·6 µg/ml respectively. The LD_{50} in mice has been given as 40 mg/kg administered intravenously.

Aszalos *et al.*, *German Patent*, 2,139,261 (1972)

TUNICAMYCIN
M.p. 234–235°C (dec.)

Streptomyces lysosuperficus produces this antibiotic when grown under aerobic conditions on a medium containing glucose, yeast extract, gluten meal and inorganic salts at 27°C and pH 6·8 for 4 days. The compound is extracted from the culture broth by adsorption on activated carbon, eluted with $CHCl_3$ and purified by chromatography on a silica gel column. Extraction of the cells with pyridine, CH_3OH or $(CH_3)_2CO$ also yields the antibiotic. Tunicamycin is a white microcrystalline powder and is dextrorotatory with a specific rotation of $[\alpha]_D^{25} + 52°$ (c 0·5, pyridine) and gives an ultraviolet spectrum in CH_3OH with absorption maxima at 205 and 260 nm. It has a molecular weight of approximately 870. The antibiotic is stable towards alkalies but is readily hydrolysed by acids, particularly HCl. The antiviral activity of the compound is completely inhibited by potassium periodate.

Tunicamycin is active against gram-positive bacteria, yeasts and fungi, especially *Bacillus* species and *Piricularia oryzae*. It suppresses the occurrence of lesions on tobacco mosaic virus-infected leaf discs, inhibits the multiplication of the virus *in vivo* in the leaves of *Nicotiana tabacum*, and inhibits herpes simplex virus and Newcastle disease virus in cultured cells.

Takasuki *et al.*, *J. Antibiotics* (Japan), **24**, 215 (1971)
Arima, Tamura, Takasuki, *Japanese Patent*, 7,329,156 (1973)

TUOROMYCIN
See α-Rubromycin

TYROCIDIN
Dubos first described an antibiotic substance derived from *Bacillus brevis* in 1939, naming it tyrothricin. This was later shown to be composed of two dissimilar groups of antibiotics, the gramicidins (q.v.) and the tyrocidins. Most of the bacteriological examination has been carried out on the mixture of tyrocidins which is assayed by a number of methods including hemolysis of rat red blood cells, suppression of acid production by *Streptococcus lactis*, turbidimetric with *Micrococcus conglomeratus* and serial dilution with *Streptococcus fecalis* and *S. hemolyticus*.

Inhibition concentrations (μg/ml) have been determined by a number of workers *in vitro*: *Eberthella typhi* (500); *Escherichia coli* (500); *Neisseria gonorrheae* (0·01); *Pasteurella tularensis* (100); *Past. tularensis avir.* (25); *Salmonella schottmuelleri* (250); *Shigella dysenteriae* (50); *Staphylococcus aureus* (50); *Streptococcus fecalis* (5·0); hemolytic streptococci (1·0); meningococci (1·0) and pneumococci (1·0).

Similar inhibition dilutions ($\times 1000$) have been measured by Stokes *et al.*; *Achorion schoenleinii* (20); *Eberthella typhi* (1·2); *Escherichia coli* (1·2); *Microsporon gypseum* (10); *Neisseria catarrhalis* (1·6); *Salmonella paratyphi* (1·2); *Staphylococcus aureus* (40); *Streptococcus hemolyticus* (1000) and *Trichophyton gypseum* (10).

Clinically, tyrocidin is used as a topical agent in infections due to pneumococcus, staphylococcus and streptococcus in skin and eye infections and ulcers. Resistant strains occur, however, following therapy with this antibiotic.

The LD_{50} in mice and rats is 15 mg/kg (intravenous), 40–60 mg/kg (intraperitoneal) and 1000 mg/kg (oral).

Dubos, *J. Exper. Med.*, **70**, 1 (1939)
Dubos, *Proc. Soc. Exptl. Biol. Med.*, **40**, 311 (1939)
Dubos, *J. Pediat.*, **19**, 588 (1941)
Hotchkiss, Dubos, *J. Biol. Chem.*, **141**, 155 (1941)
Goldstein, *Chem. Abstr.*, **43**, 3884 (1949)
Battersby, Craig, *J. Amer. Chem. Soc.*, **74**, 4019, 4023 (1952)

TYROCIDIN A
$C_{66}H_{87}O_{13}N_{13}$
M.p. Indefinite

```
    L-Val────L-Orn
   /              \
  L-Tyr          L-Leu
   |              |
  L-Glu·NH_2     D-Phe
   |              |
  L-Asp·NH_2     L-Pro
   \              /
    D-Phe────L-Phe
```

One of the components of tyrocidin, this cyclic polypeptide forms a cyrstalline hydrochloride, m.p. 240–242°C and $[\alpha]_D^{25} - 111°$ (c 1·37, EtOH). The salt is readily soluble in aqueous CH_3OH or EtOH, slightly soluble in CH_3OH, EtOH, insoluble in $CHCl_3$, $(CH_3)_2CO$ and Et_2O.

Battersby, Craig, *J. Amer. Chem. Soc.*, **74**, 4019, 4023 (1952)
Structure
Paladini, Craig, *J. Amer. Chem. Soc.*, **76**, 688 (1954)
Ohno *et al.*, *Bull. Chem. Soc., Japan*, **39**, 1738 (1966)

TYROCIDIN B
$C_{68}H_{88}O_{13}N_{14}$
M.p. Indefinite

Tyrocidin C

```
        L-Val────L-Orn
       /              \
    L-Tyr            L-Leu
      |                |
   L-Glu·NH₂         D-Phe
      |                |
   L-Asp·NH₂         L-Pro
       \              /
        D-Phe────L-Try
```

A further constituent of tyrocidin, this antibiotic also has a decapeptide structure, that given above being based upon a study of the hydrolysis products.

King, Craig, *J. Amer. Chem. Soc.*, **77**, 6624, 6627 (1955)

TYROCIDIN C
$C_{70}H_{88}O_{13}N_{15}$
M.p. Indefinite

```
        L-Val────L-Orn
       /              \
    L-Tyr            L-Leu
      |                |
   L-Glu·NH₂         D-Phe
      |                |
   L-Asp·NH₂         L-Pro
       \              /
        D-Try────L-Try
```

A third cyclic polypeptide isolated from the tyrocidin complex, the structure of this antibiotic is the same as that of the preceding compound but with the D-phenylalanine moiety being replaced by D-tryptophan.

Ruttenberg *et al.*, *Biochemistry*, **4**, 11 (1965)

TYROTHRICIN
See Tyrocidin

UMBRINOMYCIN
M.p. Indefinite

Streptomyces umbrinus elaborates diumycin and this antibiotic when cultured in an aqueous medium containing glucose, dehydrated potato and soybean flour, together with inorganic salts at 25°C under submerged aerobic conditions. The broth is then adjusted to pH 3·0, filtered, and the mycelium extracted with CH_3OH, concentrated *in vacuo* to leave an aqueous suspension and then re-extracted with an organic solvent and chromatographed to separate the two antibiotics. Umbrinomycin is composed of at least two active components and is active against gram-positive bacteria.

Meyers *et al.*, *S. African Patent*, 6,707,652 (1968)

UNDECYLPRODIGININE
$C_{25}H_{35}N_3O$

An unclassified species of *Streptomyces* elaborates this pigment which has the structure shown above based upon chemical analysis and spectroscopic evidence. It possesses antimalarial activity.

Gerber., *J. Antibiotics* (Japan), **28**, 194 (1975)

URFAMYCIN
See Thiamphenicol

USNIC ACID
$C_{18}H_{16}O_7$
M.p. 204°C

Usnic acid is derived from several species of lichens, e.g. *Cetraria islandica*, *Cladonia alpestris*, *C. cristatella*, *C. leptoclada*, *C. sylvatica*, *Ramalina reticulata* and *Usnea barbata*. The antibiotic substance is obtained by fermentation of the fungal symbiont on a synthetic medium or by extracting the lichens with boiling $(CH_3)_2CO$, concentrating the extract until crystallization occurs. When purified it forms yellow needles or rhombic crystals which sublime at 205°C/5 mm. It is readily soluble in sodium hydroxide and sodium carbonate solutions, slightly soluble in CH_3OH, EtOH, isoPrOH and petroleum ether, insoluble in H_2O. The D-form has a specific rotation of $[\alpha]_D^{20}$ + 495° ($CHCl_3$) and the L-form of −452° ($CHCl_3$). The ultraviolet spectrum in $CHCl_3$ has absorption maxima at 226–230 and 284 nm.

Usnic acid is assayed by cylinder plate with *Bacillus subtilis* as the test organism. Stoll, Brack and Renz have determined the following inhibition dilutions (× 10,000) *in vitro*: *Eberthella typhi* (>0·25); *Escherichia coli* (>0·25); *Mycobacterium phlei* (20); *Myco. smegmatis* (20–25); *Myco. tuberculosis bovis* (64); *Myco. tuberculosis hominis* (8·0–100); *Myco. tuberculosis avium* (32); *Penicillium notatum* (>0·25); *Staphylococcus aureus* (10–25) and *Streptococcus pyogenes* (12·5–16).

When examined *in vivo* in guinea pigs experimentally infected with tuberculosis infections, a dose of 15 mg/kg per day of the sodium salt, given orally, results in some improvement, but experiments in humans have proved inconclusive. The antibiotic is relatively toxic, 1·5–2·0 mg proving lethal to mice when administered subcutaneously.

Curd, Robertson, *J. Chem. Soc.*, 894 (1937)
Schopf, Ross, *Ann. Chem.*, **546**, 1 (1941)
Burkholder, Evans, *Bull. Torrey Bot. Club.*, **72**, 157 (1945)
Marshak, *Publ. Health Rep.*, **62**, 3 (1947)
Stoll, Renz, Brack, *Experientia*, **3**, 111, 115 (1947)
Marshak, Barry, Craig, *Science*, **106**, 394 (1947)
Castle, Kubsch, *Arch. Biochem.*, **23**, 158 (1949)
Kupchan, Kopperman, *Experientia*, **31**, 625 (1975)

USTIN
$C_{19}H_{15}O_5Cl_3$
M.p. 184–186°C

Aspergillus ustus elaborates an antibiotic substance which has been separated into at least three components either by countercurrent distribution or by fractionating according to solubility in neutral, sodium bicarbonate or sodium carbonate solution. The major fraction, soluble in sodium carbonate, is normally designated as ustin and has the melting point given above. It has an ultraviolet spectrum with a single absorption maximum at 325 nm. It is insoluble in H_2O, dilute acids and cyclohexane, soluble in sodium carbonate, sodium hydroxide, EtOH, Et_2O, C_6H_6 and $(CH_3)_2CO$.

Ustin is assayed by serial dilution with *Mycobacterium tuberculosis* as the test organism. It is active against staphylococci and streptococci but not against gram-negative bacteria and *Escherichia coli*. At a dilution of 1:150,000–500,000 it inhibits both *Mycobacterium ranae* and *Myco. tuberculosis*. It is only moderately toxic, 6–8 mg of the crude preparation being tolerated by mice when administered intraperitoneally.

Kurung, *Science*, **102**, 11 (1945)
Hogeboom, Craig, *J. Biol. Chem.*, **162**, 363 (1946)
Doering *et al.*, *J. Amer. Chem. Soc.*, **68**, 725 (1946)

VALIDAMYCIN A
$C_{20}H_{35}O_{13}N$
M.p. *ca.* 135°C (*dec.*)

Streptomyces hygroscopicus produces a number of closely related antibiotics. This compound is also formed by chemical or enzymatic hydrolysis of validamycins C, E or F, by incorporating the latter antibiotics in a nutrient medium and fermenting with *Endomyces decipens* IFO 0102 at 28°C for 6 days. Validamycin A is an amorphous white powder which decomposes at the melting point. It has a specific rotation of $[\alpha]_D^{24} + 110°$ (c 1.0, H_2O). The hydrochloride has m.p. 95°C (*dec.*) and the acetate, also crystalline, m.p. 100°C (*dec.*). Two of the hydrolysis products have been fully characterized: validatol with m.p. 119–121°C; $[\alpha]_D - 39°$ (c 1.0, H_2O), shown to be 1-hydroxyethylcyclohexane-2:3:4-triol and validamine (1-amino-5-hydroxymethylcyclohexane-2:3:4-triol), characterized as the hydrochloride with m.p. 229–232°C (*dec.*); $[\alpha]_D + 57.4°$ (c 1.0, 1.0 *N*-HCl). The antibiotic is a pesticide, particularly active against *Pellicularia sasakii*.

    Horii, Iwasa, Kameda, *J. Antibiotics* (Japan), **24**, 57 (1971)
    Horii *et al.*, *ibid.*, **24**, 59 (1971)
    Iwasa *et al.*, *ibid.*, **24**, 107, 119 (1971)
    Horii, Kameda, Kawahara, *ibid.*, **25**, 48 (1972)
    Horii, Kameda, *Japanese Patent*, 7,334,103 (1973)
Structure
    Horii, Kameda, *J. Chem. Soc., Chem. Commun.*, 747 (1972)

VALIDAMYCIN B
$C_{20}H_{35}O_{14}N$
M.p. Indefinite

A second antibiotic produced by *Streptomyces hygroscopicus*, validamycin B is also an amorphous powder having no definite melting point. It is dextrorotatory with a specific rotation of $[\alpha]_D^{24} + 102°$ (c 1.0, H_2O) and yields a crystalline acetate, m.p. 155°C (*dec.*).

    Iwasa *et al.*, *J. Antibiotics* (Japan), **24**, 107 (1971)
    Iwasa *et al.*, *ibid.*, **24**, 119 (1971)
    Horii, Kameda, Kawahara, *ibid.*, **25**, 48 (1972)

VALIDAMYCIN C
$C_{26}H_{45}O_{18}N$
M.p. Indefinite

Also elaborated by *Streptomyces hygroscopicus*, this antibiotic is an amorphous white powder which is dextrorotatory having a specific rotation of $[\alpha]_D$ + 132·9° (c 1·0, H_2O).

Horii, Kameda, Kawahara, *ibid.*, **25**, 48 (1972)

VALIDAMYCIN D
$C_{20}H_{35}O_{13}N$
M.p. Indefinite

A further amorphous antibiotic produced by *Streptomyces hygroscopicus*, validamycin D has a specific rotation of $[\alpha]_D$ + 169·3° (c 1·0, H_2O).

Horii, Kameda, Kawahara, *J. Antibiotics* (Japan), **25**, 48 (1972)

VALIDAMYCIN E
$C_{26}H_{45}O_{18}N$
M.p. Indefinite

This antibiotic from *Streptomyces hygroscopicus* is an isomer of validamycin C (q.v.). It has a specific rotation of $[\alpha]_D$ + 148·2° (c 1·0, H_2O).

Horii, Kameda, Kawahara, *J. Antibiotics* (Japan), **25**, 48 (1972)

VALIDAMYCIN F
$C_{26}H_{45}O_{18}N$
M.p. Indefinite

A further isomer of validamycin C, this antibiotic from *Streptomyces hygroscopicus* has a specific rotation of $[\alpha]_D$ + 130·7° (c 1·0, H_2O). It also possesses some activity against *Pellicularia sasakii*.

Horii, Kameda, Kawahara, *J. Antibiotics* (Japan), **25**, 48 (1972)

VALIDOXYLAMINE A
$C_{14}H_{25}O_8N$
M.p. Indefinite

Streptomyces hygroscopicus var. *limoneus* elaborates two closely related antibiotics. This particular substance, separated from the accompanying antibiotics by chromatography, has a specific rotation of $[\alpha]_D$ + 170° (c 1·0, H_2O).

Horii, Kameda, Kawahara, *J. Antibiotics* (Japan), **25**, 48 (1972)

VALIDOXYLAMINE B
$C_{14}H_{25}O_9N$
M.p. Indefinite

An antibiotic from *Streptomyces hygroscopicus* var. *limoneus*, validoxylamine B is also dextrorotatory with a specific rotation of $[\alpha]_D$ + 130·7° (c 1·0, H_2O).

Horii, Kameda, Kawahara, *J. Antibiotics* (Japan), **25**, 48 (1972)

VALINOMYCIN
$C_{54}H_{90}O_{18}N_6$
M.p. 187°C

```
D-Val—L-Lac—L-Val—D-Hyv—D-Val—L-Lac
  ↑                                ↓
D-Hyv—L-Val—L-Lac—D-Val—D-Hyv—L-Val
```

A macrocyclic polypeptide antibiotic, valinomycin forms colourless crystals when purified by extraction from the culture filtrate of a number of *Streptomyces* species and recrystallized from di-*iso*butyl ether. It is dextrorotatory with a specific rotation of $[\alpha]_D$ + 32·8° (c 1·25, C_6H_6). Valinomycin has a marked effect upon the mitachondria of yeasts, increasing the rate of respiration and potassium ion absorption in both *Endomyces magnusii* (resistant to the antibiotic) and *Saccharomyces carlsbergensis* (sensitive to valinomycin). It has also been shown to stimulate lysine uptake by *Staphylococcus aureus* but does not affect the uptake of glutamate and has only a transient effect with glycine and isoleucine. When applied topically or subconjunctivally, the antibiotic decreased intraocular pressure in normal rabbit or monkey eyes, this effect lasting for more than 3 weeks. In rabbit eyes it also causes severe corneal edema and there is an increase in protein in the aqueous humor 1 day after treatment although these effects tend to disappear after 3 to 7 days.

Brockmann, Schmidt-Kastner, *Chem. Ber.*, **88**, 57 (1955)
Brockmann, Geeren, *Annalen*, **603**, 217 (1957)
Shemyakin *et al.*, *Tetrahedron Lett.*, 1921 (1963)
Brockmann *et al.*, *Naturwiss.*, **50**, 689 (1963)
McDonald, *Antibiotics*, **2**, 268 (1967)
Murav'eva *et al.*, *Mitokhondrii, Biokhim. Ultrastrukt. Mater. Vses. Simp. Biokhim. Mitokhondrii 7th*, 80 (1971)
Niven, Hamilton, *Fed. Eur. Biochem. Soc.., Lett.*, **37**, 244 (1973)
Lee, Lam, *Ann. Ophthalmol.*, **5**, 33 (1973)
Murav'eva *et al.*, *Biokhimiya*, **38**, 845 (1973)
Haynes *et al.*, *Mol. Pharmacol.*, **10**, 381 (1974)
Sweeney, *Plant. Physiol.*, **53**, 337 (1974)

VANCOCIN
See Vancomycin

VANCOMYCIN (*Vancocin*)

This antibiotic substance has been isolated from a strain of *Streptomyces orientalis* growing in Indian and Indonesian soil. Analysis indicates a molecular weight of about 3300 and a nitrogen content of approximately 7 per cent with 16–17 per cent carbohydrate. It has been obtained as the hydrochloride, a white amorphous solid with no definite melting point and giving an ultraviolet spectrum in H_2O with a single absorption maximum at 282 nm. This salt is freely soluble in H_2O, moderately so in dilute CH_3OH but insoluble in $(CH_3)_2CO$, Et_2O and the higher alcohols. It has been found that low concentrations of urea tend to increase the solubility in neutral aqueous solutions. Both sodium chloride and ammonium sulphate precipitate the antibiotic from acid solutions.

Vancomycin is used as an antimicrobial, the normal intravenous dose being 500 mg in slow infusion. Side effects include fever, rashes and loss of hearing. The LD_{50} in mice is 400 mg/kg when administered intravenously.

McCormick *et al.*, *Antibiotics Annual*, 606 (1955–56)
Nishimura, *Ann. Rept. Shionogi Res. Lab.*, **1**, 479 (1957)
Higgins *et al.*, *Antibiotics Annual*, 906 (1957–58)
Eli Lilly & Co., *British Patent*, 795,289 (1958)
Eli Lilly & Co., *U.S. Patent*, 3,067,099 (1962)
Marshall, *J. Med. Chem.*, **8**, 18 (1965)

VARIABILIN
$C_{25}H_{34}O_4$

This recently discovered antibiotic from *Ircinia variabilis* must not be confused with the alkaloid variabiline isolated from *Ocotea variabilis*. The structure of this antibiotic has been established from chemical and spectroscopic investigations.

Faulkner, *Tetrahedron Lett.*, 3821 (1973)

VARIACYCLOMYCIN A
$C_{27}H_{23}O_{11}N$
M.p. Indefinite

Actinomyces olivovariabilis produces two antibiotics which are extracted from the culture filtrate with AcOEt and separated and purified by chromatography on an alumina column. Variacyclomycin A may be characterized as the hexaacetate, m.p. 300°C; $[\alpha]_D^{20} + 48°$ which is prepared by reduction of variacyclomycin B with ascorbic acid in pyridine followed by acetylation with acetic anhydride. The antibiotic is active against a number of gram-positive bacteria.

Gromova *et al.*, *Antibiotiki*, **19**, 486 (1974)

VARIACYCLOMYCIN B
$C_{27}H_{21}O_{11}N$
M.p. Indefinite

A second antibiotic isolated from cultures of *Actinomyces olivovariabilis*, this compound may also be prepared by oxidation of the preceding antibiotic with potassium ferricyanide. Exhaustive reduction with zinc powder yields anthracene. Variacyclomycin B is characterized as the tetraacetate, m.p. 280°C, forming a dimethoxy derivative with m.p. 175°C, and the tetramethoxy compound, m.p. 180°C. Like the accompanying antibiotic, variacyclomycin B is active against a range of gram-positive bacteria.

Gromova *et al.*, *Antibiotiki*, **19**, 486 (1974)

VARIAMYCIN
$C_{52}H_{76}O_{24}$
M.p. Indefinite

Cultures of *Actinomyces olivovariabilis* species nova, when grown aerobically in a nutrient medium containing sources of carbon and nitrogen and inorganic salts, yield this glycosidic antibiotic. The structure has been established from chemical and spectroscopic evidence.

Zhdanovich *et al.*, *Soviet Patent*, 309,601 (1972)
Zhdanovich *et al.*, *British Patent*, 1,314,983 (1973)

VARIOTIN (Pecilocin)
$C_{17}H_{25}O_3N$
M.p. 41·5–42·5°C

This antibiotic has been isolated from cultures of *Paecilomyces variotus* var. *antibioticus*. It forms hygroscopic white needles of the hydrate when crystallized from Et_2O-light petroleum and gives an ultraviolet spectrum consisting of a single absorption maximum at 320 nm. Dehydration of the hydrate furnishes a yellow oil. Variotin is active against a range of fungi. Pecilocin is the name which has been approved by the General Medical Council for this antibiotic.

Takeuchi, Yonehara, *J. Antibiotics* (Japan), **14A**, 44 (1961)
Takeuchi, Yonehara, *ibid.*, **17A**, 267 (1964)
Takeuchi, Yonehara, *Tetrahedron Lett.*, 5197 (1966)

VEBECILLIN
See Penicillin V

VENTURICIDIN
$C_{43}H_{71}O_{12}N$
M.p. Indefinite

A complex antibiotic isolated from *Streptomyces* species, particularly *S. Griseolus* and *S. xanthophaeus*, venturicidin crystallizes from CH_3OH–H_2O or AcOEt-petroleum ether as colourless needles. It is dextrorotatory with a specific rotation of $[\alpha]_D + 114°$ (c 1·0, $CHCl_3$). The antibiotic is soluble in BuOH, $CHCl_3$ and AcOEt. It has a weak activity against bacteria but is markedly active against a range of pathogenic fungi.

Rhodes *et al.*, *Nature*, **192**, 952 (1961)

VENTURICIDIN A
$C_{41}H_{67}O_{11}N$
M.p. 141–142°C

Venturicidin is produced, together with the following antibiotic, from cultures of *Streptomyces aureofaciens* Duggar. It has also been isolated from

Venturicidin B

Streptomyces hygroscopicus A-130 grown on a medium of glucose and soybean flour, being obtained by extraction of the cells with $(CH_3)_2CO$ and chromatography on a silica gel column. Venturicidin A forms small, colourless needles from $CHCl_3$—Et_2O and is dextrorotatory with a specific rotation of $[\alpha]_D + 119°$ (c 0·5, $CHCl_3$). The ultraviolet spectrum in light petroleum shows an absorption maximum at 206 nm and shoulders at 247 and 300 nm. Two secondary and one tertiary hydroxyl groups are present and the compound forms a crystalline diacetate, m.p. 169–171°C. The antibiotic is active against plant pathogenic fungi.

Brufani et al., *Helv. Chim. Acta*, **51**, 1293 (1968)
Tsuji, Wakisaka, *Japanese Patent*, 7,322,689 (1973)
Structure
Brufani et al., *Experientia*, **27**, 604 (1971)
Brufani et al., *Helv. Chim. Acta*, **55**, 2329 (1972)

VENTURICIDIN B
$C_{40}H_{66}O_{10}$
M.p. 145–149°C

Venturicidin B is structurally related to the preceding antibiotic and is also produced by *Streptomyces aureofaciens* Duggar. The specific rotation is $[\alpha]_D + 100°$ (c 0·847, $CHCl_3$). Three secondary hydroxyl groups are present and the antibiotic forms a triacetate as colourless needles with m.p. 150–152°C. It is active against fungi but not against yeasts and therefore finds some use in viticulture. Its use has also been suggested as a food preservative and disinfectant.

Brufani et al., *Helv. Chim. Acta*, **51**, 1293 (1968)
Zaehner, Keller, *U.S. Patent*, 3,636,198 (1972)
Structure
Brufani et al., *Experientia*, **27**, 604 (1971)
Brufani et al., *Helv. Chim. Acta*, **55**, 2329 (1972)

VENTURICIDIN X
$C_{39}H_{64}O_{11}$

This antibiotic, unlike the two preceding compounds, is not a glycoside. It is produced by cultivating *Streptomyces aureofaciens* Tu 342 (NRRL 3399) in an aqueous nutrient medium under aerobic conditions at 33–37°C and separating from the accompanying venturicidin B by solvent extraction and Craig distribution. Catalytic reduction furnishes the tetrahydro derivative. It also finds some use in viticulture being effective against fungi but not against yeasts.

Zaehner, Keller, *U.S. Patent*, 3,636,198 (1972)

VERDAMICIN I
$C_{20}H_{39}N_5O_6$

Produced by *Micromonospora grisea*, this aminoglycoside antibiotic is present in the culture medium together with antibiotic G-418, gentamicin A and sisomicin. The antibiotic is formed by using an inoculum of a pre-culture of the organism in a medium containing dextrin, soybean meal, dextrose and $CaCO_3$ and incubating at 30°C with stirring and aeration for approximately

90 hours. The broth is filtered and the antibiotic isolated by chromatography on an ion-exchange resin and finally purified by silica gel column chromatography.

Weinstein, Wagman, Marquez, U.S. Patent, 3,988,316 (1976)

VERMICULINE
$C_{21}H_{28}O_7$
M.p. 175–177°C (dec.)

An antibiotic elaborated by *Penicillium vermiculatum* Dangeard, vermiculine forms colourless crystals from AcOEt. It is laevorotatory having a specific rotation of $[\alpha]_D^{20} - 12.5°$ (c 1.0, $CHCl_3$). The original formula of $C_{10}H_{12}O_4$ and structure 6-acetyl-5-oxacyclonon-2-ene-1:4-dione has been shown to be incorrect. The compound is unusually stable towards acids and shows a resistance to isomerization of the endocyclic double bone. Single cyrstal X-ray diffraction has revealed that the structure is the dilactone shown above. Vermiculine is active against gram-positive and gram-negative bacteria.

Fuska, Menec, Kuhr, *J. Antibiotics* (Japan), **25**, 208 (1972)
Structure
Sedmera *et al.*, *Tetrahedron Lett.*, 1347 (1973)
Revised structure
Boeckman, Fayos, Clardy, *J. Amer. Chem. Soc.*, **96**, 5954 (1974)

VERNAMYCIN A
M.p. 193–195°C (dec.)
Streptomyces loidensis ATCC 11,415 elaborates this macrocyclic antibiotic which is not a peptide compound. It has a specific rotation of $[\alpha]_D^{25} - 206°$ (c 1.0, CH_3OH) and gives an ultraviolet spectrum in CH_3OH with absorption maxima at 210–230 and 270 nm. It is readily soluble in CH_3OH, EtOH, glacial AcOH and dimethylformamide, slightly so in Et_2O, AcOEt, $(CH_3)_2CO$, C_6H_6, BuOH and *iso*PrOH and insoluble in H_2O and hexane. It has found some use in medicine as an antimicrobial.

Donovick *et al.*, *U.S. Patent*, 2,990,325 (1961)

VERNAMYCIN B
In addition to the preceding antibiotic, *Streptomyces loidensis* ATCC 11,415 also produces a complex of peptide lactones from which the following have been isolated and characterized. The complex itself possesses antimicrobial properties.

VERNAMYCIN B_α (*Ostreogrycin B, Mikamycin B*)
$C_{44}H_{52}O_{10}N_8$
Dec. 130–135°C

A component of vernamycin B, this antibiotic forms colourless crystals which decompose without melting. It has a specific rotation of $[\alpha]_D^{25} - 72°$ and gives an ultraviolet spectrum in CH_3OH with an absorption maximum at 231 nm. It is freely soluble in CH_3OH, EtOH, *iso*PrOH, BuOH, $(CH_3)_2CO$, AcOEt, Et_2O, dioxan, dimethylformamide, AcOH and C_6H_6, but only slightly soluble in H_2O and hexane. Like the parent substance, this antibiotic is active against gram-positive and some gram-negative bacteria.

Donovick *et al.*, *U.S. Patent*, 2,990,325 (1961)
Structure
Bodansky, Ondetti, *Antimicrobial Agents & Chemotherapy*, 360 (1963)

VERNAMYCIN B_β (*Ostreogrycin B_2*)
$C_{43}H_{50}O_{10}N_8$
Dec. 131–135°C

A further constituent of vernamycin B, the chemical and physical properties of this antibiotic are very similar to those of varnamycin B.

Donovick et al., U.S. Patent, 2,990,325 (1961)
Structure
  Bodanszky, Ondetti, *Antimicrobial Agents & Chemotherapy*, 360 (1963)

VERNAMYCIN B$_\gamma$ (*Ostreogrycin B$_1$*)
$C_{42}H_{48}O_{10}N_8$
Dec. 130–135°C

A third component of vernamycin B, this antibiotic forms colourless crystals from EtOH. The solubility in organic solvents is similar to that of vernamycin B$_\alpha$.

Donovick et al., U.S. Patent, 2,990,325 (1961)
Structure
  Bodanszky, Ondetti, *Antimicrobial Agents & Chemotherapy*, 360 (1963)

VERNAMYCIN B$_\delta$
$C_{41}H_{46}O_{10}N_8$
Dec. 132–135°C

A further crystalline polypeptide antibiotic separated from vernamycin B, produced by *Streptomyces loidensis*, the structure of this substance has been deduced by chemical and spectroscopic methods.

Donovick et al., U.S. Patent, 2,990,325 (1961)
Structure
  Bodanszky, Ondetti, *Antimicrobial Agents & Chemotherapy*, 360 (1963)

VERRUCARIN A
$C_{27}H_{34}O_9$
M.p. >330°C

One of a number of antibiotics isolated from *Myrothecium verrucaria*, this substance crystallizes as colourless plates which do not melt below 330°C. It is dextrorotatory with a specific rotation of $[\alpha]_D + 260°$ (CHCl$_3$) and $[\alpha]_D + 208°$ (dioxan). The ultraviolet spectrum in EtOH exhibits a single absorption maximum at 260 nm. When hydrolysed, the antibiotic furnishes muconic acid, verrucarinolactone and verrucarol. The latter, $C_{15}H_{22}O_4$, forms colourless crystals, m.p. 155–156°C; $[\alpha]_D - 39°$ (c 1·0, CHCl$_3$) and yields an acetate, m.p. 148–150°C; $[\alpha]_D - 17°$.

Härri et al., *Helv. Chim. Acta*, **45**, 839 (1962)
Gutzwiller, Tamm, *ibid.*, **45**, 1726 (1962)
Gutzwiller, Tamm, *ibid.*, **46**, 1786 (1963)

VERRUCARIN B
$C_{27}H_{32}O_9$
M.p. >330°C
Also produced by *Myrothecium verrucaria*, verrucarin B forms colourless needles when crystallized from $Et_2O-(CH_3)_2CO$ which do not melt below 330°C. The substance is dextrorotatory with specific rotations of $[\alpha]_D^{23} + 147°$ (c 1·06, C_6H_6) and $[\alpha]_D^{23} + 94°$ (c 0·99, $CHCl_3$). The ultraviolet spectrum in EtOH consists of a single absorption maximum at 258·5 nm. This antibiotic possesses antifungal and cytostatic activity.

Härri *et al.*, *Helv. Chim. Acta*, **45**, 839 (1962)

VERRUCARIN C
M.p. 223–224°C
A minor constituent of cultures of *Myrothecium verrucaria*, this antibiotic has been separated from the accompanying antibiotics by means of countercurrent distribution.

Härri *et al.*, *Helv. Chim. Acta*, **45**, 839 (1962)

VERRUCARIN D
M.p. 127–128°C
A further antibiotic isolated from cultures of *Myrothecium verrucaria*, verrucarin D forms colourless crystals when purified by recrystallization from EtOH.

Härri *et al.*, *Helv. Chim. Acta*, **45**, 839 (1962)

VERRUCARIN E
$C_7H_9O_2N$
M.p. 90·5–91°C
Myrothecium verrucaria also elaborates this antibiotic which forms colourless needles from $Et_2O-(CH_3)_2CO$. The ultraviolet spectrum has absorption maxima at 198 and 249 nm and an inflexion at 270 nm. The structure is 3-acetyl-4-hydroxymethylpyrrole. The acetate has been obtained as colourless needles from $Et_2O-(CH_3)_2CO$ with m.p. 102°C.

Härri *et al.*, *Helv. Chim. Acta*, **45**, 839 (1962)
Fetz, Tamm, *ibid.*, **49**, 349 (1966)
Revised structure and synthesis
Pfäffli, Tamm, *Helv. Chim. Acta*, **52**, 1911 (1969)
Biosynthesis
Pfäffli, Tamm, *Helv. Chim. Acta*, **52**, 1921 (1969)

VERRUCARIN F
M.p. 237–238°C
Also obtained from *Myrothecium verrucaria*, this antibiotic forms colourless crystals from EtOH. It is slightly laevorotatory with a specific rotation of $[\alpha]_D^{23} - 1° \pm 3·5°$ (c 0·643, pyridine). The ultraviolet spectrum consists of three absorption maxima at 202, 233 and 308 nm.

Härri *et al.*, *Helv. Chim. Acta*, **45**, 839 (1962)

VERRUCARIN G
M.p. 118°C and 131–135°C
This antibiotic from *Myrothecium verrucaria* has a double melting point and is best crystallized from CH_3OH containing a trace of $CHCl_3$ when the melting point is raised somewhat to 142–144°C. The substance is almost certainly optically inactive with $[\alpha]_D^{23} - 0° \pm 2°$. In EtOH, the ultraviolet spectrum has absorption maxima at 208, 254 and 300 nm.

Härri *et al.*, *Helv. Chim. Acta*, **45**, 839 (1962)

VERRUCARIN H
See Roridin H

VERRUCARIN K
$C_{28}H_{38}O_8$
M.p. 177–178°C
Myrothecium verrucaria NRRL 3003 elaborates this antibiotic when cultured in a medium containing glucose, malt extract, Bacto yeast, peptone and inorganic salts at 27°C for 4 days. It is isolated by extraction of the broth and purification by chromatography. The antibiotic forms colourless needles from Et_2O-pentane and has a specific rotation of $[\alpha]_D^{23} - 27°$ (c 1·3, $CHCl_3$).

Tamm, Sigg, Härri, *Swiss Patent*, 436, 570 (1967)

VERTICILLIN A
$C_{30}H_{28}O_6N_6S_4$
M.p. 199–213°C or 202–217°C (dec.)
Several species of *Verticillium* yield this sulphur-containing antibiotic which has the structure given above. When crystallized from $CHCl_3$ it forms pale yellow plates with the lower melting point while from pyridine it furnishes yellow needles having the higher melting point. From tetrahydrofuran it is obtained as an amorphous yellow powder, m.p. 203–214°C.

It is strongly dextrorotatory with $[\alpha]_D + 703 \cdot 7°$ and in dioxan gives an ultraviolet spectrum with an absorption maximum at 306 nm.

Katagiri et al., *J. Antibiotics* (Japan), **23B**, 420 (1970)
Minato, Matsumoto, Katayama, *Chem. Commun.*, 44 (1971)

VERTICILLIN B
$C_{30}H_{28}O_7N_6S_4$
M.p. 254–256°C

A further dimeric antibiotic isolated from a species of *Verticillium*, this compound crystallizes as pale yellow prisms from $CHCl_3$ and has a specific rotation of $[\alpha]_D + 704 \cdot 7°$ (c 0·493, dioxan). The diacetate has also been prepared, m.p. 200°C (*dec.*).

Minato, Matsumoto, Katayama, *J. Chem. Soc., Perkin I*, 1819 (1973)

VERTICILLIN C
$C_{30}H_{28}O_7N_6S_5$
M.p. 230–235°C (*dec.*)

A third antibiotic obtained from a *Verticillium* species, this compound forms a pale yellow amorphous powder from aqueous CH_3OH. It is strongly dextrorotatory like the two preceding antibiotics with a specific rotation of $[\alpha]_D + 765°$ (c 0·506, dioxan).

Minato, Matsumoto, Katayama, *J. Chem. Soc., Perkin I*, 1819 (1973)

VERTISPORIN
$C_{29}H_{36}O_{10}$
M.p. 176–183°C

A macrocyclic antibiotic, vertisporin has been isolated from cultures of *Verticimonosporium diffractum* strains TM-2098 and TM-2492. It yields colourless crystals and is dextrorotatory having a specific rotation of $[\alpha]_D^{26} + 62\cdot5°$. The ultraviolet spectrum is ethanolic solution consisting of a single absorption maximum at 216 nm. The structure given on p. 455 has been elucidated from chemical analysis and a study of the infrared, NMR and mass spectra. Vertisporin in fungistatic inhibiting *Trichophyton asteroides* at a concentration of 10 micrograms/millilitre and also possesses cytotoxic properties, the cytotoxic effect (ED_{50}) for Hela cells being 0·001 micrograms/millilitre.

Hayakawa et al., *J. Antibiotics* (Japan), **28**, 550 (1975)

VICEMYCETIN
See Thiamphenicol

VINACETIN
M.p. 157–158°C
Elaborated by a species of *Streptomyces* related to *S. albosporeus*, this antibiotic is obtained as a brown powder in the impure form and is purified by recrystallization from Et_2O—$CHCl_3$ when it yields yellow platelets. Vinacetin is soluble in CH_3OH, $(CH_3)_2CO$, AcOEt and butyl acetate, slightly soluble in H_2O and insoluble in Et_2O and petroleum ether. It is also soluble in dilute alkalies giving a violet colour. The antibiotic gives a positive $FeCl_3$, Molisch and Fehling's reaction and negative ninhydrin, Millon and Sakaguichi tests. It is more stable and active at pH 5·0 than at pH 7·0.

Vinacetin is active against gram-positive bacteria, particularly *Corynebacterium diphtheriae* and *Staphylococcus citreus* and also against mycobacteria. It is inactive against fungi and gram-negative bacteria. At a dosage of 5 mg/15 g mouse, the antibiotic has no toxic effect when given either intraperitoneally or intravenously but a dose of 10 mg proves fatal.

Omachi, *J. Antibiotics* (Japan), **6A**. 73 (1953)

VINACTIN A
The preparation vinactin isolated from *Streptomyces vinaceus*, and which may be identical with viomycin (q.v.), has been separated into three components. This antibiotic is a polypeptide and consists of the aminoacids alanine, aspartic acid, glutamic acid, glycine, lysine and serine. It is highly active against mycobacteria and also against a number of both gram-positive and gram-negative bacteria and rickettsiae. No information regarding its toxicity has been published.

Mayer et al., *12th Intern. Congr. Pure Appl. Chem.*, New York, 283 (1951)

VIOCIN
See Viomycin

VIOLACEIN
$C_{42}H_{35}O_6N_5$
M.p. Indefinite
An antibacterial and antiprotozoal substance, violacein is elaborated by *Chromobacterium violaceum*. It is obtained by surface growth on a medium containing meat extract, lactose and peptone incubated for 14 days at 22°C. At the end of this period, the bacterial cells are separated by centrifuging, extracted with $(CH_3)_2CO$, the extract concentrated *in vacuo*, cooled to yield a semi-crystalline material, the precipitate filtered and purified by extraction first with $CHCl_3$ and then Et_2O, the extracts discarded and the residue dissolved in pyridine, the filtrate concentrated and cooled after the addition of $CHCl_3$. The material is then dried *in vacuo* over a drying agent, preferably phosphorus pentoxide. Violacein forms black-violet needles or elongated crystals which decompose without melting. It forms a violet solution in EtOH in which it is slightly soluble.

Violacein is bactericidal to *Staphylococcus aureus* even at concentrations as low as 0·001 per cent. Lichstein and Van de Sand have determined typical inhibition concentrations (per cent) *in vitro*: *Bacillus anthracis* (0·002); *B. mesentericus* (0·002); *B. subtilis* (0·0005); *Brucella abortus* (>0·01); *Clostridium welchii* (>0·01); *Corynebacterium diphtheriae* (0·005); *Eberthella typhi* (>0·03); *Escherichia coli* (>0·03); *Hemophilus pertussis* (>0·01); *Neisseria catarrhalis* (>0·01); *Penicillium notatum* (>0·01); *Proteus vulgaris* (>0·03); *Saccharomyces cerevisiae* (>0·0005); *Serratia marcescens* (>0·03); *Staphylococcus albus* (0·002); *Staph. aureus* (0·002); *Streptococcus hemolyticus* (0·001); *Strep. viridans* (0·001) and *Trichophyton rubrum* (0·01).

The antibiotic is virtually inactive *in vivo*, affording no protection to mice against a massive infective dose of pneumococcus II although there were indications of a delayed death rate when a smaller infective dose was administered. Violacein is relatively non-toxic, mice tolerating a dose of 1–2 mg administered intraperitoneally.

Singh, *Nature*, **149**, 168 (1942)
Singh, *Ann. Appl. Biol.*, **29**, 18 (1942)
Strong, *Science*, **100**, 287 (1944)

Lichstein, Van de Sand, *J. Inf. Diseases*, **76**, 47 (1945)
Lichstein, Van de Sand, *J. Bact.*, **52**, 145 (1946)

VIOLAMYCIN

Streptomyces violaceus IMET JA 6844 yields a mixture of antibiotics, violamycins A and B, when cultivated aerobically with stirring in a common nutrient medium at 28°C for 3–4 days. The mycelium is extracted with CH_3OH, the extract concentrated, and then re-extracted with BuOH. The crude material is obtained by the addition of petroleum ether. It may be separated into the two components and also from the antibiotically-inactive chromophores, violamycinones A and B, by chromatography. The antibiotics, and the mixture, have cancerostatic activity and inhibit the growth of *Mycoplasma gallisepticus* and *M. hyorhinis*.

Fleck *et al.*, *East German Patent*, 100,494 (1973)
Fleck *et al.*, *German Patent*, 2,243,554 (1974)

VIOMYCIN (*Celiomycin, Florimycin, Tuberactinomycin B, Viocin*)
$C_{25}H_{43}O_{10}N_{13}$

Viomycin is an antibiotic produced by *Streptomyces puniceus* var. *Floridae* and was originally given the empirical formula $C_{23}H_{36}O_8N_{12}$. It forms purple crystals, is a strong base and is freely soluble in H_2O. In medicine it is normally employed as the sulphate, purple crystals, m.p. 280°C (*dec.*); $[\alpha]_D^{25} - 32°$ (c 1·0, H_2O). This salt gives an ultraviolet spectrum with absorption maxima at 239 and 268 nm in 0·1 *N*-HCl and at 219, 282 nm in 0·1 *N*-NaOH. It is comparatively soluble in H_2O but insoluble in common organic solvents.

In medicine, its main use is as an antimicrobial agent and also as an antituberculous agent. The normal dose of the sulphate is 1 g. Among the side effects which may occur are disturbances of the eighth cranial nerve and renal irritation. A number of workers have shown that although acylation of the hydroxyl groups has no effect on the activity, any change in the terminal amino groups brings about inactivity.

Marsh *et al.*, *U.S. Patent*, 2,633,445 (1953)
Freaney, *ibid.*, 2,828,245 (1958)
Kitagawa *et al.*, *J. Antibiotics* (Japan), **25**, 429 (1972)
Kitagawa *et al.*, *Chem. Pharm. Bull.*, **20**, 2176 (1972)
Tyc *et al.*, *Polish Patent*, 67,161 (1973)
Kitagawa *et al.*, *Chem. Pharm. Bull.*, **22**, 1827 (1974)
Structure
Kitagawa *et al.*, *Progr. Antimicrob. Anticancer Chemother.*, *Proc. Int. Congr. Chemother.*, *6th*, **2**, 1027 (1969)
Bycroft *et al.*, *Experientia*, **27**, 501 (1971)
Yoshioka *et al.*, *Tetrahedron Lett.*, 2043 (1971)
Bycroft, *Chem. Commun.*, 660 (1972)
Noda *et al.*, *J. Antibiotics* (Japan), **25**, 427 (1972)
Bycroft *et al.*, *J. Chem. Soc.*, *Perkin I*, 827 (1972)

VIRENOMYCIN

This antibiotic has been obtained from cultures of *Streptomyces virens* strains 3831 and 3931/183, the latter giving the higher yield. The antibiotic is produced primarily in the mycelium and the preferred medium for strain 3831/183 contains glycerol, soybean meal, NaCl, $CaCO_3$ and $(NH_4)_2SO_4$. Tests with experimental animals have shown that virenomycin given subcutaneously at a dose of 200–700 mg/kg six times daily inhibited lymphadenosis N1C/Li tumour development in mice by 55–60 per cent. A dose of 100–200 mg/kg given orally six times daily reduced tumour development by 5–70 per cent. However, virenomycin had no effect on lymphosarcoma, Sarcoma 180 or Garding-Passi melanoma.

Gauze *et al.*, *Antibiotiki*, **22**, 963 (1977)

VIRGIMYCIN
See Staphylomycin

VIRGINIAMYCIN
See Staphylomycin

VIRGINIAMYCIN M

This antibiotic compound from cultures of *Streptomyces virginiae* is a mixture of virginiamycins M_1 and M_2, the latter being the 2:3-dihydro

Virginiamycin S

derivatives of the former compound. Virginiamycin M interferes with the initiation and elongation of peptide chains in cell-free systems and also increases DNA in the liver and spleen of chickens but only at high doses. It is reversibly bound to plasma proteins, 0·6–2·8 µg/ml of the antibiotic being found in human plasma some 1–4 hours following the intake of an oral dose of 500 mg of virginiamycin M. It has also been shown to block the preferential message translation of bacteriophage 2C which lyses *Bacillus subtilis*, i.e. the means by which the virus halts host-macromolecular formation and the synthesis of DNA. It is possible that the antibiotic inhibits the synthetis and function of virus-dictated proteins.

Van Dijck, Van Braekel, *Chemotherapy*, **14**, 109 (1969)
Cocito, *J. Gen. Microbiol.*, **57**, 195 (1969)
Crooy, De Neys, *J. Antibiotics* (Japan), **25**, 371 (1972)
Cocito, Voorman, Bosch, *Biochim. Biophys. Acta*, **340**, 285 (1974)
Petkova, *Zhivonovud. Nauki.*, **11**, 79 (1974)

VIRGINIAMYCIN S
$C_{42}H_{47}O_{10}N_7$

Streptomyces virginiae also elaborates this antibiotic which is the major component of a number of similar antibiotics, separated on silica gel with $CHCl_3$—CH_3OH. The individual constituents are described below. They all possess antibacterial activity although this is lower than with virginiamycin S itself. Virginiamycin S and its components have a synergistic effect upon virginiamycin M.

Crooy, De Neys, *J. Antibiotics* (Japan), **25**, 371 (1972)
Vanderhaeghe, Janssen, Compernolle, *Verh. Kon. Vlaam. Acad. Geneesk., Belg.*, **34**, 209 (1972)
Petkova, *Zhivonovud. Nauki.*, **11**, 79 (1974)

VIRGINIAMYCIN S₁
$C_{42}H_{47}O_{10}N_7$

An isomer of the preceding antibiotic, this substance is obtained by thin-layer chromatography on silica gel which separates it from the accompanying antibiotics of the virginiamycin S complex.

Vanderhaeghe, Janssen, Compernolle, *Verh. Kon. Vlaam. Acad. Geneesk., Belg.*, **34**, 209 (1972)

VIRGINIAMYCIN S₂
$C_{42}H_{49}O_{10}N_7$

A minor component of the virginiamycin S complex, virginiamycin S₂ is the secondary alcohol corresponding to virginiamycin S as the ketone. The structure has been determined by chemical and spectroscopic methods.

Vanderhaeghe, Janssen, Compernolle, *Verh. Kon. Vlaam. Acad. Geneesk., Belg.*, **34**, 209 (1972)

VIRGINIAMYCIN S₃
$C_{43}H_{49}O_{11}N_7$

Also present in the virginiamycin S antibiotic complex, this substance has the structure given above. It is less active against gram-positive bacteria than virginiamycin S itself.

Vanderhaeghe, Janssen, Compernolle, *Verh. Kon. Vlaam. Acad. Geneesk., Belg.*, **34**, 209 (1972)

VIRIDICATIN
$C_{15}H_{11}O_2N$
M.p. 268°C

This antibiotic has been isolated from *Penicillium viridicatum* and from various strains of *P. cyclopium*. It crystallizes as lustrous needles from CH_3OH or EtOH, subliming at 160–170°C in high vacuum. Viridicatin is soluble in cold aqueous $2N$-KOH and glacial AcOH, sparingly so in dilute mineral acids, concentrated HCl and cold organic solvents, insoluble in H_2O or aqueous sodium bicarbonate. It behaves as a very weak acid and forms a series of salts and derivatives including monoacetylviridicatin, m.p. 200–201°C; the O,O-dimethyl derivative, m.p. 86–87°C; the O,N-dimethyl compound, m.p. 197–200°C; the sodium salt, *dec.* 260–265°C and the 3:5-dinitrobenzoate, m.p. 238°C.

Viridicatin is active against *Mycobacterium tuberculosis* at a dilution of 1:15,000.

Cunningham, Freeman, *Biochem. J.*, **53**, 328 (1953)
Bracken *et al.*, *ibid.*, **57**, 587 (1954)
Biosynthesis
Luckner, *Tetrahedron Lett.*, 1035 (1962)
Luckner, Mothes, *Arch. Pharm.*, **296**, 18 (1963)
Synthesis
Eistert, Selzer, *Z. Naturforsch.*, **17B**, 202 (1962)

α-VIRIDIN
$C_{20}H_{16}O_6$
Dec. 208–217°C

This fungistatic antibiotic, isolated from *Trichoderma viride* and originally believed to be a single substance, has recently been separated into two isomers. This isomer crystallizes from dilute AcOH as colourless needles and is laevorotatory with a specific rotation of $[\alpha]_D^{20} - 213.4°$ ($CHCl_3$). In EtOH it gives an ultraviolet spectrum with two absorption maxima at 241 and 304.5 nm. The diacetate yields colourless crystals with m.p. 145–150°C. α-viridin is soluble in H_2O and $CHCl_3$, only sparingly so in CS_2 or CCl_4 and virtually insoluble in Et_2O. The aqueous solution rapidly loses its activity unless acidified to pH 3.0.

α-Viridin is assayed by the inhibition of spore germination of the conidia of *Botrytis allii*, one unit being equivalent to 0.005 µg/ml. It has little activity against bacteria but is highly fungicidal. The following concentrations for inhibition of spore germination of various fungi (µg/ml) *in vitro* have been determined by Brian and his coworkers: *Aspergillus niger* (3.1); *Botrytis allii* (0.005); *Cladosporium herbarum* (0.2); *Colleotrichum lini* (0.003); *Fusarium caeruleum* (0.003); *F. culmorum* (0.2); *Penicillium digitatum* (0.2); *P. expansum* (6.25); *P. notatum* (0.2); *Stachybotrys atra* (6.25); *Trichoderma viride* (>50) and *Trichothecium roseum* (0.05).

Brian, McGowan, *Nature*, **156**, 144 (1945)
Brian *et al.*, *Ann. Appl. Biol.*, **33**, 190 (1946)
Vischer, Howland, Raudnitz, *Nature*, **165**, 528 (1950)

β-VIRIDIN
$C_{20}H_{16}O_6$
Dec. 140°C

This isomer of the preceding antibiotic also occurs in cultures of *Trichoderma viride*. It forms colourless needles when crystallized from CH_3OH and has $[\alpha]_D^{20} + 50\cdot7°$ ($CHCl_3$). The ultraviolet spectrum in EtOH has absorption maxima at 241·5 and 304 nm. It possesses similar antifungal properties to those given for α-viridin.

Brian *et al.*, *Ann. Appl. Biol.*, **33**, 190 (1946)
Vischer, Howland, Raudnitz, *Nature*, **165**, 528 (1950)

VIRIDOGRISEIN
See Etamycin

VIRILEMYCIN A
$C_{40}H_{67}O_{11}N$
M.p. 107–108°C

An antibiotic produced by a number of *Streptomyces* species represented by *Streptomyces* strain 5900 (FERM-P 1053) when cultivated aerobically in a common nutrient medium at 25–32°C for 3–6 days. The antibiotic may be extracted from the cells and the culture broth with $(CH_3)_2CO$, re-extracted with AcOEt and precipitated by hexane. Purification is carried out by chromatography with silica gel and Sephadex LH-20. The compound is best crystallized from $CHCl_3$ or CH_3OH when it forms colourless plates. It is dextrorotatory with a specific rotation of $[\alpha]_D^{25} + 69°$ ($CHCl_3$). The culture filtrate also contains small amounts of virilemycins B and C which have not been extensively examined. Virilemycin A is active against a number of gram-positive bacteria and has LD_{50} in mice of 250 mg/kg given intravenously.

Aizawa *et al.*, *Japanese Patent*, 7,348,688 (1973)

VISCOSIN
$C_{36}H_{66}O_{10}N_6$
M.p. 270–273°C (*dec.*)

This polypeptide antibiotic is elaborated by *Pseudomonas viscosa* and forms a colourless microcrystalline powder which is soluble in CH_3OH, EtOH, $(CH_3)_2CO$, $CHCl_3$ and alkaline phosphate buffer solutions, but virtually insoluble in H_2O. It is laevorotatory having a specific rotation of $[\alpha]_D^{20} - 168\cdot3°$. The structure has been established as (−)-3-hydroxydecanoyl-L-leucylglycylseryl-valylthreonyl-L-leucine.

Kochi *et al.*, *Bact. Proc.*, 29 (1951)
Ohno, Tajima, Toki, *J. Agr. Chem. Soc., Japan*, **27**, 665 (1953)
Toki, Ohno, *Nippon Nogei-Kagaku Kaishi*, **29**, 370 (1955)

VIVICIL
See Fluvomycin

VULGAMYCIN (*Enterocin*)
$C_{22}H_{20}O_{10}$
M.p. 166–168°C

An antibiotic elaborated by *Streptomyces hygroscopicus* strain A-5294, this substance forms colourless crystals and is laevorotatory with a specific rotation of $[\alpha]_D^{21} - 11°$ (c 1·0, MeOH). It gives an ultraviolet spectrum in MeOH having absorption maxima at 250 and 283 nm. Vulgamycin is active against gram-negative bacteria. It has been shown to be identical with enterocin.

Aizawa *et al.*, *Abstr. Agr. Chem. Soc. Japan*, 83 (1975)
Identity with enterocin
Miyairi *et al.*, *J. Antibiotics* (Japan), **29**, 227 (1976)
Structure
Seto *et al.*, *Tetrahedron Lett.*, 4367 (1976)

X

XANTHOBACIDIN

Bacillus subtilis elaborates this antibiotic which has been isolated from the culture medium. It is soluble in H_2O and the lower alcohols and is highly effective against *Xanthomonas*. Chemical and physical data have shown that xanthobacidin is not identical with known antibiotics.

Huang, Chang., *Bot. Bull. Acad. Sin.*, **16**, 137 (1975)

XANTHOCIDIN

$C_{11}H_{16}O_5$
M.p. 185°C (*dec.*)

A number of *Streptomyces* species elaborate this antibiotic which gives colourless crystals from $CHCl_3$. It has a specific rotation of $[\alpha]_D^{25} + 16.7°$ and gives an ultraviolet spectrum in CH_3OH with a single absorption maximum at 227 nm. The structure has been shown to be 4:5-dihydroxy-4-*iso*propyl-4-methyl-2-methylene-3-oxocyclopentane-1-carboxylic acid.

Asahi, Nagatsu, Suzuki, *J. Antibiotics* (Japan), **19**, 195 (1966)
Structure
Asahi, Suzuki, *Agr. Biol. Chem.*, **34**, 325 (1970)

XANTHOCILLIN X

$C_{18}H_{12}O_2N_2$
Dec. ca. 210°C

Penicillium notatum produces a complex, xanthocillin, which is composed of at least two antibiotics. Xanthocillin X is the predominant component, present to the extent of 70 per cent. It crystallizes from EtOH as yellow needles and from AcOEt as yellow rhombs. Both forms char at about 210°C without melting. The antibiotic is insoluble in H_2O, $CHCl_3$, C_6H_6 and light petroleum and soluble to the extent of 1 per cent in dioxan, EtOH, Et_2O and $(CH_3)_2CO$. It forms a dipotassium salt which is freely soluble in H_2O.

The structure has been established as 1:4-bis(*p*-hydroxyphenyl)-2:3-di*iso*nitrilo-1:3-butadiene.

Rothe, *Pharmazie*, **5**, 190 (1950)
Structure
Hagedorn, Tönjes, *Pharmazie*, **11**, 409 (1956)
Hagedorn, Tönjes, *ibid.*, **12**, 567 (1957)
Hagedorn *et al.*, *Ber.*, **93**, 1584 (1960)
Synthesis
Hagedorn, Eholzer, *Angew. Chem.*, **74**, 215 (1962)

XANTHOCILLIN Y

This antibiotic is a minor constituent of the complex produced by *Penicillium notatum*. At present very little has been reported concerning its structure.

Rothe, *Pharmazie*, **5**, 190 (1950)

XANTHOCILLIN Y_1

$C_{18}H_{12}O_3N_2$

Isolated from *Penicillium notatum*, the structure of this antibiotic has recently been shown to be that given above.

Achenbach, Strittmatter, Kohl, *Chem. Ber.*, **105**, 3061 (1972)

XANTHOCILLIN Y_2

$C_{18}H_{12}O_4N_2$

A further antibiotic isolated from cultures of *Penicillium notatum*, the structure of this compound is very similar to that of the preceding substance containing an additional phenolic hydroxyl group in the molecule.

Achenbach, Strittmatter, Kohl, *Chem. Ber.*, **105**, 3061 (1972)

XANTHOCYCLINE

$C_{29}H_{38}O_8N_8$

A semi-synthetic antibiotic of the tetracycline class, this compound is active in decreasing the adjuvant properties of endotoxin in the immune response when given intraperitoneally to mice at a dose of 50μg/ml 2 days before

XANTHOMYCIN A

$C_{23}H_{29-31}O_7N_3$
M.p. Indefinite

An antibiotic substance, xanthomycin, was first isolated from an unclassified *Streptomyces* species, a strain of type S-94, and subsequently from *S. pseudogriseolus* present in the soil of Nagano prefecture, Japan. This material was then shown to consists of at least two components, xanthomycins A and B. The mixture is obtained by submerged culture in shaker flasks, the culture medium containing corn steep liquor solids, dextrin, soybean meal and inorganic salts incubated for 4–5 days at 25°C. The yield after this period is 5000–8000 *Staphylococcus aureus* units, the yield dropping sharply after 5 days. The substance is isolated by treating the culture filtrate with activated carbon, the cake being washed with BuOH in H_2O and the activity eluted with 0·1 N-HCl saturated with BuOH. After concentrating *in vacuo*, the eluate is neutralized with sodium hydroxide, filtered, extracted with $CHCl_3$ and the active material removed from the organic extract with water at pH 2·0. Purification is carried out by precipitation of the picrate or reineckate followed by countercurrent distribution of the hydrochloride. Xanthomycin A is precipitated as the reineckate which is dissolved in CH_3OH, decomposed with HCl, the precipitate dissolved in anhydrous CH_3OH, reprecipitated with Et_2O and dried *in vacuo*. Xanthomycin A forms an orange-yellow amorphous powder which is strongly basic when pure. The ultraviolet spectrum in EtOH exhibits absorption maxima at 288 and 460 nm. In dilute acids the solutions are bright yellow and a reddish-pink in dilute alkalies. Although this colour change is reversible, all antibiotic activity is destroyed during this treatment. Among the hydrolysis products that have been identified are methylamine, ammonia and ethanolamine. The hydrochloride is crystalline, forming yellow-orange plates and is dextrorotatory with a specific rotation of $[\alpha]_D^{25} + 115°$ (c 0·4, H_2O). In 0·1 N-HCl, this salt gives an ultraviolet spectrum with absorption maxima at 265 and 345 nm. The reineckate forms long orange needles with m.p. 165–170°C (*dec.*). The antibiotic is stable in acid solution and gives negative Molisch, ninhydrin and Sakaguchi reactions.

Xanthomycin is assayed by turbidimetric and serial dilution with *Staphylococcus aureus* as the test organism. The salts of xanthomycin A have the following potencies based upon these tests: reineckate, 490,000 units/mg, picrate 293,500 units/mg and the hydrochloride, 670,000 units/mg. Thorne and Peterson have determined the following inhibition dilutions (× 1,000,000) *in vitro* for the picrate: *Bacillus albolactis* (0·4); *B. brevis* (4·0); *B. cereus* (2·4); *B. fusiformis* (800); *B. megatherium* (4·0); *B. mesentericus* (4·0); *B. mycoides* (28); *B. subtilis* (240); *Escherichia coli* (2·4); *Micrococcus flavescens* (200); *Micro. subcitreus* (24·); *Salmonella gallinarum* (2·4); *Serratia marcescens* (4·0); *Staphylococcus albus* (2400) and *Staph. aureus* (300).

Xanthomycin A hydrochloride is highly toxic, the LD_{50} in mice being approximately 3·2 μg administered intravenously.

Thorne, Peterson, *J. Biol. Chem.*, **176**, 413 (1948)
Mold, Bartz, *J. Amer. Chem. Soc.*, **72**, 1847 (1950)
Okami, *J. Antibiotics* (Japan), **8A**, 126 (1955)
Rao, Peterson, *J. Amer. Chem. Soc.*, **76**, 1335, 1338 (1954)
Peterson, van Tamelen, *ibid.*, **77**, 4327 (1955)

XANTHOMYCIN B

M.p. Indefinite

This antibiotic is present to the extent of between 10 and 35 per cent of the antibiotic mixture obtained from *Streptomyces* S-94 and *S. pseudogriseolus*. It may be separated from xanthomycin A by virtue of the fact that the reineckate is non-crystallizable. It has similar physical properties to those of the preceding antibiotic and the picrate gives an almost identical spectrum *in vitro*. The purest preparation so far prepared also has a toxicity identical with that of xanthomycin A hydrochloride in mice.

Thorne, Peterson, *J. Biol. Chem.*, **176**, 413 (1948)
Mold, Bartz, *J. Amer. Chem. Soc.*, **72**, 1847 (1950)
Okami, *J. Antibiotics* (Japan), **8A**, 126 (1955)
Roa, Peterson, *J. Amer. Chem. Soc.*, **76**, 1335, 1338 (1954)
Peterson, van Tamelen, *ibid.*, **77**, 4327 (1955)

XANTHOTHRICIN

See Toxoflavin

---

administration of sheep erythrocytes. No effect is observed if the compound is administered 24 hours after immunization.

Slavcheva, *Izv. Mikrobiol. Inst. Bulg. Akad. Nauk.*, **23**, 111 (1972)

XYLOSTASIN
$C_{17}H_{34}O_{10}N_4$
M.p. 150–180°C (*dec.*)

A new antibiotic, xylostasin has been isolated from cultures of *Bacillus* species Y-399 (ATCC 21,932) when aerobically cultivated in a common nutrient medium at 28°C and pH 7·5 for 66 hours. Both the parent antibiotic and its sulphate are active against gram-positive and gram-negative bacteria and have an extremely low toxicity, being useful against bacterial infections such as bronchopneumonia, pyelitis, tonsillitis and urinary tract infections.

Horii *et al.*, *German Patent*, 2,326,943 (1974)

YAKUSIMYCIN A

Streptomyces species H-827 elaborates three closely related antibiotics when aerobically fermented in a medium normally used for Actinomycete culture, optimum conditions being 24–30°C for 1–3 days. The cells are then extracted with $(CH_3)_2CO$ at pH 6·0 and the culture filtrate with AcOEt. The solvents are then removed by evaporation under reduced pressure and the antibiotic separated and purified by chromatography on a silica gel column. Yakusimycin A forms a white, amorphous powder having no definite melting point. It is active against a range of gram-positive bacteria.

Aizawa et al., *Japanese Patent*, 7,330,398 (1973)

YAKUSIMYCIN B

M.p. Indefinite
This antibiotic is also produced by *Streptomyces* species H-827 and separated from the accompanying substances by chromatography on alumina or silica gel. It also forms a white, amorphous powder and has a similar antibiotic activity to yakusimycin A.

Aizawa et al., *Japanese Patent*, 7,330,398 (1973)

YAKUSIMYCIN C

$C_{47}H_{59}O_{12}N_7$
M.p. Indefinite
A third antibiotic obtained from cultures of *Streptomyces* species H-827, this depsipeptide compound is crystalline, insoluble in H_2O but freely soluble in AcOEt. It is synergistic with yakusimycin A and active against *Sarcina lutea* and *Staphylococcus aureus*. The LD_{50} in mice is 200 mg/kg when given intraperitoneally.

Aizawa et al., *Japanese Patent*, 7,310,294 (1973)

YAMACILLIN

$C_{24}H_{23}N_3O_6S$
A semi-synthetic antibiotic, yamacillin has the structure given above. It possesses potent bactericidal activity against *Escherichia coli*, *Micrococcus lutea* and *Staphylococcus aureus*, being more active than either amoxicillin or cephalexin. It is active against *E. coli* at a concentration of 6·25 micrograms/millilitre bringing about elongation of the bacteria and inhibition of cell wall formation. At a concentration of 62·5 micrograms/millilitre cell lysis occurs.

Nishino, *Shinyaku To Chiryo*, **219**, 14 (1977)
Anon., *ibid.*, **219**, 15 (1977)

YAZUMYCIN A

See Racemomycin A

YAZUMYCIN C

See Racemomycin C

YEMENIMYCIN

M.p. 212–214°C
A recently discovered antibiotic, yemenimycin is produced by *Streptomyces* AS-Y-52 cultivated in a medium containing starch and inorganic salts at 28°C for 6 days. The antibiotic is isolated from both the mycelium and culture broth by extraction with an organic solvent and crystallized from $CHCl_3$ when it forms pale yellowish-buff needles. It is freely soluble in $CHCl_3$, $(CH_3)_2CO$, AcOEt and butyl acetate, moderately soluble in CH_3OH, EtOH and BuOH but insoluble in H_2O and petroleum ether. Chemical and spectroscopic evidence shows that it is a polypeptide. Yemenimycin inhibits the growth of gram-positive bacteria. The minimum inhibitory concentration against *Bacillus*, *Candida*, *Microsporum*, *Staphylococcus* and *Trichophyton* species is 0·006–0·78 μg/ml.

Shimi, Dewedar, Abdallah., *J. Antibiotics* (Japan), **24**, 283 (1971)

Z

ZERVACIN I
See Zervamicin I

ZERVACIN II
See Zervamicin II

ZERVAMICIN (*Zervacin I*)
$C_{70}H_{114}O_{21}N_4$
M.p. 220°C (*dec.*)

Emericellopsis salmosynnemata produces two complex antibiotics when grown on a common nutrient medium with aeration. This compound forms a microcrystalline powder and is dextrorotatory with a specific rotation of $[\alpha]_D^{25} + 16°$ (c 1·0, CH_3OH). It is soluble in CH_3OH, EtOH and $(CH_3)_2CO$. Zervamicin is active against gram-positive bacteria.

Argoudelis, Dietz, Johnson, *J. Antibiotics* (Japan), **27**, 321 (1974)

ZERVAMICIN II (*Zervacin II*)
$C_{93}H_{152}O_{20}N_{19}$
M.p. 257°C (*dec.*)

A second highly complex antibiotic isolated from cultures of *Emericellopsis salmosynnemata*, this compound is an amorphous powder. It is slightly dextrorotatory with a specific rotation of $[\alpha]_D^{25} + 4·5°$ (c 1·0, CH_3OH) and has an antibiotic spectrum similar to that of the preceding substance.

Argoudelis, Dietz, Johnson, *J. Antibiotics* (Japan), **27**, 321 (1974)

ZORBAMYCIN
$C_{56}H_{100}O_{24}N_{18}S_2Cu$
M.p. Indefinite

A copper-containing antibiotic isolated from cultures of *Streptomyces bikiniensis* var. *zorbonensis*, zorbamycin is obtained as an amorphous blue powder. It has been characterized as the hydrochloride which is dextrorotatory with a specific rotation of $[\alpha]_D^{25} + 247°$ (c 0·6, H_2O), giving an ultraviolet spectrum in CH_3OH with absorption maxima at 244, 298 and 309 nm with a shoulder at 290 nm. In the visible spectrum there is an absorption maximum at 600 nm. The antibiotic is active against a wide range of gram-positive and gram-negative bacteria and fungi. Zorbamycin appears to belong to the phleomycin group of antibiotics.

Argoudelis, Bergy, Pyke, *J. Antibiotics* (Japan), **24**, 543 (1971)

ZORBAMYCIN B
M.p. Indefinite

A further complex antibiotic isolated from *Streptomyces bikiniensis* var. *zorbonensis*, the structure of this compound is not firmly established. It forms a blue powder and is active against a number of gram-positive and gram-negative bacteria and fungi.

Argoudelis, Bergy, Pyke, *J. Antibiotics* (Japan), **24**, 543 (1971)

ZORBAMYCIN C
M.p. Indefinite

Also produced by *Streptomyces bikiniensis* var. *zorbonensis*, this antibiotic appears to have a structure similar to that of zorbamycin, yielding a blue powder with no definite melting point. It has an antibiotic spectrum similar to those of the two accompanying antibiotics.

Argoudelis, Bergy, Pyke, *J. Antibiotics* (Japan), **24**, 543 (1971)

ZORBONOMYCIN
$C_{59}H_{97}O_{24}N_{19}S_2Cu$
M.p. Indefinite

A further group of copper-containing antibiotics is elaborated by *Streptomyces bikiniensis* var. *zorbonensis*, grown on a common medium containing assimilable sources of carbon and nitrogen and inorganic salts at 18–40°C for 2–10 days. The mixture of antibiotics is isolated by adsorption on an ion exchange resin, eluting with an organic solvent and freeze-drying the product. Further purification is carried out by column chromatography. Zorbonomycin is dextrorotatory with a specific rotation of $[\alpha]_D^{25} + 247°$ (c 0·58, H_2O). It is probable that this compound is identical with zorbamycin.

Upjohn Co., *British Patent*, 1,277,150 (1972)

ZORBONOMYCIN B
$C_{58}H_{88}O_{25}N_{19}S_2Cu$
M.p. Indefinite
A further component of the antibiotic complex elaborated by *Streptomyces bikinensis* var. *zorbonensis*. This compound is isolated by adsorbing the activity of the broth on activated carbon or an ion exchange resin, eluting, and freeze-drying the elute. It is separated from zorbonomycin by column chromatography. Like the accompanying antibiotics, it is active in inhibiting the growth of gram-positive and gram-negative bacteria and various fungi.

Upjohn Co., *British Patent*, 1,277,150 (1972)

ZYGOSPORIN A
M.p. 268–270°C
A crystalline antibiotic, zygosporin A is produced by the cultivation of *Zygosporium masonii* or *Z. mycophilum* under aerobic conditions for 50–150 hours at 25–32°C. The antibiotic is obtained primarily from the mycelium and recrystallization from $(CH_3)_2CO$ yields zygosporin A as colourless needles. It has an inhibitory action against a variety of abscesses.

Hayakawa *et al.*, *British Patent*, 1,160,846 (1969)

ZYGOSPORIN D
$C_{28}H_{35}O_5N$
A further member of the group of antibiotic compounds produced by *Zygosporium masonii* ATCC 20,011 when cultivated in a potato-starch medium at 28°C for 3 days. The antibiotic possesses antitumour and anti-inflammatory properties.

Minato, Matshushima, *Japanese Patent*, 7,223,394 (1972)

ZYGOSPORIN E
$C_{30}H_{37}O_5N$
A further antibiotic elaborated by *Zygosporium masonii* ATCC 20,011. This compound has a similar biological action to those of the preceding antibiotic.

Minato, Matshushima, *Japanese Patent*, 7,223,394 (1972)

ZYGOSPORIN F
$C_{32}H_{39}O_7N$
Isolated from the culture filtrate of *Zygosporium masonii* ATCC 20,011, by extraction with AcOEt, this compound is separated from the associated antibiotics by chromatography. It is active against transplantable tumours and is also an anti-inflammatory agent.

Minato, Matshushima, *Japanese Patent*, 7,223,394 (1972)

ZYGOSPORIN G
$C_{30}H_{37}O_5N$
Zygosporium masonii ATCC 20,011 also furnishes this antibiotic when grown in a potato-starch medium at 28°C for 3 days, the culture filtrate being extracted with AcOEt and chromatographed. Like the preceding compounds it has antitumour and anti-inflammatory properties.

Minato, Matshushima, *Japanese Patent*, 7,223,394 (1972)

R 615.329 G548e 1979   Glasby, John S. John Ste
Encyclopaedia of antibiotics /

0 1901 0024879 7
Carson Library, Lees-McRae College

PRIMA... LIBRARY OF